Cognitive and Brain Plasticity: Current Research

Cognitive and Brain Plasticity: Current Research

Editor: Ronnie Turner

MURPHY & MOORE
www.murphy-moorepublishing.com

www.murphy-moorepublishing.com

MURPHY & MOORE

Cataloging-in-Publication Data

Cognitive and brain plasticity : current research / edited by Ronnie Turner.
p. cm.
Includes bibliographical references and index.
ISBN 978-1-63987-116-2
1. Neuroplasticity. 2. Cognitive neuroscience. 3. Developmental neurobiology. 4. Neuropsychology.
5. Neurophysiology. I. Turner, Ronnie.
QP363.3 .C64 2022
612.82--dc23

Murphy & Moore Publishing,
1 Rockefeller Plaza,
New York City, NY 10020, USA

ISBN 978-1-63987-116-2 (Hardback)

Contents

Preface

The adaptive changes in the patterns of cognition that are related to the brain activity are known as cognitive plasticity. Brain plasticity, also known as neuroplasticity, refers to the changes on a non-neuron level that can be stimulated by experience. Neuroplasticity encompasses the potential of neural networks in the brain to change through growth and reorganization. A few of its examples are changes in the circuit and network resulting from environmental influences, learning a new ability, psychological stress and practice. The changes may range from individual neuron pathways that make new connections, to systematic adjustments like cortical remapping. The degree of plasticity is higher in the developing brain than the adult brain. The various studies that are constantly contributing towards advancing technologies and evolution of this field are examined in detail in this book. Also included herein is a detailed explanation of the various concepts of cognitive and brain plasticity. This book will help the readers in keeping pace with the rapid changes in this field.

This book has been the outcome of endless efforts put in by authors and researchers on various issues and topics within the field. The book is a comprehensive collection of significant researches that are addressed in a variety of chapters. It will surely enhance the knowledge of the field among readers across the globe.

It gives us an immense pleasure to thank our researchers and authors for their efforts to submit their piece of writing before the deadlines. Finally in the end, I would like to thank my family and colleagues who have been a great source of inspiration and support.

Editor

1

Computer-Based Cognitive Training for Executive Functions after Stroke

Renate M. van de Ven[1], Jaap M. J. Murre[1], Dick J. Veltman[2] and Ben A. Schmand[1,3]*

[1] *Department of Psychology, Brain and Cognition, University of Amsterdam, Amsterdam, Netherlands,* [2] *Department of Psychiatry, VU University Medical Center, Amsterdam, Netherlands,* [3] *Department of Medical Psychology, Academic Medical Centre, University of Amsterdam, Netherlands*

Edited by:
Louis Bherer,
PERFORM Centre at Concordia University, Canada

Reviewed by:
Claude Alain,
Rotman Research Institute, Canada
Sean Commins,
National University of Ireland Maynooth, Ireland

****Correspondence:***
Renate M. van de Ven
r.m.vandeven@uva.nl

Background: Stroke commonly results in cognitive impairments in working memory, attention, and executive function, which may be restored with appropriate training programs. Our aim was to systematically review the evidence for computer-based cognitive training of executive dysfunctions.

Methods: Studies were included if they concerned adults who had suffered stroke or other types of acquired brain injury, if the intervention was computer training of executive functions, and if the outcome was related to executive functioning. We searched in MEDLINE, PsycINFO, Web of Science, and The Cochrane Library. Study quality was evaluated based on the CONSORT Statement. Treatment effect was evaluated based on differences compared to pre-treatment and/or to a control group.

Results: Twenty studies were included. Two were randomized controlled trials that used an active control group. The other studies included multiple baselines, a passive control group, or were uncontrolled. Improvements were observed in tasks similar to the training (near transfer) and in tasks dissimilar to the training (far transfer). However, these effects were not larger in trained than in active control groups. Two studies evaluated neural effects and found changes in both functional and structural connectivity. Most studies suffered from methodological limitations (e.g., lack of an active control group and no adjustment for multiple testing) hampering differentiation of training effects from spontaneous recovery, retest effects, and placebo effects.

Conclusions: The positive findings of most studies, including neural changes, warrant continuation of research in this field, but only if its methodological limitations are addressed.

Keywords: working memory, attention, restitution, retraining, acquired brain injury, brain training, executive functions, computer-based

INTRODUCTION

Stroke, resulting from brain hemorrhage or infarction, commonly results in cognitive impairments such as aphasia, neglect, reduced processing speed, impaired attention, and executive dysfunction (e.g., Cumming et al., 2013). Even though cognition can improve during the first year after stroke (Desmond et al., 1996; Tham et al., 2002; del Ser et al., 2005), cognitive impairment frequently persists long after. More than 60% of stroke survivors still reported mild to severe cognitive impairment up to 10 years after stroke (Maaijwee et al., 2014; Middleton et al., 2014). Furthermore, cognitive impairments continue to deteriorate in 11% of stroke survivors during the first year after stroke (Tham et al., 2002). Therefore, rehabilitation efforts to ameliorate these cognitive impairments are essential.

Guidelines for neurorehabilitation are mainly focused on compensational strategy training (Cicerone et al., 2011). These strategies do not aim to restore brain functions (i.e., restitution), but aim to compensate for the lost function by using remaining intact functions. In this approach, residual plasticity of the brain throughout adulthood, which may enable restitution of the impaired function, is ignored (e.g., Kelly et al., 2006; Takeuchi and Izumi, 2015).

Robertson and Murre (1999) postulated that depending on the amount of remaining connectivity, different types of intervention are needed, notably restitution or compensation. Mildly damaged brain networks might reconnect by everyday life activities, and no special intervention is necessary. Severely affected brain networks may not be able to reconnect at all. Therefore, in severe cases compensational interventions are required that make use of preserved networks. For moderately affected networks, restitution-based interventions may be needed to stimulate the relevant parts of the impaired network.

Restitution focused treatments commonly consist of massed frequent repetition or stimulation of the affected function (Hamzei et al., 2006). They have proven to be effective in the domains of language, motor function, and vision (e.g., Kurland et al., 2010; Thrane et al., 2014). For other cognitive domains, such as attention and executive function, restitution training may consist of, for example, training reaction speed. Conversely, compensation interventions may consist of, for example, time management training to teach the patient to take more time for task execution. One type of restitution-based interventions use computer tasks aimed at training of damaged networks.

To date it is not yet clear whether restitution-based computer training can improve attention, working memory, and executive functions. In healthy adults, training effects have been contradictory (e.g., Owen et al., 2010; Anguera et al., 2013; Corbett et al., 2015), but a recent meta-analysis concluded that cognition can be improved (Toril et al., 2014). A systematic review of 10 studies in stroke patients concluded that restitution- and compensation-based interventions improved executive functions (Poulin et al., 2012). Even though the review by Poulin et al. did not only focus on restitution-based computerized training programs, their review does provide ground to further evaluate these restitution-based training programs.

This systematic review provides an overview of the evidence concerning the effects of computer-based restitution rehabilitation after stroke and other acquired brain damage to restore executive functioning. The term executive function includes a spectrum of cognitive functions, all revolving around control of one's behavior. This includes mental set shifting (i.e., changing from one set of task rules to another), information updating, and inhibition of prepotent but inappropriate responses (Miyake et al., 2000). For this review we considered working memory and divided (or selective) attention as part of the executive domain. Training programs that only focused on vigilance, tonic alertness, and sustained attention without any divided or selective attention tasks were not included.

METHODS

Search Strategies

We performed this systematic review according to the Preferred Reporting Items for Systematic Reviews and Meta-Analyses (PRISMA, Moher et al., 2009) statement. We searched in MEDLINE, PsycINFO, Web of Science, and The Cochrane Library. The search terms entered were a combination of three search areas that defined (1) the population as adults who had suffered a stroke or acquired brain injury, (2) the intervention as executive function computer training, and (3) the outcome as executive functioning. The complete search strategy can be found in Supplementary Material 1.

Inclusion and Exclusion Criteria

We considered articles in English, limited to humans, and published before the 12th of May 2015. Included participants were adults who had suffered stroke or other acquired brain injury. Computer training had to be the main intervention with a focus to improve working memory, attention related to executive functioning, or executive functioning.

Studies of strategy education or virtual reality training were excluded. Study protocols and dissertations were not considered. The selection of studies was first based on screening of title and abstract, followed by reading of the full text of the remaining studies (see flowchart in **Figure 1**). When in doubt, selection was discussed until consensus was reached.

Rating of Methodological Quality

The quality of the included studies was evaluated based on recommendations for reporting trials of the Consolidated Standards of Reporting Trials (CONSORT) statement (see **Table 1**). For each study, we also extracted the authors; year of publication; population; control group; training and its focus, duration, and setting; outcome measures and their significance level; the presence of adjustments for multiple testing; whether performance on training was related to outcome measures; use of ecologically valid measures; and potential conflicts of interest (see **Tables 2–4**). Treatment effect was evaluated based on statistically significant differences compared to pre-treatment and/or to a control group. Whenever adjustment for multiple testing was not performed and p-values were provided, we adjusted the reported p-values with Bonferroni-Holm correction. Similarly, for studies that did adjust but provided sufficient information to calculate the unadjusted p-value, **Tables 2–4** show tasks that would be significant *without* the adjustment. Due to the heterogeneity of the outcome measures, it was not possible to perform a meta-analysis.

RESULTS

We reviewed 1469 titles and abstracts; 63 studies were reviewed based on full-text. Twenty studies satisfied inclusion and

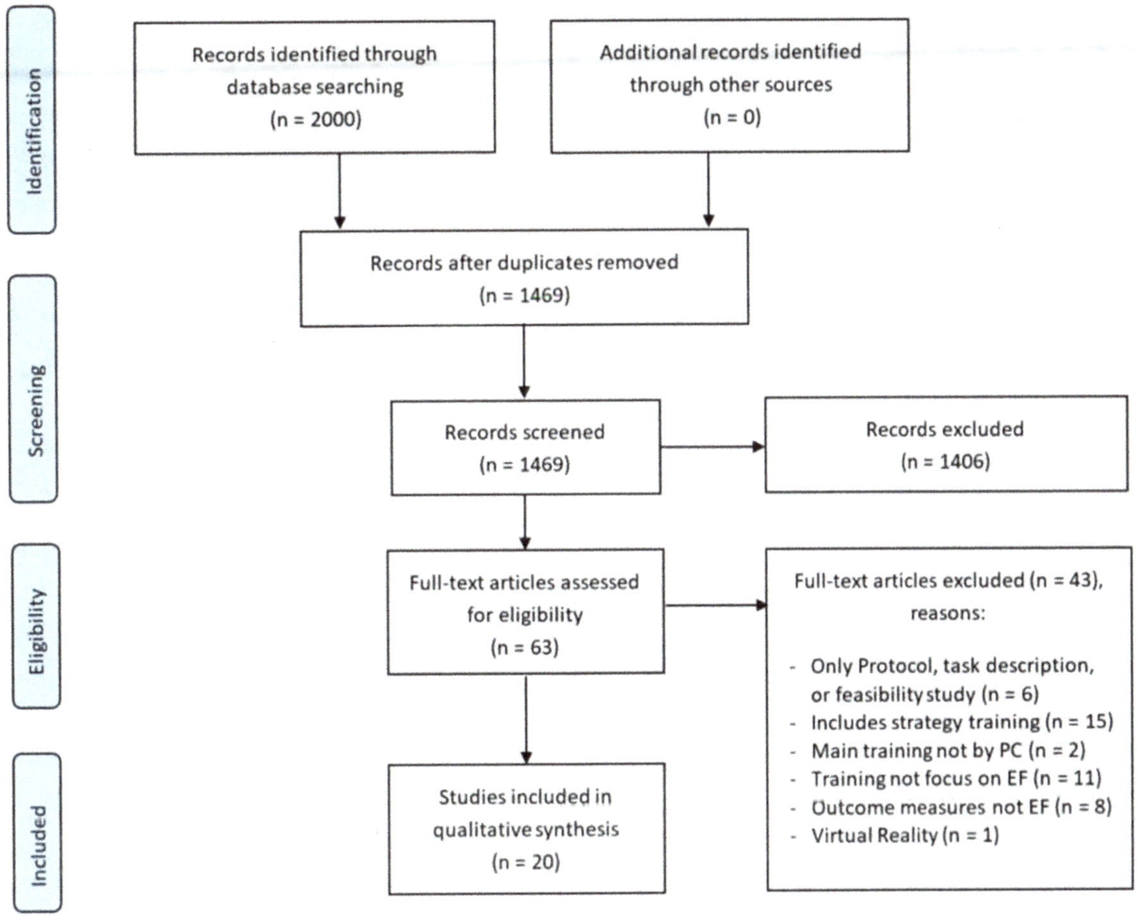

FIGURE 1 | PRISMA flow diagram (Moher et al., 2009) of study identification process.

exclusion criteria for this systematic review (see **Figure 1**). An overview of the data extracted is listed in **Tables 2–4**.

The included studies consisted of nine randomized controlled trials (RCT), six single case studies, four uncontrolled trials of which two used multiple baselines (i.e., multiple measurement time-points before training onset), and one retrospective study. Two studies used an active control group (i.e., the control group received an alternative, but supposedly ineffective training), and seven studies used a passive control group (i.e., the control group did not receive anything in addition to care as usual). The median sample size was 32 (range: 1–75). Two studies had a single subject design (i.e., $n = 1$). Two studies used the same sample (Akerlund et al., 2013; Björkdahl et al., 2013). Five studies included post-acute patients, six included chronic patients, and nine included a combination of both.

Scores on the selected CONSORT statement criteria ranged from 7 to 11.5 out of maximum 16 (see **Table 1**). Setting of training (e.g., given at home or in the rehabilitation center with or without supervision) was described in 11 studies. In all but two studies (Chen et al., 1997; De Luca et al., 2014) reports of training duration included the scheduled number of sessions per week. The median *planned* number of hours of training was 15.6 (range: 4.5–60). Only three studies included the *actual* number of training hours performed by the participants (Gray et al., 1992; Westerberg et al., 2007; Lundqvist et al., 2010).

Blinding of assessors was done in three studies, but the participants were never blinded. Description of outcome measures commonly included the name of the task, but not which specific task parameter was used (e.g., raw scores or scaled scores, response times or number of errors). One study did not use statistical methods to evaluate its results (van Vleet et al., 2015). Potential harms of the training were evaluated in two studies. One study reported no harms (Westerberg et al., 2007); the other reported mental fatigue, headache, and eye irritation (Fernandez et al., 2012).

Four studies adjusted for multiple statistical testing (Chen et al., 1997; Sturm et al., 1997, 2003; Spikman et al., 2010), and one corrected part of the statistical tests (Lundqvist et al., 2010). None of the studies correlated improvements on outcome measures with progression of performance during the training. Four studies examined performance on the training tasks itself, which improved in all studies (Westerberg et al., 2007; Lundqvist et al., 2010; Zickefoose et al., 2013; van Vleet et al., 2015). Two studies reported conflicts of interest (Ruff et al., 1994; Westerberg

TABLE 1 | Study quality based on the CONSORT statement.

	Study	Working memory				Attention								Multi modal							Imaging
		Akerlund et al., 2013	**Björkdahl et al., 2013**	**Lundqvist et al., 2010**	**Westerberg et al., 2007**	**Gauggel and Niemann, 1996**	**Hauke et al., 2011**	**Ponsford and Kinsella, 1988**	**Prokopenko et al., 2013**	**Sturm et al., 1997**	**Sturm et al., 2003**	**van Vleet et al., 2015**	**Zickefoose et al., 2013**	**Chen et al., 1997**	**De Luca et al., 2014**	**Fernandez et al., 2012**	**Gray et al., 1992**	**Ruff et al., 1994**	**Spikman et al., 2010**	**Lin et al., 2014**	**Nordvik et al., 2012**
	Design	**B**	**B**	**B**	**B**	**C**	**C**	**C**	**B**	**G**	**C**	**E**	**C**	**F**	**B**	**G**	**A**	**D**	**A**	**B**	**C**
	Total score	**11**	**9.5**	**9.5**	**11.5**	**7.5**	**8.5**	**8.5**	**10.5**	**8.5**	**9.5**	**7**	**9.5**	**7**	**9.5**	**8.5**	**8.5**	**7.5**	**9.5**	**9**	**7**
Methods	Eligibility criteria participants	+	+	+	+	+	−	+	+	+	+	+	+	+	+	+	+	+	+	+	−
	Setting data collection	+	+	+	+	−	±	±	+	+	+	+	±	+	±	+	±	±	±	±	±
	Intervention description	+	+	+	+	±	+	+	+	+	+	±	+	−	±	±	+	±	±	±	±
	Outcome description	+	+	+	±	±	±	±	±	+	+	±	+	±	±	+	±	+	+	±	±
	Determination of N	−	−	−	−	−	−	−	−	−	−	−	−	−	−	−	−	−	−	−	−
	Randomization	+	+	+	+	−	n.a.	+	+	−	±	−	+	−	+	−	+	+	+	+	n.a.
	Blinding	−	−	−	−	−	n.a.	−	±	−	−	−	−	−	−	−	−	−	±	±	n.a.
	Statistical methods used	+	+	+	+	+	+	+	+	+	+	−	±	+	+	+	+	±	+	+	±
Results	N per group	+	+	+	+	+	+	+	+	+	+	+	+	+	+	+	+	+	+	±	+
	Attrition per group	±	−	+	+	+	+	±	+	±	±	+	+	n.a.	+	±	+	±	±	−	+
	Recruitment dates	+	+	−	−	−	+	−	−	±	−	−	−	+	+	+	−	−	−	+	−
	Termination reason	−	−	−	−	−	−	−	−	−	−	−	−	n.a.	−	−	−	−	−	−	−
	Baseline characteristics table	+	−	−	+	+	+	+	+	−	+	+	+	−	+	−	+	−	+	+	+
	N per analysis	+	±	+	+	+	+	±	+	+	+	+	+	+	±	−	−	+	+	+	+
	Extend of results reports	±	+	±	+	±	±	±	±	±	±	−	±	±	±	±	±	±	±	±	+
	Harms	−	−	−	+	−	−	−	−	−	−	−	−	−	−	+	−	−	−	−	−

Akerlund et al. (2013) and Björkdahl et al. (2013) used the same dataset; A, RCT with active control group (CG); B, RCT with passive CG; C, single case, multiple baseline; D, uncontrolled, multiple baseline; E, single case, matched controlled; F, Retrospective, case matched controlled; G, uncontrolled, pre-post; +, reported; ±, partially sufficient; -, not sufficient; n.a., not applicable.

TABLE 2 | An overview of working memory training studies.

Study (focus)	Population	Sample size	Training (focus)	Duration training (actual mean)	Setting	Outcome measures	Significance of comparisons of pre-training (t_0), post-training (t_1), and follow-up (t_2): Within Ss				Between Ss			Multiple testing adjusted	Ecological valid measure	Train. improv. Evaluated	Reported conflicts of interest
							t_1–t_0		t_2–t_0	t_2–t_1	t_1–t_0	t_2–t_0	t_2–t_1				
							CG	IG									
Akerlund et al., 2013 (WM, cognitive function, psychological health)	ABI, post-acute - chronic	$N = 38$: IG = 20 CAU = 18, cross-over	QM, Cogmed (WM)	30–45 min, 5 d/w, 5 w = 15,6 h (unkn.)	Rehab.; Coach feed-back 1/w	Dig Span	–	+	+	–	–	±	–	No	Yes, question-naire	No	None
						Dig Span rev.	–	+	+	–	–	+	–				
						Span board	–	–	–	–	–	–	–				
						Span board rev.	+	–	–	–	–	–	–				
						WM composite	+	+	+	–	–	–	–				
						BNIS	–	+	+	–	±	–	–				
						DEX	–	–	–	–	–	–	–				
						HADS anx.	–	–	–	–	–	–	–				
						HADS depr.	–	–	+	–	–	–	–				
Björkdahl et al., 2013 (WM, ADL)	See Akerlund et al.	See Akerlund et al.	QM, Cogmed (WM)	See Akerlund et al.	See Akerl. et al.	AMPS-motor	–	–	±	±	×	–	×	No	Yes, question-naires	No	None
						AMPS-process	–	–	–	–	×	–	×				
						RBMT-II	–	–	–	–	×	–	×				
						FIS	–	±	–	–	×	–	×				
						WM quest.	–	×	+	×	×	±	×				
Lundqvist et al., 2010 (complex WM, QoL and health)	ABI, chronic (≥ 1 y post onset)	$N = 21$: IG = 10 pCG = 11, cross-over	QM, Cogmed (WM)	45–60 min, 5 d/w, 5 w = 22 h [actual train sessions = 21–25 d (M = 23.2; SD = 1.6)]	Rehab.; Coach feed-back 1/w	PASAT	–	+[a]	+	.	.	.	.	Yes, Bonferroni correct. for tasks not for question-naires	Yes, question-naires	Yes, but not related to outcome measures	None
						LSPAN	–	+[a]	+	.	.	.	.				
						Picture Span	–	+[a]	+	.	.	.	.				
						Block Span forw.	–	+[a]	+	.	.	.	.				
						Block Span rev	–	+[a]	+	.	.	.	.				
						CWIT inh./swtch.	–	+[a]	+	.	.	.	.				
						COPM - perform.	.	.	+	.	.	.	.				
						COPM - satisfy	.	.	+	.	.	.	.				
						EQ-5D	.	.	–	.	.	.	.				
						Health VAS	.	.	±	.	.	.	.				
Westerberg et al., 2007 (visuo-spatial and auditory WM)	first stroke, chronic (1–3 y post onset)	$N = 18$: IG = 9 pCG = 9	QM, Cogmed (WM)	40 min, 5 d/w, 5 w = 16.7 h [actual train sessions M = 23 d (SD = 2.2)]	Home; Coach feed-back 1/w by phone	Digit span	.	.	.	.	+	.	.	No	Yes, question-naire	Yes, but not related to outcome measures	Yes, stock holders in company of software used
						Span board	.	.	.	.	±	.	.				
						Word list learning	.	.	.	.	–	.	.				
						Word list learning DR	.	.	.	.	–	.	.				

(Continued)

TABLE 2 | Continued

Study (focus)	Population	Sample size	Training (focus)	Duration training (actual mean)	Setting	Outcome measures	Significance of comparisons of pre-training (t_0), post-training (t_1), and follow-up (t_2)							Multiple testing adjusted	Ecological valid measure	Train. improv. Evaluated	Reported conflicts of interest
							Within Ss				Between Ss						
							t_1–t_0		t_2–t_0	t_2–t_1	t_1–t_0	t_2–t_0	t_2–t_1				
							CG	IG									
						PASAT	.	.	.	.	+	.	.				
						Ruff 2 & 7 SAT	.	.	.	.	+	.	.				
						Stroop - time	.	.	.	.	–	.	.				
						Stroop - raw	.	.	.	.	–	.	.				
						Raven's PM	.	.	.	.	–	.	.				
						CFQ	.	.	.	.	+	.	.				

+, significant (sign.) and survives adjustment for multiple testing (Bonferroni-Holm adjustment is based on the number of outcome measures used at that time-point); ±, sign. but doesn't survive adjustment; -, not sign.; ×, not included in analysis;., not mentioned in methods; a, post measure was 4 weeks after training completion.

Train. improv., training improvements; Ss, subjects; IG, intervention group; (p)CG, (passive) control group; CAU, care as usual; N, sample size; y, years; w, weeks; d/w, days per week; h, hours; min, minutes; WM, working memory; ADL, activities of daily living; QoL, quality of life; ABI, acquired brain injury; unkn., unknown; M, mean; SD, standard deviation; rehab., rehabilitation center; correct., correction.

Abbreviations neuropsychological tests: Rev., reversed; BNIS, Barrow Neurological Institute Screen for Higher Cerebral Functions; DEX, Dysexecutive Questionnaire; HADS, Hospital Anxiety and Depression Scale; anx., anxiety; depr., depression; AMPS, Assessment of Motor and Process Skills; RBMT, Rivermead Behavioral Memory Test; FIS, Fatigue Impact Scale; quest., questionnaire; PASAT, Paced Auditory Serial Attention Test; LSPAN, Listening Span Test; forw., forward; CWIT inh./swtch., Color Word Interference Test inhibition/switching; COPM, Canadian Occupational Performance Measure; perform., performance; EQ-5D, EuroQol 5D; VAS, visual analog scale; DR, delayed recall; SAT, Selective Attention Test; PM, progressive matrices; CFQ, Cognitive Failures Questionnaire.

TABLE 3A | An overview of attention training studies with double baseline measurement.

Study	Population	Sample size	Training (focus)	Duration training (actual mean)	Setting	Outcome measures	Significance of comparisons of pre-training (t_0), second baseline (t_{0b}), post-training (t_1), and follow-up (t_2)							Multiple testing adjusted	Ecological valid measure	Train. improv. Evaluated	Reported conflicts of interest
							Within Ss				Between Ss						
							t_{0b}–t_0	t_1–t_0	t_2–t_0	t_2–t_1	t_1–t_0	t_2–t_0	t_2–t_1				
Gauggel et al., 1996	ABI, post-acute - chronic (4–16 m post onset) with deficit in ≥2/3 NPA att. tasks	$N = 4$	Hierarchical (alertness, RT, vigilance, suppress interference, selective and divided att.)	30–40 min, 5 d/w, 2–4 w = 12.5 h (unkn.)	Unkn.	Attention:								No	No, only global question-naire	No	Not reported
						WDG	*[a]	–	.	.	.	.	.				
						Numb. connect.	*[a]	*[a]	.	.	.	.	.				
						D2	–	*[a]	.	.	.	.	.				
						WMS:											
						Logical mem.	–	–	.	.	.	.	.				
						Assoc. learning	–	–	.	.	.	.	.				
						CFT - Rey	–	–	.	.	.	.	.				
						LPS (IQ)	–	–	.	.	.	.	.				
						Sat. w Life Scale	*[a]	–	.	.	.	.	.				
						CES-D	–	–	.	.	.	.	.				
Hauke et al., 2011	Brainstem encephalitis, chronic (4.5 y post onset)	$N = 1$	CogniPlus (alertness)	45 min, 5 d/w, 3 w = 11 h (unkn.)	Unkn.	Intrinsic alert.	–	*	.	-	.	.	.	No	Yes, question-naire of att. deficit	No	Not reported
						Focused att.	*	*		- -	.	.	.				
						Vigilance	*	*	.	-	.	.	.				
						Divided att.:											
						Audio	*	*	.	- -	.	.	.				
						Visual	*	*	.	-	.	.	.				
						subj. att. (FEDA)	.	*	.	-	.	.	.				
Ponsford et al., 1988	Very severe HI, post-acute (<9 m post onset) with deficit in SoP	$N = 15$ (10 comple-ted)	Unkn. (speed of visual RT, visual search, selective att.)	15 times 30 min, 3 w = 7.5 h (unkn.)	Rehab.?	Four-choice RT	↑	–	↑	.	.	.	.	No	Yes, clerical task	No	Not reported
						SDMT	↑	–	↑	.	.	.	.				
						2-letter cancel.	↑	–	↑	.	.	.	.				
						Similarities	.	–	*	.	.	.	.				
						subj. Att. Beh.	↑	–	*	.	.	.	.				
						Clerical task	.	–	–	.	.	.	.				

(Continued)

TABLE 3A | Continued

Study	Population	Sample size	Training (focus)	Duration training (actual mean)	Setting	Outcome measures	Significance of comparisons of pre-training (t_0), second baseline (t_{0b}), post-training (t_1), and follow-up (t_2): Within Ss				Between Ss			Multiple testing adjusted	Ecological valid measure	Train. improv. Evaluated	Reported conflicts of interest
							t_{0b}–t_0	t_1–t_0	t_2–t_0	t_2–t_1	t_1–t_0	t_2–t_0	t_2–t_1				
Sturm et al., 2003	ABI, post-acute - chronic (3 m - 13 y post onset) with att. deficits in ≥2 att. domains	$N = 33$: 9: alertness 7: vigilance 11: selective att. 6: divided att.	AIXTENT (either alertness, vigilance, selective, or divided att.) + CAU (but no other att. therapies)	14 times 1 h = 14 h (unkn.)	Rehab.	TAP:								Yes, Bonferroni correct.	No	No	Not reported
						Alertness:											
						Phasic	-*	+[b]	.	.	.	.	.				
						Intrinsic	-*	+[b]	.	.	.	.	.				
						Vigilance:											
						Error	-*	-*	.	.	.	.	.				
						Omission	-*	+[b]	.	.	.	.	.				
						Selective att.:											
						Error	-*	-*	.	.	.	.	.				
						RT	-*	-*	.	.	.	.	.				
						Divided att.:											
						Omission	+	+[b]	.	.	.	.	.				

*+, significant (sign.) and survives adjustment for multiple testing (Bonferroni-Holm adjustment is based on the number of outcome measures used at that time-point); -, not sign.; *, sign. but unknown whether it would survive adjustment; -*, not sign. but unknown whether it would be sign. without adjustment; - -, sign; decrease ↑, improvement but not statistically tested;., not mentioned in methods; a, max 1/4 of patients sign. improved; b, max 1/4 training programs resulted in sign. improvement.*

Train. improv., training improvements; Ss, subjects; N, sample size; y, years; m, months; w, weeks; d/w, days per week; h, hours; min, minutes; ABI, acquired brain injury; NPA, Neuropsychological assessment; att., attention; HI, head injury; SoP, speed of processing; RT, reaction time; unkn., unknown; CAU, care as usual; rehab., rehabilitation center; correct., correction.

Abbreviations neuropsychological tests: WDG, Wiener Determination Apparatus; Numb. connect., Number Connection Test; WMS, Wechsler Memory Scale; mem., memory; Assoc., Associated; CFT, Complex Figure Test; LPS, Leistungsprüfsystem; Sat. w Life Scale, Satisfaction with Life Scale; CES-D, Center for Epidemiologic Studies Depression Scale; alert., alertness; subj. att. (FEDA), subjective attention (Fragebogen erlebter Defizite der Aufmerksamkeit); SDMT, Symbol Digit Modalities Test; 2-letter cancel., Two-letter cancellation task; subj. Att. Beh., Rating Scale of Attentional Behaviors; TAP, Test of Attentional Performance.

TABLE 3B | An overview of attention training studies with single baseline measurement.

Study	Population	Sample size	Training (focus)	Duration training (actual mean)	Setting	Outcome measures	Significance of comparisons of pre-training (t_0), post-training (t_1), and follow-up (t_2)							Multiple testing adjusted	Ecological valid measure	Train. improv. Evaluated	Reported conflicts of interest
							Within Ss				Between Ss						
							$t_1–t_0$		$t_2–t_0$	$t_2–t_1$	$t_1–t_0$	$t_2–t_0$	$t_2–t_1$				
							CG	IG									
Prokopenko et al., 2013	Stroke, acute–post-acute (<2 w) with mild cognitive impairments to mild dementia	$N = 43$: IG = 24 CAU = 19	Neuropsychological computer training (sustained, selective, divided, and alternating att.)	30 min, 7 d/w, 2 w = 15 h (unkn.)	Rehab.	Schulte's tables	±	±	.	.	±	.	.	No	Yes, question-naires but not specific about EF	No	None
						Clock drawing	–	±	.	.	±	.	.				
						MMSE	–	±	.	.	–	.	.				
						MoCA	±	±	.	.	–	.	.				
						FAB	–	±	.	.	±	.	.				
						HADS anx.	–	–	.	.	×	.	.				
						HADS depr	–	–	.	.	×	.	.				
						IADL	–	–	.	.	×	.	.				
						SS-QOL-2	–	–	.	.	×	.	.				
						PGIS	=	↑	.	.	×	.	.				
						CGIS	×	×	.	.	×	.	.				
van Vleet et al., 2015	Mild TBI, chronic (2–12 y) with Executive dysfunc.	$N = 5$: IG = 3 CG = 2 (contact matched)	TAPAT (tonic and phasic alertness)	9 times 36 min, 3 w = 4.5 h (unkn.)	Home?	EF:	Ratio pts clinically sign. improved:							N.a., no stat. analyses	No	Yes, but not related to outcome measures	Not reported
						ACT-18s	0/2	2/3	.	.	.	.	.				
						ACT-36s	0/2	0/3	.	.	.	.	.				
						TMT-B	1/2	2/3	.	.	.	.	.				
						verb. Fluency	0/2	2/3	.	.	.	.	.				
						LNS	0/2	2/3	.	.	.	.	.				
						Att. blink	0/2	3/3	.	.	.	.	.				
						PCL:											
						Concentration	×	2/3	.	.	.	.	.				
						Hyper-vigilance	×	1/3									
						Training – acc.	0/2	3/3	.	.	.	.	.				
						Training - FT	0/2	1/3	.	.	.	.	.				

(Continued)

TABLE 3B | Continued

Study	Population	Sample size	Training (focus)	Duration training (actual mean)	Setting	Outcome measures	Significance of comparisons of pre-training (t_0), post-training (t_1), and follow-up (t_2)							Multiple testing adjusted	Ecological valid measure	Train. improv. Evaluated	Reported conflicts of interest
							Within Ss				Between Ss						
							t_1–t_0		t_2–t_0	t_2–t_1	t_1–t_0	t_2–t_0	t_2–t_1				
							CG	IG									
Sturm et al., 1997	Unilateral stroke, post-acute—chronic (2 m-3 y post stroke) with att. deficits in ≥2 att. domains	$N = 38$: No control	AIXTENT (either alertness, vigilance, selective, or divided att.)	14 times 1 h = 14 h (unkn.)	Rehab.	TAP:								Yes, Bonfer-roni correct.	No	No	Not reported
						Alertness:											
						no warning	.	+[a]	.	.	.	.	.				
						warning	.	-*	.	.	.	.	.				
						Vigilance - hits	.	+[a]	.	.	.	.	.				
						Vigilance - RT	.	-*	.	.	.	.	.				
						Selective att.:											
						Error	.	–	.	.	.	.	.				
						RT	.	+[a]	.	.	.	.	.				
						Divided att.:											
						Error	.	+[a]	.	.	.	.	.				
						RT	.	+[a]	.	.	.	.	.				
Zickefoose et al., 2013	Severe TBI, chronic (≥3 y post injury)	$N = 4$: A-B-A-C-A design; B first: $n = 2$, C first: $n = 2$	B: Hierarchically-based Attention Process Training (att.; 4 w) C: Lumosity (att.; 4 w)	Per training 20 times 30 min in 1 m = 20 h (unkn.)	Unknw. (researcher was present)	Training	.	*	.	.	.	.	.	No	No	Yes, but not related to outcome measures	None
						TEA	.	?	.	.	.	.	.				
						Att. probe	.	?	.	.	.	.	.				

+, significant (sign.) and survives adjustment for multiple testing (Bonferroni-Holm adjustment is based on the number of outcome measures used at that time-point); ±, sign. but doesn't survive adjustment; -, not sign.; *, sign. but unknown whether it would survive adjustment; -*, not sign. but unknown whether it would be sign. without adjustment; ↑, improvement but not statistically tested; =, no improvement but not statistically tested; ?, not conclusive; ×, not included in analysis;., not mentioned in methods; a, max 2/4 training programs resulted in sign. improvement.

Train. improv., training improvements; Ss, subjects; IG, intervention group; CG, control group; CAU, care as usual; N, sample size; y, years; m, months; w, weeks; d/w, days per week; h, hours; min, minutes; TBI, traumatic brain injury; dysfunc., dysfunction; att., attention; unkn., unknown; rehab., rehabilitation center; n.a., not applicable; stat., statistical; correct., correction; EF, executive functioning.

Abbreviations neuropsychological tests: MMSE, Mini-Mental State Examination; MoCA, Montreal Cognitive Assessment; FAB, Frontal Assessment Battery; HADS, Hospital Anxiety and Depression Scale; anx., anxiety; depr., depression; IADL, Instrumental Activities of Daily Living Scale; SS-QOL-2, Stroke Specific Quality of Life Scale; PGIS, Patients' Global Impressions Scale; CGIS, Clinical Global Impressions Scale; ACT, auditory consonant trigrams; TMT, Trail Making Test; verb., verbal; LNS, letter number sequencing; PCL, Post-Traumatic Stress Disorder Checklist; acc., accuracy; RT, reaction time; TAP, Test of Attentional Performance; TEA, Test of Everyday Attention.

TABLE 4A | An overview of combined working memory and attention training study with double baseline measurement.

Study	Population	Sample size	Training (focus)	Duration training (actual M)	Setting	Outcome measures	Significance of comparisons of pre-training (t_0), second baseline (t_{0b}), post-training (t_1), and follow-up (t_2)							Multiple testing adjusted	Ecological valid measure	Train. improv. Evaluated	Reported conflicts of interest
							Within Ss				Between Ss						
							t_{0b}–t_0	t_1–t_0	t_2–t_0	t_2–t_1	t_1–t_0	t_2–t_0	t_2–t_1				
Ruff et al., 1994	Severe head injury, post-acute—chronic (> 6 m post onset)	$N = 15$: no control	THINKable (attention, memory)	2 h/d, ??? w = 2 × 20 = 40 h (unkn.)	Rehab.	Pc Attention	.	±	×	×	×	×	×	No	Yes	No	Yes, research was supported by company that developed the training
						Pc Memory I	.	–	×	×	×	×	×				
						Pc Memory II	.	±	×	×	×	×	×				
						Pc Memory III	.	–	×	×	×	×	×				
						Ruff 2 & 7 SAT	.	–	×	×	×	×	×				
						Digit symbol	.	+	×	×	×	×	×				
						Cont. perf. I	.	–	×	×	×	×	×				
						Cont. perf. II	.	–	×	×	×	×	×				
						RAVLT - direct	.	±	×	×	×	×	×				
						RAVLT - delayed	.	–	×	×	×	×	×				
						Corsi - direct	.	=	×	×	×	×	×				
						Corsi - delayed	.	–	×	×	×	×	×				
						WMS:											
						Information	.	–	×	×	×	×	×				
						Orientation	.	–	×	×	×	×	×				
						Mental control	.	±	×	×	×	×	×				
						Logical memory	.	±	×	×	×	×	×				
						Digits forward & backward	.	–	×	×	×	×	×				
						Visual reprod.	.	–	×	×	×	×	×				
						Assoc. learning	.	–	×	×	×	×	×				
						Subj att. - self	.	–	×	×	×	×	×				
						Subj att. - proxy	.	±	×	×	×	×	×				
						Subj mem. - self	.	±	×	×	×	×	×				
						Subj mem.-proxy	.	+	×	×	×	×	×				
						Beck depr.	.	–	×	×	×	×	×				

+, significant and survives adjustment for multiple testing (Bonferroni-Holm adjustment is based on the number of outcome measures used at that time-point); ±, significant but doesn't survive adjustment; -, not significant; ×, not included in analysis;., not mentioned in methods.

M, mean; Train. improv., training improvements; Ss, subjects; N, sample size; m, months; w, weeks; h/d, hours per day; h, hours; unkn., unknown; rehab., rehabilitation center.

Abbreviations neuropsychological tests: Pc, personal computer; SAT, Selective Attention Test; Cont. perf., Continuous performance; RAVLT, Rey Auditory Verbal Learning Test; WMS, Wechsler Memory Scale; reprod., reproduction; Assoc., Associated; Subj., subjective; att., attention; mem., memory; depr., depression.

TABLE 4B | An overview of combined working memory and attention training studies with single baseline measurement.

Study	Population	Sample size	Training (focus)	Duration training (actual M)	Setting	Outcome measures	Significance of comparisons of pre-training (t_0), post-training (t_1), and follow-up (t_2)							Multiple testing adjusted	Ecological valid measure	Train. improv. Evaluated	Reported conflicts of interest
							Within Ss				Between Ss						
							t_1–t_0		t_2–t_0	t_2–t_1	t_1–t_0	t_2–t_0	t_2–t_1				
							CG	IG									
Chen et al., 1997	CHI, post-acute–chronic (M = 15.9 m)	N = 40: IG = 20 CAU = 20	Bracy Process Approach (att., visual-spatial orientation, memory, problem-solving)	Differed per participant (unkn.)	Rehab.	Verbal IQ	+	+	.	.	×	.	.	Yes, p <.004 with Bonferroni correct.	No	No	Not reported
						Performance IQ	+	+	.	.	×	.	.				
						Full scale IQ	+	+	.	.	×	.	.				
						WAIS-R:											
						Information	(+)/-	+	.	.	×	.	.				
						Vocabulary	–	+	.	.	×	.	.				
						Digit span	(+)/-	+	.	.	×	.	.				
						Arithmetic	–	–	.	.	×	.	.				
						Comprehension	–	–	.	.	–	.	.				
						Similarities	(+)/-	+	.	.	×	.	.				
						Picture compl.	+	+	.	.	×	.	.				
						Picture arrange.	+	+	.	.	×	.	.				
						Block design	+	+	.	.	–	.	.				
						Object assem.	+	+	.	.	–	.	.				
						Digit symbol	+	+	.	.	×	.	.				
						Category test	(+)/-	+	.	.	–	.	.				
						TMT-A	+	+	.	.	–	.	.				
						TMT-B	+	+	.	.	–	.	.				
						WCST	(+)/-	+	.	.	–	.	.				
						Mental control	–	–	.	.	–	.	.				
						Digit span forw.	–	(+)/-	.	.	–	.	.				
						Digit span rev.	(+)/-	+	.	.	–	.	.				
						Logical mem.	–	+	.	.	–	.	.				
						Logical mem. DR	(+)/-	+	.	.	–	.	.				
						Visual reprod.	–	+	.	.	–	.	.				
						Visual reprod DR	(+)/-	–	.	.	–	.	.				
						Paired assoc.	×	×	.	.	×	.	.				
						Paired assoc. DR	×	×	.	.	×	.	.				

(Continued)

TABLE 4B | Continued

Study	Population	Sample size	Training (focus)	Duration training (actual M)	Setting	Outcome measures	Significance of comparisons of pre-training (t_0), post-training (t_1), and follow-up (t_2)							Multiple testing adjusted	Ecological valid measure	Train. improv. Evaluated	Reported conflicts of interest
							Within Ss				Between Ss						
							t_1–t_0		t_2–t_0	t_2–t_1	t_1–t_0	t_2–t_0	t_2–t_1				
							CG	IG									
De Luca et al., 2014	Severe brain injury, post-acute phase (3–6 m post onset)	$N = 34$: IG + CAU = 15 CAU = 19	Based on several web-based programs (memory, EF, abilities of thinking)	??? min, 3 d/w, 8 w (unkn.)	Rehab.?	MMSE	−	+	×	.	+	×	.	No	Yes, question-naires but not specific about EF	No	Not reported
						LCF	±	+	×	.	+	×	.				
						RML	−	+	×	.	+	×	.				
						RAVLT - direct	−	+	×	.	+	×	.				
						RAVLT - delayed	−	+	×	.	+	×	.				
						Att. Matrices	−	+	×	.	+	×	.				
						CV Fluency	−	+	×	.	±	×	.				
						LV Fluency	−	+	×	.	+	×	.				
						Constr. Apraxia	±	±	×	.	+	×	.				
						Barthel Index	+	+	×	.	−	×	.				
						ADL	±	+	×	.	±	×	.				
						IADL	±	+	×	.	±	×	.				
						HRS anx.	−	−	×	.	±	×	.				
						HRS depr.	−	+	×	.	±	×	.				
Fernandez et al., 2012	ABI (Stroke or TBI), mostly chronic (1-5 y post onset)	$N = 50$ no control	RehaCom software package (divided att., concentration, RT, audio and visual memory)	50 min, 5 d/w, 12 w = 50 h (unkn.)	Lab, 4 at a time with presence two specialists	MMSE	.	−	.	.	.	.	.	No	No	No	Not reported
						WMS:											
						Information	.	*	.	.	.	.	.				
						Orientation	.	*	.	.	.	.	.				
						Mental control	.	*	.	.	.	.	.				
						Logical memory	.	*	.	.	.	.	.				
						Digits forward and backward	.	*	.	.	.	.	.				
						Visual reprod.	.	*	.	.	.	.	.				
						Assoc. learning	.	*	.	.	.	.	.				
						Mem. quotient	.	*	.	.	.	.	.				
						TMT-A	.	*	.	.	.	.	.				
						TMT-B	.	−	.	.	.	.	.				

(Continued)

TABLE 4B | Continued

Study	Population	Sample size	Training (focus)	Duration training (actual M)	Setting	Outcome measures	Significance of comparisons of pre-training (t_0), post-training (t_1), and follow-up (t_2)							Multiple testing adjusted	Ecological valid measure	Train. improv. Evaluated	Reported conflicts of interest
							Within Ss				Between Ss						
							t_1–t_0		t_2–t_0	t_2–t_1	t_1–t_0	t_2–t_0	t_2–t_1				
							CG	IG									
Gray et al., 1992	mild-severe ABI, post-acute—chronic (7 w–10 y) with attention deficits	$N = 31$: IG = 17 aCG = 14 (recreational computing without time pressure)	Unkn. (att. involved in processes of control)	14 times 75 min, 2 d/w = 17.5 h (15.35h)	Rehab.?	Digit span forw.	×	×	×	×	–	–	.	No	No, only a psycho-logical well-being measure but not specific about EF	No	Not reported
						Digit span rev.	×	×	×	×	–	±	.				
						PASAT:											
						Total	–	±	×	±	–	+	.				
						Longest string	–	–	±	±	–	±	.				
						Info proc. rate	–	±	×	+	±	±	.				
						Arithmetic	–	±	×	×	–	±	.				
						WCST error	×	×	×	×	–	–	.				
						WCST pers. error	×	×	×	×	–	–	.				
						Finger tapping	×	×	×	×	–	–	.				
						Word fluency	×	×	×	×	–	–	.				
						Letter cancel.:											
						Time	×	×	×	×	×	×	.				
						Error	×	×	×	×	–	–	.				
						Picture compl.	×	×	×	×	±	–	.				
						Time estimation	×	×	×	×	–	–	.				
						Logical mem.	×	×	×	×	–	–	.				
						Logical mem. DR	×	×	×	×	–	–	.				
						Rey - copy	×	×	×	×	–	–	.				
						Rey - delayed	×	×	×	×	–	–	.				
						Neale accuracy	×	×	×	×	×	×	.				
						Comprehension	×	×	×	×	–	–	.				
						Block design	×	×	×	×	–	±	.				
						Similarities	×	×	×	×	–	–	.				
						GHQ-28	–	–	–	–	–	–	.				

(Continued)

TABLE 4B | Continued

Study	Population	Sample size	Training (focus)	Duration training (actual M)	Setting	Outcome measures	Significance of comparisons of pre-training (t_0), post-training (t_1), and follow-up (t_2)							Multiple testing adjusted	Ecological valid measure	Train. improv. Evaluated	Reported conflicts of interest
							Within Ss				Between Ss						
							t_1–t_0		t_2–t_0	t_2–t_1	t_1–t_0	t_2–t_0	t_2–t_1				
							CG	IG									
Lin et al., 2014	Stroke, post-acute (6–10 m) with EF and memory deficit	*N* = 34: IG = 16 pCG = 18	RehaCom software package (EF, memory)	1 h, 6 d/w, 10 w = 60 h (unkn.)	Rehab.?	WMS:								Not for NPA MRI *p* was set to < 0.005	No	No	None
						Information	–	–	.	.	×	.	.				
						Orientation	–	–	.	.	×	.	.				
						Mental control	–	+	.	.	×	.	.				
						Logical memory	–	+	.	.	×	.	.				
						Digits forward and backward	–	±	.	.	×	.	.				
						Visual reprod.	–	+	.	.	×	.	.				
						Assoc. learning	–	+	.	.	×	.	.				
						Memory quotient	–	+	.	.	×	.	.				
						TMT-A	–	+	.	.	×	.	.				
						TMT-B	–	–	.	.	×	.	.				
						Corr. between MRI & NPA	–	+	.	.	.	.	.				
						MRI	+	+	.	.	.	.	.				
Spikman et al., 2010	ABI, post-acute—chronic (3 m–39 y post onset) with dysexecutive complaints	*N* = 75: PC = 37 strategy training = 38	Cogpack (reaction speed, att., memory, planning)	20–24 times 1 h, 2 d/w, in 3 m = 22 h (unkn.)	Rehab.	Role Resum. List	+	+	+	–	- -	- -	- -	Yes, Bonferroni Holm correct.	Yes	No	Not reported
						DEX patient	+	+	+	×	–	–	.				
						DEX proxy	+	+	–*	×	–	–	.				
						DEX therapist	+	+	+	×	- -	–	.				
						Ex. Obser. Scale	+	+	+	×	- -	- -	.				
						QOLIBRI satisfac	+	+	–*	×	–	–	.				
						QOLIBRI burden	+	+	–*	×	–	–	.				
						BADS	+	+	+	×	–	–	.				
						TMT-B/A	–*	–*	–*	×	–	–	.				
						Stroop 3/2	–*	–*	+	×	–	–	.				
						ToL	+	+	–*	×	–	–	.				
						RAVLT - direct	+	+	×	×	–	×	.				
						RAVLT - delayed	–*	–*	×	×	–	×	.				

(Continued)

TABLE 4B | Continued

Study	Population	Sample size	Training (focus)	Duration training (actual M)	Setting	Outcome measures	Significance of comparisons of pre-training (t_0), post-training (t_1), and follow-up (t_2)							Multiple testing adjusted	Ecological valid measure	Train. improv. Evaluated	Reported conflicts of interest
							Within Ss				Between Ss						
							t_1–t_0		t_2–t_0	t_2–t_1	t_1–t_0	t_2–t_0	t_2–t_1				
							CG	IG									
						Tx Satisf. Scale	.	.	.	.	.	.	–				
						Tx Goal Attain.	.	.	.	.	- -[a]	.	- -				
						Ex. Secret. Task	.	.	.	.	.	.	–				

+, significant (sign.) and survives adjustment for multiple testing (Bonferroni-Holm adjustment is based on the number of outcome measures used at that time-point); ±, sign. but doesn't survive adjustment; -, not sign.; (+)/-, not sign. but would be without adjusting; *, sign. but unknown whether it would survive adjustment; –*, not sign. but unknown whether it would be sign. without adjustment; - -, CG is sign better than IG; ×, not included in analysis;., not mentioned in methods; a, not measured at baseline.

M, mean; Train. improv., training improvements; Ss, subjects; IG, intervention group; CG, control group; aCG, active control group; pCG passive control group; CAU, care as usual; strat., strategy group; PC, personal computer; N, sample size; y, years; m, months; w, weeks; d/w, days per week; h, hours; min, minutes; CHI, closed head injury; ABI, acquired brain injury; TBI, traumatic brain injury; EF, executive functioning; att., attention; RT, reaction time; unkn., unknown; rehab., rehabilitation center; NPA, neuropsychological tests; correct., correction.

Abbreviations neuropsychological tests: WAIS-R, Wechsler Adult Intelligence Scale revised; compl., completion; arrange., arrangement; assem., assembly; TMT, Trail Making Test; WCST, Wisconsin Card Sorting Test; forw., forward; rev., reversed; mem., memory; DR, delayed recall; reprod., reproduction; assoc., associated; MMSE, Mini-Mental State Examination; LCF, Levels of Cognitive Functioning; RML, Reversal Motor Learning; RAVLT, Rey Auditory Verbal Learning Test; Att. Matrices, Attentive Matrices; CV, Category Verbal; LV, Letter Verbal; Constr., Constructional; (I)ADL, (Instrumental) Activities of Daily Living Scale; HRS, Hamilton Rating Scale; anx., anxiety; depr., depression; WMS, Wechsler Memory Scale; PASAT, Paced Auditory Serial Attention Test; proc., processing; pers., perseverative; cancel., cancelation; GHQ-28, General Health Questionnaire; corr., correlation; Role Resum. List, Role Resumption List; DEX, Dysexecutive Questionnaire; Ex. Obser. Scale, Executive Observation Scale; QOLIBRI, Quality of Life after Brain Injury; satisfac, satisfaction; BADS, Behavioural Assessment of the Dysexecutive Syndrome; ToL, Tower of London; Tx Satisf. Scale, Treatment Satisfaction Scale; Tx Goal Attain., Treatment Goal Attainment; Ex. Secret. Task, Executive Secretarial Task.

et al., 2007), six studies reported no conflicts of interest, and 12 studies did not report on this. The extracted studies evaluated working memory training, attention training, or both. We will now discuss the evidence of these training programs in more detail.

Working Memory Training

Working memory is the storage of information for a short period of time such that it can be manipulated (Baddeley, 1992). It is important for many other cognitive functions such as planning, problem solving, and learning. It is crucial for everyday functioning, which is one of the reasons that it is the focus of many training studies (Westerberg et al., 2007; Lundqvist et al., 2010; Akerlund et al., 2013; Björkdahl et al., 2013). The most common computerized working memory training currently used is Cogmed QM (from Cogmed Systems AB, Stockholm, Sweden; now published by Pearson Assessment and Information B.V.).

Cogmed Training

The Cogmed training consists of five 30–40 min sessions per week during 5 weeks. Thus, a total of about 15 h of training is provided. It includes both audio (verbal) and visual (visuospatial) working memory tasks, which always require a motor response. Task difficulty is adapted to the performance of the trainee, and positive feedback is given immediately. It is a computer-based program that can either be done at the rehabilitation center (Lundqvist et al., 2010; Akerlund et al., 2013; Björkdahl et al., 2013) or at home (Westerberg et al., 2007). A coach monitors the progression of the trainee and contacts the trainee once per week to provide individual feedback. A detailed description of each task used in the training can be found elsewhere (Westerberg et al., 2007).

Objective Improvements of Working Memory

The training resulted in improvements on most objective working memory tasks used (Westerberg et al., 2007; Lundqvist et al., 2010; Akerlund et al., 2013) and the effects remained stable during three (Akerlund et al., 2013) or 5 months after training completion (Lundqvist et al., 2010; see **Table 2** for an overview). The tasks used to evaluate the training were all fairly similar to the training tasks and included verbal and visuospatial tasks, but some tasks were dissimilar to the training. This is important, because improvements only on tasks that are similar to the training (i.e., near transfer effect) are less likely to contribute to improvements in daily living than improvements that also generalize to tasks that are dissimilar to the training (i.e., far transfer effects). Far transfer was observed for complex working memory tasks that involved more than just remembering the stimuli (Lundqvist et al., 2010). These improvements in the intervention group ($n = 21$) were not observed in the passive control group ($n = 11$), but the two groups were not directly compared. The improved performance of one of these complex working memory tasks remained significant 5 months after training completion.

Objective Improvements in Untrained Cognitive Tasks

Objective improvements were not only observed on working memory tasks. General cognitive performance, as measured by an elaborate screening, significantly improved after training, also in comparison to the control group (Akerlund et al., 2013).

Improvements in other cognitive domains were mixed. Attention, which is closely related to working memory, also benefited from working memory training (Westerberg et al., 2007). Conversely, performance on a non-trained reasoning task did not improve significantly more than in the control group (Westerberg et al., 2007). The effect of the working memory training on inhibition appears somewhat inconclusive. Improvement on the Stroop color-word interference task was not significantly greater than in the control group (Westerberg et al., 2007). In another study, however, scores on the inhibition and switching condition of the slightly different Color Word Interference Test (CWIT) significantly improved after the training and remained stable 20 weeks after training completion (Lundqvist et al., 2010). This task seems to involve more working memory than the Stroop task, as it requires not only inhibiting a preferred response, but also switching between two task sets (i.e., mentioning the color of the ink vs. mentioning the letters of the word). This may explain why improvement of working memory could benefit CWIT performance and, thus, may not reflect improved inhibition *per se*.

Subjective Improvements

Working memory training also seems to improve subjective functioning in daily life. Improvements were seen in subjective ratings of working memory and in the effects of fatigue on daily living (Björkdahl et al., 2013), subjective cognitive functioning (Westerberg et al., 2007), and (satisfaction with) occupational performance (Lundqvist et al., 2010). It did not specifically improve subjective executive functioning (Akerlund et al., 2013). Effects of the training on health related quality of life were inconsistent as a significant improvement was only found for one of two questionnaires (Lundqvist et al., 2010).

However, all these studies used a control group that received either no training (Westerberg et al., 2007; Lundqvist et al., 2010) or care as usual (Akerlund et al., 2013; Björkdahl et al., 2013). Factors such as social contact or placebo effects may have accounted for the reported results. Nevertheless, Westerberg and colleagues reported that the effect of the training on the subjective measure of cognitive functioning was mostly in items related to attention and not in more general items. This suggests that it was a real training effect. Future studies should include an active control group that receives a mock training to control for placebo effects.

The question is, however, whether a placebo effect should be seen as irrelevant. The subjective experience of participants is important as this may improve their mood and self-confidence. Indeed, mood seemed to improve after working memory training (Akerlund et al., 2013). Furthermore, as Lundqvist suggested, following the structured training program may prepare individuals for returning back to work as they need to adhere to appointments and schedules in both instances.

Limitations of Working Memory Training Studies

Apart from the lack of appropriate control groups, another limitation of most of these studies is that they did not adjust for multiple statistical testing (Westerberg et al., 2007; Akerlund et al., 2013; Björkdahl et al., 2013), or only for part of the statistical tests (Lundqvist et al., 2010). An overview of which tasks would survive adjustment for multiple testing can be found in **Table 2**.

If multiple testing and comparisons with appropriate control groups were taken into account, some effects would disappear. From the objective working memory measures, only digit span backwards appeared to be significantly improved immediately after training (Westerberg et al., 2007; Akerlund et al., 2013) and at 3 months follow-up (Akerlund et al., 2013). The objective improvements of attention would remain significant and thus seem promising (Westerberg et al., 2007). Of the subjective measures, only subjective cognitive improvement tended to remain significant (Westerberg et al., 2007). In the study by Björkdahl et al. (2013) none of the between-group comparisons of subjective measures remained significant after adjusting for multiple testing, suggesting that these effects were not robust.

In two out of three studies there was no effect of the training on the visuospatial working memory task after adjustment for multiple testing (Westerberg et al., 2007; Akerlund et al., 2013). The visuospatial tasks used in the training may not have been sufficiently challenging to elicit transfer effects.

Lundqvist et al. (2010) and Westerberg et al. (2007) reported improved performance on training tasks. If improvements in cognition are due to the training, there needs to be a substantial correlation between the two. However, none of the studies related the improvements of the outcome measures to the improvement observed during the training.

Conclusion of Working Memory Training Studies

In sum, there is preliminary evidence that Cogmed can improve performance on tasks that are similar to the training (near transfer) and tasks that are dissimilar to the training (far transfer). This is the case for both objective working memory and attention. It also seems to improve subjective cognitive functioning. Moreover, the effect of the training has been shown for verbal working memory but not for visual working memory. Nevertheless, all studies described so far suffered from methodological limitations, to which we will return in the discussion section.

Attention Training

AixTent Training

Training programs aimed at improving attention are more diverse than those aimed at working memory (see **Table 3A** for an overview of attention studies with double baseline and **Table 3B** for studies with single baseline). One commonly used training is AixTent, which consists of separate training modules that can be combined. The modules focus on phasic alertness, vigilance, selective attention, or divided attention. Responses can be given with two response keys that can also be operated with only one hand. All tasks were designed to be game-like, and task difficulty is automatically adapted to the performance of the participant. Feedback is given during and at the end of a training session.

The phasic alertness training task requires controlling the speed of a vehicle to avoid hitting obstacles. The vigilance training tasks include identifying damaged objects in a production line and identifying changes in airplane movements on a flight radar. The selective attention training tasks requires to respond quickly when previously defined objects appear on the screen and to ignore others. The divided attention training task requires to monitor three parameters (both visual and auditory) and press whenever either of these parameters fall outside a certain range (Sturm et al., 1997).

Specific vs. Non-Specific Attention Training

AixTent was used in two studies that examined whether attention training should be specifically aimed at the impaired domain or whether general attention training could also result in improvements of a specific attention domain. Participants received the training for one of at least two attention domains that were impaired. Thus, the affected target domain received specific training, whereas the other received a non-specific training. After adjusting for multiple testing, the training improved only (Sturm et al., 2003) or mostly (Sturm et al., 1997) the target domain. This does not imply that the training resulted only in near transfer, as the tasks used for the training differed from the outcome measures. Moreover, the vigilance training improved selective attention, and the basic alertness training improved more complex selective and divided attention (Sturm et al., 1997). Thus, some far transfer effects to other domains seemed to be present. The authors concluded that attention training should be specific. This may in particular be the case when cognitive functions are hierarchical, where more basic functions should be trained first followed by more complex cognitive functions.

Basic Attention Training

These results (Sturm et al., 1997, 2003) also suggest that improvements in basic cognitive functions may generalize toward improving more complex cognitive functions but not the other way around. This implication indeed seemed to hold (at least partially) in a single case study and in a small matched control study of a basic alertness training (Hauke et al., 2011; van Vleet et al., 2015). In the single case study, the training effect was largest for alertness, that is, for the attention domain being trained (Hauke et al., 2011). During the multiple baseline assessments there was no improvement of alertness, suggesting the effect was specific to the training period. Training this basic attention domain not only improved alertness, but also focused attention, vigilance, and divided attention (both visual and auditory). These improvements remained stable 6 months after training completion. The participant also reported subjective improvements of attention to a normal level. She reported lower levels of fatigue, but still not at a normal level.

All improvements were observed already within six or eight training sessions, and subsequently, performance remained stable, suggesting that a few sessions suffice to train attention. Alternatively, placebo effects may have been present as only three training sessions already had a significant effect on alertness. Moreover, the significant improvements in the attention domains not being trained were already observed during the baseline period. Thus, it is impossible to separate the effect of the basic attention training in these more complex attention domains.

Basic attention training also resulted in improvements of non-trained executive functioning in a small matched control study (van Vleet et al., 2015). Three mild TBI patients with complaints of executive functioning received 4.5 h of alertness training. Clinically significant improvements (z-score difference > 1) were found on the individual level. All three patients clinically improved on two or three of the five executive functioning tasks and on an attention task. Conversely, one of the two control participants improved on only one of the five executive functioning tasks. These two small studies did not provide *p*-values (Hauke et al., 2011) or did not perform statistical testing (van Vleet et al., 2015). Thus, evaluation of the effects after adjustment for multiple testing could not be performed.

Hierarchical Attention Training

The above findings suggest that training basic attention may result in improvement of more complex attention and executive functioning. The effect of a hierarchical approach to attention training was examined in four patients who suffered an acquired brain injury (Gauggel and Niemann, 1996). During the first week of the study alertness was trained, followed by vigilance training and selective attention training, and in the last week divided attention was trained.

Participants were studied within 3–16 months post onset, and two already showed improvements during the baseline phase. It was, therefore, impossible to conclude whether the improvement after training of these two participants on an attention task was due to the hierarchical training. The effect of training did not generalize to ratings of life satisfaction and depressive feelings, or to non-trained cognitive domains.

The inconclusive results of this small study are not in line with the previous studies. Since this study presented the training in a hierarchical manner, one would expect clear improvement in attention and maybe even in other cognitive domains. The training duration of 12.5 h may have been insufficient as multiple training tasks were used. No outcome measures related to executive functioning were included. Thus, it is impossible to determine whether a hierarchical approach results in improvements of executive functioning.

Training of Multiple Attention Domains

Several other studies that also used tasks from multiple attention domains, but which did so for each training session in a non-hierarchical way, showed mixed results. Tasks used to train attention can be either basic or can be made more interesting by adding graphics and by integrating them into a game-like environment (such as AixTent). Zickefoose et al. (2013) compared both of these types of attention training within one study. Their sample consisted of four participants who had suffered a severe traumatic brain injury (TBI) at least 3 years ago. Within an A-B-A-C-A design, participants first started with 20 half-hour sessions of either the basic Attention Process Training-3 or several game-like attention tasks of the Lumosity website. Next, they followed 20 sessions of the other training.

Participants improved on the training tasks; they especially enjoyed Lumosity and were motivated to continue the training. Improvements were only observed in a subset of the non-trained tasks. One of the attention tasks appeared to suffer from a ceiling effect. One participant significantly improved after both training programs, whereas the other three participants showed both improvements and decrements in performance. Nevertheless, when there was an improvement, it was not only in basic attention but also in the more complex divided attention. The patterns of improvement revealed that generalization effects in this study, if any, were not very convincing. The authors suggested that the effects could be larger for less severely affected patients or for those receiving training early after injury. In addition, similar to Gauggel and Niemann (1996), the training occurred two times per week for 4 weeks, giving a total of 20 h, which may have been too short for generalization to occur.

In a RCT, Prokopenko et al. (2013) trained post-acute stroke patients with mild cognitive impairment and mild dementia. They based their training on several tasks used in neuropsychological assessments and kept the graphics of the training simple. Two weeks of training, focused on improving attention and visual and spatial abilities, apparently resulted in near transfer effects. After the training, participants in the intervention group ($n = 24$) scored significantly higher than the care-as-usual control group ($n = 19$) on tasks that closely resembled tasks used in the training.

Far transfer effects, however, were only observed in one out of seven tasks (a screening of executive functioning). Instrumental activities of daily living, mood, and quality of life did not improve (Prokopenko et al., 2013). None of the significant near and far transfer effects would survive adjustment for multiple testing. The measures that did not improve were very general and may have been insensitive to training effects. Furthermore, even though relatively long compared to other attention training programs, this training was still short. It only involved 15 h spread over 2 weeks and over training tasks of multiple attention domains, and the training tasks were not very attractive, which may have influenced participants' motivation. Nevertheless, only the intervention group reported subjective improvement of symptoms after the 2-week period, based on a rating of training satisfaction.

One study did not find any training effects. Ten patients who were within 9 months post severe head injury followed a speed of processing training that consisted of simple reaction time tasks, some of which involved the inhibition of responses (Ponsford and Kinsella, 1988). At a group level, the training did not add to the effect of spontaneous recovery. In half of the participants there only appeared to be a training effect when the therapist gave feedback about performance on the training tasks. This suggests that giving insight into the participant's performance, and thereby potentially increasing their motivation for the training, is important.

The training duration was 7.5 h in total, which is nearly half as long as the attention training programs we discussed so far. In addition, multiple tasks were used in the training, thus the training may not have been long enough to result in improvements. Another study that did show some effect of training with multiple tasks had at least 15 h of training (Prokopenko et al., 2013). In addition, the participants of Ponsford and Kinsella's study suffered very severe head injury, so that their brain damage may have been too severe for restitution training to be effective.

A strong point of the study by Ponsford and Kinsella is that they used an appropriate method to control for effects of spontaneous recovery. They did not only use a multiple baseline design, but they also investigated whether the *increase* in performance was larger during the training period than during the baseline period. The lack of training effect after correcting for spontaneous recovery underscores the necessity of adequate control groups or multiple baseline measurements.

Conclusion of Attention Training Studies

Based on the results of these studies, it is still unclear what an attention training should consist of to be effective. Neither the Attention Process Training-3 nor Lumosity training proved to be superior to the other (Zickefoose et al., 2013). Participants preferred the graphically stimulating Lumosity training, compared with the basic training. This indicates the importance to adjust training environments to the preferences of the trainee. Graphics can make the training more interesting. However, our experience in clinical practice is that, for example, flashing graphics and sounds may be distracting for certain patients. This potential trade-off should be investigated further.

Training is most effective in the attention domain that is specifically trained (Sturm et al., 1997, 2003; Hauke et al., 2011; Prokopenko et al., 2013; van Vleet et al., 2015). Attention may be seen as a hierarchy, in which training of basic attention can improve more complex attention. It is not clear yet whether training complex before basic attention can result in overloaded basic attention and consequently in deteriorated performance, as was suggested by Sturm et al. (1997, 2003). It is also not clear whether a hierarchical training would be superior to a training that either focuses on one attention domain or that combines several attention domains per session (Gauggel and Niemann, 1996; Prokopenko et al., 2013).

Several types of attention training transferred to at least some executive function tasks (Sturm et al., 1997; Hauke et al., 2011; Prokopenko et al., 2013; Zickefoose et al., 2013; van Vleet et al., 2015), but not to an abstraction task (Ponsford and Kinsella, 1988). Ecologically valid measures were not often included (Sturm et al., 1997, 2003; Zickefoose et al., 2013) or were only very general (Gauggel and Niemann, 1996; van Vleet et al., 2015). Of these ecologically valid measures, objective attention (Ponsford and Kinsella, 1988), subjective IADL (Prokopenko et al., 2013), and life satisfaction (Gauggel and Niemann, 1996; Prokopenko et al., 2013) did not significantly improve. Only subjective attention improved (Hauke et al., 2011), whereas results for mood were inconclusive (Gauggel and Niemann, 1996; Prokopenko et al., 2013; van Vleet et al., 2015). Finally, it is important to provide feedback to the participant (Ponsford and Kinsella, 1988). Except for Sturm et al. (1997, 2003) and Prokopenko et al. (2013), studies did not correct for multiple testing and did not provide p-values. Thus, we were unable to take into account any distortions due to multiple statistical testing.

Limitations

The inter-individual differences in training outcomes may be due to factors such as lesion characteristics. None of the studies determined the extent of brain damage. One would expect that not everybody benefits equally from restitution-based training, assuming it depends on the residual functionality of the network being trained (Robertson and Murre, 1999). The study that included very severe head injury patients (Ponsford and Kinsella, 1988) did not reveal any transfer effects of the training, whereas the studies that included mild brain injury patients showed some transfer effects (e.g., Prokopenko et al., 2013; van Vleet et al., 2015). Future studies should, therefore, include imaging measures that can provide insight into the severity of damage to brain networks. Other limitations will be outlined in the discussion section.

Combined Working Memory and Attention Training

Non-specific training may result in beneficial effects when the aim is not to train one specific domain. Most studies that combined several cognitive domains included attention and working memory games (see **Table 4A** for an overview of a combined training study with double baseline and **Table 4B** for studies with single baseline). A variety of programs were used. One program used by two studies was RehaCom.

RehaCom

The RehaCom training consists of several graphical games that adapt to the performance of the participant and use a variety of stimuli such as playing cards. The training focusses on several cognitive domains. First, selective attention tasks where, for example a particular image needs to be found amongst several distracter images. Second, working memory tasks included to click on the playing cards that were shown before; at higher levels the cards need to be reproduced in reversed order. Finally, executive function was trained via divided attention tasks such as control the speed of a car while listening to the radio; or buying items from a shopping list while the purchases must fit within a certain budget.

Non-Specific Training

The two studies that evaluated RehaCom found generalizing effects to nearly all tasks used. Training improved performance on seven working memory tasks (both auditory and visual) and an attention task (Fernandez et al., 2012; Lin et al., 2014). Even though the authors did not adjust for multiple testing, the effect found by Lin et al. (2014) would remain significant if adjusted. No improvements were observed in the control group (n = 18), which received no training (Lin et al., 2014). However, the two groups were not directly compared, and Fernandez and colleagues did not include a control group. Thus, the results may be due to factors other than the training. Although these two studies used training programs of 50–60 h that included executive function tasks, there were no significant improvements on a task that is frequently used to measure executive function (i.e., the Trail Making Task version B). Both studies only used one outcome measure to assess executive function, which may have been insufficient to capture the spectrum of executive functioning.

A RCT using a similar, non-specific, 8-week training did reveal significant improvements on two tasks measuring executive function (De Luca et al., 2014). Participants who completed this training ($n = 15$) improved on 13 of the 14 outcome measures. This included objective neuropsychological measures of executive functioning, attention, and memory. It also included subjective functional and behavioral scales for daily living (De Luca et al., 2014). These improvements, except for one scale measuring functional performance in everyday life, were significantly larger than in a control group ($n = 19$), which received care as usual. Even though the authors did not adjust for multiple testing, 12 outcome measures (including the executive function measure) would survive adjustment for multiple testing. This suggests that the training resulted in improvements that generalized to untrained tasks.

As the study sample consisted of post-acute patients who had suffered severe brain injury, these positive results do not agree with the studies discussed earlier that failed to reveal (conclusive) transfer of training effects after severe brain injury (Ponsford and Kinsella, 1988; Zickefoose et al., 2013). De Luca and colleagues did not provide detailed information about the training or session duration. It is, therefore, impossible to evaluate which elements of the training resulted in these positive effects. For the subjective outcome measures it should be kept in mind that the control group received less attention, whereas the intervention group received 24 extra sessions, which may have contributed to a larger placebo effect.

Spikman et al. (2010) evaluated a 20-h Cogpack training ($n = 37$) and compared it to a multifaceted strategy training ($n = 38$). They found improvements in objective and subjective executive functioning in both groups. A far transfer effect was also observed in short-term memory and in subjective quality of life. All but the subjective quality of life improvements remained significant 6 months after training completion. These results were adjusted for multiple testing, which suggests that effects were likely to be true effects. Nevertheless, the Cogpack computer-training group never improved significantly more than the comparison group. Conversely, immediately after training, the strategy group improved more than the computer-training group on two executive function scales. These were, however, both rated by the therapist who was not blind to treatment condition. Neither of the training programs showed improvements in two tasks commonly used to measure inhibition or executive functioning. This was similar to what was found by Fernandez et al. (2012) and Lin et al. (2014). These two tasks may have been less vulnerable to retest effects than the other two executive function tasks that did show improvements after the training.

Both groups were equally satisfied with training, reported less executive dysfunction 6 months after the training, and felt that they started to participate again in social and vocational life. There was no evidence that the Cogpack computer training resulted in better outcome compared to strategy training. However, since improvements were observed in both groups a waiting list control group would be necessary to confirm whether the effects were specific to the training. Nevertheless, even if the improvements were mere retest effects, they may have had a positive effect on the participants' mood and motivation to continue a rehabilitation program.

In sum, training that combines memory and attention tasks resulted in transfer to working memory and attention tasks that were not trained. The extent of these training effects on executive function remains unclear as most studies included only one executive function task (Fernandez et al., 2012; Lin et al., 2014). The studies that did include multiple executive function tasks, did find improvements on most of these tasks (Spikman et al., 2010; De Luca et al., 2014), but the results of Spikman and colleagues were also found in their comparison group.

More Specific Training

Two studies used training programs that were primarily focused on one cognitive domain. The main focus of the training used in the RCT by Gray et al. (1992) was attention; we report this training in this section as it also included set shifting. The training consisted of approximately 14 sessions of 1–1.5 h, resulting in about 15 h of training ($n = 17$). The active control group ($n = 14$) could play computer games of their choice that did not involve time pressure, and they trained 12.7 h on average.

Twenty-one outcome measures were used, but only two significant group differences were found. Moreover, these effects disappeared when time since onset of brain injury and premorbid IQ were taken into account. Thus, the authors failed to find any far transfer effects immediately after training. However, 6 months after training completion, the experimental group did show a significant improvement compared to the control group on several tasks that were similar to the focus of the training. This effect remained after controlling for premorbid IQ and time since onset. The authors suggested that these improvements were already visible immediately after training but only reached significance at follow-up. They concluded that the training only had an effect on targeted functions but failed to generalize to cognitive functions that were not trained. This study stresses the importance of follow-up measurements.

Although the training included several executive functioning tasks, the experimental group did not improve significantly more on these tasks than the control group. Both groups showed large variability in baseline scores on the executive functioning task similar to the training. Perhaps the study lacked sufficient statistical power to reveal a significant improvement. Furthermore, as the control group could freely choose the computer tasks, it was unclear which they performed and whether these tasks improved cognition.

Another study that used a specific training consisted of either memory tasks or attention tasks (Ruff et al., 1994). These two training programs were compared in a multiple baseline design with 15 participants who had suffered severe head injury. However, both groups were pooled for statistical analyses, so that unfortunately training specific effects could not be identified. Results revealed that a proxy, who knew that their acquaintance followed the training, rated significant improvements in both attention and memory. Participants themselves rated that they significantly improved in memory, but not in attention. The training also improved objective short-term memory performance but failed to influence long-term memory. Depression scores did not consistently change after the training.

The authors did not include a control group, nor did they adjust for multiple testing. Only the effect on a processing speed task and the proxy ratings on memory would remain significant if they would have been adjusted. As the training tasks were not described, it is impossible to evaluate the results in light of the training. Moreover, the absence of executive function outcome measures makes it impossible to conclude whether the effects generalized to executive functions.

Hierarchical Training

In a retrospective study a hierarchical computer training was evaluated in closed head injury patients (Chen et al., 1997). The training started with basic cognitive functions and subsequently focused on more complex functions. Due to the retrospective nature of this study, training duration and interval between training and follow-up differed between participants. No differences were found between the care-as-usual group ($n = 20$) and the computer-training group ($n = 20$) in four composite scores of the cognitive domains on which the training focused. Nevertheless, when evaluating each task separately, the computer-training group gained significantly on 20 tasks compared with a mere 10 tasks in the care-as-usual group after adjusting for multiple testing (see **Table 4B** for measures that would be significant without adjustment). This included an executive function task, an attention task, and some memory tasks. Participants were not randomly assigned to groups, and the groups differed significantly in time since onset and length of treatment. Even though these two variables were added as covariates, still other factors may have influenced the treatment effects.

Conclusions and Limitations of Combined Working Memory and Attention Training

Training programs combining attention, working memory, and other executive function tasks did not show consistent objective executive functioning improvements. This may be due to the small number of tasks used in some studies to measure executive functioning, to the large variability of baseline scores on these tasks, and to the often small sample sizes and ensuing low statistical power of these studies.

Subjective executive function improvements were noted by the participants themselves and by their proxies and therapists (Spikman et al., 2010). Other subjective improvements were reported for attention and memory (Ruff et al., 1994), everyday life functioning (De Luca et al., 2014), and quality of life (Spikman et al., 2010). Effects on mood were inconclusive; whereas reductions in anxiety were found, psychological well-being did not improve (Gray et al., 1992) and depression levels were only reduced in one of two studies in which it was measured (De Luca et al., 2014). Except for depression, these subjective ratings were never measured in more than one study. Thus, replication is clearly needed. Moreover, studies that included an active control group found improvements in both groups (Spikman et al., 2010) and did not find any group differences (Gray et al., 1992; Spikman et al., 2010). The other studies either included a passive control group or no control group at all, and thus results could be due to placebo effects.

Both objective auditory and visual memory commonly improved (Chen et al., 1997; Fernandez et al., 2012; Lin et al., 2014), but this was the case for immediate recall and rarely for delayed recall (Ruff et al., 1994; Spikman et al., 2010; De Luca et al., 2014). Similarly, objective attention also improved (Gray et al., 1992; Ruff et al., 1994; Chen et al., 1997; Fernandez et al., 2012; De Luca et al., 2014; Lin et al., 2014). Some of these effects were revealed only at the long term (Gray et al., 1992) and some effects were not significantly larger compared with the control group (Chen et al., 1997; Spikman et al., 2010). Most training programs did include a memory or attention component, and therefore, improvements in these domains were expected.

Improvements in non-trained objective outcomes were also frequently reported. General cognition improved more than in the control group (De Luca et al., 2014). Furthermore, increased participation in everyday life (Spikman et al., 2010), processing speed (Ruff et al., 1994; Chen et al., 1997), IQ, and problem solving (Chen et al., 1997) were found. Conversely, improvements of verbal reasoning were inconsistent (Gray et al., 1992; Chen et al., 1997). The within group effects were not compared with a control group (Ruff et al., 1994; Chen et al., 1997) or the effects were also found in the control group (Spikman et al., 2010). Thus, even though these results seem promising, they need to be interpreted cautiously because of the lack of proper control groups, and they need to be replicated with improved methodological designs.

In contrast to attention specific training (Ponsford and Kinsella, 1988; Zickefoose et al., 2013), the training programs including multiple cognitive domains were effective after severe brain injury (Ruff et al., 1994; De Luca et al., 2014). Training also appeared to be effective for both post-acute patients (De Luca et al., 2014; Lin et al., 2014) and for those who were in the chronic phase (Fernandez et al., 2012). Finally, stroke patients (Lin et al., 2014) as well as patients with other etiologies (Ruff et al., 1994; Chen et al., 1997; Spikman et al., 2010; Fernandez et al., 2012; De Luca et al., 2014) seemed to benefit from the training.

Neural Effects of Computer Training

Nordvik et al. (2014) emphasized that most computer-based training studies do not investigate the effects on a neural level. In their overview, they summarize evidence for both gray and white matter changes after training certain skills in the healthy population (Nordvik et al., 2014). Within the stroke population, imaging is rarely used as an outcome measure. However, recently two studies reported both functional and structural changes in the brain after restitution-based training. One of these studies included strategy education as part of their training (Nordvik et al., 2012). Even though this study, therefore, does not fulfill our inclusion criteria, we still report it here, because the main elements of the training were two types of computer training, and because such imaging studies are sparse.

In a single case study, both a general computer training (focusing on five cognitive domains) and the specific Cogmed working memory training, were combined with a weekly session which included discussions about possible strategy use. Structural white matter connectivity measures changed during the training period and were stable when the participant was not training (Nordvik et al., 2012). Visual inspection of the data revealed that both training programs improved working memory. The connectivity measure correlated with working memory.

Functional connectivity also changed after the training used by Lin et al. (2014). As mentioned before, both working memory and attention improved after this training. This improvement was related to increased functional connectivity of several brain areas. The control group did not show any improvements in working memory, attention, or executive function after the training. The regional functional connectivity of this group did, however, significantly decrease after the period without training, but these changes did not correlate with cognitive performance. Although changes in functional connectivity were observed in both groups, this suggests that these changes were only related to the training effects in the intervention group and not in the control group.

It is important to note that brain changes can occur even when no behavioral changes are measurable. As both increased and decreased activity can be interpreted positively (i.e., increased communication vs. more parsimonious and efficient communication, respectively), one should preferably have a clear a-priori hypothesis and include healthy aged matched controls. Using non-invasive brain imaging is still relatively new in the field of brain training, which will be able to provide more insight into its effectiveness.

DISCUSSION

Summary of Results

In this review we aimed to determine whether computer-based restitution training can improve executive functions. Two of the studies we reviewed were of high quality because they were RCTs with active control groups and a sufficiently large sample size (Gray et al., 1992; Spikman et al., 2010). The intervention training groups in these studies did not improve more than the active control groups.

All other studies suffered from important methodological limitations. Consequently, their more positive results should be interpreted with caution. Results from the RCTs that included passive control groups, thus not correcting for potential placebo effects, revealed that training resulted in near transfer effects (Westerberg et al., 2007; Lundqvist et al., 2010; Akerlund et al., 2013; Prokopenko et al., 2013). Far transfer effects were also found, but mostly in tasks that were somehow related to the trained cognitive function (Westerberg et al., 2007; Lundqvist et al., 2010; Akerlund et al., 2013; Prokopenko et al., 2013; De Luca et al., 2014; Lin et al., 2014). Subjective improvements were not conclusively demonstrated but transfer was observed in several studies (Westerberg et al., 2007; Lundqvist et al., 2010; Björkdahl et al., 2013; De Luca et al., 2014). Spikman et al. (2010) found similar results within their intervention group (thus without comparing it to the active control group).

Effects on executive function remain inconclusive. Four studies found no improvements (Ponsford and Kinsella, 1988; Fernandez et al., 2012; Akerlund et al., 2013; Lin et al., 2014), five found improvements in part of the measures (Gray et al., 1992; Chen et al., 1997; Westerberg et al., 2007; Spikman et al., 2010; Zickefoose et al., 2013), and seven found improvements in all of their executive function outcome measures (Sturm et al., 1997, 2003; Lundqvist et al., 2010; Hauke et al., 2011; Prokopenko et al., 2013; De Luca et al., 2014; van Vleet et al., 2015). These effects were usually based on only one or two tasks. One particular working memory and attention measure (i.e., Paced Auditory Serial Addition Test; PASAT (Gronwall, 1977)) showed training effects in all three studies that included this task as an outcome measure (Gray et al., 1992; Westerberg et al., 2007; Lundqvist et al., 2010). This concerned studies of working memory training and studies of combined working memory and attention training. The PASAT seems to be a sensitive task to training effects and is suitable to be included in future studies. Three studies did not evaluate training effects on executive functioning (Ruff et al., 1994; Gauggel and Niemann, 1996; Björkdahl et al., 2013).

Six studies evaluated long-term outcome (Ponsford and Kinsella, 1988; Gray et al., 1992; Lundqvist et al., 2010; Spikman et al., 2010; Akerlund et al., 2013; Björkdahl et al., 2013). Transfer effects mostly remained stable several months after training. In the RCT with an active control group of Gray and colleagues, the only significant effects were observed at long-term follow-up. Only two studies evaluated the neural effects of training (Nordvik et al., 2012; Lin et al., 2014). They found that both structural and functional changes were related to training improvement.

What are the Effective Elements of Training, and Who Benefits?

It remains unclear which patients benefit from training and which training elements are essential. Positive results were observed in both severe and mildly affected patients in both the post-acute or the chronic phase. One study did not find any effects in a very severely affected post-acute sample (Ponsford and Kinsella, 1988). Both specific and general training programs seemed to be effective. Nevertheless, improvements were largest in the domain of the training itself, and results suggest that the function being trained should at least partially be targeted on the task where transfer is desired. The two hierarchical training programs failed to be effective, perhaps due to their methodological limitations. Training can be either basic or provided in a game-like environment. Participants showed a slight preference for the game-like training, not surprisingly, so training should be adjusted to the personal preferences of the patient. Finally, it is important to provide feedback.

Limitations of the Reviewed Studies

Lack of Control Groups and Blinding

The lack of proper control groups is one of the most important limitations of the studies reviewed here. Including a proper control group is important because spontaneous recovery can occur, and retest effects are common, especially for executive functioning tasks. A meta-analysis of attention training (not necessarily by computer) revealed that effect sizes of studies without control groups were always larger than effect sizes of studies with control groups (Park and Ingles, 2001). Similarly, transfer effects were absent in the current review when compared to an active control group (Gray et al., 1992; Spikman et al., 2010). Without proper controls it is impossible to draw conclusions about the nature of any effects. A passive control group will only correct for retest effects and spontaneous recovery, but not for placebo effects. An active control group controls for both placebo effects and Hawthorne effects (i.e., effects of being involved in something new and receiving attention). Nonetheless, the training interventions of the two active control groups used by Gray and Spikman were both potentially effective themselves, suggesting that both the experimental and the control training resulted in transfer effects. On the basis of our review we recommend that both an active control group and a passive control group should be included.

Placebo effects, for that matter, are not necessarily an objectionable phenomenon. Even if just being involved in something new results in placebo effects, it may improve the patients' quality of life, and motivate them for other types of rehabilitation. Long-term evaluation, which is currently lacking in most studies, is necessary to determine whether short-term training or placebo effects indeed benefit the patient.

Some may consider the use of control groups as controversial from an ethical point of view, because a potentially beneficial training is withheld from patients. Alternatively, multiple baseline measures, especially if baseline duration varies between participants, could filter out some of the effects of spontaneous recovery and retesting (as done by Ponsford and Kinsella, 1988). Also, the methodology of single-subject designs has improved considerably over the last decade, and it deserves to be applied more often (Dugard et al., 2011).

Blinding of both assessor and participant is another important factor for reliable assessment of outcomes. Only three studies blinded the assessors, and none of the studies reported that the participants were blinded. Blinding of the participants is of course difficult, but can be achieved when mock training is included. This is challenging, because the line between an effective training and a convincing control training is very thin.

Incomplete Training Descriptions

Most studies did not report the mean training time. In studies that did report the actual training time, this often differed from the training time as previously planned by protocol (e.g., Gray et al., 1992). Training duration and frequency are important in order to conclude whether behavioral improvements may be ascribed to the training, and whether neural changes may be likely. The median planned training duration of the reviewed studies was 15.6 h. This seems rather brief to obtain stable behavioral changes. The number of repetitions achieved within this time frame may also be insufficient for neural changes to occur (Kimberley et al., 2010).

The setting of the training was hardly ever described. In healthy elderly, training effects were smaller when training was done at home than when it was done in a group setting on site (Lampit et al., 2014). Face to face instructions also resulted in longer training sessions (Cruz et al., 2014) and in larger improvements (Man et al., 2006), than when they were given online and training was done at home. These factors could not be evaluated in the current review. The lack of description of the specific outcome parameters used, of relating the outcomes to training performance, of reports on conflicts of interest, and of evaluation of possible harmful effects of the training, all complicate evaluation of training effects. Without a clear description of all training tasks, it is impossible to determine whether an effect is evidence for far or near transfer.

Statistical Considerations

Only four studies adjusted for multiple statistical testing. Currently, there is no consensus whether this correction is necessary for pre-planned analyses (Rothman, 1990; Curran-Everett, 2000; Glickman et al., 2014). Confirmatory studies need to correct for multiple tests that concern the same research question; exploratory studies are not required to do so (Bender and Lange, 2001). In any case, it seems advisable to report unadjusted *p*-values and confidence intervals, and interpret the results in light of the number of statistical tests performed, especially when many tests are done. Replication studies are needed with the same outcome measures that previously have shown transfer effects, to allow drawing firm conclusions. The reviewed studies hardly ever used the same training program or outcome measures, and thus replication is still lacking.

The sample sizes used in the studies were small. Only three studies had more than 20 participants per group, one of which did not include a control group. None of the studies reported an a-priori sample size calculation to determine the sample size needed to reveal clinically significant effects. It is likely that effect sizes in this research field are small or moderate at best (e.g., Corbett et al., 2015). Thus, the studies reviewed here may have been underpowered, in which case, however, one might ask whether such small effects are still clinically relevant. For better insight into the clinical relevance of training interventions, future studies should report effect sizes.

Outcome Measures

Executive functioning was usually measured with only one task. As this is a very broad concept, a single task may not be enough to capture potential effects on executive functioning. The large variation of baseline performance on executive function tasks may mask potential individual improvements, which also remain undetected with small sample sizes.

Ecologically valid measures were rarely used. If used, they mostly consisted of subjective ratings and questionnaires. Ecologically valid measures are needed to evaluate real life benefits. Imaging was used in only two studies, and it was thus rarely possible to assess the training effects at the neural level. Results from imaging were promising, supporting the inclusion of imaging as an outcome measure in future studies.

Selection Bias

Another issue is possible selection bias. Most likely, patients only participated if they had at least some affinity with computers. Patients were recruited via rehabilitation centers, and sometimes from only one center. The latter may reduce the generalizability of the results. The exclusion rate was not often reported, but in the Akerlund study it was very high (e.g., >50%) which again reduces generalizability.

Limitations of This Review

There are several limitations to this review, most of which are inherent to the novelty of the field. First, due to heterogeneity of outcome measures it was not possible to perform a meta-analysis. Second, we could not assess the risk of bias. It is possible, and maybe even likely, that publication biases exist in this field of research. Selection bias in the studies was also not assessed. The acquired brain injury population is very heterogeneous with many different outcome and impairment patterns. Studies used strict inclusion criteria, which reduces generalizability. Third, we excluded virtual reality studies. Virtual reality often involves the use of the whole body, which makes is difficult to distil whether the effect is due to cognitive retraining or to the physical exercise involved. A recent systematic review of virtual reality studies concluded that it can be effective in improving cognition (Larson et al., 2014). With virtual reality it is possible to safely recreate real life situations. This may, therefore, be a good future way for repeated practice of certain tasks requiring executive functions.

Strength of This Review

Computers are now widely available and there is a trend to do brain training in many patient populations. It is important to establish whether the effectiveness of restitution-based computer programs can be confirmed. Our review added to the results of the previously performed systematic review (Poulin et al., 2012) because we systematically evaluated 20 studies that provided restitution-based training. Results of our review can be used to improve the methodology of future studies.

CONCLUSION

Most studies we reviewed suffered from methodological limitations. Samples were mostly small, appropriate control groups were often absent, and adjustment for multiple testing was rarely done. Consequently, it is difficult to draw firm conclusions about the effectiveness of training. With the current study designs, the effects reported may be due—at least in part—to spontaneous recovery, retest effects, or placebo effects.

Effects were most often reported on non-trained tasks that measured the function being trained. There were also reports of far transfer to non-trained tasks, but these tasks still mostly included some part of the function being trained. Training often increased subjective functioning, which is probably very important to motivate patients to continue following rehabilitation and to work on improvements. Overall, the results of these studies warrant continuation of research to determine whether restorative training methods can improve cognitive functioning. Computer training can easily be done at home, which is a cost effective way of improving motivation and subjective functioning, and hopefully of objective functioning after acquired brain injury.

The most important methodological improvements for future studies are that these should have larger sample sizes, both a stimulating but non-effective active control group and a passive control condition. Training periods should be longer and more stimulating training tasks adjusted to the preference and the ability level of the trainee should be used. Studies should also evaluate predictors of training outcome such as time since injury and symptom severity. Multiple outcome measures per cognitive domain without ceiling effects and with satisfactory ecological validity should be used. Long-term effects need to be evaluated and results should be replicated. The interpretation of the results should be in light of training progression and after appropriate adjustment for multiple testing. Effect sizes should be reported in order to evaluate clinical significance of results.

In this field it is a challenge to conduct well designed and sufficiently powered studies due to low budgets available, limited number of available patients, heterogeneity of the population, and ethical considerations. With this in mind, the currently reviewed studies provide valuable insights and emphasize the need of carefully designed RCTs for the future.

AUTHOR CONTRIBUTIONS

Conception and design of the work: RV, JM, BS. Data acquisition: RV. Data analysis: RV, BS. Interpretation of data: RV, JM, DV, BS. Drafting and revising the work: RV, JM, DV, BS. Final approval of the version to be published: RV, JM, DV, BS. Agreement to be accountable for all aspects of the work: RV, JM, DV, BS.

ACKNOWLEDGMENTS

This project is part of the research program "*Treatment of cognitive disorders based on functional brain imaging*" funded by the Netherlands Initiative Brain and Cognition, a part of the Organization for Scientific Research (NWO) under grant number 056-14-013. We thank Janneke Staaks for the search strategy assistance.

REFERENCES

Akerlund, E., Esbjornsson, E., Sunnerhagen, K. S., and Björkdahl, A. (2013). Can computerized working memory training improve impaired working memory, cognition and psychological health? *Brain Inj.* 27, 1649–1657. doi: 10.3109/02699052.2013.830195

Anguera, J. A., Boccanfuso, J., Rintoul, J. L., Al-Hashimi, O., Faraji, F., Janowich, J., et al. (2013). Video game training enhances cognitive control in older adults. *Nature* 501, 97. doi: 10.1038/nature12486

Baddeley, A. (1992). Working memory. *Science* 255, 556–559. doi: 10.1126/science.1736359

Bender, R., and Lange, S. (2001). Adjusting for multiple testing - when and how? *J. Clin. Epidemiol.* 54, 343–349. doi: 10.1016/S0895-4356(00)00314-0

Björkdahl, A., Akerlund, E., Svensson, S., and Esbjornsson, E. (2013). A randomized study of computerized working memory training and effects on functioning in everyday life for patients with brain injury. *Brain Inj.* 27, 1658–1665. doi: 10.3109/02699052.2013.830196

Chen, S. H., Thomas, J. D., Glueckauf, R. L., and Bracy, O. L. (1997). The effectiveness of computer-assisted cognitive rehabilitation for persons with traumatic brain injury. *Brain Inj.* 11, 197–209. doi: 10.1080/026990597123647

Cicerone, K. D., Langenbahn, D. M., Braden, C., Malec, J. F., Kalmar, K., Fraas, M., Ashman, T. (2011). Evidence-based cognitive rehabilitation: Updated review of the literature from 2003 through 2008. *Arch. Phys. Med. Rehabil.*, 92, 519–530. doi:10.1016/j.apmr.2010.11.015

Corbett, A., Owen, A., Hampshire, A., Grahn, J., Stenton, R., Dajani, S., et al. (2015). The effect of an online cognitive training package in healthy older adults: an online randomized controlled trial. *J. Am. Med. Dir. Assoc.* 16, 990–997. doi: 10.1016/j.jamda.2015.06.014

Cruz, V. T., Pais, J., Alves, I., Ruano, L., Mateus, C., Barreto, R., et al. (2014). Web-based cognitive training: patient adherence and intensity of treatment in an outpatient memory clinic. *J. Med. Internet Res.* 16, 130–140. doi: 10.2196/jmir.3377

Cumming, T. B., Marshall, R. S., and Lazar, R. M. (2013). Stroke, cognitive deficits, and rehabilitation: still an incomplete picture. *Int. J. Stroke* 8, 38–45. doi: 10.1111/j.1747-4949.2012.00972.x

Curran-Everett, D. (2000). Multiple comparisons: philosophies and illustrations. *Am. J. Physiol. Regul. Integr. Comp. Physiol.* 279, R1–R8.

del Ser, T., Barba, R., Morin, M. M., Domingo, J., Cemillan, C., Pondal, M., et al. (2005). Evolution of cognitive impairment after stroke and risk factors for delayed progression. *Stroke* 36, 2670–2675. doi: 10.1161/01.STR.0000189626.71033.35

De Luca, R., Calabro, R. S., Gervasi, G., De Salvo, S., Bonanno, L., Corallo, F., et al. (2014). Is computer-assisted training effective in improving rehabilitative outcomes after brain injury? A case-control hospital-based study. *Dis. Health J.* 7, 356–360. doi: 10.1016/j.dhjo.2014.04.003

Desmond, D., Moroney, J., Sano, M., and Stern, Y. (1996). Recovery of cognitive function after stroke. *Stroke* 27, 1798–1803. doi: 10.1161/01.STR.27.10.1798

Dugard, P., File, P., and Todman, J. (2011). *Single-Case and Small-N Experimental Designs: A Practical Guide to Randomization Tests, 2nd Edn.* Hove; Sussex; New York: Routledge.

Fernandez, E., Bringas, M. L., Salazar, S., Rodriguez, D., Garcia, M. E., and Torres, M. (2012). Clinical impact of RehaCom software for cognitive rehabilitation of patients with acquired brain injury. *MEDICC Rev.* 14, 32–35. doi: 10.1590/S1555-79602012000400007

Gauggel, S., and Niemann, T. (1996). Evaluation of a short-term computer-assisted training programme for the remediation of attentional deficits after brain injury: a preliminary study. *Int. J. Rehabil. Res.* 19, 229–239. doi: 10.1097/00004356-199609000-00004

Glickman, M. E., Rao, S. R., and Schultz, M. R. (2014). False discovery rate control is a recommended alternative to bonferroni-type adjustments in health studies. *J. Clin. Epidemiol.* 67, 850–857. doi: 10.1016/j.jclinepi.2014.03.012

Gray, J. M., Robertson, I., Pentland, B., and Anderson, S. (1992). Microcomputer-based attentional retraining after brain damage: a randomised group controlled trial. *Neuropsychol. Rehabil.* 2, 97–115. doi: 10.1080/09602019208401399

Gronwall, D. M. A. (1977). Paced auditory serial-addition task: measure of recovery from concussion. *Percept. Mot. Skills* 44, 367–373. doi: 10.2466/pms.1977.44.2.367

Hamzei, F., Liepert, J., Dettmers, C., Weiller, C., and Rijntjes, M. (2006). Two different reorganization patterns after rehabilitative therapy: an exploratory study with fMRI and TMS. *Neuroimage* 31, 710–720. doi: 10.1016/j.neuroimage.2005.12.035

Hauke, J., Fimm, B., and Sturm, W. (2011). Efficacy of alertness training in a case of brainstem encephalitis: clinical and theoretical implications. *Neuropsychol. Rehabil.* 21, 164–182. doi: 10.1080/09602011.2010.541792

Kelly, C., Foxe, J. J., and Garavan, H. (2006). Patterns of normal human brain plasticity after practice and their implications for neurorehabilitation. *Arch. Phys. Med. Rehabil.* 87, S20–S29. doi: 10.1016/j.apmr.2006.08.333

Kimberley, T. J., Samargia, S., Moore, L. G., Shakya, J. K., and Lang, C. E. (2010). Comparison of amounts and types of practice during rehabilitation for traumatic brain injury and stroke. *J. Rehabil. Res. Dev.* 47, 851–861. doi: 10.1682/JRRD.2010.02.0019

Kurland, J., Baldwin, K., and Tauer, C. (2010). Treatment-induced neuroplasticity following intensive naming therapy in a case of chronic wernicke's aphasia. *Aphasiology* 24, 737–751. doi: 10.1080/02687030903524711

Lampit, A., Hallock, H., and Valenzuela, M. (2014). Computerized cognitive training in cognitively healthy older adults: a systematic review and meta-analysis of effect modifiers. *PLoS Med.* 11:e1001756. doi: 10.1371/journal.pmed.1001756

Larson, E. B., Feigon, M., Gagliardo, P., and Dvorkin, A. Y. (2014). Virtual reality and cognitive rehabilitation: a review of current outcome research. *NeuroRehabilitation* 34, 759–772. doi: 10.3233/NRE-141078

Lin, Z., Tao, J., Gao, Y., Yin, D., Chen, A., and Chen, L. (2014). Analysis of central mechanism of cognitive training on cognitive impairment after stroke: Resting-state functional magnetic resonance imaging study. *J. Int. Med. Res.* 42, 659–668. doi: 10.1177/0300060513505809

Lundqvist, A., Grundstrom, K., Samuelsson, K., and Ronnberg, J. (2010). Computerized training of working memory in a group of patients suffering from acquired brain injury. *Brain Inj.* 24, 1173–1183. doi: 10.3109/02699052.2010.498007

Maaijwee, N. A. M. M., Schaapsmeerders, P., Rutten-Jacobs, L. C. A., Arntz, R. M., Schoonderwaldt, H. C., van Dijk, E. J., et al. (2014). Subjective cognitive failures after stroke in young adults: prevalent but not related to cognitive impairment. *J. Neurol.* 261, 1300–1308. doi: 10.1007/s00415-014-7346-3

Man, D. W. K., Soong, W. Y. L., Tam, S. F., and HuiChan, C. W. Y. (2006). Self-efficacy outcomes of people with brain injury in cognitive skill training using different types of trainer-trainee interaction. *Brain Inj.* 20, 959–970. doi: 10.1080/02699050600909789

Middleton, L. E., Lam, B., Fahmi, H., Black, S. E., McIlroy, W. E., Stuss, D. T., et al. (2014). Frequency of domain-specific cognitive impairment in sub-acute and chronic stroke. *NeuroRehabilitation* 34, 305–312.

Miyake, A., Friedman, N. P., Emerson, M. J., Witzki, A. H., Howerter, A., and Wager, T. D. (2000). The unity and diversity of executive functions and their contributions to complex "frontal lobe" tasks: a latent variable analysis. *Cogn. Psychol.* 41, 49–100. doi: 10.1006/cogp.1999.0734

Moher, D., Liberati, A., Tetzlaff, J., Altman, D. G., and The PRISMA Group (2009). Preferred reporting items for systematic reviews and meta-analyses: The PRISMA Statement. *PLoS Med.* 6:e1000097. doi: 10.1371/journal.pmed1000097

Nordvik, J. E., Schanke, A., Walhovd, K., Fjell, A., Grydeland, H., and Landro, N. I. (2012). Exploring the relationship between white matter microstructure and working memory functioning following stroke: a single case study of computerized cognitive training. *Neurocase* 18, 139–151. doi: 10.1080/13554794.2011.568501

Nordvik, J. E., Walle, K. M., Nyberg, C. K., Fjell, A. M., Walhovd, K B., Westlye, L. T., et al. (2014). Bridging the gap between clinical neuroscience and cognitive rehabilitation: The role of cognitive training, models of neuroplasticity and advanced neuroimaging in future brain injury rehabilitation. *NeuroRehabilitation* 34, 81–85. doi: 10.3233/NRE-131017

Owen, A. M., Hampshire, A., Grahn, J. A., Stenton, R., Dajani, S., Burns, A. S., et al. (2010). Putting brain training to the test. *Nature* 465. 775–778. doi: 10.1038/nature09042

Park, N. W., and Ingles, J. L. (2001). Effectiveness of attention rehabilitation after an acquired brain injury: a meta-analysis. *Neuropsychology* 15, 199–210. doi: 10.1037/0894-4105.15.2.199

Ponsford, J. L., and Kinsella, G. (1988). Evaluation of a remedial programme for attentional deficits following closed-head injury. *J. Clin. Exp. Neuropsychol.* 10, 693–708. doi: 10.1080/01688638808402808

Poulin, V., Korner-Bitensky, N., Dawson, D. R., and Bherer, L. (2012). Efficacy of executive function interventions after stroke: a systematic review. *Top. Stroke Rehabil.* 19, 158–171. doi: 10.1310/tsr1902-158

Prokopenko, S. V., Mozheyko, E. Y., Petrova, M. M., Koryagina, T. D., Kaskaeva, D. S., Chernykh, T. V., et al. (2013). Correction of post-stroke cognitive impairments using computer programs. *J. Neurol. Sci.* 325, 148–153. doi: 10.1016/j.jns.2012.12.024

Robertson, I. H., and Murre, J. M. J. (1999). Rehabilitation of brain damage: brain plasticity and principles of guided recovery. *Psychol. Bull.* 125, 544–575. doi: 10.1037/0033-2909.125.5.544

Rothman, K. J. (1990). No adjustments are needed for multiple comparisons. *Epidemiology* 1, 43–46. doi: 10.1097/00001648-199001000-00010

Ruff, R. M., Mahaffey, R., Engel, J., Farrow, C., Cox, D., and Karzmark, P. (1994). Efficacy study of THINKable in the attention and memory retraining of traumatically head-injured patients. *Brain Inj.* 8, 3–14. doi: 10.3109/02699059409150954

Spikman, J. M., Boelen, D. H. E., Lamberts, K. F., Brouwer, W. H., and Fasotti, L. (2010). Effects of a multifaceted treatment program for executive dysfunction after acquired brain injury on indications of executive functioning in daily life. *J. Int. Neuropsychol. Soc.* 16, 118–129. doi: 10.1017/S1355617709991020

Sturm, W., Fimm, B., Cantagallo, A., Cremel, N., North, P., Passadori, A., et al. (2003). Specific computerized attention training in stroke and traumatic brain-injured patients: a european multicenter efficacy study. *Zeitschrift Fur Neuropsychol.* 14, 283–292. doi: 10.1024/1016-264X.14.4.283

Sturm, W., Willmes, K., Orgass, B., and Hartje, W. (1997). Do specific attention deficits need specific training? *Neuropsychol. Rehabil.* 7, 81–103. doi: 10.1080/713755526

Takeuchi, N., and Izumi, S. (2015). Combinations of stroke neurorehabilitation to facilitate motor recovery: perspectives on hebbian plasticity and homeostatic metaplasticity. *Front. Hum. Neurosci.* 9:349. doi: 10.3389/fnhum.2015.00349

Tham, W., Auchus, A. P., Thong, M., Goh, M. L., Chang, H. M., Wong, M. C., et al. (2002). Progression of cognitive impairment after stroke: one year results from a longitudinal study of singaporean stroke patients. *J. Neurol. Sci.* 203, 49–52. doi: 10.1016/S0022-510X(02)00260-5

Thrane, G., Friborg, O., Anke, A., and Indredayik, B. (2014). A meta-analysis of constraint-induced movement therapy after stroke. *J. Rehabil. Med.* 46, 833–842. doi: 10.2340/16501977-1859

Toril, P., Reales, J. M., and Ballesteros, S. (2014). Video game training enhances cognition of older adults: a meta-analytic study. *Psychol. Aging* 29, 706–716. doi: 10.1037/a0037507

van Vleet, T. M., Chen, A., Vernon, A., Novakovic-Agopian, T., and D'Esposito, M. T. (2015). Tonic and phasic alertness training: a novel treatment for executive control dysfunction following mild traumatic brain injury. *Neurocase* 21, 489–498. doi: 10.1080/13554794.2014.928329

Westerberg, H., Jacobaeus, H., Hirvikoski, T., Clevberger, P., Ostensson, M. L., Bartfai, A., et al. (2007). Computerized working memory training after stroke - A pilot study. *Brain Inj.* 21, 21–29. doi: 10.1080/026990506011 48726

Zickefoose, S., Hux, K., Brown, J., and Wulf, K. (2013). Let the games begin: a preliminary study using attention process training-3 and LumosityTM brain games to remediate attention deficits following traumatic brain injury. *Brain Inj.* 27, 707–716. doi: 10.3109/02699052.2013.775484

2

Training on Working Memory and Inhibitory Control in Young Adults

Maria J. Maraver[1], M. Teresa Bajo[1] and Carlos J. Gomez-Ariza[2]*

[1] Department of Experimental Psychology – Research Center for Mind, Brain and Behavior, University of Granada, Granada, Spain, [2] Department of Psychology, University of Jaen, Jaen, Spain

Edited by:
Soledad Ballesteros,
National University of Distance Education, Spain

Reviewed by:
Marco Calabria,
Pompeu Fabra University, Spain
Erika Borella,
University of Padua, Italy

***Correspondence:**
Maria J. Maraver
mjmaraver@ugr.es

Different types of interventions have focused on trying to improve Executive Functions (EFs) due to their essential role in human cognition and behavior regulation. Although EFs are thought to be diverse, most training studies have targeted cognitive processes related to working memory (WM), and fewer have focused on training other control mechanisms, such as inhibitory control (IC). In the present study, we aimed to investigate the differential impact of training WM and IC as compared with control conditions performing non-executive control activities. Young adults were divided into two training (WM/IC) and two (active/passive) control conditions. Over six sessions, the training groups engaged in three different computer-based adaptive activities (WM or IC), whereas the active control group completed a program with low control-demanding activities that mainly involved processing speed. In addition, motivation and engagement were monitored through the training. The WM-training activities required maintenance, updating and memory search processes, while those from the IC group engaged response inhibition and interference control. All participants were pre- and post-tested in criterion tasks (*n*-back and Stroop), near transfer measures of WM (Operation Span) and IC (Stop-Signal). Non-trained far transfer outcome measures included an abstract reasoning test (Raven's Advanced Progressive Matrices) and a well-validated experimental task (AX-CPT) that provides indices of cognitive flexibility considering proactive/reactive control. Training results revealed that strongly motivated participants reached higher levels of training improvements. Regarding transfer effects, results showed specific patterns of near transfer effects depending on the type of training. Interestingly, it was only the IC training group that showed far transfer to reasoning. Finally, all trained participants showed a shift toward a more proactive mode of cognitive control, highlighting a general effect of training on cognitive flexibility. The present results reveal specific and general modulations of executive control mechanisms after brief training intervention targeting either WM or IC.

Keywords: executive control, cognitive training, working memory, inhibitory control, plasticity, transfer

INTRODUCTION

Executive Functions (EFs) refer to a variety of cognitive and brain mechanisms thought to be in charge of regulating the dynamics of human cognition and behavior in changing environments (Burgess, 1997; Smith and Jonides, 1999; Miyake et al., 2000; Jurado and Rosselli, 2007). In an influential empirical work, Miyake et al. (2000; see also Miyake and Friedman, 2012) used latent variables analyses to show that, despite their unity indicated by shared features, three different EFs emerged from performance in a variety of tasks: (i) *Switching*, which involves shifting flexibly between tasks or mental sets; (ii) *Inhibitory Control* (IC), which refers to overriding dominant or prepotent responses; and (iii) *Updating* of information maintained in Working Memory (WM). WM is usually defined as a cognitive system for temporarily storing and managing information that is necessary for undertaking complex cognitive tasks, and it is thought to play a key role in guiding goal-oriented behavior and novel problem solving (Braver et al., 2008; Unsworth, 2010; Wiley and Jarosz, 2012). As WM is thought to have limited capacity, the ability to update and disengage from information in this system is considered a core component of cognitive control and self-regulation (Miyake and Shah, 1999; Braver and Cohen, 2001).

Although there is some disagreement over the exact nature of EFs and their precise neural substrates (Miyake et al., 2000; Braver and Cohen, 2001; Kane and Engle, 2002; Banich, 2009), substantial evidence supports the fact that EFs play an essential role in learning and academic achievement (Bull and Scerif, 2001; St Clair-Thompson and Gathercole, 2006), knowledge acquisition (Blair and Razza, 2007; Danielsson et al., 2010), metacognition (Fernandez-Duque et al., 2000) as well as emotional and self-regulation (Barkley, 2001; Hofmann et al., 2012). The large role that EFs seem to play in efficient cognition and in successful behavior regulation has led researchers to develop interventions aimed at improving executive functioning, even in the short term. Brain plasticity is at the basis of the proposal that cognitive functioning can be enhanced by means of training. The basic idea is that during cognitive training, participants repeatedly activate neural regions involved in the training tasks (Olesen et al., 2004; Buschkuehl et al., 2012; Hussey and Novick, 2012; Hsu et al., 2014) enhancing, thus, the cognitive function supported by the specific neural region. As a consequence, training effects would generalize and transfer to non-trained tasks that also involve the targeted training domain, and the underlying trained brain areas (*near transfer*) (Lee et al., 2007; Thorell et al., 2009; Borella et al., 2014; Beauchamp et al., 2016). Furthermore, training effects could go beyond the trained domain and show benefits in measures considerably different from the training task, as long as they were associated with the trained process and shared comparable neural circuits (*far transfer*) (Jaeggi et al., 2008; Borella et al., 2010; Loosli et al., 2012; Dahlin, 2013). Similarly, at the behavioral level, transfer effects could be expected in potentially related cognitive functions, and lead to enhanced performance in a variety tasks that, although untrained, share the same cognitive mechanism than the targeted trained processes (Morrison and Chein, 2011). Although plenty of studies have found near transfer effects after training WM, IC, or attention, far transfer effects are still limited and inconclusive (Thorell et al., 2009; Spierer et al., 2013; Sprenger et al., 2013; Enge et al., 2014; Schwaighofer et al., 2015; Melby-Lervåg et al., 2016).

Training studies differ in the type of EFs targeted by the training tasks. WM has traditionally been the target for many cognitive training programs due to its well-known central role in cognition and its relationship with high-level abilities (Klingberg et al., 2005; Morrison and Chein, 2011; Jaeggi et al., 2013). Several studies have demonstrated positive effects of WM training in different age groups (Borella et al., 2010; Söderqvist et al., 2012; Jaeggi et al., 2013) with transfer to trained and untrained domains such as mathematical performance (Dahlin, 2013; Bergman-Nutley and Klingberg, 2014), reading abilities (Chein and Morrison, 2010; Dahlin, 2010; Loosli et al., 2012; Karbach et al., 2015), or reasoning and fluid intelligence (Klingberg et al., 2005; Borella et al., 2010; Jaušovec and Jaušovec, 2012; Au et al., 2014; but see Chooi and Thompson, 2012; Harrison et al., 2013; Redick et al., 2013 for failures to find far transfer effects after WM training; and Melby-Lervåg and Hulme, 2013; Bogg and Lasecki, 2015; Schwaighofer et al., 2015; Dougherty et al., 2016 for reviews).

Some other studies have focused on training IC processes (Spierer et al., 2013). Although several of these studies have failed to find behavioral transfer effects after training IC (Thorell et al., 2009; Berkman et al., 2014; Enge et al., 2014), others have found positive near and far transfer effects after task-switching training across the lifespan of healthy individuals (Karbach and Kray, 2009), training-related benefits in fluid intelligence scores in children after executive control training (Rueda et al., 2005, 2012; Liu et al., 2015), and near transfer effects in normal developing children (Dowsett and Livesey, 2000) or with executive control deficits (Kray et al., 2012). In addition to the behavioral effects, brain activity studies have reported different activation patterns in the brain network associated with IC: namely, increased activation in the right inferior frontal gyrus after training response inhibition in young adults (Berkman et al., 2014); or a more adult-like pattern of EEG markers (dorsolateral prefrontal negativity linked to the anterior cingulate gyrus) in 6-year-old children after a 5-day training with tasks involving conflict resolution (Rueda et al., 2005).

While, with some exceptions, studies focusing on either WM or executive control training show transfer effects (see Karbach and Verhaeghen, 2014 for a meta-analysis with studies that trained WM, switching and IC in older adults), to date very few studies have directly compared the effects of WM and IC training across tasks (see Thorell et al., 2009 for a comparison between WM and IC training in preschoolers). Thus, the main aim of the present study was to directly compare near and far transfer effects of two different training programs targeting either WM or IC processes. The direct comparison of these two types of programs is theoretically interesting since, according to some proposals, WM and IC seem to represent two separate EFs and may therefore have separate effects (Miyake et al., 2000). In addition, we also aimed to carefully control some factors that have been subject to criticism in previous training studies.

As mentioned, despite the studies showing positive results after training in young adults, its effectiveness is still controversial and far transfer effects are not always obtained (Schwaighofer et al., 2015; Melby-Lervåg et al., 2016). Results stemming from different training studies need to be carefully interpreted with special attention to methodological differences that could account for the diversity of findings. Thus, for example, training procedures targeting specific cognitive abilities (such as WM or IC) allow for more restricted attributions on training-derived transfer effects (Borella et al., 2010; Rueda et al., 2012; Jaeggi et al., 2013) than complex procedures that include multiple cognitive domains (memory, attention, IC, reasoning, etc), which seem to be less specific, and often yield more limited transfer effects (Schmiedek et al., 2010; Baniqued et al., 2014, 2015; Dovis et al., 2015; Hardy et al., 2015). Moreover, although many studies have used single training tasks (Rueda et al., 2005; Loosli et al., 2012; Carretti et al., 2013; Jaeggi et al., 2013), the potential generalization of the training might be enhanced by the use of different tasks recruiting the particular targeted process. Switching between multiple tasks targeting the same process during training might promote cognitive flexibility by adapting general processes and strategies, and thus, preventing the use of very specific task-strategies that would more likely be implemented when training is based on just one single task (Schmidt and Bjork, 1992; Bherer et al., 2005; Dahlin et al., 2008; Schwaighofer et al., 2015). Finally, the presence and type of control groups is an essential requirement to dissociate the effectiveness of training (Mohr et al., 2009; Dougherty et al., 2016; Melby-Lervåg et al., 2016). Thus, passive control groups (PC) may allow researchers to keep track of simple practice effects, while active control (AC) groups may enable them to uncover the specificity of different cognitive training procedures by maintaining similar levels of motivation and reducing the possibility of placebo effects (Boot et al., 2013; Dougherty et al., 2016).

Hence, in the present study we explored potential transfer effects of two executive-control training programs in young adults. We used a procedure that attempted to maximize generalization (by using multiple activities within each trained process) and to control for practice and motivation (by including active and passive control groups and by capturing motivational variables during training). Specifically, we compared a group of participants trained in working memory (WMT) to a group trained in inhibitory control (ICT). Both groups were trained with three different training activities during six sessions spread across 2 weeks. Importantly, the training procedures were adaptive and increased executive control demands. We included passive (PC) and active (AC) control groups in the study. AC performed the same training protocol as their experimental counterparts, but they engaged in activities that relied on perceptual abilities and progressively increased their speed demands, without increments in executive load (Peng et al., 2012; Takeuchi and Kawashima, 2012; Lawlor-Savage and Goghari, 2016). The batteries of training activities used here were designed from the Cognitive Training Program of the University of Granada (PEC-UGR[1]), which included a number of tasks that could be adapted and combined. We designed these batteries considering both the neural basis of the cognitive processes underlying the activities and the logic of the experimental procedures traditionally used to evaluate executive control. As for the ICT group, the training included versions of (i) the Stroop task in which participants had to select coins/numbers contained in congruent or incongruently sized bags; (ii) the Conflict resolution task, where a sample of animals was presented and participants were asked to search for a target match from a set of distractors displaying congruent/incongruent shaped/colored animals; and (iii) the Go/No-Go and Stop-Signal tasks, in which participants had to respond to matching shapes (a robot and a screw), and stop their response when faced with a rusted-looking shape. Regarding WMT, participants performed versions of (i) the *n*-back task, in which participants had to monitor sequences of open/closed windows from a six-window display presentation, and press a key whenever the open window was the same as the window *n* trials back; (ii) WM updating, that consisted of the serial presentation of objects of different sizes that were introduced in boxes. Participants were asked to recall the 2 to 6 largest/smallest elements from the series; and (iii) Dual Span tasks, in which participants were asked to recall the shape and color of an increasing number of animals and then ask to select the animal that matched one of the study animals from a set of distractors. Participants were evaluated before and after training with two criterion tasks (*n*-back and Stroop), with near transfer WM (Operation Span) and IC (Stop-Signal) tasks, as well as with far transfer non-verbal reasoning (Raven's Advanced Progressive Matrices). In addition, we included a far transfer task (AX-CPT; the AX version of the Continuous Performance Test) to explore whether WM and IC training might change the adjustment of distinct executive control strategies (proactive versus reactive), which have been proposed to support cognitive flexibility[2] (Braver et al., 2009; Burgess et al., 2011; Braver, 2012).

Also of relevance, in the present study we also aimed to explore the role of individual differences on training and transfer performance. This represents a recent and unexplored issue that may be important in predicting the benefits of training (Könen and Karbach, 2015). In this sense, previous studies have already reported that at baseline, reasoning predicts training achievement (Bürki et al., 2014). Furthermore, individuals' improvement during training has been shown to be a relevant predictor of transfer effects in young adults (Jaeggi et al., 2011) as well as in children and older adults (Zinke et al., 2013; Wang et al., 2014). Thus, in order to explore the potential role of individual differences in training success, predictors of training improvement and transfer gains were analyzed (Könen and Karbach, 2015).

Based on the key assumption that generalization to non-trained tasks could occur whenever there is cognitive and neural overlap between the trained processes and those engaged in the outcome measures (Woodworth and Thorndike, 1901; Persson and Reuter-Lorenz, 2008; Hussey and Novick, 2012), we expected the two experimental groups to exhibit differential and specific

[1]The Cognitive Training Program (PEC-UGR) has been developed by the collaboration between professors M. Teresa Bajo and M. Rosario Rueda from the School of Psychology of the University of Granada.

[2]Proactive control refers to an "early selection" control mode that anticipates and prevents interference before it occurs, while reactive control implies a "late correction" strategy that detects and solves interferences once it is already present (Braver et al., 2009; Braver, 2012; Morales et al., 2013). The AX-CPT is a sensitive and reliable experimental task widely used to explore individual differences in the use of proactive and reactive control strategies (Braver, 2012; Chiew and Braver, 2014). Hence, we used it to assess whether the participants' control mode changes with training. While young adults tend to rely on a proactive control strategy while performing the AX-CPT (Braver et al., 2009; Morales et al., 2013), training could somehow modulate the way they faced the task, which systematically required goal maintenance, interference detection and conflict resolution.

enhanced post-training performance (for related findings, see Chein and Morrison, 2010; Foy and Mann, 2014). Thus, we expected that, after training, the WMT group would outperform the ICT group on the *n*-back and Operation Span tasks, which involved WM maintenance demands. On the other hand, due to the greater reliance on conflict resolution for the ICT group than for the WMT group, we predicted better performance after IC training in the Stroop and Stop-Signal tasks relative to the WMT group.

Regarding the active control group, which went through progressive response speed demands, we expected benefits in response times after training. Processing speed, even at a low demand level, may lead to changes in performance mainly driven by the fact that participants' responses could become faster after the training (Peng et al., 2012; Takeuchi and Kawashima, 2012; Lawlor-Savage and Goghari, 2016).

As for the AX-CPT, which provided an index of the control strategy deployed by the participants, we hypothesized that the two executive control-training programs would make participants more dependent on proactive control relative to control conditions. This hypothesis is based on the assumption that the high executive control demands of both training programs would encourage participants to focus on contextual cues and, hence, to enhanced reliance on cue processing (rather than probe processing) on the AX-CPT task. If so, both types of training would lead to maximize the typical proactive strategy deployed by young healthy adults. However, we also expected the WM training, which specifically focuses on monitoring and maintenance, to have a stronger impact on proactivity than IC training.

Finally, on the basis of either the close relationship between matrix problem resolution, WM (Colom et al., 2004; Friedman et al., 2006; Harrison et al., 2015) and executive control (Dempster and Corkill, 1999; Engle and Kane, 2004; Jarosz and Wiley, 2012; Shipstead et al., 2015) and the results of some previous training studies (Jaeggi et al., 2008; Karbach and Kray, 2009; Rueda et al., 2012; Au et al., 2014), we expected to find better post-training performance in the reasoning test in the two experimental groups than in the active and passive control conditions.

MATERIALS AND METHODS

Participants

Participants were recruited via physical ads in the University of Granada requiring the fulfillment of the following conditions: (i) be aged between 18 and 30 years old; (ii) not to have any major medical or psychological condition; (iii) be committed to undertake at least four experimental sessions in the lab, which could be extended to 10. One hundred and twelve undergraduate students were selected to take part in the present study ($M_{age} = 20.51$ years; $SD_{age} = 1.74$; range = 18 – 25; 83 females). After pre-testing, they were randomly assigned to one of the four groups making up the study: ICT, ($N = 32$; $M_{age} = 20.41$ years; $SD_{age} = 1.88$; 23 females), WMT ($N = 32$; $M_{age} = 20.31$ years; $SD_{age} = 1.57$; 23 females), active control (AC, $N = 24$; $M_{age} = 20.75$ years; $SD_{age} = 1.32$; 18 females), or passive control (PC, $N = 24$; $M_{age} = 20.67$ years; $SD_{age} = 2.16$; 19 females). There were no significant differences either in age ($p = 0.76$; $\eta_p^2 = 0.01$) or in gender distribution ($p = 0.92$; $\eta_p^2 = 0.00$). At the end of the study, the participants were economically compensated for their involvement. None of the participants withdrew from the study although they were informed they could do so if they wished. This study was approved and carried out in accordance with the recommendations of the Research Ethics Committees of the University of Granada, with written informed consent from all subjects. All participants were provided with information about the study and gave written informed consent in accordance with the Declaration of Helsinki (World Medical Association, 2013).

Procedure

The cognitive training schedule consisted of two (pre- and post-training) testing sessions and six training sessions distributed over 2 weeks, with three training sessions per week. Therefore, the total length of the study extended for approximately 4 weeks. In the testing sessions all of the participants were evaluated for: (i) criterion tasks (*n*-back and Stroop); (ii) WM (Operation Span) and IC (Stop-Signal) as near transfer measures; and (iii) adjustment of proactive/reactive cognitive control (AX-CPT) and abstract reasoning (Raven's Advanced Progressive Matrices) as far transfer measures. We created two random task orders for evaluation that were counterbalanced across participants. The training and active control groups engaged in three different activities during each session (20 min per activity). The order of the activities in each training session was also counterbalanced over all participants. The resulting total training time for each activity was 120 min. The passive control group only performed the evaluation sessions and continued with their regular college activity during the 2 weeks between pre- and post-training.

Participants worked in individual cabins although an experimenter continuously supervised the procedure and was available to attend to any request. Every two training sessions participants were to complete a motivation questionnaire (Alonso-Tapia and de la Red Fadrique, 2007; Colom et al., 2013) in which they were asked for their: (i) involvement in the program; (ii) perceived difficulty of the activity levels; (iii) perceived challenge of improving over the levels; and iv) expectations for their achievement. They had to rate each of the four statements on a scale ranging from 0 (very low) to 10 (very high). In the last training session, they were asked for a general evaluation of the training program and their satisfaction with the experimental procedure.

Executive Control Training

We used the online training program from the University of Granada (PEC-UGR) that included different game-like activities organized in levels of increasing difficulty. Training difficulty was adaptive in order to maintain activities as a constant challenge (Klingberg et al., 2005; Brehmer et al., 2011; Karbach et al., 2015). Also, participants received feedback on whether their performance was correct or not (Katz et al., 2014). Activity levels were built up over runs of trials. Whenever participants succeeded in three runs they went forward to the next level and if they failed two runs, they went back to the previous level. Details of each of the three activities per training group are detailed below.

Inhibitory Control Training

Stroop-like

This activity was modeled on the Steinhauser and Hübner's (2009) complex Stroop task, which involved both conflict resolution and switching. The task was implemented in a scenario where bags of different sizes containing amounts of money had to be put into a treasure chest. Participants had to select the bag with the largest (gold in color) or the smallest (silver in color) number of items, with the number of bags increasing over the levels. The size of the bags could be either congruent or incongruent with the amount inside. An example of a congruent trial is one in which the stimuli were a big bag containing seven golden coins (correct choice) and a small bag containing five golden coins. In an example of an incongruent trial the stimuli could be a small bag containing six golden coins (correct choice) and a big bag containing three golden coins. Difficulty increased by changing the ratio of congruent/incongruent trials (0; 0.25; 0.50; 0.75), so that the larger the proportion of congruent trials, the harder the choice for incongruent trials. At higher levels, switching was manipulated by changing the color of the items from gold to silver between trials within the same round. Times to respond and inter-stimuli intervals were also progressively reduced with each level. The dependent variable was a relative index of conflict resolution [(RT in incongruent trials – RT in congruent trials)/RT in congruent trials].

Conflict resolution task

The scenario of this activity was an ocean where a sample of sea animals was displayed in the upper part of the screen and a group of animal buttons was shown in the lower part. The buttons set size was always sample $n + 1$ and it was progressively increased over the levels from 2 to 6. Participants had to select, as fast as possible, the animal of the buttons that had the same shape and color as one of the animals in the sample (match trials). If there was an animal whose shape matched but the color did not, they had to click on the different button (no-match trials). An example of match trial could be one in which the sample stimuli included "blue turtle – yellow starfish – brown crab" and the button choices included "pink turtle – yellow starfish (correct choice) – red crab – gray dolphin." On the other hand, a no-match trial could be one displaying as sample "blue turtle – yellow starfish – brown crab" and the button choices containing "pink turtle – green starfish – red crab – gray dolphin (correct choice)." The percentage of match trials was manipulated (0.25; 0.5; 0.75) so that the higher this ratio, the stronger the tendency to respond. Difficulty was also manipulated with the similarity of the color between the sample and the choice of the buttons. When colors were limited (a different color between the target and the possible options), the choice got harder since the color of the distractors had to be inhibited. The time to respond and inter-stimuli intervals were also reduced over the levels. The parameter distribution across the levels was manipulated following the procedures used in Rueda et al. (2005, 2012). As in the previous activity, the dependent variable was the score in the relative index of conflict.

Go/No Go-like

This was a matching-to-sample activity based on the shape of the items: a robot was the target and a screw was the sample. Participants had to respond when the shape of the robot and the screw matched (Go trials: i.e., a squared robot and a squared screw on its top) and inhibit their response when the shapes did not match (No-Go – shape trials: i.e., a circled robot and a squared screw on its top). At higher levels, there was an extra difficulty because the response had to be also inhibited when the screw was rusted (No-Go – color trials: i.e., a squared robot and a rusted squared screw on its top), even if its shape matched that of the robot. The proportion of Go trials (0.10; 0.20; 0.50; 0.80; 0.90) was manipulated together with the additional No-Go color trials ratio (from 0 to 0.30). The higher the proportion of Go trials, the stronger the tendency to respond with greater IC being required to succeed. The manipulation of the parameters was conducted following similar procedures regarding Go/No Go trials proportion (Benikos et al., 2013b) and reaction times deadlines (Benikos et al., 2013a). As in the previous activities, the maximum time to respond was reduced when levels increased (Benikos et al., 2013a). In this case, false alarms and omission errors were the dependent variables.

Working Memory Training

N-back

Participants had to monitor, maintain and continuously update the items throughout a sequence of elements. Participants were presented with a six-window house and had to detect coincidence between positions (opening/closing of the windows), sounds, or the combination of both modalities. They had to give their response pressing a button whenever the position of the opening window, its sound or both, matched the one that was presented as n positions-back in the sequence. Increments in n-back (from 1 to 8) were implemented after participants had completed the n-back level with single (position or sound) and dual (position plus sound) modality levels. As for the dependent variables, we considered the achieved n-back level and the sum of errors in each session.

WM search

This was a matching-to-sample activity based on the shape and color of the items sequentially displayed: animals on one screen as the sample, and a group of animal buttons after a retention interval. Participants were presented with a matrix to be maintained in memory composed of animals with different shapes and colors displayed in an open field (i.e., memory matrix, "brown bear – red eagle – purple snake"). After a retention time of 5000 ms, participants performed a memory test in which they had to select as fast as possible the animal on the buttons that had the same shape and color of one of the previously retained animals (i.e., button choices, "orange bear – red eagle (correct choice) – yellow snake – blank button"). If none of the animals on the buttons had the same shape and color, they had to select the blank button (i.e., button choices, "orange bear – green eagle–

yellow snake – blank button (correct choice)"). The number of to-be-maintained items increased from 1 to 8 over the levels. The number of elements recalled (set size) was the dependent variable.

WM updating

This task was adapted from the word updating task from Palladino and Cornoldi (2001). Participants were presented with a group of numbered boxes. Items of different categories (food, objects, animals, or clothing) were sequentially displayed. For each trial, items from only one category were relevant and introduced into the boxes (i.e., animals). Participants were asked to recall the larger (or smaller) element(s) by selecting the box or boxes in which they were introduced (i.e., Rule: recall the smallest animal; Items presented: apple – cat – trousers – bee (correct choice) – chair – elephant). Maintenance and updating in WM were involved in this activity. The memory load was manipulated by increasing the number of elements to recall (from 1 to 7), the number of distractors that belong to the target category (from 1 to 7), and the number of distractors from different categories (from 2 to 20). The program randomly changed the rule from big to small keeping an equal proportion of the trials within a level. The dependent variable was the number of items successfully recalled.

Active Control

Speed comparison

In this matching-to-sample activity, participants were presented with a group of sea animals in the upper half of the screen and another group of animals in the lower half, and they were asked to find as fast as possible which animal in the lower part was present in the upper part of the screen. In all of the trials, the target was presented in the sample, which increased from 2 to 6. Times were reduced within each sample size, so that whenever one element was added to the sample the time to respond started at a higher level at the beginning and was progressively reduced. Response time was the dependent variable.

Speed visual search

For this speed of processing task, participants were presented with a plate of soup with 10 elements (digits and letters) and they had to find one element contained in the soup out of four different possible options. The number of elements to be found and the possible options remained constant so that the difficulty of the levels was only determined by the speed of the responses over the levels. Average reaction time per session was the dependent variable in this case.

Speed categorization

This activity required participants to categorize groups of figures while progressively reducing the time to do so over the levels. Participants saw three groups of figures and two boxes to classify them according to different rules (size, color, shape, or quantity). The rule to be applied for categorizing them was always displayed in the upper left corner of the screen so that it trained the response time throughout the levels. As in the two previous activities, we considered reaction time as the dependent variable.

Transfer Tasks

Stroop

The scenario of this task was similar to the one used for training, where participants were presented with different-sized bags and they had to select one with the largest (or smallest) amount inside. The bags were either congruent or incongruent in size. The switching component was manipulated by changing the color of the coins and the consequent response rule from the largest (gold) to the smallest (silver). The number of bags presented (from 2 to 7), the proportion of incongruent trials (0, 0.25 or 0.50), the proportion of switching trials (0, 0.25, 0.50, 0.75), the inter-stimuli interval (from 1500 to 600 ms) and the maximum time to respond (from 3000 to 3600, this increased as a function of the number of bags) was manipulated across blocks of trials (levels). Inter-stimuli intervals were designed considering the average ITI used in the study by Steinhauser and Hübner (2009); the maximum and minimum intervals limited a wider range than the one parametrized for the training so that enough room was left to observe a possible benefit in response time. The dependent variable (conflict score) was calculated as a relative index from (Incongruent trials RT – Congruent trials RT)/Congruent trials RT, for hits. Stimuli were presented randomly both in pre- and post-training testing sessions.

N-back

In this WM task, participants had to retain the spatial position of a sequence of elements over nine blocks of increasing memory load. Participants had to give a response any time an element matched the position of an element presented *n* (from 1 to 8) position-back. The length of the sequence in a block increased parallel to the memory load, from 6 to 20. The maximum time to respond and the inter-stimuli interval was, respectively, 2000 and 1000 for the first four blocks, and 1500 and 800 for the four last ones. *N*-back level and errors (omissions and commissions) were considered as dependent variables. The order of the stimuli in the sequence was randomized in pre- and post-testing.

Stop-Signal

We used this task of response inhibition with the standard parameters of the software STOP-IT (Verbruggen et al., 2008). Participants had to respond with the keyboard as fast as possible to two different stimuli (circles or square) presented in the center of the screen. In 25% of the trials, participants faced an auditory stop-signal (750 Hz, 75 ms) that was presented briefly after the visual stimuli onset and required the response to the current stimulus to be withdrawn. The task comprised of 32 practice trials and three blocks with 64 experimental trials each. The trials were displayed on a black screen and were composed of a 250 ms fixation point (white +), the stimuli presentation (a white square or circle) during 1250 ms and a fixed inter-stimuli interval of 2000 ms. Stimuli were randomized in pre- and post-testing, and in all cases the stop signal was presented with a variable stop-signal delay (SSD). Although initially it was set to 250 ms, it was continuously adjusted. When the inhibition was successful it was reduced 50 ms and if not, increased in 50 ms, so that according to the performance the software tried to maintain a stopping probability of 50%. We considered the Stop-Signal Reaction Time

(SSRT) as a measure of motor inhibition efficiency (Verbruggen and Logan, 2008; Verbruggen et al., 2008; Morales et al., 2013).

Operation Span (O-Span)

We used the Spanish adapted version of the procedure developed by Turner and Engle (1989) (Turner and Engle, 1989; Tokowicz et al., 2004; Redick et al., 2012). It was a dual memory span task that required participants to verify mathematical operations while trying to remember sets of words of increasing set sizes. Each trial was composed of a simple solved mathematical equation [i.e., $(14/2) + 2 = 9$] presented for 3750 ms that participants had to verify and mark as correct or not by pressing one out of two keys on the keyboard. Afterward, a word was presented for 1250 ms to be maintained in memory. Operation-word pairs were presented in increasing set sizes from 2 to 6. After each set, participants had to recall and type the words. While the order of recall was not important, they were told to avoid writing the last word presented first in order to prevent recency effects. The task comprised of 18 trials (three trials per set size) and the testing procedure was repeated until the end. We developed parallel versions of the task by randomizing the order of the stimuli presented that were counterbalanced across sessions and participants. Two parallel versions were created and counterbalanced for pre- and post-testing by randomizing the equation-word pairing. Special care was taken to avoid a similar pairing set size distribution between the two versions.

AX-CPT

We used the same version of the task as Morales et al. (2013) did to explore the adjustment of proactive/reactive cognitive control. In each trial participants were presented with five letters for 300 ms each (cue - three distractors - probe) in the center of a black screen, with a fixed inter-stimuli interval of 1000 ms. Cue and probe stimuli were presented in red font while distractors were presented in white. Participants were instructed to respond "yes" whenever they saw an A in the first position (cue) followed by an X in the fifth position (probe). Participants were asked to respond "no" to any other cue-probe combination and to the distractors (items in positions 2 to 4). The task was composed of a 10 trials practice phase and an experimental block of 100 trials, which were presented randomly both in pre- and post-testing. The target trials (AX) were the most frequent ones (70%) and the rest of the trials (cue - distractor: AY; distractor - probe; BX or neither cue nor probe: BY) occurred in a 10% of the remaining cases. Proactive and reactive control adjustment can be assessed by considering the proportion of errors in AY and BX type trials (Braver et al., 2009; Morales et al., 2013; Chiew and Braver, 2014).

Raven's Advanced Progressive Matrices (RAPM)

We used the computerized version of the set II of this test as a standardized measure of fluid intelligence (Raven, 1990). Participants had to solve visual analogy problems of increasing difficulty. A 3×3 matrix of patterns was presented and they had to a missing pattern of a matrix, from eight different response alternatives. We counterbalanced two parallel versions of the test over sessions with 18 matrices for the pre- and post-testing as used by Jaeggi et al. (2013). Participants had to complete the task as fast and accurately as possible with a 20 min time restriction. The dependent variable was the proportion of correct matrices answered and the reaction times of the hits.

RESULTS

Training Effects

To determine the significance of the training improvement in each activity, we compared the performance in the first training session with that of the final training session (sixth session). Thus, for all tasks repeated-measures analyses of variance (ANOVAs) were conducted on the specific dependent variables for the task (conflict score, errors, reactions times, or memory load) with training session (first vs. sixth) as the within-subject independent variable.

ICT Group

For the Stroop-like task, the reaction times from 20 participants (10 from ICT and 10 from WMT) were not registered due to a software coding error and consequently they could not be included in the analyses. The ANOVA yielded a reliable difference in the relative conflict effect [(incongruent-congruent)/congruent hits RT] from the first to the last training session [$M_{s1} = 0.52$, $SD_{s1} = 0.24$; $M_{s6} = 0.33$, $SD_{s6} = 0.19$; $F(1,21) = 5.94$; $p = 0.02$; $\eta_p^2 = 0.22$]. The conflict effect was also reduced from the first to the last training session in the Conflict resolution task, although the difference did not reach statistical significance [$M_{s1} = 0.48$, $SD_{s1} = 0.34$; $M_{s6} = 0.39$, $SD_{s6} = 0.25$; $F(1,31) = 1.71$; $p = 0.20$; $\eta_p^2 = 0.05$]. For the Go/No-Go task we analyzed both omission errors and false alarms. The results of these analyses showed that participants reduced their average omission errors [$M_{s1} = 3.50$, $SD_{s1} = 2.68$; $M_{s6} = 1.43$, $SD_{s6} = 2.01$; $F(1,31) = 13.11$; $p < 0.01$; $\eta_p^2 = 0.30$], while the reduction of false alarms was not reliable [$M_{s1} = 3.90$, $SD_{s1} = 3.50$; $M_{s6} = 3.25$, $SD_{s6} = 2.70$; $F < 1$; $p = 0.40$; $\eta_p^2 = 0.02$].

WMT Group

For all the WM-training tasks (*n*-back, WM search and WM updating), we compared the memory set size recalled from the first to the last training sessions. The increment in set size recalled was statistically significant for all the three activities trained: *n*-back [$M_{s1} = 1.13$, $SD_{s1} = 0.17$; $M_{s6} = 2.60$, $SD_{s6} = 0.57$; $F(1,31) = 190.92$; $p < 0.01$; $\eta_p^2 = 0.75$]; WM Search [$M_{s1} = 2.21$, $SD_{s1} = 0.17$; $M_{s6} = 4.92$, $SD_{s6} = 1.07$; $F(1,31) = 198.32$; $p < 0.01$; $\eta_p^2 = 0.76$] and WM Updating [$M_{s1} = 1.00$, $SD_{s1} = 0.06$; $M_{s6} = 3.20$, $SD_{s6} = 0.63$; $F(1,31) = 390.95$; $p < 0.01$; $\eta_p^2 = 0.86$].

AC Group

Note that this group did not change the level of executive demands, which was held constant throughout the training sessions. Although, they went forward over levels, so their impression was that they were training, the changes from one level to the next were the progressive reduction of presentation speed and response-time. Hence, we compared the speed of the participants' responses (ms) from the first to the last session for the three activities. The results of this comparison yielded statistically significant differences for Speed Comparison [$M_{s1} = 5075.87$, $SD_{s1} = 437.75$; $M_{s6} = 3539.04$, $SD_{s6} = 656.75$; $F(1,23) = 89.62$; $p < 0.01$; $\eta_p^2 = 0.66$]; Speed Visual Search [$M_{s1} = 22555.57$, $SD_{s1} = 864.64$; $M_{s6} = 3585.23$, $SD_{s6} = 534.92$; $F(1,23) = 8096.82$; $p < 0.01$; $\eta_p^2 = 0.99$] and Speed Categorization [$M_{s1} = 24987.26$, $SD_{s1} = 62.39$; $M_{s6} = 13731.60$, $SD_{s6} = 194.22$; $F(1,23) = 374.22$; $p < 0.01$; $\eta_p^2 = 0.89$].

Training Slopes

The training program PEC-UGR enabled us to create many training levels by using all possible combinations of task parameters (i.e., proportion of congruent/incongruent trials; target-distractor similarity; memory load; response times; etc.). Nonetheless, because the tasks differed in the number of to-be-manipulated parameters, the number of training levels varied across activities. Consequently, in order to put together the trained activities and to compare how far participants from the different groups went in the training, we standardized the level of achievement for each participant by dividing the average level reached in a given activity by the number of levels possible in the activity. Thus, **Figure 1** represents the relative level achieved in each activity and each training session for the three trained groups.

To quantify participants' training improvement over the six sessions of training, we calculated the slope of a linear regression model using the standardized average level in each training session and activity per participant (Katz et al., 2014; Wang et al., 2014). In order to compare the training achievements of the different groups (**Figure 1**), slopes of the three training tasks for each group were averaged. A one-way ANOVA showed a main effect of group [$F(2,85) = 16.26$; $p < 0.01$; $\eta_p^2 = 0.27$], as the average slope for the AC ($M = 12.23$; $SD = 1.34$) was significantly larger than the one for the ICT ($M = 8.68$; $SD = 2.92$; $p < 0.01$) and the WMT ($M = 8.05$; $SD = 1.78$; $p < 0.01$) groups. This is consistent with the fact that active control activities were significantly easier that the executive control ones, facilitating the advancement through the activity levels. The slopes of the two experimental training groups did not differ one from each other ($p = 0.76$).

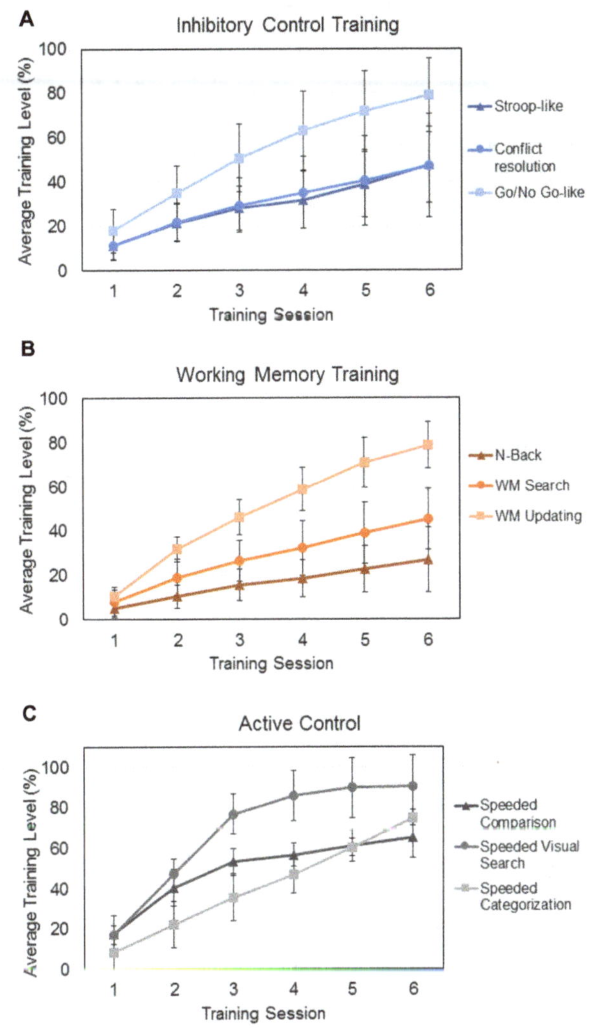

FIGURE 1 | Training improvement over the six training sessions for the three different groups that complete training procedures: (A) Inhibitory Control Training, **(B)** Working Memory Training, **(C)** Active Control. In all the cases, *y*-axes represent the average relative level achieved in each session and training activity. Error bars represent standard deviations.

Correlations at Pre-test

To check for relationships between the cognitive functions tested at baseline, Pearson correlations were run on the pre-test scores for all the participating groups as a whole. These analyses showed that WM-related measures were correlated: those participants with a higher combined score in the O-Span task showed fewer intrusions in the O-Span ($r = -0.34$; $p < 0.01$) and fewer errors in the *n*-back task ($r = -0.19$; $p = 0.03$). Additionally, participants with a larger BSI showed fewer intrusions in the O-Span task ($r = -0.20$; $p = 0.03$).

Finally, RAPM scores significantly correlated with errors in the *n*-back ($r = -0.21$; $p = 0.10$) and with the combined score from the O-Span task ($r = 0.31$; $p < 0.01$).

Transfer Results

Table 1 summarizes the descriptive data of the outcome measures, including statistical comparisons for the session effects (pre vs. post) in each of the groups. We also calculated standardized gains subtracting the pre-test scores from the post-test (the opposite for reaction times and errors) and divided by the standard deviation of the entire sample (Colom et al., 2013; Jaeggi et al., 2013; Redick et al., 2013; Borella et al., 2014). One-way ANOVAs were performed for each variable in order to compare standardized gains between the groups. The participants who were excluded at pre-test due to missing data were also excluded from analyses of performance after the training.

Stroop

We obtained a relative conflict score from the difference in reaction times between incongruent and congruent trials. There were no pre-test differences between the groups [$F(3,88) = 1.86$;

TABLE 1 | Descriptive statistics for outcome measures: Mean and standard deviations for the outcome measures in the pre- and post-testing.

		Pre-test		Post-test		Pre–Post effects		Standardized Gain	
Variables	***N***	***M***	***SD***	***M***	***SD***	***p***	***d***	***M***	***SD***
Stroop: Conflict effect ((Incongruent – Congruent)/Congruent) hits RT (ms)									
IC Training	21	0.12	0.20	0.01	0.03	0.02*	0.76	0.61	1.01
WM Training	22	0.14	0.21	0.09	0.14	0.32	0.28	0.25	0.99
Active Control	24	0.04	0.07	0.05	0.04	0.62	−0.17	−0.05	0.50
Passive Control	24	0.04	0.18	0.07	0.30	0.70	−0.12	−0.13	1.72
N−back: level									
IC Training	32	1.55	0.82	1.72	0.95	0.28	0.19	0.07	1.05
WM Training	32	1.78	0.83	2.43	0.75	0.00*	0.82	0.75	1.23
Active Control	24	1.95	0.80	2.12	0.94	0.44	0.19	0.19	1.21
Passive Control	24	1.66	0.96	1.41	0.58	0.20	−0.31	−0.28	1.09
N-back: errors									
IC Training	32	8.51	4.77	8.51	5.48	1.00	0.00	0.12	1.28
WM Training	32	9.81	4.40	6.34	3.80	0.00*	0.84	0.79	1.26
Active Control	24	9.95	3.74	9.70	2.64	0.76	0.07	0.05	0.93
Passive Control	24	4.62	1.78	4.20	1.44	0.38	0.25	0.09	0.53
Stop-Signal: SSRT (ms)									
IC Training	30	280.47	39.02	255.54	53.56	0.00*	0.53	0.54	0.97
WM Training	31	266.29	51.68	254.66	36.19	0.28	0.26	0.25	1.30
Active Control	21	258.96	48.16	244.30	51.59	0.10	0.29	0.32	0.87
Passive Control	22	254.55	39.36	239.30	37.17	0.19	0.39	0.33	1.17
O-Span Index: Words recalled × Equations hits									
IC Training	32	0.59	0.10	0.66	0.12	0.00*	0.63	0.52	0.68
WM Training	32	0.59	0.18	0.66	0.19	0.00*	0.37	0.45	0.82
Active Control	24	0.55	0.13	0.60	0.13	0.00*	0.38	0.19	0.28
Passive Control	24	0.58	0.12	0.61	0.10	0.24	0.27	0.18	0.77
O-Span: Intrusions									
IC Training	32	2.31	1.71	1.78	1.66	0.10	0.32	0.20	0.87
WM Training	32	2.46	1.81	1.34	1.42	0.00*	0.69	0.55	0.92
Active Control	24	3.00	2.91	2.70	2.31	0.46	0.11	0.14	0.94
Passive Control	24	2.50	1.61	2.87	2.29	0.44	−0.18	−0.18	1.15
AX-CPT: BSI (AY-BX)/(AY+BX)									
IC Training	28	0.42	0.13	0.50	0.17	0.01*	0.52	0.48	1.03
WM Training	30	0.39	0.17	0.51	0.14	0.00*	0.77	0.66	1.26
Active Control	23	0.40	0.18	0.45	0.17	0.15	0.28	0.33	1.08
Passive Control	23	0.39	0.19	0.36	0.32	0.72	−0.11	−0.15	2.04
RAPM: Hits									
IC Training	32	0.44	0.18	0.51	0.18	0.01*	0.38	0.36	0.77
WM Training	32	0.43	0.20	0.47	0.17	0.34	0.21	0.20	1.18
Active Control	24	0.47	0.20	0.49	0.18	0.44	0.10	0.14	0.91
Passive Control	24	0.48	0.15	0.42	0.17	0.06	−0.37	−0.32	0.76
RAPM: Hits RT (s)									
IC Training	32	35.75	12.94	33.87	15.50	0.49	0.13	0.12	0.98
WM Training	32	34.42	16.63	31.38	15.92	0.15	0.18	0.19	0.76
Active Control	24	42.32	17.13	40.51	15.27	0.55	0. 11	0.11	0.93
Passive Control	24	34.44	15.55	32.24	16.44	0.48	0.13	0.14	0.95

Significance p-values and effect sizes (Cohen's d) estimators are reported for the Repeated-Measures ANOVAs including session as a within subject variable (pre-test and post-test values) and group as a between-subject effect in each of the four groups. Standardized gains were computed as (Mpost – Mpre)/(SDpre) for hits and as (Mpre – Mpost)/(SDpre) for errors and reaction times.

$p = 0.14$; $\eta_p^2 = 0.05$]. The ANOVA on the standardized gains failed to show a reliable effect of group, $F(3,88) = 1.76$; $p = 0.16$; $\eta_p^2 = 0.05$. As can be observed in **Table 1**, however, it was only the ICT group that was able to significantly reduce their conflict scores after completing the training.

N-back

The *n*-back level and the number of errors were considered in this task. There were no differences in the baseline *n*-back level before training [$F(3,108) = 1.39$; $p = 0.24$; $\eta_p^2 = 0.03$]. However, a one-way ANOVA revealed differences in the number of errors at pre-test [$F(3,108) = 10.02$; $p < 0.01$; $\eta_p^2 = 0.21$], whereby the PC group committed significantly fewer errors than the other three groups (all *ps* < 0.01). **Table 1** shows that only the WMT group showed a reliable increase in the number of items that could be maintained/updated in WM and a reduction in the number of errors committed after the training. The ANOVA performed on the standardized gains scores revealed a statistically significant effect of group for *n*-back level: [$F(3,108) = 4.06$; $p < 0.01$; $\eta_p^2 = 0.10$]. *Post hoc* comparisons for the *n*-back level indicated that the only reliable difference was between the PC and the WMT groups ($p < 0.01$) whereas the pairwise comparisons between the remaining groups were not significant (ICT-WMT: $p = 0.11$; ICT-AC: $p = 1.00$; ICT-CP: $p = 1.00$; WMT-AC: $p = 0.42$; PC-AC: $p = 0.89$). In the case of errors, and because we found differences between groups at pre-test, we checked whether there were group differences in the standardized gains as *n*-back errors committed at pre-test were introduced as a covariate. The analysis of covariance (ANCOVA) revealed a reliable effect of the covariate [$F(3,107) = 59.06$; $p < 0.01$; $\eta_p^2 = 0.35$] but also a significant effect of group [$F(3,107) = 5.28$; $p < 0.01$; $\eta_p^2 = 0.13$]. Further analyses showed that there was a statistically significant difference between the AC and WMT groups ($p = 0.01$), and between the two control groups ($p < 0.01$). None of the other comparisons showed reliable differences (ICT-WMT: $p = 0.39$; ICT-AC: $p = 0.89$; ICT-CP: $p = 0.14$; WMT-CP: $p = 1.00$).

Stop-Signal

We used the software ANALYZE-IT provided by Verbruggen et al. (2008) to determine the impact of training on inhibition. The SSRT is an index of pure response inhibition and the program calculates it by subtracting the SSD from the untrimmed RT mean. Following the criteria of Verbruggen, we removed five participants (one ICT, one WMT, one AC, and two PC participants) from the analysis, since they had an overall probability of responding on stop trials significantly below or above 50% in both pre- and post-test. The groups did not differ in SSRT at pre-test [$F(3,104) = 1.85$; $p = 0.14$; $\eta_p^2 = 0.05$]. As for response inhibition, while the corresponding ANOVA did not revealed a reliable effect of group [$F(3,104) < 1$; $\eta_p^2 = 0.01$], the only reliable pre–post reduction of SSRT was in the ICT group (**Table 1**). Note that there were training-related effects neither on hits nor on the RTs of Go trials[3]. Thus, training effects were only evident in the SSRT as an index of response inhibition, but not in the other variables that assess basic task performance. This is important since it shows that transfer is specific to the executive control trained process.

Operation Span

For the O-Span task, we considered the number of words recalled (storage capacity) and the averaged accuracy of equations (ongoing processing) multiplied, and resulting as a combined index of dual processing. For the calculation, we used a partial credit load scoring approach (PCL, Conway et al., 2005), which considered the average proportion of correctly recalled words from all set sizes, regardless of whether the set size group was perfectly recalled or not.

A one-way ANOVA on the combined scores (words recalled and equations accuracy) showed that there were no differences between the groups at pre-test [$F(3,108) = 0.42$; $p = 0.73$; $\eta_p^2 = 0.01$]. Particularly, there was a reliable pre–post enhancement in the three training groups, with the greatest effect size in the ICT group (**Table 1**). The ANOVA comparing the groups' standardized gains failed to show reliable differences however, $F(3,108) = 1.76$; $p = 0.15$; $\eta_p^2 = 0.04$.

Finally, intrusions were also considered as a measure of updating in WM (low intrusion corresponding to successful updating). In this case, only the WMT group was able to significantly reduce the number of intrusions in the dual task (**Table 1**). The one-way ANOVA confirmed a reliable effect of group, $F(3,108) = 2.73$; $p = 0.04$; $\eta_p^2 = 0.07$. The *post hoc* comparisons showed that the only reliable difference involved the WMT and the PC groups ($p = 0.03$).

AX-CPT

To assess the tendency toward proactive/reactive control, we calculated the Behavioral Shift Index (BSI)[4] introduced by Braver et al. (2009) and Chiew and Braver (2014). Larger BSIs stands for a greater tendency toward proactive control, whereas smaller BSIs indicate a tendency toward reactive control. Invalid trials, which included no responses and trials with responses times below 100 or above 1000 ms, were 6.1% out of the trial total. Eight participants were removed from the analysis because they had more than 10% of invalid trials in pre- and post-test. The four groups were comparable in BSI at pre-test [$F(3,100) = 0.21$; $p = 0.88$; $\eta_p^2 = 0.01$].

The one-way ANOVA on BSI standardized gains failed to show a group effect [$F(3,100) = 1.60$; $p = 0.19$; $\eta_p^2 = 0.04$]. Nonetheless, the pre-post analyses only showed a reliable effect in both ICT and WMT groups, which exhibited larger BSI after the training (**Table 1**, $ps \leq 0.01$).

Raven's Advanced Progressive Matrices

There were no differences between the groups at pre-test in either hit rates [$F(3,108) = 0.44$; $p = 0.72$; $\eta_p^2 = 0.01$], or reaction times [$F(3,108) = 1.47$; $p = 0.22$; $\eta_p^2 = 0.03$]. As shown in **Table 1**, however, the ICT was the only group that exhibited a pre–post increase in hit rates. The one-way ANOVA confirmed an effect of group, $F(3,108) = 2.63$; $p = 0.05$; $\eta_p^2 = 0.06$), which was mainly accounted for by the difference between the ICT and PC groups (*post hoc* comparison with $p = 0.04$). No effects were found in hit reaction times.

---

[3]No reliable differences in pre–post effects were observed on hits ($ps > 0.33$) or RTs ($ps > 0.56$) in Go trials for the ICT, WMT or AC groups. The PC group showed a worse performance with a lower hit rate [$M_{pre} = 95.71$, $SD_{pre} = 4.76$; $M_{post} = 91.77$, $SD_{post} = 4.56$; $F(1,21) = 8.06$; $p = 0.01$; $\eta_p^2 = 0.27$]; and slower RTs [$M_{pre} = 753.21$, $SD_{pre} = 156.80$; $M_{post} = 832.54$, $SD_{post} = 168.07$; $F(1,21) = 11.75$; $p = 0.00$; $\eta_p^2 = 0.35$] in the post-test.

[4]This index is based on the formula (AY − BX)/(AY + BX) for errors and reaction times. Trials where errors were equal to 0 were corrected [(errors + 0.5)/frequency of trials + 1].

Predictors for Training Improvement and Transfer

We were also interested in exploring which of the cognitive abilities tested at the baseline level predicted the magnitude of training improvement. We ran linear regression analyses with the average training slope as the outcome, and all the measures at the pre-testing stage as predictors. Only for the experimental training groups, RAPM scores significantly predicted the global training improvement ($R^2 = 0.12$; $p = 0.01$; $\beta = 0.86$). We also looked at whether pre-test performance on the reasoning test predicted transfer gains after training. However, there was not a reliable relationship between RAPM scores before training and any of the gain scores on the transfer tasks. Reasoning scores at pre-test only predicted reasoning scores at post-test ($R^2 = 0.24$; $p < 0.01$; $\beta = 0.45$).

Going a step further we also looked at whether the magnitude of training improvement predicted transfer gains. We ran linear regression analyses in each training group, setting the standardized gains in the different transfer tasks as the criterion and the average training slope as the predictor variable. In the ICT group, higher training improvements predicted larger gains in the relative conflict score of the Stroop task ($R^2 = 0.29$; $p < 0.01$; $\beta = 0.19$) and larger gains in the RAPM ($R^2 = 0.12$; $p = 0.04$; $\beta = 0.09$). No reliable regressions emerged for the WMT and the AC groups (all with *ps* > 0.15).

On the whole trained sample, the analyses showed that the level participants were able to achieve in the training activities only predicted performance in the criterion tasks; namely, conflict in Stroop ($R^2 = 0.12$; $p < 0.01$; $\beta = 0.13$) and errors in the *n*-back task ($R^2 = 0.05$; $p = 0.03$; $\beta = -0.10$).

Motivation Results

In order to account for the motivational factors during training, every two sessions we asked participants about their: (i) involvement in the program; (ii) perceived difficulty of the activity levels; (iii) perceived challenge of improving over the levels; (iv) expectations for their achievement (Alonso-Tapia and de la Red Fadrique, 2007; Colom et al., 2013). We averaged all the variables across the three measurement points and explored their distribution across groups. One-way ANOVAs failed to show group differences in any of the four motivational variables: implication [(AC: $M = 9.09$; $SD = 0.85$; ICT: $M = 9.03$; $SD = 0.94$; WMT: $M = 8.98$; $SD = 0.92$); $F < 1$; $p = 0.90$, $\eta_p^2 = 0.00$]; perceived difficulty [(AC: $M = 6.31$; $SD = 1.46$; ICT: $M = 6.11$; $SD = 1.76$; WMT: $M = 6.25$; $SD = 1.49$); $F < 1$; $p = 0.8$, $\eta_p^2 = 0.00$]; perceived challenge to improve [(AC: $M = 7.15$; $SD = 1.46$; ICT: $M = 7.31$; $SD = 1.47$; WMT: $M = 7.28$; $SD = 1.52$); $F < 1$; $p = 0.91$, $\eta_p^2 = 0.00$] and expectations to improve [(AC: $M = 7.28$; $SD = 1.58$; ICT: $M = 7.76$; $SD = 1.20$; WMT: $M = 7.94$; $SD = 1.07$); $F(2,85) = 1.91$; $p = 0.15$; $\eta_p^2 = 0.04$]. Then, we calculated partial correlations controlling for group between the four motivation variables and the global training slope. We only found a modest correlation between the training slope and the perceived challenge ($r = 0.25$; $p = 0.04$), so that those participants who perceived the training as more challenging were the ones who tended to improve the most.

In order to explore whether participant's motivation modulated training improvement, we averaged the four motivation variables and calculated a global motivation score (AC: $M = 6.81$; $SD = 0.69$; ICT: $M = 6.99$; $SD = 0.75$; WMT: $M = 6.99$; $SD = 0.54$). A one-way ANOVA showed no differences between the groups in general motivation, $F < 1$; $p = 0.54$; $\eta_p^2 = 0.01$. However, because we wanted to more precisely examine whether the motivation level was related to the participants' training achievement, we split all the executive control trained participants by the median of the global score ($Md = 6.95$) to differentiate between high and low motivated participants. A one-way ANOVA with motivation (high and low) as the factor and global training slope of ICT and WMT participants as the dependent variable showed motivation levels to be statistically significant, $F(1,62) = 5.55$; $p = 0.02$; $\eta_p^2 = 0.08$); with high motivated participants exhibiting a higher training slope ($M = 9.39$; $SD = 2.65$) than less motivated participants ($M = 7.82$; $SD = 2.66$).

To explore whether motivation predicted transfer, multiple linear regression models were run setting the standardized gains in the transfer tasks as criterion variables, the four motivational variables measured during training as predictor variables, and considering the two training groups as a whole. The level of motivation predicted transfer to the O-Span task in the two experimental training groups ($R^2 = 0.15$; $p = 0.03$), so that those who felt more involved ($\beta = 0.28$; $p = 0.03$) and those who perceived the training as less difficult ($\beta = -0.31$; $p = 0.02$) had larger gains after training.

Lastly, we compared the transfer gains in those participants who were highly motivated from the experimental groups (ICT: $n = 17$; WMT: $n = 15$) with those who were highly motivated in the active control group ($n = 12$). Most likely due to the small sample sizes, only a marginal statistical effect was found on the standardized gains of one of the two criterion tasks. Specifically, in the *n*-back task the WMT participants had larger gains ($M = 0.92$; $SD = 0.99$) than the ICT ($M = 0.13$; $SD = 1.07$) and the AC participants ($M = 0.19$; $SD = 0.96$), [$F(2,31) = 2.80$; $p = 0.07$; $\eta_p^2 = 0.12$].

DISCUSSION

The main goal of the present study was to directly compare the effectiveness of two specific process-based EFs training programs (WM and IC) in young adults. These two programs were based on the assumption of the highly influential "Unity and Diversity" model of EFs proposed by Miyake et al. (2000). The main feature of this model is that the EFs system could be partitioned into overlapping (unity) and yet distinct (diversity) components (inhibition, shifting, and WM updating). A logical conclusion drawn from the assumption of diversity is that EFs training could specifically be targeted to one of these functions with transfer effects showing some degree of specificity and commonality. The results of the present experiment generally support this assumption.

Thus, regarding the improvement in the criterion tasks – structurally similar to the trained ones – our results support the specificity of EFs training on the basis of the specific benefits observed at post-test. Only the WMT group showed pre–post enhancement in the n-back task (n-back level and errors) and only the ICT group exhibited reduced conflict scores in the Stroop task after training. Even though some previous studies have shown benefits in the Stroop task following WM training (Borella et al., 2010; Chein and Morrison, 2010; Schweizer et al., 2011), we failed to observe a reliable effect of WMT over conflict resolution. Hence, the results concerning the criterion tasks point to straightforward training-specific effects.

In relation to near transfer effects, we also observed specific training benefits for the WMT group in the non-trained WM task (O-Span). Particularly, for the O-Span task only the WMT group showed a benefit in suppressing memory intrusions; consistent with previous studies showing the relationship between high WMC and more efficient intrusions suppression in span tasks (Rosen and Engle, 1998; Turley-Ames and Whitfield, 2003; Borella et al., 2008). Similarly, the ICT group was the only group that specifically showed a benefit in response inhibition (SSRT), indicating that adaptive training in conflict resolution tasks improves performance in other tasks also thought to require conflict resolution mechanisms (for related results, see Logan and Burkell, 1986; Manuel et al., 2013; Berkman et al., 2014; Enge et al., 2014; Dovis et al., 2015). Together with the results found with the criterion tasks, the near transfer results also support the idea that training on either WM or IC leads to specific performance benefits in tasks related to the training (Simons et al., 2016).

However, and despite this specificity, the two EFs-trained groups also showed some common features regarding near transfer effects. Thus, both WMT and ICT groups improved dual performance (Equations accuracy × Words recalled) in the O-Span task [related findings of improved complex span scores have been reported after simple, complex span and visual search training, (Harrison et al., 2013); rehearsal strategy training (Turley-Ames and Whitfield, 2003) or task switching training (Karbach and Kray, 2009)], suggesting that dual tasking may require both WM capacity and IC mechanisms (Towse et al., 2000; Smith et al., 2001; Unsworth, 2010; Chein et al., 2011). Hence, IC seem to be demanded not only in the training activities practiced by our ICT group but also in the WM updating tasks that required suppression of irrelevant information and that were extensively practiced by the WMT group. This might be indicating the relationship between WM and IC at the behavioral level, and be suggestive of the degree to which trained and transfer processes may overlap in their underlying neuro-cognitive networks. Kane and Engle (2002) proposed that dorsolateral prefrontal cortex could play a role in WM capacity in contexts providing potential interference (and requiring attentional control). Conway et al. (2003) and Gray et al. (2003) agree that in WM span tasks regions in the prefrontal cortex are activated when an executive control mechanism is recruited to reduce interference during the maintenance and manipulation of information.

It is, however, puzzling that we also observed a training effect for the active control group in the O-Span task, which did not differ from that obtained by the WMT group. Note that, although the AC group did not increase the cognitive load over the training levels, we used activities that involved increasing difficulty by augmenting the speed of processing. Thus, as also predicted, it is possible that the positive effect for this control group stemmed from the overarching time-limited nature of the tasks. Increasing speed of processing could have led to more efficient processing and maintenance in WM that would result in better performance in the O-Span task. Unsworth et al. (2009) reported a negative correlation between processing speed and WM maintenance, suggesting that participants who processed quickly recalled more items that those who worked slowly. Similarly, faster speed processing has been proposed to reduce the possibility of items being forgotten, and less time for rehearsing or refreshing processes (Towse et al., 2000; Hudjetz and Oberauer, 2007; Unsworth et al., 2009).

Regarding far transfer effects, we also found common and diverse features in our trained groups. We included two tasks (AX-CPT and RAPM) that did not directly capture WM or IC: the AX-CPT was used to explore whether training effects might change the control strategy used by the participants, and Raven's matrices to explore whether WM and IC training transferred to a more general complex domain such as abstract reasoning. The AX-CPT is widely used to explore the dynamic adjustment of cognitive control strategies and it has shown to be very sensitive to individual differences in cognitive control (Braver et al., 2009; Burgess et al., 2011; Braver, 2012). Proactive control requires goal maintenance and is related to paying attention to contextual cues in order to effectively solve interference while keeping the monitored cues in mind (Rush et al., 2006). In this version of the task, the use of a proactive control strategy was encouraged since the context was highly predictive (the A cue precedes the X target in 70% of the trials); hence, a control mode that involves sustained maintenance of task-relevant information would lead to a high success rate, albeit it would lead to errors in trials where the cue was A but the probe was not X (AY trials; 10% of the trials). Thus, enhanced proactive control is expected to increase AY errors and reduce BX errors, with the BSI tending to larger values since the cue in BX trials does not signal a "yes" response. Usually, because it is the most efficient strategy, young adults exhibit behavioral performance and brain activity (sustained lateral PFC activation) consistent with a predominant proactive control strategy (Braver, 2012; Morales et al., 2013).

Interestingly, results from our experiment regarding the BSI (an index signaling changes toward proactive control) in the AX-CPT suggested a higher reliance on proactive control for WM and IC trained participants compared to active and passive control groups. Previous studies have already reported the malleability of cognitive control mechanisms engaged in the AX-CPT due to experience-based conditions such as bilingualism (Morales et al., 2013, 2015) or different kinds of training interventions: task-strategy training made older adults (Paxton et al., 2006) and people with schizophrenia (Braver et al., 2009; Edwards et al., 2009) more prone to engage in proactive control; indeed, more similar to adults-like performance than before training. Previous studies have also reported proactive shifts in cortical regions as the lateral PFC after strategy (Braver et al., 2009) and IC training (Berkman et al., 2014), suggesting the possibility that the lateral PFC might serve to anticipate upcoming control demands across a range of executive control domains. Our results replicate and extend these findings by showing behavioral shifts toward proactive processing in both ICT and WMT (even though numerically larger in the WMT group), suggesting again some common executive resources for inhibitory and WM processes.

In contrast, the results of the non-verbal reasoning (RAPM) task showed some degree of specificity. Specifically, we observed a benefit for the ICT group but not for the WMT group. The question of whether cognitive training could improve fluid intelligence is a recurrent controversial area of research with considerable number of studies reporting data against (Shipstead et al., 2012; Melby-Lervåg and Hulme, 2013) and in favor of it (Morrison and Chein, 2011; Au et al., 2014). Results of our ICT group join others showing better reasoning performance after training. Karbach and Kray (2009) reported improved performance in a composite measure of reasoning after four sessions of task-switching training in children, young and older adults compared to an active control group (Karbach and Kray, 2009). Similarly, Rueda et al. (2005) found benefits in a measure of reasoning after 5 and 10 days (Rueda et al., 2012) of executive-control training in pre-school children when compared to control groups (but see Thorell et al., 2009 and Enge et al., 2014 for failures to show such positive effects).

However, our WMT group did not show benefits in abstract reasoning. Although fluid intelligence and WM share common variance (Colom et al., 2004; Oberauer et al., 2005; Friedman et al., 2006; Harrison et al., 2015) and EFs have been related to reasoning operations (Dempster and Corkill, 1999; Engle and Kane, 2004; Jarosz and Wiley, 2012; Shipstead et al., 2015) it is possible that our participants did not reach the level of difficulty needed to show far transfer. In support of this interpretation, the results of the regression analyses showed that training improvement only predicted transfer to abstract reasoning for the ICT group, which suggests that the training levels achieved by the WMT group did not reach high enough demand levels to promote transfer. Previous studies reporting positive training effects have normally used single but highly demanding tasks, such as the dual *n*-back task (Jaeggi et al., 2008, 2010, 2013) and/or participants attained high levels of performance over training, such as *n*-back levels of over 3 (Jaeggi et al., 2008, 2013). Note that, in average, our WMT participants reached an *n*-back level below three and performed a single *n*-back task. Hence, and considering the fact that we trained more than one task, it is possible that the level of difficulty was below that needed to show far transfer effects with WM training.

Together, the observed transfer effects allow us to claim that it was the ICT group that showed the most consistent pattern of enhanced performance across tasks. While there might be more than a single reason behind this finding, we favor the idea that the benefit for the ICT group is not related to differences in cognitive demands or motivational aspects between the two training programs. As previously noted, the training levels achieved by the WMT group could have not been demanding enough to lead to stronger overall transfer.

An additional and interesting point addressed in the present work was to look at individual differences regarding training and transfer effects. This is an issue that remains to be explored in deep (Könen and Karbach, 2015). In line with previously reported studies (Bürki et al., 2014), we have found that abstract reasoning was a meaningful predictor of training improvement, indicating that people with higher reasoning scores benefited more from training. Furthermore, training improvement constituted a relevant predictor of transfer to the criterion tasks for the two experimental trained groups, and particularly in the case of the ICT group a predictor for transfer to reasoning and conflict reduction. This pattern of results highlights the importance of considering individual differences before training because they might influence how well they do during training and how much benefit they can take from it (Könen and Karbach, 2015).

In addition to the more important theoretical issues related to brain plasticity and transfer, a secondary aim of our study was methodological in nature. Previous training studies have been criticized for the suitability of the control conditions, for not considering motivational factors, or for the use of single training tasks (Jaeggi et al., 2013; Redick et al., 2013; Melby-Lervåg et al., 2016). In our study, we took these factors into account by using different tasks to train the target processes (and to increase the probability of generalization), by introducing two different control conditions (active and passive), and by considering motivational variables associated with training. Thus, the active control group engaged in tasks essentially requiring processing speed (for related approaches see Goldin et al., 2014; Lawlor-Savage and Goghari, 2016), in order to keep participants' motivation and engagement similar to those from the experimental groups. Importantly, all trained participants (including the AC group) showed a meaningful improvement in the specifically trained process (IC, WM and processing speed). In fact, the AC group showed larger training slopes than the two experimental groups (**Figure 1**). Note again that control activities were mainly perceptual and successive levels did not engage greater executive load but only faster responses with a low constant cognitive effort.

Also of relevance, the motivation questionnaire revealed similar levels of implication, perceived difficulty, perceived challenge and expectations during training for the three trained groups, indicating that transfer differences among the groups were not due to differences in motivation or perceived difficulty. Interestingly, while motivation cannot easily account for the differences between the training and control groups, it was a factor that predicted training improvement in the experimental groups, so that highly motivated participants – those that were more involved and perceived the training as less difficult – showed larger improvements across the training sessions than less-motivated participants. Thus, and consistent with previous studies, motivation this result highlights the importance of considering individual motivation through training, since it is related to greater improvements that could result in greater transfer effects (Mather and Carstensen, 2005; Jaeggi et al., 2013; Katz et al., 2014). Apart from motivation, it would be of interest in future studies the inclusion of additional self-reporting assessments regarding individual differences in beliefs about the fixed or malleable nature of cognition (Jaeggi et al., 2013), expectancy and perceived improvement (Boot et al., 2011).

It must be noted that the present research is not without limitations. First, and despite the specific benefits found in the within-group comparisons, the lack of group effects in some of the standardized gain measures suggests caution in the interpretation of the results. Null effects in the gain comparisons may reflect the lack of statistical power but also inflated variability among groups. In a recent meta-analysis, Melby-Lervåg et al. (2016) established that training studies with large effect sizes normally included small sample sizes (less than 20 participants per training condition) and untreated (passive) control groups, which produces biases toward significant – but low powered – results (Enge et al., 2014; Melby-Lervåg et al., 2016). In the present study, we used samples that were all over 20 participants per condition and we included a passive control group as well as an active control group. Second, the present training schedule covered 2 weeks, which is in the lower end of the range of the current training studies (from 2 to 14 weeks; Morrison and Chein, 2011). Hence, it is yet to be explored the magnitude of the transfer effects when training is extended over a longer period of time. Similarly, our study is blind regarding possible long-term effects since we did not follow them up in time. Future studies should address this issue because the value of training interventions essentially relies on the durability of training-induced results. Finally, we recognize that transfer effects in studies with young healthy samples are limited as long as they might be optimally functioning at pre-testing, leaving not enough room for meaningful improvements with training. Hence, studies with children and older adults could be more sensitive to training-related changes than studies with young people (Kelly et al., 2014; Spencer-Smith and Klingberg, 2015; Weicker et al., 2016).

In closing, and despite the existing limitations, our results lead us to suggest that executive-control training may modulate cognitive abilities in young people. The malleability of EFs challenges the long-standing assumption that cognitive abilities remain fixed over time. Training cognition is not a new concept (Jolles and Crone, 2012; Boot and Kramer, 2014; Schubert et al., 2014), but the idea that training and experience can generalize to tasks and domains beyond those trained is still controversial. In this sense, our results, while being modest and at the task level – rather than at the construct level – are promising and support substantial plasticity of cognitive control mechanisms by means of training. Interestingly, the results also suggest that there is some specificity in the consequences of the trained processes so that transfer occurs only when the specific trained process is tapped by the transfer task and domain. This opens the possibility that training in applied settings may be specific to the process needed for a specific domain, or to the impaired process due to deficient brain functioning. Also, this is suggestive of setting the ambitious goal of exploring the potential benefit of executive control training for everyday activities (Simons et al., 2016). Before this, further research would need to address the potential effects of executive-control training over brain structure and dynamics. Analyzing structural and functional brain profiles may provide further insight into why specific interventions may be more successful for certain individuals, and help characterize the overlap between training tasks and tests that show training-related transfer.

AUTHOR CONTRIBUTIONS

This work is part of the thesis dissertation of the first author (MM). The authors developed the concept of the study together. MM contributed to the design of training tasks, data collection and analyses, and manuscript writing. MB in collaboration with M. R. Rueda designed the online program PEC-UGR. MB and CG-A supervised the process of accomplishing the study, and wrote, reviewed and approved the final version of the manuscript.

ACKNOWLEDGMENTS

We would like to thank M. J. Ruiz for his help in data collection, and R. Garcia-Ortega and D. Lopez-Padial for his technical support with the online training program PEC-UGR.

REFERENCES

Alonso-Tapia, J., and de la Red Fadrique, I. (2007). Evaluar "para" el aprendizaje, aprender para estar motivado: el orden de los factores sí afecta al producto. *REOP* 18, 241–253.

Au, J., Sheehan, E., Tsai, N., Duncan, G. J., Buschkuehl, M., and Jaeggi, S. M. (2014). Improving fluid intelligence with training on working memory: A meta-analysis. *Psychon. B Rev.* 105, 6829–6833. doi: 10.3758/s13423-014-0699-x

Banich, M. T. (2009). Executive Function: The search for an integrated account. *Curr. Dir. Psychol. Sci.* 18, 89–94. doi: 10.1111/j.1467-8721.2009.01615.x

Baniqued, P. L., Allen, C. M., Kranz, M. B., Johnson, K., Sipolins, A., Dickens, C., et al. (2015). Working memory, reasoning, and task switching training: Transfer effects, limitations, and great expectations? *PLoS ONE* 10:e0142169. doi: 10.1371/journal.pone.0142169

Baniqued, P. L., Kranz, M. B., Voss, M. W., Lee, H., Cosman, J. D., Severson, J., et al. (2014). Cognitive training with casual video games: points to consider. *Front. Psychol.* 4:1010. doi: 10.3389/fpsyg.2013.01010

Barkley, R. (2001). The executive functions and self-regulation: an evolutionary neuropsychological perspective. *Neuropsychol. Rev.* 11, 1–29. doi: 10.1023/A:1009085417776

Beauchamp, K. G., Kahn, L. E., and Berkman, E. T. (2016). Does inhibitory control training transfer?: Behavioral and neural effects on an untrained emotion regulation task. *Soc. Cogn. Affect. Neur.* 2016, 1–9. doi: 10.1093/scan/nsw061

Benikos, N., Johnstone, S. J., and Roodenrys, S. J. (2013a). Varying task difficulty in the Go/Nogo task: The effects of inhibitory control, arousal, and perceived effort on ERP components. *Int. J. Psychophysiol.* 87, 266–272. doi: 10.1016/j.ijpsycho.2012.08.005

Benikos, N., Johnstone, S. J., and Roodenrys, S. J. (2013b). Short-term training in the Go/Nogo task: behavioural and neural changes depend on task demands. *Int. J. Psychophysiol.* 87, 301–312. doi: 10.1016/j.ijpsycho.2012.12.001

Bergman-Nutley, S., and Klingberg, T. (2014). Effect of working memory training on working memory, arithmetic and following instructions. *Psychol. Res.* 78, 869–877. doi: 10.1007/s00426-014-0614-0

Berkman, E. T., Kahn, L. E., and Merchant, J. S. (2014). Training-induced changes in inhibitory control network activity. *J. Neurosci.* 34, 149–157. doi: 10.1523/jneurosci.3564-13.2014

Bherer, L., Kramer, A. F., Peterson, M. S., Colcombe, S., Erickson, K., and Becic, E. (2005). Training effects on dual-task performance: are there age-related differences in plasticity of attentional control? *Psychol. Aging.* 20, 695–709. doi: 10.1037/0882-7974.20.4.695

Blair, C., and Razza, R. P. (2007). Relating effortful control, executive function, and false belief understanding to emerging math and literacy ability in kindergarten. *Child Dev.* 78, 647–663. doi: 10.1111/j.1467-8624.2007.01019.x

Bogg, T., and Lasecki, L. (2015). Reliable gains? Evidence for substantially underpowered designs in studies of working memory training transfer to fluid intelligence. *Front. Psychol.* 5:1589. doi: 10.3389/fpsyg.2014.01589

Boot, W. R., Blakely, D. P., and Simons, D. J. (2011). Do action video games improve perception and cognition? *Front. Psychol.* 2:226. doi: 10.3389/fpsyg.2011.00226

Boot, W. R., and Kramer, A. F. (2014). The brain-games conundrum: does cognitive training really sharpen the mind? *Cerebrum* 2014:15.

Boot, W. R., Simons, D. J., Stothart, C., and Stutts, C. (2013). The pervasive problem with placebos in psychology: why active control groups are not sufficient to rule out placebo effects. *Perspect. Psychol. Sci.* 8, 445–454. doi: 10.1177/1745691613491271

Borella, E., Carretti, B., Cantarella, A., Riboldi, F., Zavagnin, M., and De Beni, R. (2014). Benefits of training visuospatial working memory in young-old and old-old. *Dev. Psychol.* 50, 714–727. doi: 10.1037/a0034293

Borella, E., Carretti, B., and De Beni, R. (2008). Working memory and inhibition across the adult life-span. *Acta Psychol.* 128, 33–44. doi: 10.1016/j.actpsy.2007.09.008

Borella, E., Carretti, B., Riboldi, F., and De Beni, R. (2010). Working memory training in older adults: evidence of transfer and maintenance effects. *Psychol. Aging.* 25, 767–778. doi: 10.1037/a0020683

Braver, T. S. (2012). The variable nature of cognitive control: A dual-mechanisms framework. *Trends Cogn Sci.* 16, 106–113. doi: 10.1016/j.tics.2011.12.010

Braver, T. S., and Cohen, J. D. (2001). Working memory, cognitive control, and the prefrontal cortex: computational and empirical studies. *Cogn. Process.* 2, 25–55.

Braver, T. S., Gray, J. R., and Burguess, G. C. (2008). "Explaining the many varieties of working memory variation: Dual mechanisms of cognitive control," in *Variation in Working Memory*, eds A. Conway, C. Jarrold, M. Kane, A. Miyake, and J. Towse (Oxford: Oxford University Press), doi: 10.1093/acprof:oso/9780195168648.003.0004

Braver, T. S., Paxton, J. L., Locke, H. S., and Barch, D. M. (2009). Flexible neural mechanisms of cognitive control within human prefrontal cortex. *Proc. Natl. Acad. Sci.U.S.A.* 106, 7351–7356. doi: 10.1073/pnas.0808187106

Brehmer, Y., Rieckmann, A., Bellander, M., Westerberg, H., Fischer, H., and Bäckman, L. (2011). Neural correlates of training-related working- memory gains in old age. *Neuroimage* 58, 1110–1120. doi: 10.1016/j.neuroimage.2011.06.079

Bull, R., and Scerif, G. (2001). Executive functioning as a predictor of children's mathematics ability: inhibition, switching, and working memory. *Dev. Neuropsychol.* 19, 273–293. doi: 10.1207/s15326942dn1903

Burgess, G. C., Gray, J. R., Conway, A. R., and Braver, T. S. (2011). Neural mechanisms of interference control underlie the relationships between Fluid intelligence and working memory span. *J. Exp. Psychol. Gen.* 140, 674–692. doi: 10.1037/a0024695

Burgess, P. (1997). "Theory and methodology in executive function research," in *Methodology of Frontal and Executive Function*, ed. P. Rabbitt (Hove: Psychology Press).

Bürki, C., Ludwig, C., Chicherio, C., and de Ribaupierre, A. (2014). Individual differences in cognitive plasticity: an investigation of training curves in younger and older adults. *Psychol. Res.* 78, 821–835. doi: 10.1007/s00426-014-0559-3

Buschkuehl, M., Jaeggi, S. M., and Jonides, J. (2012). Neuronal effects following working memory training. *Dev. Cogn. Neurosci.* 2, 167–179. doi: 10.1016/j.dcn.2011.10.001

Carretti, B., Borella, E., Zavagnin, M., and De Beni, R. (2013). Gains in language comprehension relating to working memory training in healthy older adults. *Int. J. Geriatr. Psychiatry* 28, 539–546. doi: 10.1002/gps.3859

Chein, J. M., Moore, A. B., and Conway, A. R. (2011). Domain-general mechanisms of complex working memory span. *Neuroimage* 54, 550–559. doi: 10.1016/j.neuroimage.2010.07.067

Chein, J. M., and Morrison, A. B. (2010). Expanding the mind's workspace: training and transfer effects with a complex working memory span task. *Psychon. B Rev.* 17, 193–199. doi: 10.3758/PBR.17.2.193

Chiew, K. S., and Braver, T. S. (2014). Dissociable influences of reward motivation and positive emotion on cognitive control. *Cogn. Affect. Behav. Nerosci.* 14, 509–529. doi: 10.3758/s13415-014-0280-0

Chooi, W. T., and Thompson, L. (2012). Working memory training does not improve intelligence in healthy young adults. *Intelligence* 40, 531–542. doi: 10.1016/j.intell.2012.07.004

Colom, R., Rebollo, I., Palacios, A., Espinosa, M. J., and Killonen, P. C. (2004). Working memory is (almost) perfectly predicted by g. *Intelligence.* 32, 277–296. doi: 10.1016/j.intell.2003.12.002

Colom, R., Román, F. J., Abad, F. J., Shih, P. C., Privado, J., Froufe, M., et al. (2013). Adaptive n-back training does not improve fluid intelligence at the construct level: gains on individual tests suggest that training may enhance visuospatial processing. *Intelligence* 41, 712–727. doi: 10.1016/j.intell.2013.09.002

Conway, A. R. A., Kane, M. J., Bunting, M. F., Hamrick, D. Z., Wilhelm, O., and Engle, R. W. (2005). Working memory span tasks: a methodological review and user's guide. *Psychon. Bull. Rev.* 12, 769–786. doi: 10.3758/BF03196772

Conway, A. R. A., Kane, M. J., and Engle, R. W. (2003). Working memory capacity and its relation to general intelligence. *Trends Cogn. Sci.* 7, 547–552. doi: 10.1016/j.tics.2003.10.005

Dahlin, E., Neely, A. S., Larsson, A., Bäckman, L., and Nyberg, L. (2008). Transfer of learning after updating training mediated by the striatum. *Science* 320, 1510–1512. doi: 10.1126/science.1155466

Dahlin, K. I. E. (2010). Effects of working memory training on reading in children with special needs. *Read Writ.* 24, 479–491. doi: 10.1007/s11145-010-9238-y

Dahlin, K. I. E. (2013). Working memory training and the effect on mathematical achievement in children with attention deficits and special needs. *J. Educ. Learn.* 2, 118–133. doi: 10.5539/jel.v2n1p118

Danielsson, H., Henry, L., Rönnberg, J., and Nilsson, L. G. (2010). Executive functions in individuals with intellectual disability. *Res. Dev. Disab.* 31, 1299–1304. doi: 10.1016/j.ridd.2010.07.012

Dempster, F. N., and Corkill, A. J. (1999). Interference and inhibition in cognition and behavior: unifying themes for educational psychology. *Educ. Psychol. Rev.* 11, 1–88. doi: 10.1023/A:1021992632168

Dougherty, M. R., Hamovitz, T., and Tidwell, J. W. (2016). Reevaluating the effectiveness of n-back training on transfer through the Bayesian lens: support for the null. *Psychon. Bull. Rev.* 23, 306–316. doi: 10.3758/s13423-015-0865-9

Dovis, S., Van Der Oord, S., Wiers, R. W., and Prins, P. J. M. (2015). Improving executive functioning in children with ADHD: training multiple executive functions within the context of a computer game. A randomized double-blind placebo controlled trial. *PLoS ONE* 10:e0121651. doi: 10.1371/journal.pone.0121651

Dowsett, S. M., and Livesey, D. J. (2000). The development of inhibitory control in preschool children: effects of "executive skills" training. *Dev. Psychobiol.* 36, 161–174. doi: 10.1002/(SICI)1098-2302(200003)36:2<161::AID-DEV7>3.0.CO;2-0

Edwards, B. G., Barch, D. M., and Braver, T. S. (2009). Improving prefrontal cortex function in schizophrenia through focused training of cognitive control. *Front. Hum. Neurosci.* 4:32. doi: 10.3389/fnhum.2010.00032

Enge, S., Behnke, A., Fleischhauer, M., Küttler, L., Kliegel, M., and Strobel, A. (2014). No evidence for true training and transfer effects after inhibitory control training in young healthy adults. *J. Exp. Psychol. Learn.* 40, 987–1001. doi: 10.1037/a0036165

Engle, R. W., and Kane, M. J. (2004). "Executive attention, working memory capacity, and a two-factor theory of cognitive control," in *The Psychology of Learning and Motivation*, ed. B. Ross (New York, NY: Elsevier), 145–199.

Fernandez-Duque, D., Baird, J., and Posner, M. I. (2000). Executive attention and metacognitive regulation. *Conscious Cogn.* 9(2 Pt 1), 288–307. doi: 10.1006/ccog.2000.0447

Foy, J. G., and Mann, V. A. (2014). Adaptive cognitive training enhances executive control and visuospatial and verbal working memory in beginning readers. *Int. Educ. Res.* 2, 19–43. doi: 10.12735/ier.v2i2p19

Friedman, N. P., Miyake, A., Corley, R. P., Young, S. E., DeFries, J. C., and Hewitt, J. K. (2006). Not all executive functions are related to intelligence. *Psychol. Sci.* 17, 172–179. doi: 10.1111/j.1467-9280.2006.01681.x

Goldin, A. P., Hermida, M. J., Shalom, D. E., Elias Costa, M., Lopez-Rosenfeld, M., Segretin, M. S., et al. (2014). Far transfer to language and math of a short software-based gaming intervention. *Proc. Natl. Acad. Sci. U.S.A.* 111, 6443–6448. doi: 10.1073/pnas.1320217111

Gray, J. R., Chabris, C. F., and Braver, T. S. (2003). Neural mechanisms of general fluid intelligence. *Nat. Neurosci.* 6, 316–322. doi: 10.1038/nn1014

Hardy, J. L., Nelson, R. A., Thomason, M. E., Sternberg, D. A., Katovich, K., Farzin, F., et al. (2015). Enhancing cognitive abilities with comprehensive training: a large, online, randomized, active- controlled trial. *PLoS ONE* 10:e0134467. doi: 10.1371/journal.pone.0134467

Harrison, T. L., Shipstead, Z., and Engle, R. W. (2015). Why is working memory capacity related to matrix reasoning tasks? *Mem. Cogn.* 43, 389–396. doi: 10.3758/s13421-014-0473-3

Harrison, T. L., Shipstead, Z., Hicks, K. L., Hambrick, D. Z., Redick, T. S., and Engle, R. W. (2013). Working memory training may increase working memory capacity but not fluid intelligence. *Psychol. Sci.* 42, 2409–2419. doi: 10.1177/0956797613492984

Hofmann, W., Schmeichel, B. J., and Baddeley, A. D. (2012). Executive functions and self-regulation. *Trends Cogn. Sci.* 16, 174–180. doi: 10.1016/j.tics.2012.01.006

Hsu, N. S., Novick, J. M., and Jaeggi, S. M. (2014). The development and malleability of executive control abilities. *Front. Behav. Neurosci.* 8:221. doi: 10.3389/fnbeh.2014.00221

Hudjetz, A., and Oberauer, K. (2007). The effects of processing time and processing rate on forgetting in working memory: testing four models of the complex span paradigm. *Mem. Cognit.* 35, 1675–1684. doi: 10.3758/BF03193501

Hussey, E. K., and Novick, J. M. (2012). The benefits of executive control training and the implications for language processing. *Front. Psychol.* 3:158. doi: 10.3389/fpsyg.2012.00158

Jaeggi, S. M., Buschkuehl, M., Jonides, J., and Perrig, W. J. (2008). Improving fluid intelligence with training on working memory. *Pro. Natl. Acad. Sci. U.S.A.* 105, 6829–6833. doi: 10.1073/pnas.0801268105

Jaeggi, S. M., Buschkuehl, M., Jonides, J., and Shah, P. (2011). Short- and long-term benefits of cognitive training. *Proc. Natl. Acad. Sci. U.S.A.* 108, 10081–10086. doi: 10.1073/pnas.1103228108

Jaeggi, S. M., Buschkuehl, M., Shah, P., and Jonides, J. (2013). The role of individual differences in cognitive training and transfer. *Mem. Cogn.* 42, 464–480. doi: 10.3758/s13421-013-0364-z

Jaeggi, S. M., Studer-Luethi, B., Buschkuehl, M., Su, Y. F., Jonides, J., and Perrig, W. J. (2010). The relationship between n-back performance and matrix reasoning - implications for training and transfer. *Intelligence* 38, 625–635. doi: 10.1016/j.intell.2010.09.001

Jarosz, A. F., and Wiley, J. (2012). Why does working memory capacity predict RAPM performance? A possible role of distraction. *Intelligence* 40, 427–438. doi: 10.1016/j.intell.2012.06.001

Jaušovec, N., and Jaušovec, K. (2012). Working memory training: Improving intelligence - Changing brain activity. *Brain Cogn.* 79, 96–106. doi: 10.1016/j.bandc.2012.02.007

Jolles, D. D., and Crone, E. (2012). Training the developing brain: a neurocognitive perspective. *Front. Hum. Neurosci.* 6:76. doi: 10.3389/fnhum.2012.00076

Jurado, M. B., and Rosselli, M. (2007). The elusive nature of executive functions: a review of our current understanding. *Neuropsychol. Rev.* 17, 213–233. doi: 10.1007/s11065-007-9040-z

Kane, M. J., and Engle, R. W. (2002). The role of prefrontal cortex in working-memory capacity, executive attention, and general fluid intelligence: an individual-differences perspective. *Psychon. B Rev.* 9, 637–671. doi: 10.3758/BF03196323

Karbach, J., and Kray, J. (2009). How useful is executive control training? Age differences in near and far transfer of task-switching training. *Dev Sci.* 12, 978–990. doi: 10.1111/j.1467-7687.2009.00846.x

Karbach, J., Strobach, T., and Schubert, T. (2015). Adaptive working-memory training benefits reading, but not mathematics in middle childhood. *Child Neuropsychol.* 21, 285–301. doi: 10.1080/09297049.2014.899336

Karbach, J., and Verhaeghen, P. (2014). Making working memory work: a meta-analysis of executive-control and working memory training in older adults. *Psychol. Sci.* 25, 2027–2037. doi: 10.1177/0956797614548725

Katz, B., Jaeggi, S., Buschkuehl, M., Stegman, A., and Shah, P. (2014). Differential effect of motivational features on training improvements in school-based cognitive training. *Front. Hum. Neurosci.* 8:242. doi: 10.3389/fnhum.2014.00242

Kelly, M. E., Loughrey, D., Lawlor, B. A., Robertson, I. H., Walsh, C., and Brennan, S. (2014). The impact of cognitive training and mental stimulation on cognitive and everyday functioning of healthy older adults: a systematic review and meta-analysis. *Ageing Res. Rev.* 15, 28–43. doi: 10.1016/j.arr.2014.02.004

Klingberg, T., Fernell, E., Olesen, P. J., Johnson, M., Gustafsson, P., Dahlström, K., et al. (2005). Computerized training of working memory in children with ADHD–a randomized, controlled trial. *J. Am. Acad. Child Adolesc. Psychiatry* 44, 177–186. doi: 10.1097/00004583-200502000-00010

Könen, T., and Karbach, J. (2015). The benefits of looking at intraindividual dynamics in cognitive training data. *Front. Psychol.* 6:615. doi: 10.3389/fpsyg.2015.00615

Kray, J., Karbach, J., Haenig, S., and Freitag, C. (2012). Can task-switching training enhance executive control functioning in children with attention deficit/-hyperactivity disorder? *Front Hum Neurosci.* 5:180. doi: 10.3389/fnhum.2011.00180

Lawlor-Savage, L., and Goghari, V. M. (2016). Dual N-back working memory training in healthy adults: A randomized comparison to processing speed training. *PLoS ONE* 11:e0151817. doi: 10.1371/journal.pone.0151817

Lee, Y., Lu, M., and Ko, H. (2007). Effects of skill training on working memory capacity. *Learn. Instr.* 17, 336–344. doi: 10.1016/j.learninstruc.2007.02.010

Liu, Q., Zhu, X., Ziegler, A., and Shi, J. (2015). The effects of inhibitory control training for preschoolers on reasoning ability and neural activity. *Sci. Rep.* 5:14200. doi: 10.1038/srep14200

Logan, G. D., and Burkell, J. (1986). Dependance and independance in responding to double stimulation: a comparison of stop, change, and dual-task paradigms. *J. Exp. Psychol.* 12, 549–563. doi: 10.1037/0096-1523.12.4.549

Loosli, S. V., Buschkuehl, M., Perrig, W. J., and Jaeggi, S. M. (2012). Working memory training improves reading processes in typically developing children. *Child Neuropsychol.* 18, 62–78. doi: 10.1080/09297049.2011.575772

Manuel, A. L., Bernasconi, F., and Spierer, L. (2013). Plastic modifications within inhibitory control networks induced by practicing a stop-signal task: an electrical neuroimaging study. *Cortex* 49, 1141–1147. doi: 10.1016/j.cortex.2012.12.009

Mather, M., and Carstensen, L. L. (2005). Aging and motivated cognition: the positivity effect in attention and memory. *Trends Cogn. Sci.* 9, 496–502. doi: 10.1016/j.tics.2005.08.005

Melby-Lervåg, M., and Hulme, C. (2013). Is working memory training effective? A meta-analytic review. *Dev. Psychol.* 49, 270–291. doi: 10.1037/a0028228

Melby-Lervåg, M., Redick, T., and Hulme, C. (2016). Working memory training does not improve performance on measures of intelligence or other measures of "far transfer": Evidence from a meta-analytic review. *Perspect. Psychol. Sci.* 11, 512–534. doi: 10.3837/tiis.0000.00.000

Miyake, A., and Friedman, N. (2012). The nature and organization of individual differences in executive functions: four general conclusions. *Curr. Dir. Psychol. Sci.* 21, 8–14. doi: 10.1177/0963721411429458

Miyake, A., Friedman, N. P., Emerson, M. J., Witzki, H., Howerter, A., and Wager, T. D. (2000). The unity and diversity of executive functions and their contributions to complex "Frontal Lobe" tasks: A latent variable analysis. *Cogn. Psychol.* 41, 49–100. doi: 10.1006/cogp.1999.0734

Miyake, A., and Shah, P. (eds) (1999). *Models of Working Memory: Mechanisms of Active Maintenance and Executive Control.* Cambridge: Cambridge University Press.

Mohr, D. C., Spring, B., Freedland, K. E., Beckner, V., Arean, P., Hollon, S. D., et al. (2009). The selection and design of control conditions for randomized controlled trials of psychological interventions. *Psychother. Psychosom.* 78, 275–284. doi: 10.1159/000228248

Morales, J., Gómez-Ariza, C. J., and Bajo, M. T. (2013). Dual mechanisms of cognitive control in bilinguals and monolinguals. *J. Cogn. Psychol.* 25, 531–546. doi: 10.1080/20445911.2013.807812

Morales, J., Yudes, C., Gómez-Ariza, C. J., and Bajo, M. T. (2015). Bilingualism modulates dual mechanisms of cognitive control: evidence from ERPs. *Neuropsychology* 66, 157–169. doi: 10.1016/j.neuropsychologia.2014.11.014

Morrison, A. B., and Chein, J. M. (2011). Does working memory training work? The promise and challenges of enhancing cognition by training working memory. *Psychon. B Rev.* 18, 46–60. doi: 10.3758/s13423-010-0034-0

Oberauer, K., Schulze, R., Wilhelm, O., and Süss, H. M. (2005). Working memory and intelligence–their correlation and their relation: comment on Ackerman, Beier, and Boyle (2005). *Psycol. Bull.* 131, 61–65. doi: 10.1037/0033-2909.131.1.61

Olesen, P. J., Westerberg, H., and Klingberg, T. (2004). Increased prefrontal and parietal activity after training of working memory. *Nat. Neurosci.* 7, 75–79. doi: 10.1038/nn1165

Palladino, P., and Cornoldi, C. (2001). Working memory and updating processes in reading comprehension. *Mem. Cogn.* 29, 344–354. doi: 10.3758/BF03194929

Paxton, J. L., Barch, D. M., Storandt, M., and Braver, T. S. (2006). Effects of environmental support and strategy training on older adults' use of context. *Psychol. Aging.* 21, 499–509. doi: 10.1037/0882-7974.21.3.499

Peng, H., Wen, J., Wang, D., and Gao, Y. (2012). The impact of processing speed training on working memory in old adults. *J. Adult Dev.* 9, 150–157. doi: 10.1007/s10804-012-9142-6

Persson, J., and Reuter-Lorenz, P. (2008). Gaining control: training executive function and far transfer of the ability to resolve interference. *Psychol. Sci.* 19, 881–888. doi: 10.1111/j.1467-9280.2008.02172.x

Raven, J. C. (1990). *Advanced Progressive Matrices: Sets I, II.* Oxford: Oxford Univeristy Press.

Redick, T. S., Broadway, J. M., Meier, M. E., Kuriakose, P. S., Unsworth, N., Kane, M. J., et al. (2012). Measuring working memory capacity with automated complex span tasks. *Eur. J. Psychol. Assess.* 28, 164–171. doi: 10.1027/1015-5759/a000123

Redick, T. S., Shipstead, Z., Harrison, T. L., Hicks, K. L., Fried, D. E., Hambrick, D. Z., et al. (2013). No evidence of intelligence improvement after working memory training: a randomized, placebo-controlled study. *J. Exp. Psychol. Gen.* 142, 359–379. doi: 10.1037/a0029082

Rosen, V. M., and Engle, R. W. (1998). Working memory capacity and suppression. *J. Mem. Lang.* 39, 418–436. doi: 10.1006/jmla.1998.2590

Rueda, M. R., Checa, P., and Combita, L. M. (2012). Enhanced efficiency of the executive attention network after training in preschool children: immediate changes and effects after two months. *Dev. Cogn. Neurosci.* 2, 192–204. doi: 10.1016/j.dcn.2011.09.004

Rueda, M. R., Rothbart, M. K., Mccandliss, B. D., Saccomanno, L., and Posner, M. I. (2005). Training, maturation, and genetic influences on the development of executive attention. *Proc Natl. Acad. Sci. U.S.A.* 102, 14931–14936. doi: 10.1073/pnas.0506897102

Rush, B. K., Barch, D. M., and Braver, T. S. (2006). Accounting for cognitive aging: context processing, inhibition or processing speed? *Neuropsychol. Dev. Cogn. B Aging Neuropsychol. Cogn.* 13, 588–610. doi: 10.1080/13825580600680703

Schmidt, R., and Bjork, R. (1992). New conceptualizations of practice: common principles in three paradigms suggest new concepts for training. *Psychol. Sci.* 3, 207–217. doi: 10.1111/j.1467-9280.1992.tb00029.x

Schmiedek, F., Lövden, M., and Lindenberger, U. (2010). Hundred days of cognitive training enhance broad cognitive abilities in adulthood: findings from the COGITO study. *Front. Aging Neurosci.* 2:27. doi: 10.3389/fnagi.2010.00027

Schubert, T., Strobach, T., and Karbach, J. (2014). New directions in cognitive training: on methods, transfer, and application. *Psychol. Res.* 78, 749–755. doi: 10.1007/s00426-014-0619-8

Schwaighofer, M., Fischer, F., and Bühner, M. (2015). Does working memory training transfer? A meta-analysis including training conditions as moderators. *Educ. Psychol.* 50, 138–166. doi: 10.1080/00461520.2015.1036274

Schweizer, S., Hampshire, A., and Dalgleish, T. (2011). Extending brain-training to the affective domain: increasing cognitive and affective executive control through emotional working memory training. *PLoS ONE* 6:9. doi: 10.1371/journal.pone.0024372

Shipstead, Z., Harrison, T. L., and Engle, R. W. (2015). Working memory capacity and the scope and control of attention. *Atten. Percept. Psychophys.* 77, 1863–1880. doi: 10.3758/s13414-015-0899-0

Shipstead, Z., Redick, T. S., and Engle, R. W. (2012). Is working memory training effective? *Psychol. Bull.* 138, 628–654. doi: 10.1037/a0027473

Simons, D. J., Boot, W. R., Charness, N., Gathercole, S. E., Chabris, C. F., Hambrick, D. Z., et al. (2016). Do "brain-training" programs work? *Psychol. Sci. Public Interest.* 17, 103–186. doi: 10.1177/1529100616661983

Smith, E. E., Geva, A., Jonides, J., Miller, A., Reuter-Lorenz, P., and Koeppe, R. (2001). The neural basis of task-switching in working memory: effects of performance and aging. *Proc. Natl. Acad. Sci. U.S.A.* 98, 2095–2100. doi: 10.1073/pnas.98.4.2095

Smith, E. E., and Jonides, J. (1999). Storage and executive processes in the frontal lobes. *Science* 283, 1657–1661. doi: 10.1126/science.283.5408.1657

Söderqvist, S., Nutley, S. B., Ottersen, J., Grill, K. M., and Klingberg, T. (2012). Computerized training of non-verbal reasoning and working memory in children with intellectual disability. *Front. Hum. Neurosci.* 6:271. doi: 10.3389/fnhum.2012.00271

Spencer-Smith, M., and Klingberg, T. (2015). Benefits of a working memory training program for inattention in daily life: a systematic review and meta-analysis. *PLoS ONE* 10:e0119522. doi: 10.1371/journal.pone.0119522

Spierer, L., Chavan, C. F., and Manuel, A. L. (2013). Training-induced behavioral and brain plasticity in inhibitory control. *Front. Hum. Neurosci.* 7:427. doi: 10.3389/fnhum.2013.00427

Sprenger, A. M., Atkins, S. M., Bolger, D. J., Harbison, J. I., Novick, J. M., Chrabaszcz, J. S., et al. (2013). Training working memory: limits of transfer. *Intelligence* 41, 638–663. doi: 10.1016/j.intell.2013.07.013

St Clair-Thompson, H. L., and Gathercole, S. E. (2006). Executive functions and achievements in school: shifting, updating, inhibition, and working memory. *Q. J. Exp. Psychol.* 59, 745–759. doi: 10.1080/17470210500162854

Steinhauser, M., and Hübner, R. (2009). Distinguishing response conflict and task conflict in the stroop task: evidence from ex-gaussian distribution analysis. *J. Exp. Psychol. Hum. Percept. Perform.* 35, 1398–1412. doi: 10.1037/a0016467

Takeuchi, H., and Kawashima, R. (2012). Effects of processing speed training on cognitive functions and neural systems. *Rev. Neurosci.* 23, 289–301. doi: 10.1515/revneuro-2012-0035

Thorell, L. B., Lindqvist, S., Bergman Nutley, S., Bohlin, G., and Klingberg, T. (2009). Training and transfer effects of executive functions in preschool children. *Dev. Sci.* 12, 106–113. doi: 10.1111/j.1467-7687.2008.00745.x

Tokowicz, N., Michael, E. B., and Kroll, J. F. (2004). The roles of study-abroad experience and working-memory capacity in the types of errors made during translation. *Biling. Lang. Cogn.* 7, 255–272. doi: 10.1017/S13667289040 01634

Towse, J. N., Hitch, G. J., and Hutton, U. (2000). On the interpretation of working memory span in adults. *Mem. Cogn.* 28, 341–348. doi: 10.3758/BF031 98549

Turley-Ames, K. J., and Whitfield, M. M. (2003). Strategy training and working memory task performance. *J. Mem. Lang.* 49, 446–468. doi: 10.1016/S0749-596X(03)00095-0

Turner, M. L., and Engle, R. W. (1989). Is working memory capacity task dependent? *J. Mem. Cogn.* 28, 127–154. doi: 10.1016/0749-596X(89)90040-5

Unsworth, N. (2010). Interference control, working memory capacity, and cognitive abilities: a latent variable analysis. *Intelligence* 38, 255–267. doi: 10.1016/j.intell.2009.12.003

Unsworth, N., Redick, T. S., Heitz, R. P., Broadway, J. M., and Engle, R. W. (2009). Complex working memory span tasks and higher-order cognition: a latent-variable analysis of the relationship between processing and storage. *Memory* 17, 635–654. doi: 10.1080/09658210902998047

Verbruggen, F., and Logan, G. (2008). Response inhibition in the stop-signal pardigm. *Trends Cogn. Sci.* 12, 418–424. doi: 10.1016/j.tics.2008.07.005

Verbruggen, F., Logan, G. D., and Stevens, M. (2008). STOP-IT: windows executable software for the stop-signal paradigm. *Behav. Res. Methods* 40, 479–483. doi: 10.3758/BRM.40.2.479

Wang, Z., Zhou, R., and Shah, P. (2014). Spaced cognitive training promotes training transfer. *Front. Hum. Neurosci.* 8:207. doi: 10.3389/fnhum.2014.00217

Weicker, J., Villringer, A., and Thöne-Otto, A. (2016). Can impaired working memory functioning be improved by training? A meta-analysis with a special focus on brain injured patients. *Neuropsychology* 30, 190–212. doi: 10.1037/neu0000227

Wiley, J., and Jarosz, A. (2012). Working memory capacity, attentional focus, and problem solving. *Curr. Dir. Psychol. Sci.* 21, 258–262. doi: 10.1177/0963721412447622

Woodworth, R. S., and Thorndike, E. L. (1901). The influence of improvement in one mental function upon the efficiency of other functions. *Psychol. Rev.* 8, 247–261. doi: 10.1037/h0074898

World Medical Association (2013). World medical association declaration of helsinki: ethical principles for medical research involving human subjects. *JAMA* 310, 2191–2194. doi: 10.1001/jama.2013.281053

Zinke, K., Zeintl, M., Rose, N. S., Putzmann, J., Pydde, A., and Kliegel, M. (2013). Working memory training and transfer in older adults: effects of age, baseline performance, and training gains. *Dev. Psychol.* 50, 304–315. doi: 10.1037/a0032982

3

Have Standard Tests of Cognitive Function been Misappropriated in the Study of Cognitive Enhancement?

Iseult A. Cremen [1] and Richard G. Carson [1,2]*

[1] Trinity College Institute of Neuroscience and School of Psychology, Trinity College Dublin, Dublin, Ireland, [2] School of Psychology, Queen's University Belfast, Belfast, United Kingdom

Edited by:
Claudia Voelcker-Rehage, Technische Universität Chemnitz, Germany

Reviewed by:
Giuliana Lucci, IRCCS Santa Lucia of Rome, Italy
Elizabeth A. L. Stine-Morrow, University of Illinois at Urbana-Champaign, United States

***Correspondence:**
Iseult A. Cremen
cremeni@tcd.ie

In the past decade, there has emerged a vast research literature dealing with attempts to harness brain plasticity in older adults, with a view to improving cognitive function. Since cognitive training (CT) has shown restricted utility in this regard, attention has increasingly turned to interventions that use adjunct procedures such as motor training or physical activity (PA). As evidence builds that these have some efficacy, it becomes necessary to ensure that the outcome measures being used to infer causal influence upon cognitive function are subjected to appropriate critical appraisal. It has been highlighted previously that the choice of specific tasks used to demonstrate transfer to the cognitive domain is of critical importance. In the context of most intervention studies, standardized tests and batteries of cognitive function are de rigueur. The argument presented here is that the latent constructs to which these tests relate are not usually subject to a sufficient level of analytic scrutiny. We present the historical origins of some exemplar tests, and give particular consideration to the limits on explanatory scope that are implied by their composition and the nature of their deployment. In addition to surveying the validity of these tests when used to appraise intervention-related changes in cognitive function, we also consider their neurophysiological correlates. In particular, we argue that the broadly distributed brain activity associated with the performance of many tests of cognitive function, extending to the classical motor networks, permits the impact of interventions based on motor training or PA to be better understood.

Keywords: aging, physical activity, coordination training, motor fitness, brain imaging

INTRODUCTION

A compelling body of evidence indicates that the aging brain's structure and function can be altered by factors amenable to intervention in later life, such as physical activity (PA) and social enhancement (for review see Ballesteros et al., 2015). As a result, the research literature now documents a multitude of attempts to harness the brain's capability for adaptive reorganization and change i.e., "neuroplasticity". The majority of these endeavors aim to improve "cognition". It is readily apparent that this term encompasses a wide range of putative capabilities. Expressed in the language of cognitive science, these may include: executive function, memory, attention and processing speed. In the context of many intervention studies, standardized tests and batteries are employed to operationalize these elements and examine the degree to which they are amenable to directed change. The argument presented herein is that the latent constructs to which such tests relate are not usually subject to a sufficient level of analytic scrutiny. Relatedly, empirical evidence to the effect that a specific intervention has an impact upon a particular measure of cognitive function does not necessarily lend support in terms relevant to how an older adult functions in daily life (e.g., Simons et al., 2016). Ecological validity is frequently defined as the extent to which results obtained in controlled experimental settings apply to real-world naturalistic settings (Tupper and Cicerone, 1990). In order for interventions to be deemed truly effective therefore, the benefits should generalize to functions germane to everyday life, such as competence and autonomy, and not simply the specific tasks upon which one is trained or tested (Lövdén et al., 2010). With respect to many of the tests that are employed to evaluate interventions to improve cognition, ecological validity is bound by the limits on explanatory scope that are implied by their composition (as distinct from their customary interpretation). This limitation notwithstanding, with the widespread availability of neuroimaging, it is further becoming apparent that the neurophysiological correlates of test performance are frequently at odds with those that are assumed by their adherents. Beyond highlighting the challenges posed by these considerations, we examine how they permit the seemingly positive impact of some forms of PA upon tests of cognitive function to be better understood.

SEEKING TO IMPROVE COGNITIVE FUNCTION IN OLDER ADULTS

Of the approaches that have been applied in an effort to improve cognitive function in older adults, the most common are cognitive training (CT) and PA. The former typically encompasses games or exercises designed to challenge specific cognitive skills. In contrast, PA interventions use exercise and movement program to improve physical capability, with the expectation that there will also be a positive impact in the cognitive domain (Bamidis et al., 2014). In relation to CT, although meta-analytic reviews have shown small improvements on measures of intermediate transfer of training gains to untrained tasks, there is little evidence of transfer to "real world" cognitive skills (Lampit et al., 2014; Melby-Lervåg et al., 2016; Simons et al., 2016). As Druin Burch noted: "Doing something repeatedly can make you better at it, which is not the same as saying it makes you better" (Burch, 2014, p.2).

PA interventions, in the forms of aerobic exercise and resistance training, appear to yield somewhat more consistent positive effects upon cognitive function in older adults (Colcombe and Kramer, 2003; Smith et al., 2010). Classes of PA that place greater explicit emphasis upon the generation of coordinated movement (and allude to a concept of "motor fitness") are now receiving particular attention (e.g., Voelcker-Rehage et al., 2011; Forte et al., 2013; Berryman et al., 2014; Moreau et al., 2015; Johann et al., 2016). In some cases the rationale for such approaches includes an emphasis on the "cognitive" demands of coordinated goal-directed movement, such as anticipatory planning and mapping sensation to action (Voelcker-Rehage et al., 2010). As the boundaries between variants of "cognitive" and "physical" training become blurred, it is an opportune moment to consider critically the nature of outcome measures used to infer causal influence upon cognitive function.

Necessarily the choice of task(s) used to demonstrate transfer of training related adaptations to the cognitive domain is of critical importance, as it determines the weight of the inferences that can be drawn. In view of this dependency, it has been recommended that multiple measures should be used to minimize measurement error and provide reliable and accurate estimates of the target construct (e.g., Shipstead et al., 2012; Moreau et al., 2016). In many cases, standardized tests and batteries (e.g., CAMDEX, Cogstate, The NIH Toolbox Cognition Battery) are de rigueur. Such selections are designed to ensure that the measurement instruments have been validated, are widely used and accepted, and permit comparisons across multiple studies. In the majority of cases however, these tests were devised to achieve an aim radically distinct from that of measuring enhancements in the cognitive functioning of older adults. We offer a perspective that includes an historical dimension, a delineation of limits on inference, and is informed by contemporary developments in neuroimaging. In examining the ecological and construct validity of prototypical tests, prudence necessarily emerges in relation to that which may be construed from their use (Heinrichs, 1990; Franzen and Arnett, 1997; Chaytor and Schmitter-Edgecombe, 2003).

SOME TESTS OF COGNITION FUNCTION

We do not seek to be comprehensive with regard to the tests of cognitive function that are employed in contemporary cognitive neurorehabilitation. Instead, we discuss a small number of exemplar tests, not in an attempt to target their specific uses and/or misappropriation, but rather to highlight the limits on their explanatory scope. In addition, we draw attention to the fact that the broadly distributed brain activity associated with the performance of these tests precludes reification in terms of any discrete cognitive processes (Uttal, 2013). Indeed, the most pervasive feature of the brain activation associated with these tests is engagement of the classical motor networks. We focus on common tests used to assess three "core executive functions" (Diamond, 2013, p.135): inhibition/inhibitory control, Working memory (WM) and cognitive flexibility/set-shifting (Miyake et al., 2000; Diamond, 2013).

Response Inhibition Tasks

Response inhibition tasks are used commonly to assess a facility to suppress prepotent actions and carry out a goal-directed response (Diamond, 2013). Response inhibition is said to be a key factor in successful cognitive and motor control (Chambers et al., 2009). The Eriksen Flanker task—perhaps the most common variant, was devised by Eriksen and Eriksen (1974). It is a speeded response time task that explores the effect of "flanker" distractor stimuli on target identification reaction time (RT). RT typically increases when the target stimulus is surrounded by "incongruent" distractor stimuli—letters or shapes from the target set that require a different response. The Flanker task is included in the NIH Toolbox Cognition Battery (Gershon et al., 2013), the Attentional Network Test (ANT; Fan et al., 2002) and a variant forms part of the CANTAB battery (Attention Switching Task). It is emblematic of a class of response inhibition tests, including the Simon task, that have been used to assess a supposed ability to suppress responses that are inappropriate in a particular context.

The Flanker task appears frequently within the cognitive enhancement literature, in particular in studies exploring the associations between cognitive function and PA (e.g., Colcombe et al., 2004; Davranche et al., 2009). This footing may in itself allude to the neural processes and adaptations to which the task may be sensitive. In Colcombe et al. (2004), a 6-month aerobic exercise intervention was shown to enhance cognition in older adults—as evidenced by improvement on the Eriksen Flanker task. It is no surprise then, that this test has since been used in many other studies examining aerobic PA (e.g., McMorris et al., 2009; Weng et al., 2015), resistance training (e.g., Liu-Ambrose et al., 2012), yoga (Gothe et al., 2013) and recently in those focusing on motor fitness (e.g., Voelcker-Rehage et al., 2010; Schoene et al., 2015). It has been included as a measure of executive function; described variously as a test of selective attention, response inhibition and information processing. In light of the fundamental characteristics of the test however, and in view of the nature of the interventions that give rise to a change in the level of performance—i.e., having an emphasis upon the selection of voluntary movements, the conclusion might be drawn that it will have a high degree of sensitivity to the functional state of elements within the classical motor networks.

The prototypical design is that in which responses in the presence of congruent or incongruent flankers are each compared to responses to neutral flankers. In many studies a direct comparison is made between responses in the presence of congruent flankers and responses in the presence of incongruent flankers. In the context of both designs, the interpretation of outcomes relies upon a "subtraction logic", whereby it is assumed that the same motor output is required in each instance, and that any difference between conditions (expressed via any given dependent measure) derives from other sources. With respect to the flanker task, the resulting contrast measure is hypothesized to be a "pure" measure of response inhibition, divorced of motor influence.

In a series of brain imaging studies, all of which employed the subtraction logic, it has been shown that during performance of the Flanker task, various elements of the cortical motor network including the pre-supplementary motor areas (pre-SMA) and SMAs (Bunge et al., 2002; Taylor et al., 2007) and Brodmann area 6 (BA6) more broadly defined (Zurawska Vel Grajewska et al., 2011; Caruana et al., 2014) exhibit differential activity in the congruent and incongruent conditions. The characteristics of neural activity registered in primary motor areas also differ reliably in the context of responses made in the presence of congruent and incongruent flankers (Grent-'t-Jong et al., 2013; see also Praamstra et al., 1998, 1999; Verleger et al., 2009). On the basis of such evidence it has been proposed that the executive control nominally sampled by these tests represents an evolutionary extension of the frontal cortex-basal ganglia loops that guide resolution of (motor) response conflict, such that the role of the supporting neural mechanisms extends to a range of processes including the reorienting of attention and the updating of WM (Neubert et al., 2013).

In line with the more general argument that is advanced in this piece, it should also be noted that, while at a phenomenological level the same motor response (e.g., depression of a response key) may appear to be generated in each condition, the state of the "motor circuitry" varies systematically across conditions. This can be revealed in a number of ways. As the latency between the onset of electromyographic (EMG) activity and the start of the response movement is longer when incongruent flankers are present than when congruent flankers are present (Coles et al., 1985; Eriksen et al., 1985; Smid et al., 1990), and shorter in the congruent condition than the neutral condition (Smid et al., 1990), differences in muscle activation dynamics are implied. It can also be shown that the time course of changes in the excitability of corticospinal projections to motoneurons innervating muscles that act as an agonists in generating the manual response when incongruent flankers are present, is distinct from that associated with responses made in the presence of congruent flankers (and in control conditions; Michelet et al., 2010; see also Klein et al., 2014; Duque et al., 2016).

In the absence of additional measurements, the possibility that intervention related changes in the state of motor networks contribute to changes in the magnitude of flanker effects cannot be excluded. Thus, when drawing inferences on the basis of the flanker task, and indeed response inhibition tests more generally, it is necessary to recognize that motor function is central to their interpretation.

Working Memory Tasks

WM is frequently described in such terms as the ability to hold and manipulate information in one's mind (Baddeley and Hitch, 1994; Smith and Jonides, 1999). The *n*-back task was introduced by Kirchner (1958) to measure differences in performance between younger and older adults on a "paced" task. A light flashed on and off in sequence at one of 12 locations, and participants were required to press buttons indicating where the light had gone out *n* positions before. As *n* increased, older adults (60–84) performed more poorly on this task when compared to younger adults (18–24). This was attributed to a slowing down of "central organizing processes of the brain" (p.357). A commonly overlooked element of this original experiment was that when the time allowed for the response was increased (from 1.5 s to 4.5 s), the performance of older adults improved substantially, leading the authors to conclude "the time factor plays an important part in the results" (p. 356).

In modern variants, stimuli may be auditory, visual, or in the case of the more recently developed dual *n*-back, auditory and verbal stimuli may be presented simultaneously (Jaeggi et al., 2003). The latter version has become popular as a WM training task (Jaeggi et al., 2008). In spite of weak convergence with other measures of WM (e.g., poor correlation with operational span (OSPAN), Kane et al., 2007, and with backward digit span, Miller et al., 2009), the task has become paradigmatic in both clinical and experimental settings. It is included in popular neuropsychological test batteries (e.g., Cogstate; the Penn Computerized Neurocognitive Battery, Gur et al., 2010), and has been used as a measure of WM in a number of physical intervention studies that have sought to enhance cognitive function (e.g., Kramer et al., 2002; Hansen et al., 2004; Gothe et al., 2013). It is however rarely the case that steps are taken in an attempt to parse separately the component elements of task performance.

A strong case can be made that when the *n*-back task is used in the context of intervention studies, subtraction logic should be applied. This is borne of the recognition that the *n*-back is a dual-task with two dissociable subcomponents. These comprise a WM updating subtask—involving the "encoding, manipulation, search and selection of information in WM", and a matching subtask—requiring the comparison of a currently presented stimulus with the (previous) one already selected (Watter et al., 2001, p. 999). In most implementations of the paradigm, participants are afforded sufficient time to complete the selection of the *n*-back stimulus prior to the presentation of a new stimulus, and thus the demands of the matching subtask are in principle the same across different *n*-back variants (i.e., 0-back, 1-back, 2- back etc). Generally this characteristic simplifies the interpretation of the data derived from the *n*-back paradigm (i.e., in relation to the impact of variations in "memory load"). In the case of changes in performance arising from an intervention however, it is not possible to exclude the possibility that a decrease in RT (or increase in accuracy) obtained for a single variant (e.g., 2-back) is attributable to a change in execution of the matching subtask. To take account of this caveat, it is necessary to express the level of performance achieved in variants with presumed higher memory load (e.g., 2-back) relative to a reference condition that also includes the matching sub-task (e.g., 0-back). We are aware of very few intervention studies with a focus on motor training or PA in which this step has been taken. Indeed, in many of the studies which have reported a positive impact upon *n*-back performance, either a single *n* was included (e.g., Hansen et al., 2004; Stroth et al., 2010; Hogan et al., 2013), or in cases in which data for more than one *n* were available (e.g., Erickson et al., 2013), normalization procedures were not applied. It is notable that with only one exception of which we are aware (Weng et al., 2015), with respect to those studies in which performance measures for more than one level of *n* were included in the analysis design, differential effects (e.g., 0-back vs. 2-back) of a motor training or PA intervention have not been reported (e.g., Kramer et al., 2002; Gothe et al., 2013). In the absence of suitable contrasts or normalization procedures, it is not evident that intervention-related improvements in the performance of an *n*-back task variant can be attributed to changes in the efficiency of WM processes. It also remains to be determined whether different *n*-back variants are characterized by distinct motor signatures—in the manner of those that distinguish the various conditions of the flanker task.

Although the speeded response selection characteristics of the matching subtask, that is intrinsic to the *n*-back, make plain that significant demands are imposed on the motor system, the ramifications of this are also amenable to scrutiny in terms of neurophysiology. In two activation likelihood estimation (ALE) meta-analyses published simultaneously (Glahn et al., 2005; Owen et al., 2005), 12 brain atlas delineated areas of activation were highlighted in association with performance of the *n*-back task. In the subset of only five areas for which there was a corresponding response across the two analyses BA6 was prominent. Although it is one of the largest regions in the Brodmann scheme, and a diversity of functions would thus be anticipated, since area 6 includes premotor cortex and SMA it necessarily has a fundamental role in regulating motor output. With respect to WM tests however, engagement of the cortical motor network is not simply a unique feature of the *n*-back protocol. In a comparison of seven further meta-analyses (in addition to the two that used the *n*-back procedure), Uttal (2013) noted that forty-seven Brodmann areas were reported as being activated during WM tasks (i.e., across the nine meta-analyses). Of these 47 brain regions, only BA6 was designated as being activated in every case. Indeed, in the context of extremely large variations in regional brain activation, the detection of signal in cortical motor areas during WM tasks is one of the most robust findings (e.g., Niendam et al., 2012). It has furthermore been determined that the threshold at which motor responses to transcranial magnetic stimulation (TMS) can be obtained—which is a measure of the excitability of corticospinal projections from primary motor cortex (M1), is negatively correlated (across individuals) with performance in *n*-back tasks (Schicktanz et al., 2013; Bridgman et al., 2016). As with response inhibition tests therefore, intervention related improvements in the performance of the *n*-back test in particular, and of WM tasks in general, may be mediated, at least in part, by adaptive changes within parts of the cortical motor network.

Cognitive Flexibility Tests

The third "core" element of executive function is considered to be cognitive flexibility/set shifting. The Trail Making Test (TMT) is used frequently in this context (Butler et al., 1991; Sellers and Nadler, 1993; Rabin et al., 2005). It is variously described as measuring cognitive flexibility, processing speed, sequencing, (Arbuthnott and Frank, 2000; Bowie and Harvey, 2006; Ashendorf et al., 2013), visual search, scanning and executive functions (Tombaugh, 2004). The TMT, originally devised in 1938 and known first as "Distributed Attention" and then as Partington's "Pathway Test" (Partington and Leiter, 1949), was originally intended as a test of speed, eye-hand coordination, alertness and distributed attention. In the 1940s, its inclusion in both the Army Individual Test Battery and the Halstead-Reitan Neuropsychological Battery (HRNB, Reitan and Wolfson, 1985) ensured its continued use and propagation in a wide range of research settings. It is now included in many national longitudinal studies of aging (e.g., the Harvard Aging Brain Study, The Irish Longitudinal Study of Aging (TILDA), The Aging, Demographics and Memory Study (ADAMS), etc.).

In the first part of the test (TMT-A), lines are drawn sequentially in order to connect 25 encircled numbers distributed on a sheet of paper. In the second part (TMT-B), the requirements are similar, with the exception that the individual being tested must alternate between letters and numbers, in increasing numerical and alphabetical order (e.g., 1, A, 2, B, 3, C, etc.). Performance is expressed in terms of the time taken to complete separately each portion of the test. On the basis of associations obtained between individual scores for elements of the TMT and other psychometric tests, it has been surmised that the TMT-A draws mainly upon visuo-perceptual abilities, that the TMT-B is primarily an expression of WM and task-switching ability (Sánchez-Cubillo et al., 2009, p.448). As it has been assumed that the demands in relation to "motor speed and visual scanning" are equivalent for both parts, further scores are also often derived (Arbuthnott and Frank, 2000, p.519). Most frequently these are the TMT-B—TMT-A difference score, and the TMT-B/TMT-A ratio. It is believed that by reflecting the additional requirements of the TMT-B, these scores measure "executive control" (p.519). In view of the fact that in the prototypical variants of the task, the distance between the targets is greater in the TMT-B than the TMT-A (Gaudino et al., 1995; Bowie and Harvey, 2006), a ratio score provides the more appropriate form of normalization. Indeed, it has been argued that it is essential to employ the ratio score when the goal is to evaluate executive function (Oosterman et al., 2010).

It is perhaps surprising therefore that many of the studies that have reported a positive impact of motor training or PA have treated the TMT-A and TMT-B separately (or singly), or reported a single additive measure (Emery et al., 1998; Scherder et al., 2005; Baker et al., 2010; Nguyen and Kruse, 2012; Vaughan et al., 2014; Eggenberger et al., 2015; Tazkari, 2016; de Natale et al., 2017; Gregory et al., 2017; Jonasson et al., 2017). Notwithstanding any evidence that completion times for either part of the TMT may be correlated (across individuals) with other measures of cognitive function (e.g., Sánchez-Cubillo et al., 2009), an intervention-induced change in the performance of TMT-A or TMT-B cannot simply be attributed to an effect on a specific faculty such as cognitive flexibility or set shifting. Contingent variations in the influence of other factors that mediate the successful completion of these tasks must also be contemplated.

On a prima facie basis, the intrinsic nature of the TMT is such as to suggest that individual levels of performance will be particularly sensitive to integrity of motor function. Indeed, this much was implied in its original formulation. The neurophysiological evidence is consistent with this supposition. When variants of the TMT specifically adapted for neuroimaging are employed, for example using a "virtual stylus" (Zakzanis et al., 2005) or button box (Jacobson et al., 2011) adapted to collect responses within the confines of an fMRI scanner, the contrast between the TMT-A and TMT-B reveals differences in BOLD response in the dorsal part of M1 (Jacobson et al., 2011; see also Zakzanis et al., 2005; Kodabashi et al., 2014). With respect to a clinical population, it has been reported that the TMT-B—TMT-A difference score is correlated with upper arm central motor conduction delay (Ravaglia et al., 2002). Using the TMT-B, Allen et al. (2011) registered the presence of task-related activation in the left precentral gyrus (M1), bilateral premotor cortex and the medial pre-SMA (see also Moll et al., 2002; Horacek et al., 2006). When measured using functional near-infrared spectroscopy, bilateral activity has been detected during the TMT-B task in premotor regions (Müller et al., 2014). In a further study using the same imaging procedures, activity was also detected in the M1, with older participants exhibiting greater task related changes in O_2Hb signal strength in this brain region, and in the right premotor cortex during both variants (Hagen et al., 2014). Employing EEG-derived measures, Wölwer et al. (2012) reported associations between TMT-B task performance and the current density of M1 designated sources. In light of the evidence of cortical motor network mediation, and particularly in view of the limitations that are associated with measures derived from a single TMT variant, the explanation that intervention associated enhancements in performance of the TMT-A or TMT-B (i.e., considered separately or additively) arise from adaptations in motor function, seems most parsimonious.

In a small number of published studies focusing on motor training or PA, a TMT-B/TMT-A ratio score has been employed (Klusmann et al., 2010; Yin et al., 2014; cf, Schoene et al., 2015). In none of these cases was an effect of a motor training or PA intervention demonstrated. Null findings have also been reported in all of the studies known to us in which a TMT-B—TMT-A difference score has been used as a dependent measure (Nagamatsu et al., 2012; Forte et al., 2013; Liu-Ambrose et al., 2016; Barban et al., 2017; de Natale et al., 2017; Jonasson et al., 2017).

Given the evidence that is available presently therefore, there is no basis upon which to suppose that motor training or PA has a reliable impact upon the facets of executive function to which the TMT is thought to be specifically sensitive. While reductions in completion times have been reported for individual task variants (TMT-A or TMT-B), it is not possible to exclude the possibility that these are attributable to changes in some aspects of motor function arising from the particular mode of intervention.

CONCLUSIONS

In the cognitive sciences, when faced with the practical challenges of operationalizing a theoretical construct, the pragmatic turn is to develop an experimental paradigm to capture its key features. Subsequently however, idiosyncratic features of the methodology may become reified as the phenomenon of interest (Nosek et al., 2012)—this may be quite distinct from the construct the paradigm was developed to capture, or indeed is capable of capturing. The point is that an improvement in the performance of a test arising from therapeutic intervention does not entail that the change may be interpreted in terms of the particular facet of cognition assigned by the practitioner to the test. Thus while enhanced performance of the Eriksen Flanker task might be ascribed to an improvement in selective attention, in the absence of convergent evidence, the effect of the intervention can with equal legitimacy be attributed to adaptations related to motor function. Indeed, with respect to many interventions that are based on PA, the latter is the more parsimonious account.

As a research tradition has evolved to explore notionally different aspects of cognition ("WM", "numeracy", "executive function" and so on), measured using different paradigms, there has also emerged a tendency to treat mediating brain processes as similarly dissociable in terms of constituent functions. Thus, in an era in which brain imaging has become the tour de force of cognitive neuroscience, and with access to tools that assign activity to specific brain regions, it remains customary to discuss variations in task-dependent activation in terms of the functional localization of various aspects of cognition (Ross, 2010). Necessarily however, the roles in cognition assumed by spatially circumscribed regions of the brain are highly diverse (Anderson, 2014). This much is certainly true of many elements of the cortical motor network. Beyond the specific examples given above, there is overwhelming evidence that their engagement is an obligatory feature of cognition in general, and the performance of tests of cognitive function in particular. In circumstances—such as therapeutic interventions based on PA, in which the purpose is more effective and/or efficient motor output, functional adaptations within motor networks are anticipated. In light of the tests that are employed, there is every reason to believe that many improvements in cognition ascribed to these interventions are also accountable in these terms.

We should strive to ensure that cognitive enhancement remains, at its core, an effort to improve the quality of life for older adults, targeting functional independence and activities of daily life. "Far" transfer from physical training to test-derived measures of cognition offers promise, however the transfer may not be as "far" as is assumed, or as "far" as is required.

AUTHOR CONTRIBUTIONS

The authors together wrote the article, jointly contributed the intellectual content and gave approval to the final version of the article to be published.

REFERENCES

Allen, M. D., Owens, T. E., Fong, A. K., and Richards, D. R. (2011). A functional neuroimaging analysis of the Trail Making Test-B: implications for clinical application. *Behav. Neurol.* 24, 159–171. doi: 10.3233/BEN-2011-0278

Anderson, M. L. (2014). *After Phrenology: Neural Reuse and the Interactive Brain.* Cambridge, MA: MIT Press.

Arbuthnott, K., and Frank, J. (2000). Trail making test, part B as a measure of executive control: validation using a set-switching paradigm. *J. Clin. Exp. Neuropsychol.* 22, 518–528. doi: 10.1076/1380-3395(200008)22:4;1-0;ft518

Ashendorf, L., Swenson, R., and Libon, D. J. (2013). *The Boston Process Approach to Neuropsychological Assessment: A Practitioner's Guide.* New York, NY: Oxford University Press.

Baddeley, A. D., and Hitch, G. J. (1994). Developments in the concept of working memory. *Neuropsychology* 8, 485–493. doi: 10.1037/0894-4105.8.4.485

Baker, L. D., Frank, L. L., Foster-Schubert, K., Green, P. S., Wilkinson, C. W., McTiernan, A., et al. (2010). Effects of aerobic exercise on mild cognitive impairment: a controlled trial. *Arch. Neurol.* 67, 71–79. doi: 10.1001/archneurol.2009.307

Ballesteros, S., Kraft, E., Santana, S., and Tziraki, C. (2015). Maintaining older brain functionality: a targeted review. *Neurosci. Biobehav. Rev.* 55, 453–477. doi: 10.1016/j.neubiorev.2015.06.008

Bamidis, P. D., Vivas, A. B., Styliadis, C., Frantzidis, C., Klados, M., Schlee, W., et al. (2014). A review of physical and cognitive interventions in aging. *Neurosci. Biobehav. Rev.* 44, 206–220. doi: 10.1016/j.neubiorev.2014.03.019

Barban, F., Annicchiarico, R., Melideo, M., Federici, A., Lombardi, M. G., Giuli, S., et al. (2017). Reducing fall risk with combined motor and cognitive training in elderly fallers. *Brain Sci.* 7:19. doi: 10.3390/brainsci7020019

Berryman, N., Bherer, L., Nadeau, S., Lauzière, S., Lehr, L., Bobeuf, F., et al. (2014). Multiple roads lead to Rome: combined high-intensity aerobic and strength training vs. gross motor activities leads to equivalent improvement in executive functions in a cohort of healthy older adults. *Age (Dordr)* 36:9710. doi: 10.1007/s11357-014-9710-8

Bowie, C. R., and Harvey, P. D. (2006). Administration and interpretation of the trail making test. *Nat. Protoc.* 1, 2277–2281. doi: 10.1038/nprot.2006.390

Bridgman, A. C., Barr, M. S., Goodman, M. S., Chen, R., Rajji, T. K., Daskalakis, Z. J., et al. (2016). Deficits in GABAA receptor function and working memory in non-smokers with schizophrenia. *Schizophr. Res.* 171, 125–130. doi: 10.1016/j.schres.2016.01.008

Bunge, S. A., Hazeltine, E., Scanlon, M. D., Rosen, A. C., and Gabrieli, J. D. E. (2002). Dissociable contributions of prefrontal and parietal cortices to response selection. *NeuroImage* 17, 1562–1571. doi: 10.1006/nimg.2002.1252

Burch, D. (2014). What could computerized brain training learn from evidence-based medicine? *PLoS Med.* 11:e1001758. doi: 10.1371/journal.pmed.1001758

Butler, M., Retzlaff, P. D., and Vanderploeg, R. (1991). Neuropsychological test usage. *Prof. Psychol. Res. Pract.* 22, 510–512. doi: 10.1037/0735-7028.22.6.510

Caruana, F., Uithol, S., Cantalupo, G., Sartori, I., Lo Russo, G., and Avanzini, P. (2014). How action selection can be embodied: intracranial γ band recording shows response competition during the Eriksen flankers test. *Front. Hum. Neurosci.* 8:668. doi: 10.3389/fnhum.2014.00668

Chambers, C. D., Garavan, H., and Bellgrove, M. A. (2009). Insights into the neural basis of response inhibition from cognitive and clinical neuroscience. *Neurosci. Biobehav. Rev.* 33, 631–646. doi: 10.1016/j.neubiorev.2008.08.016

Chaytor, N., and Schmitter-Edgecombe, M. (2003). The ecological validity of neuropsychological tests: a review of the literature on everyday cognitive skills. *Neuropsychol. Rev.* 13, 181–197. doi: 10.1023/b:nerv.0000009483.91468.fb

Colcombe, S., and Kramer, A. F. (2003). Fitness effects on the cognitive function of older adults a meta-analytic study. *Psychol. Sci.* 14, 125–130. doi: 10.1111/1467-9280.t01-1-01430

Colcombe, S. J., Kramer, A. F., Erickson, K. I., Scalf, P., McAuley, E., Cohen, N. J., et al. (2004). Cardiovascular fitness, cortical plasticity, and aging. *Proc. Natl. Acad. Sci. U S A* 101, 3316–3321. doi: 10.1073/pnas.0400266101

Coles, M. G., Gratton, G., Bashore, T. R., Eriksen, C. W., and Donchin, E. (1985). A psychophysiological investigation of the continuous flow model of human information processing. *J. Exp. Psychol. Hum. Percept. Perform.* 11, 529–553. doi: 10.1037/0096-1523.11.5.529

Davranche, K., Hall, B., and McMorris, T. (2009). Effect of acute exercise on cognitive control required during an Eriksen flanker task. *J. Sport Exerc. Psychol.* 31, 628–639. doi: 10.1123/jsep.31.5.628

de Natale, E. R., Paulus, K. S., Aiello, E., Sanna, B., Manca, A., Sotgiu, G., et al. (2017). Dance therapy improves motor and cognitive functions in patients with Parkinson's disease. *NeuroRehabilitation* 40, 141–144. doi: 10.3233/NRE-161399

Diamond, A. (2013). Executive functions. *Front. Cell. Neurosci.* 64, 135–168. doi: 10.1146/annurev-psych-113011-143750

Duque, J., Petitjean, C., and Swinnen, S. P. (2016). Effect of aging on motor inhibition during action preparation under sensory conflict. *Front. Aging Neurosci.* 8:322. doi: 10.3389/fnagi.2016.00322

Eggenberger, P., Schumacher, V., Angst, M., Theill, N., and de Bruin, E. D. (2015). Does multicomponent physical exercise with simultaneous cognitive training boost cognitive performance in older adults? A 6-month randomized controlled trial with a 1-year follow-up. *Clin. Int. Aging* 10, 1335–1349. doi: 10.2147/CIA.S87732

Emery, C. F., Schein, R. L., Hauck, E. R., and MacIntyre, N. R. (1998). Psychological and cognitive outcomes of a randomized trial of exercise among patients with chronic obstructive pulmonary disease. *Health Psychol.* 17, 232–240. doi: 10.1037/0278-6133.17.3.232

Erickson, K. I., Banducci, S. E., Weinstein, A. M., Macdonald, A. W. III., Ferrell, R. E., Halder, I., et al. (2013). The brain-derived neurotrophic factor Val66Met polymorphism moderates an effect of physical activity on working memory performance. *Psychol. Sci.* 24, 1770–1779. doi: 10.1177/0956797613480367

Eriksen, C. W., Coles, M., and Morris, L. R. (1985). An electromyographic examination of response competition. *Bull. Psychon. Soc.* 23, 165–168. doi: 10.3758/bf03329816

Eriksen, B. A., and Eriksen, C. W. (1974). Effects of noise letters upon the identification of a target letter in a nonsearch task. *Percept. Psychophys.* 16, 143–149. doi: 10.3758/bf03203267

Fan, J., McCandliss, B. D., Sommer, T., Raz, A., and Posner, M. I. (2002). Testing the efficiency and independence of attentional networks. *J. Cogn. Neurosci.* 14, 340–347. doi: 10.1162/089892902317361886

Forte, R., Boreham, C. A. G., Leite, J. C., De Vito, G., Brennan, L., Gibney, E. R., et al. (2013). Enhancing cognitive functioning in the elderly: multicomponent vs. resistance training. *Clin. Interv. Aging* 8, 19–27. doi: 10.2147/CIA.s36514

Franzen, M. D., and Arnett, P. A. (1997). "The validity of neuropsychological assessment procedures," in *Biological and Neuropsychological Mechanisms: Life-Span Developmental Psychology*, eds H. W. Resse and M. D. Franzen (Mahwah, NJ: Lawrence Erlbaum Associates, Inc.,), 51–69.

Gaudino, E. A., Geisler, M. W., and Squires, N. K. (1995). Construct validity in the trail making test: what makes part B harder? *J. Clin. Exp. Neuropsychol.* 17, 529–535. doi: 10.1080/01688639508405143

Gershon, R. C., Wagster, M. V., Hendrie, H. C., Fox, N. A., Cook, K. F., and Nowinski, C. J. (2013). NIH toolbox for assessment of neurological and behavioral function. *Neurology* 80, S2–S6. doi: 10.1212/WNL.0b013e3182872e5f

Glahn, D. C., Ragland, J. D., Abramoff, A., Barrett, J., Laird, A. R., Bearden, C. E., et al. (2005). Beyond hypofrontality: a quantitative meta analysis of functional neuroimaging studies of working memory in schizophrenia. *Hum. Brain Mapp.* 25, 60–69. doi: 10.1002/hbm.20138

Gothe, N., Pontifex, M. B., Hillman, C., and McAuley, E. (2013). The acute effects of yoga on executive function. *J. Phys. Act. Health* 10, 488–495.

Gregory, M. A., Boa Sorte Silva, N. C., Gill, D. P., McGowan, C. L., Liu-Ambrose, T., Shoemaker, J. K., et al. (2017). Combined dual-task gait training and aerobic exercise to improve cognition, mobility, and vascular health in community-dwelling older adults at risk for future cognitive decline1. *J. Alzheimers Dis.* 57, 747–763. doi: 10.3233/JAD-161240

Grent-'t-Jong, T., Oostenveld, R., Jensen, O., Medendorp, W. P., and Praamstra, P. (2013). Oscillatory dynamics of response competition in human sensorimotor cortex. *Neuroimage* 83, 27–34. doi: 10.1016/j.neuroimage.2013.06.051

Gur, R. C., Richard, J., Hughett, P., Calkins, M. E., Macy, L., Bilker, W. B., et al. (2010). A cognitive neuroscience-based computerized battery for efficient measurement of individual differences: standardization and initial construct validation. *J. Neurosci. Methods* 187, 254–262. doi: 10.1016/j.jneumeth.2009.11.017

Hagen, K., Ehlis, A. C., Haeussinger, F. B., Heinzel, S., Dresler, T., Mueller, L. D., et al. (2014). Activation during the Trail Making Test measured with functional near-infrared spectroscopy in healthy elderly subjects. *Neuroimage* 85, 583–591. doi: 10.1016/j.neuroimage.2013.09.014

Hogan, C. L., Mata, J., and Carstensen, L. L. (2013). Exercise holds immediate benefits for affect and cognition in younger and older adults. *Psychol. Aging* 28, 587–594. doi: 10.1037/a0032634

Hansen, A. L., Johnsen, B. H., Sollers, J. J. III., Stenvik, K., and Thayer, J. F. (2004). Heart rate variability and its relation to prefrontal cognitive function: the effects of training and detraining. *Eur. J. Appl. Physiol.* 93, 263–272. doi: 10.1007/s00421-004-1208-0

Heinrichs, R. W. (1990). Current and emergent applications of neuropsychological assessment: problems of validity and utility. *Prof. Psychol. Res. Pract.* 21, 171–176. doi: 10.1037//0735-7028.21.3.171

Horacek, J., Dockery, C., Kopecek, M., Spaniel, F., Novak, T., Tislerova, B., et al. (2006). Regional brain metabolism as the predictor of performance on the Trail Making Test in schizophrenia. A 18FDG PET covariation study. *Neuro Endocrinol. Lett.* 27, 587–594.

Jacobson, S. C., Blanchard, M., Connolly, C. C., Cannon, M., and Garavan, H. (2011). An fMRI investigation of a novel analogue to the Trail-Making Test. *Brain Cogn.* 77, 60–70. doi: 10.1016/j.bandc.2011.06.001

Jaeggi, S. M., Buschkuehl, M., Jonides, J., and Perrig, W. J. (2008). Improving fluid intelligence with training on working memory. *Proc. Natl. Acad. Sci. U S A* 105, 6829–6833. doi: 10.1073/pnas.0801268105

Jaeggi, S. M., Seewer, R., Nirkko, A. C., Eckstein, D., Schroth, G., Groner, R., et al. (2003). Does excessive memory load attenuate activation in the prefrontal cortex? Load-dependent processing in single and dual tasks: functional magnetic resonance imaging study. *Neuroimage* 19, 210–225. doi: 10.1016/s1053-8119(03)00098-3

Johann, V. E., Stenger, K., Kersten, S., and Karbach, J. (2016). Effects of motor-cognitive coordination training and cardiovascular training on motor coordination and cognitive functions. *Psychol. Sport Exerc.* 24, 118–127. doi: 10.1016/j.psychsport.2016.01.008

Jonasson, L. S., Nyberg, L., Kramer, A. F., Lundquist, A., Riklund, K., and Boraxbekk, C.-J. (2017). Aerobic exercise intervention, cognitive performance, and brain structure: results from the physical influences on brain in aging (PHIBRA) study. *Front. Aging Neurosci.* 8:336. doi: 10.3389/fnagi.2016.00336

Kane, M. J., Conway, A. R., Miura, T. K., and Colflesh, G. J. (2007). Working memory, attention control, and the *N*-back task: a question of construct validity. *J. Exp. Psychol. Learn. Mem. Cogn.* 33, 615–622. doi: 10.1037/0278-7393.33.3.615

Kirchner, W. K. (1958). Age differences in short-term retention of rapidly changing information. *J. Exp. Psychol.* 55, 352–358. doi: 10.1037/h0043688

Klein, P. A., Petitjean, C., Olivier, E., and Duque, J. (2014). Top-down suppression of incompatible motor activations during response selection under conflict. *Neuroimage* 86, 138–149. doi: 10.1016/j.neuroimage.2013.08.005

Klusmann, V., Evers, A., Schwarzer, R., Schlattmann, P., Reischies, F. M., Heuser, I., et al. (2010). Complex mental and physical activity in older women and cognitive performance: a 6-month randomized controlled trial. *J. Gerontol. A Biol. Sci. Med. Sci.* 65, 680–688. doi: 10.1093/gerona/glq053

Kodabashi, A., Kamiya, S., Otsubo, T., Higashi, Y., Tsuji, M., Fujimoto, T., et al. (2014). Activation of brain function in a computer-based neuropsychological test estimated using fMRI. *Adv. Biomed. Eng.* 3, 72–79. doi: 10.14326/abe.3.72

Kramer, A. F., Hahn, S., McAuley, E., Cohen, N. J., Banich, M. T., Harrison, C., et al. (2002). "Exercise, aging, and cognition: healthy body healthy mind?," in *Human Factors Interventions for the Health Care of Older Adults*, eds W. A. Rogers and A. D. Fisk (Mahwah, NJ: Erlbaum), 91–120.

Lampit, A., Hallock, H., and Valenzuela, M. (2014). Computerized cognitive training in cognitively healthy older adults: a systematic review and meta-analysis of effect modifiers. *PLoS Med.* 11:e1001756. doi: 10.1371/journal.pmed.1001756

Liu-Ambrose, T., Best, J. R., Davis, J. C., Eng, J. J., Lee, P. E., Jacova, C., et al. (2016). Aerobic exercise and vascular cognitive impairment. *Neurology* 87, 2082–2090. doi: 10.1212/WNL.0000000000003332

Liu-Ambrose, T., Nagamatsu, L. S., Voss, M. W., Khan, K. M., and Handy, T. C. (2012). Resistance training and functional plasticity of the aging brain: a 12-month randomized controlled trial. *Neurobiol. Aging* 33, 1690–1698. doi: 10.1016/j.neurobiolaging.2011.05.010

Lövdén, M., Bäckman, L., Lindenberger, U., Schaefer, S., and Schmiedek, F. (2010). A theoretical framework for the study of adult cognitive plasticity. *Psychol. Bull.* 136, 659–676. doi: 10.1037/a0020080

McMorris, T., Davranche, K., Jones, G., Hall, B., Corbett, J., and Minter, C. (2009). Acute incremental exercise, performance of a central executive task and sympathoadrenal system and hypothalamic-pituitary-adrenal axis activity. *Int. J. Psychophysiol.* 73, 334–340. doi: 10.1016/j.ijpsycho.2009.05.004

Melby-Lervåg, M., Redick, T. S., and Hulme, C. (2016). Working memory training does not improve performance on measures of intelligence or other measures of "far transfer" evidence from a meta-analytic review. *Perspect. Psychol. Sci.* 11, 512–534. doi: 10.1177/1745691616635612

Michelet, T., Duncan, G. H., and Cisek, P. (2010). Response competition in the primary motor cortex: corticospinal excitability reflects response replacement during simple decisions. *J. Neurophysiol.* 104, 119–127. doi: 10.1152/jn.00819.2009

Miller, K. M., Price, C. C., Okun, M. S., Montijo, H., and Bowers, D. (2009). Is the n-back task a valid neuropsychological measure for assessing working memory? *Arch. Clin. Neuropsychol.* 24, 711–717. doi: 10.1093/arclin/acp063

Miyake, A., Friedman, N. P., Emerson, M. J., Witzki, A. H., Howerter, A., and Wager, T. D. (2000). The unity and diversity of executive functions and their contributions to complex "frontal lobe" tasks: a latent variable analysis. *Cogn. Psychol.* 41, 49–100. doi: 10.1006/cogp.1999.0734

Moll, J., de Oliveira-Souza, R. D., Moll, F. T., Bramati, I. E., and Andreiuolo, P. A. (2002). The cerebral correlates of set-shifting: an fMRI study of the trail making test. *Arq. Neuropsiquiatr.* 60, 900–905. doi: 10.1590/s0004-282x2002000600002

Moreau, D., Kirk, I. J., and Waldie, K. E. (2016). Seven pervasive statistical flaws in cognitive training interventions. *Front. Hum. Neurosci.* 10:35. doi: 10.3389/fnhum.2016.00153

Moreau, D., Morrison, A. B., and Conway, A. R. (2015). An ecological approach to cognitive enhancement: complex motor training. *Acta Psychol.* 157, 44–55. doi: 10.1016/j.actpsy.2015.02.007

Müller, L. D., Guhn, A., Zeller, J. B., Biehl, S. C., Dresler, T., Hahn, T., et al. (2014). Neural correlates of a standardized version of the trail making test in young and elderly adults: a functional near-infrared spectroscopy study. *Neuropsychologia* 56, 271–279. doi: 10.1016/j.neuropsychologia.2014.01.019

Nagamatsu, L. S., Handy, T. C., Hsu, C. L., Voss, M., and Liu-Ambrose, T. (2012). Resistance training promotes cognitive and functional brain plasticity in seniors with probable mild cognitive impairment. *Arch. Intern. Med.* 172, 666–668. doi: 10.1001/archinternmed.2012.379

Neubert, F. X., Mars, R. B., and Rushworth, M. F. (2013). "Is there an inferior frontal cortical network for cognitive control and inhibition?," in *Principles of Frontal Lobe Function* 2nd Edn., eds D. T. Stuss and R. T. Knight (Oxford: Oxford University Press), 332–352.

Nguyen, M. H., and Kruse, A. (2012). A randomized controlled trial of Tai chi for balance, sleep quality and cognitive performance in elderly Vietnamese. *Clin. Interv. Aging* 7, 185–190. doi: 10.2147/CIA.s32600

Niendam, T. A., Laird, A. R., Ray, K. L., Dean, Y. M., Glahn, D. C., and Carter, C. S. (2012). Meta-analytic evidence for a superordinate cognitive control network subserving diverse executive functions. *Cogn. Affect. Behav. Neurosci.* 12, 241–268. doi: 10.3758/s13415-011-0083-5

Nosek, B. A., Spies, J. R., and Motyl, M. (2012). Scientific utopia: II. Restructuring incentives and practices to promote truth over publishability. *Perspect. Psychol. Sci.* 7, 615–631. doi: 10.1177/1745691612459058

Oosterman, J. M., Vogels, R. L. C., van Harten, B., Gouw, A. A., Poggesi, A., Scheltens, P., et al. (2010). Assessing mental flexibility: neuroanatomical and neuropsychological correlates of the trail making test in elderly people. *Clin. Neuropsychol.* 24, 203–219. doi: 10.1080/13854040903482848

Owen, A. M., McMillan, K. M., Laird, A. R., and Bullmore, E. (2005). N back working memory paradigm: a meta analysis of normative functional neuroimaging studies. *Hum. Brain Mapp.* 25, 46–59. doi: 10.1002/hbm.20131

Partington, J. E., and Leiter, R. G. (1949). Partington's pathways test. *Psychol. Serv. Cent. J.* 1, 11–20.

Praamstra, P., Plat, E. M., Meyer, A. S., and Horstink, M. W. (1999). Motor cortex activation in Parkinson's disease: dissociation of electrocortical and peripheral measures of response generation. *Mov. Disord.* 14, 790–799. doi: 10.1002/1531-8257(199909)14:5<790:AID-MDS1011>3.0.CO;2-A

Praamstra, P., Stegeman, D. F., Cools, A. R., and Horstink, M. W. (1998). Reliance on external cues for movement initiation in Parkinson's disease. Evidence from movement-related potentials. *Brain* 121, 167–177. doi: 10.1093/brain/121.1.167

Rabin, L. A., Barr, W. B., and Burton, L. A. (2005). Assessment practices of clinical neuropsychologists in the United States and Canada: a survey of INS, NAN, and APA Division 40 members. *Arch. Clin. Neuropsychol.* 20, 33–65. doi: 10.1016/j.acn.2004.02.005

Ravaglia, S., Costa, A., Ratti, M. T., Savoldi, F., Bo, P., and Moglia, A. (2002). Cognitive impairment and central motor conduction time in chronic alcoholics. *Funct. Neurol.* 17, 83–86.

Reitan, R. M., and Wolfson, D. (1985). *The Halstead-Reitan Neuropsycholgical Test Battery: Therapy and Clinical Interpretation.* Tucson, AZ: Neuropsychological Press.

Ross, E. D. (2010). Cerebral localization of functions and the neurology of language: fact versus fiction or is it something else? *Neuroscientist* 16, 222–243. doi: 10.1177/1073858409349899

Sánchez-Cubillo, I., Periñez, J. A., Adrover-Roig, D., Rodríguez-Sánchez, J. M., Ríos-Lago, M., Tirapu, J. F. F. A., et al. (2009). Construct validity of the trail making test: role of task-switching, working memory, inhibition/interference control, and visuomotor abilities. *J. Int. Neuropsychol. Soc.* 15, 438–450. doi: 10.1017/s1355617709090626

Scherder, E. J. A., Van Paasschen, J., Deijen, J. B., Van Der Knokke, S., Orlebeke, J. F. K., Burgers, I., et al. (2005). Physical activity and executive functions in the elderly with mild cognitive impairment. *Aging Ment. Health* 9, 272–280. doi: 10.1080/13607860500089930

Schicktanz, N., Schwegler, K., Fastenrath, M., Spalek, K., Milnik, A., Papassotiropoulos, A., et al. (2013). Motor threshold predicts working memory performance in healthy humans. *Ann. Clin. Transl. Neurol.* 1, 69–73. doi: 10.1002/acn3.22

Schoene, D., Valenzuela, T., Toson, B., Delbaere, K., Severino, C., Garcia, J., et al. (2015). Interactive cognitive-motor step training improves cognitive risk factors of falling in older adults—a randomized controlled trial. *PLoS One* 10:e0145161. doi: 10.1371/journal.pone.0145161

Sellers, A. H., and Nadler, J. D. (1993). A survey of current neuropsychological assessment procedures used for different age groups. *Psychother. Priv. Pract.* 11, 47–57. doi: 10.1300/j294v11n03_10

Shipstead, Z., Redick, T. S., and Engle, R. W. (2012). Is working memory training effective? *Psychol. Bull.* 138, 628–654. doi: 10.1037/a0027473

Simons, D. J., Boot, W. R., Charness, N., Gathercole, S. E., Chabris, C. F., Hambrick, D. Z., et al. (2016). Do "brain-training" programs work? *Psychol. Sci. Public Interest* 17, 103–186. doi: 10.1177/1529100616661983

Smid, H. G., Mulder, G., and Mulder, L. J. (1990). Selective response activation can begin before stimulus recognition is complete: a psychophysiological and error analysis of continuous flow. *Acta Psychol.* 74, 169–201. doi: 10.1016/0001-6918(90)90005-z

Smith, P. J., Blumenthal, J. A., Hoffman, B. M., Cooper, H., Strauman, T. A., Welsh-Bohmer, K., et al. (2010). Aerobic exercise and neurocognitive performance: a meta-analytic review of randomized controlled trials. *Psychosom. Med.* 72, 239–252. doi: 10.1097/PSY.0b013e3181d14633

Smith, E. E., and Jonides, J. (1999). Storage and executive processes in the frontal lobes. *Science* 283, 1657–1661. doi: 10.1126/science.283.5408.1657

Stroth, S., Reinhardt, R. K., Thöne, J., Hille, K., Schneider, M., Härtel, S., et al. (2010). Impact of aerobic exercise training on cognitive functions and affect associated to the COMT polymorphism in young adults. *Neurobiol. Learn. Mem.* 94, 364–372. doi: 10.1016/j.nlm.2010.08.003

Taylor, P. C., Nobre, A. C., and Rushworth, M. F. (2007). Subsecond changes in top-down control exerted by human medial frontal cortex during conflict and action selection: a combined transcranial magnetic stimulation-electroencephalography study. *J. Neurosci.* 27, 11343–11353. doi: 10.1523/JNEUROSCI.2877-07.2007

Tazkari, R. (2016). Physical activity, aging and cognition. (Doctoral thesis, Universität Bielefeld, Germany). Available online at: https://pub.uni-bielefeld.de/publication/2901000

Tombaugh, T. N. (2004). Trail making test A and B: normative data stratified by age and education. *Arch. Clin. Neuropsychol.* 19, 203–214. doi: 10.1016/s0887-6177(03)00039-8

Tupper, D., and Cicerone, K. (1990). "Introduction to the neuropsychology of everyday life," in *The Neuropsychology of Everyday Life: Assessment and Basic Competencies*, eds D. Tupper and K. Cicerone (Boston, MA: Kluwer Academic), 3–18.

Uttal, W. R. (2013). *Reliability in Cognitive Neuroscience: A Meta-Meta-Analysis.* Cambridge, MA: MIT Press.

Vaughan, S., Wallis, M., Polit, D., Steele, M., Shum, D., and Morris, N. (2014). The effects of multimodal exercise on cognitive and physical functioning and brain-derived neurotrophic factor in older women: a randomised controlled trial. *Age Ageing* 43, 623–629. doi: 10.1093/ageing/afu010

Verleger, R., Kuniecki, M., Möller, F., Fritzmannova, M., and Siebner, H. R. (2009). On how the motor cortices resolve an inter-hemispheric response conflict: an event-related EEG potential-guided TMS study of the flankers task. *Eur. J. Neurosci.* 30, 318–326. doi: 10.1111/j.1460-9568.2009.06817.x

Voelcker-Rehage, C., Godde, B., and Staudinger, U. M. (2010). Physical and motor fitness are both related to cognition in old age. *Eur. J. Neurosci.* 31, 167–176. doi: 10.1111/j.1460-9568.2009.07014.x

Voelcker-Rehage, C., Godde, B., and Staudinger, U. M. (2011). Cardiovascular and coordination training differentially improve cognitive performance and neural processing in older adults. *Front. Hum. Neurosci.* 5:26. doi: 10.3389/fnhum.2011.00026

Watter, S., Geffen, G. M., and Geffen, L. B. (2001). The n-back as a dual-task: P300 morphology under divided attention. *Psychophysiology* 38, 998–1003. doi: 10.1111/1469-8986.3860998

Weng, T. B., Pierce, G. L., Darling, W. G., and Voss, M. W. (2015). Differential effects of acute exercise on distinct aspects of executive function. *Med. Sci. Sports Exerc.* 47, 1460–1469. doi: 10.1249/MSS.0000000000000542

Wölwer, W., Stroth, S., Brinkmeyer, J., and Gaebel, W. (2012). Electrophysiological correlates of planning and monitoring in first episode schizophrenia. *Psychiatry Res.* 203, 83–88. doi: 10.1016/j.pscychresns.2011.11.009

Yin, S., Zhu, X., Li, R., Niu, Y., Wang, B., Zheng, Z., et al. (2014). Intervention-induced enhancement in intrinsic brain activity in healthy older adults. *Sci. Rep.* 4:7309. doi: 10.1038/srep07309

Zakzanis, K. K., Mraz, R., and Graham, S. J. (2005). An fMRI study of the trail making test. *Neuropsychologia* 43, 1878–1886. doi: 10.1016/j.neuropsychologia.2005.03.013

Zurawska Vel Grajewska, B., Sim, E. J., Hoenig, K., Herrnberger, B., and Kiefer, M. (2011). Mechanisms underlying flexible adaptation of cognitive control: behavioral and neuroimaging evidence in a flanker task. *Brain Res.* 1421, 52–65. doi: 10.1016/j.brainres.2011.09.022

4

Improving Dorsal Stream Function in Dyslexics by Training Figure/Ground Motion Discrimination Improves Attention, Reading Fluency, and Working Memory

Teri Lawton[1,2]*

[1] Perception Dynamics Institute, Del Mar, CA, USA, [2] Department of Computer Science and Engineering, University of California, San Diego, La Jolla, CA, USA

Edited by:
Soledad Ballesteros, National University of Distance Education, Spain

Reviewed by:
Elvire Vaucher, Université de Montréal, Canada
Trichur Raman Vidyasagar, University of Melbourne, Australia

***Correspondence:**
Teri Lawton
tlawton@pathtoreading.com

There is an ongoing debate about whether the cause of dyslexia is based on linguistic, auditory, or visual timing deficits. To investigate this issue three interventions were compared in 58 dyslexics in second grade (7 years on average), two targeting the temporal dynamics (timing) of either the auditory or visual pathways with a third reading intervention (control group) targeting linguistic word building. Visual pathway training in dyslexics to improve direction-discrimination of moving test patterns relative to a stationary background (figure/ground discrimination) significantly improved attention, reading fluency, both speed and comprehension, phonological processing, and both auditory and visual working memory relative to controls, whereas auditory training to improve phonological processing did not improve these academic skills significantly more than found for controls. This study supports the hypothesis that faulty timing in synchronizing the activity of magnocellular with parvocellular visual pathways is a fundamental cause of dyslexia, and argues against the assumption that reading deficiencies in dyslexia are caused by phonological deficits. This study demonstrates that visual movement direction-discrimination can be used to not only detect dyslexia early, but also for its successful treatment, so that reading problems do not prevent children from readily learning.

Keywords: attention networks, reading remediation, cortical plasticity, perceptual learning, improving dorsal stream function, neural timing, dyslexia development, figure/ground motion discrimination

INTRODUCTION

Dyslexia is a multifaceted reading disability that encompasses both pronunciation-based and visual processing-based reading issues (Stein, 2001) that is characterized by severe reading and spelling problems (Vellutino et al., 2004). Reading difficulties, including people having dyslexia and attention deficits, are prevalent in the United States (US) where 65% of fourth graders and 62% of 12th graders are not proficient in reading (National Center for Educational Statistics, 2013). Previous studies have shown that reading difficulties in many children may *indeed* be prevented through early intervention (Schatschneider et al., 2004). Identification of the cognitive skills that predict subsequent reading ability can help identify children at risk for reading problems, and following appropriate training reduce the severity of their symptoms (Kevan and Pammer, 2009). Since motion detection deficits in pre-reading children predict who will develop reading problems (Boets et al., 2011), it is likely that a task to improve motion discrimination, and thereby timing, in either the auditory or visual domain will remediate reading problems, a key question addressed by this study.

Slow reading speeds are a hallmark of dyslexia (Lyon et al., 2003; Nicholson and Fawcett, 2007). Children with dyslexia are reported to have some combination of spatial (Lovegrove et al., 1980; Cornelissen et al., 1995; Stein and Walsh, 1997; Lawton, 2000, 2007, 2008, 2011; Talcott et al., 2000; Hansen et al., 2001; Stein, 2001) and/or temporal (Stanley and Hall, 1973; Bradley and Bryant, 1983; Tallal et al., 1993; Temple et al., 2003) sequencing deficits. These spatial and temporal sequencing deficits cause the letters in the words and the words on the page to appear distorted, displaced, or crowded together (Atkinson, 1991), often resulting in eyestrain and headaches (Wilkins, 1995). These spatial and temporal sequencing deficits, found when images are rapidly presented or moving, have been hypothesized to result from neural timing deficits associated with sluggish magnocellular neurons (Livingstone et al., 1991; Stein and Walsh, 1997; Vidyasagar, 1999, 2001, 2012; Lawton, 2000, 2007, 2008, 2011; Stein, 2001; Vidyasagar and Pammer, 2010; Boets et al., 2011), causing deficits in integration of information between magnocellular ("where") and parvocellular ("what") neurons. A normally functioning magnocellular pathway is sensitive to *low-contrast* achromatic patterns (Kaplan and Shapley, 1986; Sclar et al., 1990). All dyslexics exhibit high contrast thresholds for discriminating the direction of moving patterns against stationary background patterns (Lawton, 2000, 2007, 2011; Ridder et al., 2001).

Visual Timing (Magnocellular) Deficits in Dyslexics

Receiving predominantly magnocellular input (Livingstone and Hubel, 1988; Maunsell et al., 1990; Merigan and Maunsell, 1993), the dorsal stream, specialized for processing the movement and location of objects in space (Ungerleider and Mishkin, 1982; Livingstone and Hubel, 1988; Felleman and Van Essen, 1991), projects from the primary visual cortex (V1), through visual area medial temporal cortex (MT), and on to the posterior parietal cortex (PPC), a selective spatial attention area (Posner et al., 1984). This is in contrast to the ventral stream which receives both magnocellular and parvocellular inputs as it projects from V1 through area V4 and on to the infero-temporal (IT) cortex, an area specialized in extracting details relating to an object's shape and color (Ungerleider and Mishkin, 1982; Livingstone and Hubel, 1988; Felleman and Van Essen, 1991).

Dyslexics have magnocellular responses that were found to be 20–40 ms slower than typically developing observers (Livingstone et al., 1991), being 2–4 fold slower than the normal magnocellular lead time of 10 ms (Dreher et al., 1976). Some investigators hypothesize that in dyslexics a lack of synchronization in timing between magnocellular and parvocellular activations may prevent effective sequential processing, pattern analysis, and figure/ground discrimination, and hence impede development of efficient reading and attention skills (Stein and Walsh, 1997; Vidyasagar, 1999, 2001, 2012; Lawton, 2000, 2007, 2008, 2011, 2015; Stein, 2001). It is further possible that the dyslexic reader's deficit in attentional focus (Vidyasagar, 1999, 2001; Facoetti et al., 2000, 2010; Solan et al., 2001) is another consequence of sluggish magnocellular neurons, preventing the linked parvocellular neurons from isolating and sequentially processing the relevant information needed for reading (Vidyasagar, 1999, 2001; Vidyasagar and Pammer, 2010), and not from the information overload as proposed previously (Stuart et al., 2001).

Visual timing deficits resulting from sluggish magnocellular (motion-sensitive) neurons in the dorsal stream are likely to be highly involved in the dyslexic's reading deficits (Stein and Walsh, 1997; Vidyasagar, 1999, 2001; Lawton, 2000, 2007; Stein, 2001; Gori et al., 2014). Convergent evidence suggests that many dyslexic readers demonstrate impairments in tasks that require dorsal stream involvement. Dyslexics have been found to have deficits in motion perception at: (1) the retinal level (Tyler, 1974) when measured using the frequency doubling illusion (Pammer and Wheatley, 2001; Buchholz and McKone, 2004; Kevan and Pammer, 2009; Gori et al., 2014); (2) V1 measured using Visual Evoked Potentials (VEPs; Livingstone et al., 1991; Shelley-Tremblay et al., 2011); (3) V1 and MT using both fMRI brain imaging (Eden et al., 1996; Demb et al., 1998) and psychophysical tasks of movement discrimination relative to a stationary background (Lawton, 2000, 2007, 2011); (4) MT using motion coherence for direction discrimination (Cornelissen et al., 1995; Talcott et al., 2000; Hansen et al., 2001; Boets et al., 2011); (5) the lateral intraparietal cortex (LIP) and Frontal Eye Fields (FEF), anterior cortical areas activated by saccades, based on saccade and antisaccade training tasks (Fischer, 2012); and (6) parietal structures, prefrontal language systems, cerebellum, and basal ganglia (Nicholson and Fawcett, 2007). These results are consistent with the suggestion of a relationship between dorsal stream processing and reading ability, such that poor dorsal processing relates to slower timing and poor reading skills. This study demonstrates that when a figure/ground motion discrimination paradigm is used, then poor reading skills are not only associated with poor visual dorsal stream functioning, but also can be remediated rapidly by training designed to improve dorsal stream function.

The degree to which dorsal stream deficits play a *causal* role in reading failure has yet to be established (Boden and Giaschi, 2007; Kevan and Pammer, 2009). Previous results indicate that there is a relationship between dorsal stream sensitivity and reading skill found in both pre-kindergarten children before reading is learned (Kevan and Pammer, 2009) and after the emergence of reading in children (Boets et al., 2011) and adults. Intervention studies targeting dorsal stream function need to be carried out in order to establish a direct causal link from dorsal stream functioning to reading skill (Kevan and Pammer, 2009). It is possible that since visual movement-discrimination training, designed to improve dorsal stream function, caused the reading speeds of dyslexic children to increase up to 10 times faster (Lawton, 2011), training dorsal stream function may be essential for developing not only reading fluency, but also the attention networks. Therefore, this study will not only measure reading fluency, but also measure attention and both visual and auditory working memory, for the first time, using standardized tests to demonstrate the range of cortical areas affected by training aimed at improving function in the V1-MT dorsal stream areas.

The novel question addressed by this study is whether improving neural timing in the dorsal stream (by improving magnocellular function) improves reading fluency more when training is in the auditory domain to improve auditory timing (language-based), or is in the visual domain using a visual motion direction-discrimination task (improving visual timing), when compared to a traditional reading intervention, using linguistic word building that does not specifically target neural timing. The intervention we used to improve auditory timing lengthens the individual phonemes so that phonological processing improves, the length of the phonemes decreasing as the training progresses. Motion direction-discrimination training, on the other hand, measures the contrast needed for figure/ground discrimination of sinewave gratings moving left or right relative to a stationary background. These backgrounds increase task complexity by increasing the number of background spatial frequencies, background contrast, thereby activating more parvocellular neurons, with left-right movement increasing in speed as the training progresses. The motion direction-discrimination training patterns, vertical sinewave gratings (**Figure 1**), are designed to differentially activate motion-sensitive (magnocellular) neurons in the V1-MT network (Allman et al., 1985; Felleman and Van Essen, 1991; De Valois et al., 2000) relative to pattern-sensitive (parvocellular) neurons, thereby being an effective training stimulus to improve magno-parvo integration deficits at both early and higher levels of motion processing. Unlike the motion direction-discrimination training paradigm used in this study, direction-discrimination using motion coherence of random dots, differentially activates motion-sensitive neurons only in MT and at higher processing levels (Zohary et al., 1994; Braddick et al., 2001). Deficits in detecting motion coherence are rarely found in all individuals in a dyslexic sample (e.g., Talcott et al., 2013). Moreover, improvements using motion coherence direction-discrimination (Solan et al., 2004) have not been shown to be as effective a training paradigm to improve reading speed as found previously using direction-discrimination of dim vertical bars moving relative to a stationary textured background (Lawton, 2000, 2011).

This study explored the hypothesis that if sluggish magnocellular neurons underlie dyslexia, then training to improve the sensitivity and timing of magnocellular relative to parvocellular processing should improve reading fluency and attention. This study investigated whether improving dorsal stream function is more effective in remediating reading, attention, and memory problems when the intervention training improves timing in the auditory or visual domain, compared to linguistic methods for improving phonological processing. Since both the auditory timing and linguistic interventions required responses chosen from a larger number of possible responses, it is likely they require more frequent use of selective attention than the visual direction-discrimination task, providing good comparison interventions to determine whether visual training in the dorsal stream is the most effective type of training to improve attention.

MATERIALS AND METHODS

Only students who were diagnosed as being dyslexic by the Decoding Encoding Screener for Dyslexia (DESD), based on single word decoding (word identification) and encoding (spelling and writing phonetically), participated in this study. The DESD, standardized by Western Psychological Services in Los Angeles, CA, USA was clinically validated using the Woodcock-Johnson standardized reading tests (Guerin et al., 1993), as well as the Gray Oral Reading Test (GORT) and spelling subtest of the Wide Range Achievement Test (WRAT; Handford and Borsting, 2015). In this study, the severity of dyslexia, most having borderline or mild dyslexia: (scored as 1: above normal, 2: normal, 3: borderline dyslexia, 4: mild dyslexia, 5: moderately severe dyslexia, and 6: markedly below normal) was determined by combining each student's dyseidetic score from 1 to 6 (spelling problems) and dysphonetic score from 1 to 6 (pronunciation problems) on the DESD. Matched samples were created by ordering students by their severity of dyslexia using this combined score, and then randomly assigning this ordered list into one of the three groups, either the control group or one of the two treatment groups, or in year-round schools into one of two groups, control and visual direction-discrimination training.

Dyslexic second graders (7 years old) were trained on three different reading interventions to improve: (1) auditory timing; (2) visual timing; or (3) linguistic word building. Second graders were studied since they are in the middle of the developmental period to learn direction discrimination (Lawton, 2000, 2007, 2008; Wolf et al., 2000), maximizing the ease of learning this task. This study was conducted in six elementary schools in San Diego Unified School District (SDUSD), where 50% of the students were reading below proficiency, as revealed by the California Standardized Tests available on each school's website. The students spoke English fluently. This study was carried out in accordance with the recommendations of both the University of California San Diego (UCSD) IRB and The Research and Reporting Department at SDUSD with written informed consent from all subjects. All subjects gave written informed consent in accordance with the Declaration of Helsinki.

This study examined 58 children in second grade, 7.4 ± 0.4 years of age, 49% girls and 51% boys. The number of participants in Traditional Schools (TS) was seven control, six visual timing and six auditory timing students; and in year-round schools was 19 control and 20 visual timing students. Even though participants were randomly assigned from the ordered

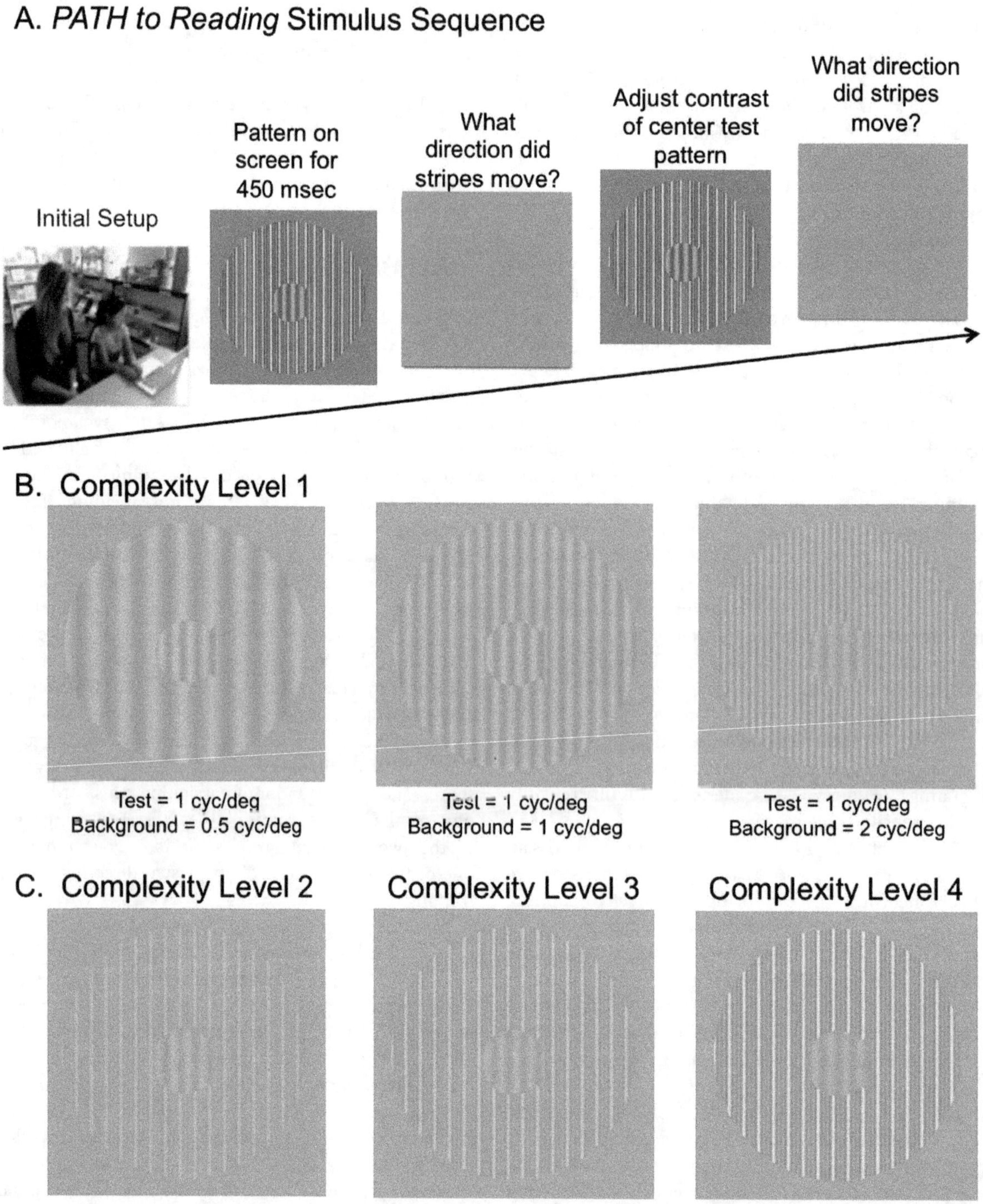

FIGURE 1 | (A) Schematic of Stimulus Presentation for *PATH to Reading* intervention. Pattern flashes on screen (shown above) while center stripes move left or right. Screen goes blank, waits for left or right arrow key to be pushed. If incorrect, short tone sounds. Pattern with same or different contrast flashes on screen while center stripes move left or right. Screen goes blank, waits for left or right arrow key to be pushed. This sequence of patterns is presented continuously until the contrast threshold for this pattern is measured. Then the next pattern combination is presented to measure next contrast threshold . . . until all 20 *PATH to Reading* patterns were presented, and the program says "Thank You" and quits. **(B)** Sample patterns at Complexity Level 1 for a background one octave lower in spatial frequency (0.5 cyc/deg) than the test frequency, equal in spatial frequency to the test frequency (1 cyc/deg), and one octave higher in spatial frequency (2 cyc/deg) than the test frequency for a 1 cyc/deg "fish shaped" test pattern. **(C)** Sample patterns at Complexity Levels 2, 3, and 4 for the center pattern in **(B)**. These patterns have multifrequency background patterns (1 cyc/deg + 2 cyc/deg + 3 cyc/deg) for a 1 cyc/deg test pattern on a 5% (Complexity Level 2), 10% (Complexity Level 3), and 20% (Complexity Level 4) contrast background. These same four complexity levels are repeated at subsequently faster speeds for each set of four complexity levels, increasing from 6.7 Hz (complexity levels 1–4) to 8 Hz (complexity levels 5–8) to 10 Hz (complexity levels 9–12) to 13.3 Hz (complexity levels 13–16), as listed in **Table 2**.

TABLE 1 | Subject baseline age and standardized scores for each group and significance levels across groups.

Baseline values	Control	PATH	FFW	*F* value	*p* value
Age	7.4 ± 0.5	7.4 ± 0.4	7.3 ± 0.2	0.39	0.82
Reading rate (words/min)	145 ± 48	136 ± 50	110 ± 30	1.73	0.15
Reading comprehension	7.2 ± 2.1	6.3 ± 2.8	5.8 ± 2.0	0.70	0.59
Blending words	8.9 ± 1.3	9.2 ± 2.7	8.8 ± 2.0	0.18	0.95
Attention (CAS)	81.7 ± 8	79.9 ± 9	77.7 ± 8	1.40	0.24
Sequential visual memory	95 ± 10	97.7 ± 13.2	96.3 ± 7.5	0.40	0.81
Sequential auditory memory	92.8 ± 9.6	92.8 ± 9.6	89.8 ± 9	0.51	0.73
NonSeq auditory memory	92.8 ± 11	91.8 ± 8	87.2 ± 8	1.10	0.36
Delayed recall	91 ± 15	94 ± 13.1	92.5 ± 12.9	0.55	0.70

Baseline values in Table 1 are mean ± SD for age and scores on tests graphed in ***Figure 2****.*

list of DESD scores into either two (year-round schedules) or three groups (TS schedules), the groups were balanced on age and baseline reading rate, attention and working memory, as shown in **Table 1**. The ethnic distribution for students in: (1) TS was 48.6% Caucasian, 25.7% Hispanic, 8.6% African American, and 17.1% Asian; and (2) Year-Round schools was 33.3% Caucasian, 28.2% Hispanic, 10.3% African American, and 28.2% Asian. These ethnicities were distributed equally among groups.

So that the training could be done by one Research Assistant (RA) for each 1–2 second graders, 40 UCSD undergraduate RAs were trained extensively at the beginning of the school year. The RAs were in charge of administering the standardized tests and reading interventions. The standardized tests were administered in a masked manner; RAs did not know whether the student was in a control or treatment group, thereby removing the possibility of experimenter effects. Moreover, parents: (1) were not aware of what group their child was in; and (2) thought that the auditory or linguistic interventions would work more effectively, since these were the traditional interventions advertised to improve reading. This fact, though anecdotal, would suggest that if any parent expectancy effects were in play, they would work against the efficacy of the visual direction-discrimination intervention. Stickers were given to students at the end of training each day for good behavior and completing the intervention correctly to reward them for paying attention to the task. Motivational strategies were used to keep the participants on task.

Experimental Design

The study was conducted for 20 weeks in four traditional schedule and 2-year-round public elementary schools in SDUSD in the morning, right before guided reading in the classroom, so that each student had plenty of practice on reading following the interventions. Twenty weeks of training was longer than used in previous studies of direction-discrimination training to improve reading fluency (Lawton, 2000, 2007, 2008, 2011), but was the minimum needed for the auditory timing training to be effective (Ostarello and De Ley, 2009). Controls were students who stayed in the classroom doing linguistic word building, when students in the treatment groups were pulled to do the visual or auditory timing interventions for 30 min, either 3 days a week for *visual timing* training or 5 days a week for *auditory timing* training. The linguistic word building intervention was a reading intervention provided by SDUSD, one aimed at improving phonics, decoding, vocabulary, reading comprehension, and reading fluency by word building exercises. Visual direction-discrimination was trained for a total of 20–30 h, depending on the time needed to complete 20 contrast thresholds, compared to 50 h of training on auditory phonemic processing. Auditory timing training was only done in schools having a traditional schedule, requested by those implementing the *auditory timing* training, since this training was found to regress in effectiveness when 4-week long vacations occur during the intervention training (Ostarello and De Ley, 2009), as occurs in the year-round schools.

At each school, the interventions were administered in a room devoted to this task on 13″ Macbook Pro computers purchased for this study. The computers were calibrated at the beginning of the school year with a Spectra Pritchard 1980A photometer to increase luminance and contrast linearly. The mean luminance was set to 125 cd/m^2 on all computers by reducing the brightness of the screen 2–3 levels. The screen brightness, volume control, and date were checked each day before beginning visual timing training. Students sat an arm's length from the screen, about 57 cm.

Standardized Tests

Standardized tests of reading fluency, phonological processing, attention, and working memory were administered one-on-one to every student in the study before and after the intervention training by trained UCSD undergraduate students. These tests were chosen as the "Gold Standard" for fast and accurate measurements of fluency-based reading, attention, and working memory skills. The standardized tests which took about 1.5 h to administer were:

1. DESD using single word reading to measure the reading grade level, and spelling eidetically and phonologically to determine the level of dyseidetic (spelling) and dysphonetic (phononetic writing) deficits took about 10 min, distributed by Western Psychological Services in Los Angeles, CA, USA;
2. A computer-based reading speed assessment, described previously (Lawton, 2007) where six words of white text on a black background were presented each time from subsequent portions of an interesting story at increasing speeds, took about 3–5 min. The words were composed of large *sans-serif* letters. Text at their reading grade level, stories from Dr. Seuss,

was used to measure reading speeds. Reading speed, measured in words/minute using a double staircase procedure, was not limited by the child's rate of speaking, as is the case for the GORT below. In addition, words/minute is a much higher resolution scale, than the 1–5 scale used to score reading rates on the GORT-3 below;

3. (GORT-3) to measure both reading comprehension and reading speed took about 20 min;
4. Comprehensive Test of Phonological Processing (CTOPP) Blending Words subtest, using CD-based delivery, to measure phonological awareness, took about 5 min;
5. Cognitive Assessment Systems (CAS) test of Attention, measured using the Stroop and Number Detection subtests, took about 10 min;
6. Test of Information Processing Skills (TIPS) to measure both sequential (remembering the letters in the correct sequence) and nonsequential (remembering the letters in any order) auditory and visual working memory, and Delayed Recall took about 15 min.

Interventions

Auditory Timing Intervention: FastForWord

The auditory timing intervention, implemented using FastForWord (FFW), developed by Scientific Learning Corporation, is designed to improve phonological processing by lengthening the phonemes until they are perceived accurately. The auditory timing intervention focuses on the building of auditory processing and oral language skills important for reading, by using acoustically-modified, digitally-generated speech: (1) frequency modulated tonal sweeps; (2) speech syllables with parametric modifications of temporal features, so format transitions were lengthened and intensified, or silent gaps were lengthened; (3) word exercises using human speech that was either parametrically modified in the temporal domain to teach students word ID, word matching, or following directions; and (4) phrases and sentences with increasingly complex grammatical structures to develop higher-level language skills, including phonology, morphology, syntax, grammar, and short-term memory. The stimuli changed adaptively, increasingly approximating normal speech, until the final levels, when normal speech was presented. This computer-based intervention is designed to build language and reading skills while strengthening the cognitive skills of memory, attention, processing, and sequencing. This auditory timing intervention was composed of seven exercises, three being done during each half-hour training session. To keep each participant challenged, but not frustrated, the exercises adapt so that the participant is successful around 80% of the time. Detailed reporting is provided to help instructors track participant performance, with alerts that let the instructor know when a participant is ready to move to the next product or when a participant is struggling and needs extra help. Individual interventions were provided for subjects who had difficulty progressing through the levels of the exercises to enable them to complete the exercises. For some subjects, occasionally the screen had to be covered, since the graphics prevented the subject from concentrating on the subtle auditory discriminations required to do *FFW* training. *FFW* was trained for 30 min, 5 days a week for 20 weeks.

Visual Timing Intervention: Motion Direction-Discrimination Training

The visual timing intervention, implemented using *PATH to Reading*, developed to remediate dorsal stream function, consisted of motion direction-discrimination training. This novel intervention (Lawton, 2000, 2007, 2008, 2011, 2015), developed by the author, and available commercially[1], will be described in sufficient detail to understand its basic components. The student sat in front of a computer monitor with a display similar to the ones in **Figure 1**. During the presentation, the bars in the "fish-shaped" window in the center of the screen formed by a sinusoidal grating, moved left or right very briefly (450 ms). The student reported which way the center pattern moved by pushing the left or right arrow key. A brief tone was presented after incorrect responses. The program adaptively changed the contrast of the test pattern in order to keep the student at 79% correct. There were also levels of difficulty introduced by making the background pattern more similar to that in the fish, by increasing the pattern's complexity level, and by increasing the number of directions of movement from one to two directions of motion.

The patterns used for this visual direction-discrimination task were designed to be optimal for activating magnocellular neurons (moving test pattern) relative to parvocellular neurons (stationary background; Lawton, 2000, 2007, 2011). In a given staircase run, the center spatial frequency (i.e., the test frequency) was either 0.25, 0.5, 1, or 2 cyc/deg. The surround grating spatial frequency was either equal to the test frequency or 1–2 octaves higher or lower than the test frequency, e.g., see **Figure 1B**. In addition to these simple backgrounds, multifrequency backgrounds were used, where the first background frequency equaled the spatial frequency of the single frequency background, having two additional background frequencies with a difference frequency equal to the test frequency. For example, the multifrequency backgrounds in **Figure 1C** are for a test frequency of 1 cyc/deg and a background frequency of 1 cyc/deg + 2 cyc/deg + 3 cyc/deg.

At the start of a session, both the test and background gratings were set to 5% contrast to ensure that the contrast of the test pattern was in the middle of the magnocellular contrast range (Kaplan and Shapley, 1986). Each time the child correctly identified the direction the fish stripes moved, the contrast of the test grating was lowered until the child answered incorrectly. Following the first incorrect response, a double-staircase procedure was used to estimate the direction-discrimination contrast threshold, which allowed measuring the contrast sensitivity, defined as the reciprocal of the contrast threshold times 100. This staircase procedure estimates the contrast needed for 79% correct responses, providing the most sensitive, repeatable measurements of contrast sensitivity (Higgins et al., 1984). A full training cycle of the direction-discrimination task required 20 threshold determinations (i.e.,

[1] www.pathtoreading.com

one for each of the four test spatial frequencies paired with each of the five background spatial frequencies).

The complexity level increased the: (1) number of sinewave components in the background from one (**Figure 1B**) to three (**Figure 1C**); (2) background contrast from 5% to 20%, (**Figure 1C**); and (3) pattern's speed of movement after every four complexity levels, increasing from 6.7 Hz up to 13.3 Hz, as shown in **Table 2**, so that the student was challenged as the training progressed. The background contrast was increased to 20% contrast to provide a background that increased parvocellular activity, since magnocellular neurons saturate at 10% contrast (Kaplan and Shapley, 1986). The 20% contrast background required students to analyze information from magnocellular activity relative to increased parvocellular activity, making the task more challenging. The order of presentation for each complexity level was chosen to gradually increase the difficulty of the task (Lawton, 2011). Therefore, as the level of complexity increased, the contrast threshold should be higher initially. Once all 16 complexity levels of the *Motion* program were completed, the student progressed onto the next program, the *MotionMemory* program. Instead of discriminating the direction one pattern moved by pushing the left or right arrow key as in the *Motion* program, *MotionMemory* requires signaling the direction that two separate patterns moved, one after the other, by pushing one of four arrow keys. Each threshold in both the *Motion* and *MotionMemory* programs required 20–40 trials to complete. A score was given to make the training more game-like. The lower the contrast threshold, the higher was the score. After learning how to do this task, children typically took about 15–20 min to complete one replication, consisting of 20 contrast thresholds. Motion direction-discrimination was trained for between 15–30 min, 3 days a week for 20 weeks.

Linguistic Word Building Intervention (Control Intervention)

A linguistic word building intervention was implemented using *Learning Upgrade* to help struggling readers at the second and third grade level overcome reading difficulties. Each course contained 60 lessons sequenced to build reading skills. The lessons featured a song-video for instruction and a game for practice with remediation. After logging onto the website, a song-video of length 1–2 min was presented which taught the word building topic through lyrics with a catchy melody and a synchronized animated visual of letters, words and pictures. A game followed the song-video, which required students to answer a series of questions through interaction. Immediate remediation through a spoken voice and animated visuals was given for each incorrect answer, followed by additional problems. When a student reached 100 points, if they had achieved higher than 75% correct, they moved on to the next lesson. If not, they repeated the lesson with the same song but varied questions in the game. When a student completed all 60 lessons, they earned a Bronze certificate which could be printed. A student then used a visual map of lessons and scores to repeat any lessons below 90% to earn a Silver certificate, and then repeated any lessons below 95% to earn a Gold certificate. When a student had earned a Gold certificate, typically in about 20–30 h of time on task, the student was finished with the course and moved to a higher course.

TABLE 2 | Stimulus characteristics at each complexity level.

Complexity level	Pattern speed (Hz)	Background frequencies	Background contrast (%)
1	6.7	Single frequency	5
2	6.7	Multi frequency	5
3	6.7	Multi frequency	10
4	6.7	Multi frequency	20
5	8	Single frequency	5
6	8	Multi frequency	5
7	8	Multi frequency	10
8	8	Multi frequency	20
9	10	Single frequency	5
10	10	Multi frequency	5
11	10	Multi frequency	10
12	10	Multi frequency	20
13	13.3	Single frequency	5
14	13.3	Multi frequency	5
15	13.3	Multi frequency	10
16	13.3	Multi frequency	20

Hypotheses

The primary hypothesis in this study is that timing interventions: either one to improve auditory timing or one to improve visual timing, would improve attention, reading, and working memory more than linguistic word building exercises. Attention is the primary outcome measure, with reading speed and comprehension, phonological processing, and working memory being secondary outcome measures that result from improved selective and sustained attention. The secondary hypotheses, based on physiological data demonstrating that 1 cyc/deg is the lowest spatial frequency channel (Blakemore and Campbell, 1969), predict that direction discrimination sensitivity improves: (1) the most for the lowest spatial frequency channel, 1 cyc/deg, which moves twice as far in the same amount of time as the higher 2 cyc/deg test pattern; (2) the least for the 0.25 cyc/deg test pattern which requires pooling across spatial frequency channels to complete the task; and (3) more when a wider background frame of reference consisting of multiple spatial frequencies that are a harmonic (multiple) of the test frequency is presented, as found in typically developing observers (Lawton, 1989).

Statistical Analyses

Change in test performance for the primary and secondary outcome measures (attention, reading speed and comprehension, working memory and phonological processing) and all secondary hypotheses were modeled using ANCOVAs controlling for age, sex, ethnicity (Caucasian, Hispanic, Asian, African-American), and school enrolled. Data was either: (1) pooled across schools having a traditional year schedule (four schools); or (2) pooled across the six schools, four having a traditional year schedule and two having a year-round schedule, with school and type of school (traditional vs. year round) included as covariates in the planned ANCOVA. ANCOVA contrast tests were used to compare change in standardized scores in controls vs. treatment groups.

A one-sample t-test was used to compare initial contrast sensitivity in the 58 dyslexics in this study to published levels in typically-developing second graders; paired t-tests were used to compare initial to final contrast sensitivity levels within each treatment group. The relationship between contrast sensitivity and the motion direction-discrimination task complexity level was assessed using 24 visual timing group students who completed all 16 levels of the *Motion* direction-discrimination training. For data from test frequencies 0.25, 0.5, 1.0, and 2.0 cyc/deg, the relationship between complexity level and contrast sensitivity was assessed using a linear mixed effects model, with hypothesis testing based on the fixed effect estimate of mean trajectory as complexity level increases, i.e., as amount of training increased. Tests investigating whether student's contrast sensitivity at specific complexity levels deviated from the overall linear trend (i.e., were higher or lower than expected) were performed by adding indicator variables for the complexity levels in question to the linear mixed effects models. Paired t-tests were used to test for significant improvement in contrast sensitivity at 0.25, 0.5, 1.0, and 2.0 cyc/deg from baseline to end of study within students trained on *PATH to Reading*. All analyses were performed using the R statistical programming language. ANCOVA models were fit using the aov function (Chambers et al., 1992), and mixed effects models were fit using the lmer function (Pinheiro and Bates, 2000). All tests were 2-sided since students could increase or decrease in academic skills, with significance level $\alpha = 0.05$ for all testing.

RESULTS

This study, examining the efficacy of visual timing vs. auditory timing vs. linguistic word building training, found significant improvements in student's attention, reading fluency, and working memory *only* following visual motion-discrimination training when compared to linguistic word building. If language-based deficits underlie dyslexia, then training to improve auditory timing should also significantly improve these academic skills, since this training was done using clever, engaging auditory exercises for twice as long, 30 min 5 times/week, compared to the training to improve visual timing, done for 15–30 min 3 times/week.

Effect of Interventions on Attention, Reading Fluency, and Working Memory

Students trained on motion direction-discrimination improved significantly more than controls, see **Table 3** and **Figure 2**, in *Attention*: **Figure 2A** (pooled data) [$t_{(44)} = 2.69$, $p = 0.009$], and **Figure 2B** TS [$t_{(21)} = 3.18$, $p = 0.004$], *Reading Speed*: **Figure 2C** (pooled data) [$t_{(44)} = 3.01$, $p = 0.004$], and **Figure 2D** TS [$t_{(21)} = 2.98$, $p = 0.007$], *Reading Comprehension*: **Figure 2E** (pooled data) [$t_{(44)} = 2.04$, $p = 0.046$], sequential *Visual Working Memory*: **Figure 2F** TS [$t_{(21)} = 2.34$, $p = 0.036$], nonsequential *Auditory Working Memory*: **Figure 2G** (pooled data) [$t_{(44)} = 2.14$, $p = 0.037$], and **Figure 2H** TS [$t_{(21)} = 2.34$, $p = 0.027$], *Delayed Recall*: **Figure 2I** TS [$t_{(21)} = 2.39$, $p = 0.026$], and *Phonological Processing* (CTOPP Blending Words): **Figure 2J** (pooled data) [$t_{(44)} = 3.52$, $p = 0.0009$], whereas students trained on improving auditory timing, implemented using *FFW*, did not improve significantly more than controls on these tasks. The significant improvements in attention by students trained on visual direction-discrimination which required less attention to complete than either the auditory or linguistic intervention, shows that visual training is more effective than auditory or linguistic training in improving the attention networks. Visual training that does not activate dorsal stream functioning at both low and high levels, e.g., motion coherence, however, is not effective in improving reading fluency (Solan et al., 2004).

Direction-discrimination training improved reading speed in the classroom from 50 to 125 words/minute on average more than found using linguistic interventions. Note that even though both the auditory and visual timing groups had only six subjects in each group in TS, the visual timing intervention improved attention, reading speed, visual and auditory working memory, and delayed recall more than found when trained on the auditory timing intervention, and significantly more than found when trained using linguistic word building, implemented using *Learning Upgrade*. This same pattern of results was found the following year, yet they were not as large in magnitude, and only reading speed, phonological processing (Blending Words subtest of the CTOPP and Auditory Working-Memory) improved significantly, since the PATH intervention had to be administered before school, instead of before guided reading. *PATH to Reading* is most effective when immediately followed by guided reading. Moreover, even though motion direction-discrimination is a visual task, it significantly improved phonological processing more than interventions using an auditory task (either auditory timing or linguistic word building). Only students trained on motion direction-discrimination improved significantly more than controls in the combined (sequential and nonsequential) auditory working memory standardized score [$t_{(44)} = 2.23$, $p = 0.03$]. Future studies with larger sample sizes are needed to determine the advantage of improving visual timing over auditory timing conclusively.

Effect of Interventions on Visual Motion Processing

Students in this study had abnormal visual motion processing, as shown by the mean baseline Contrast Sensitivity Function (CSF) for direction discrimination in **Figure 3A**. Initially participants in this study had elevated contrast thresholds for movement discrimination, averaging 2.9% $\pm$ 0.2, significantly higher [one sample $t_{(44)} = 5.81$, $p < 0.0001$] than the previously reported mean contrast threshold for typically-developing second graders of 1.35% $\pm$ 0.1 (Lawton, 2007). Direction-discrimination contrast sensitivity improved significantly only for those students who were trained on the motion direction-discrimination intervention (**Figure 3A**), improving in sensitivity three-fold

TABLE 3 | Mean increase in timing interventions (treatment effect) vs. word building intervention (controls) and the df (degrees of freedom), *t* value, and *p* value for the significant improvements only found following PATH training.

Treatment effect vs. controls	PATH	FFW	df	*t* value	*p* value
Attention—pooled data	5.7 ± 1	0.2 ± 1.6	44	2.69	0.0009
Attention—traditional schools (TS)	13.8 ± 2.2	4.9 ± 2.4	21	3.18	0.004
Reading speed (wpm)—pooled	54 ± 9	36 ± 16	44	3.01	0.004
Reading speed (wpm)—TS	125 ± 21	59 ± 23	21	2.98	0.007
Reading comprehension—pooled	1.5 ± 0.4	2.3 ± 0.8	44	2.04	0.046
Sequential visual memory—TS	13.9 ± 2.9	5.3 ± 10	21	2.34	0.036
NonSequential auditory memory—pooled	8.3 ± 1.9	6 ± 3.4	44	2.14	0.037
NonSequential auditory memory—TS	13.9 ± 3	5.3 ± 3.3	21	2.34	0.027
Delayed recall—TS	20.3 ± 4.7	10.9 ± 5.1	21	2.39	0.026
Phonological awareness—pooled	1.5 ± 0.2	1.0 ± 0.4	44	3.52	0.0009

after motion direction-discrimination training in both TS [one-sample paired $t_{(5)} = 3.694$, $p = 0.014$] and in pooled data from traditional and year-round schools, [one-sample paired $t_{(24)} = 5.618$, $p < 0.0001$]. The motion discrimination CSF increased significantly as a function of complexity level for each of the test frequency targets, shown in **Figure 3B** and **Table 4**. The

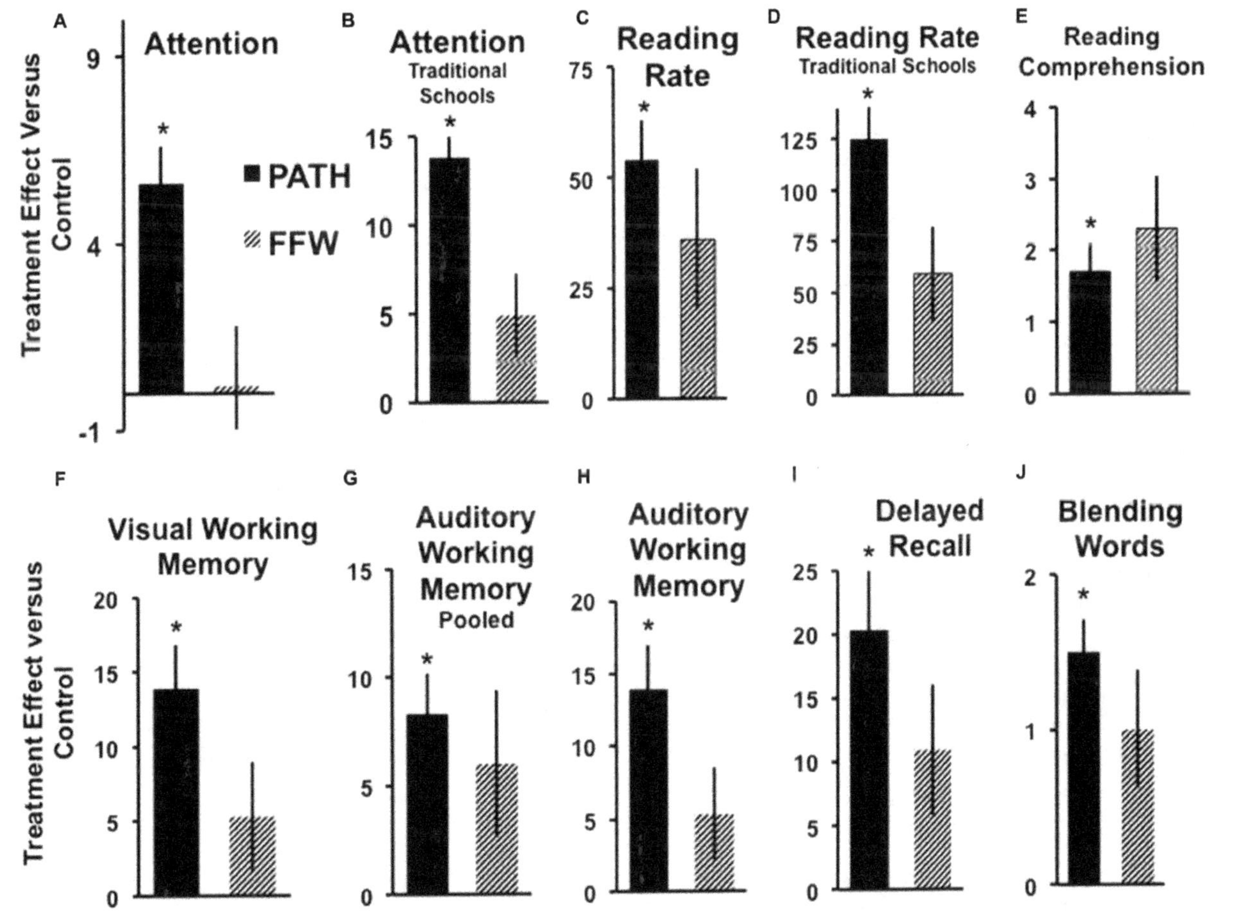

FIGURE 2 | Improvements over controls in *Attention*: (A, pooled data), *p < 0.009, (B) Traditional Schools (TS), *p < 0.004; *Reading Speed*: (C, pooled data), *p < 0.004, (D) TS, *p < 0.007; *Reading Comprehension* Gray Oral Reading Test (GORT-3): (E, pooled data), *p < 0.046; *Visual Working Memory*: (F) TS, *p < 0.036; *Auditory Working Memory*: (G, pooled data), *p < 0.037, (H) TS, *p < 0.027; *Delayed Recall*: (I) TS, *p < 0.026; and *Phonological Processing* (Blending Words): (J, pooled data), *p < 0.0009, following each intervention: [PATH to Reading (PATH): black, *FastForWord* (*FFW*): striped]. These barplots display the mean and (SE) difference in improvement of standardized scores in each treatment group compared to improvements observed in the control group. Positive bars indicate subjects in the treatment group improved more than subjects in the control group, negative bars mean control subjects improved more than those in the treatment group.

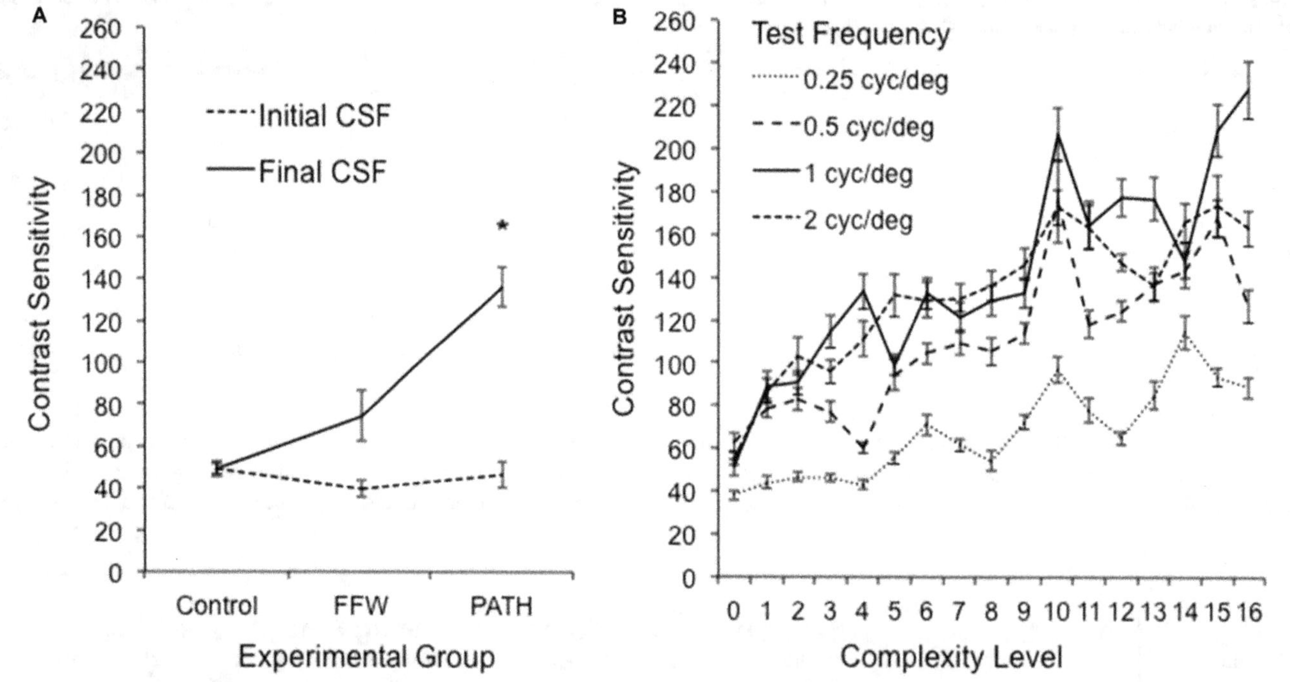

FIGURE 3 | (A) Mean and (SE) improvements in *direction-discrimination* contrast sensitivity for 1 cyc/deg test patterns at first complexity level, plotting initial contrast sensitivity function (CSF) measured at the beginning and end of intervention training, averaged over the five different background patterns, for students in the *PATH* group, *significant at $p < 0.0001$. **(B)** Pooled data from traditional and year-round schools (26 subjects). Improvements in *direction-discrimination* contrast sensitivity at increasing levels of complexity, plotting initial (0) and maximum contrast sensitivity at each level of complexity (1–16) for each of the four test frequencies: 0.25, 0.5, 1 and 2 cyc/deg. The data in this graph represent the mean and (SE) contrast sensitivity averaged across subjects trained on *PATH* in TS (6) and year-round schools (20) for subjects who completed all 16 levels of complexity in the *PATH* program.

temporal frequencies that the students could not discriminate the direction of movement before training, and had the highest contrast sensitivities following training were the 10 and 13 Hz motion (complexity levels 9–16).

When the 5% contrast background changed from being single frequency to being composed of multiple spatial frequencies (i.e., at complexity levels 2, 6, 10, and 14, described in **Table 2**), contrast sensitivity levels were higher, on average, 18.5 points relative to the general linear trend [$t_{(21)} = 2.62$, $p = 0.016$]. Conversely, when the multifrequency background pattern was presented at 20% contrast for the lowest spatial frequency target of 0.25 cyc/deg (complexity levels 4, 8, 12, and 16 in **Table 2**), contrast sensitivity was lower, being marginally significant [$t_{(21)} = -1.99$, $p = 0.06$], which is expected because at 20% contrast, the background activates parvocellular neurons more than magnocellular neurons (Kaplan and Shapley, 1986), making the task more difficult. The 0.25 cyc/deg test frequency requires pooling of contrast information over several spatial frequency channels since, as shown by Blakemore and Campbell (1969), there are no luminance-varying spatial frequency channels below 1 cyc/deg. Since the 1 cyc/deg test pattern showed the highest mean increase in contrast sensitivity, 11.2% per level of complexity, this indicates that the 1 cyc/deg test pattern, is the predominant test frequency for improving motion discrimination. Finding an increased CSF at increasing levels of complexity, thereby increasing: (1) the speed of motion, as shown in **Table 2**; and (2) the width of the background frame of reference (from single to multifrequency backgrounds) and its contrast (activating more parvocellular neurons at higher contrasts) suggests that direction-discrimination training improves the functioning of magnocellular neurons (left-right movement) relative to the functioning of parvocellular neurons (stationary background).

TABLE 4 | Mean increase in contrast sensitivity as a function of test frequency and PATH complexity level for pooled data from traditional and year-round schools.

Test frequency	Mean increase per complexity level	Standard error	$t_{(22)}$ value	*p* value
0.25 cyc/deg	4.19%	0.59%	7.11	<0.0001
0.5 cyc/deg	7.29%	0.85%	8.56	<0.0001
1 cyc/deg	11.22%	1.54%	7.26	<0.0001
2 cyc/deg	7.83%	1.35%	5.79	<0.0001

Not only was contrast sensitivity for direction-discrimination increased significantly following motion training, but also the time to discriminate the direction of motion was reduced significantly for students who did the direction-discrimination intervention. For example, for the 1 cyc/deg test frequency, the most sensitive test frequency target (see **Figure 3B**), the mean time to complete five threshold measurements decreased an average of 6 s per complexity level [mean decrease by mixed effects model analysis $t_{(22)} = 4.225$, $p = 0.004$]; mean time was 5.00 min ± 0.22 at baseline and 2.38 min ± 0.17 at complexity level 16. That is, the mean time to complete motion direction-discrimination decreased as the complexity level increased. These results show that both the: (1) sensitivity to discriminate direction-discrimination increased; and (2) time required to complete motion direction-discrimination training decreased.

DISCUSSION

The key stimulus attribute needed to detect motion discrimination deficits in dyslexics is assessed by measuring the contrast sensitivity for the direction of motion relative to a stationary background (Georgeson and Scott-Samuel, 1999). Only when the direction of motion is discriminated against a stationary background do both dysphonetic and dyseidetic dyslexics exhibit an impaired ability to discriminate the direction of motion (Lawton, 2000, 2007, 2011; Ridder et al., 2001). When the direction of movement is not judged relative to a stationary background, then some dyslexics do not exhibit motion deficits, as reviewed previously (Stein, 2001; Gori et al., 2014). Studies that have questioned whether magnocellular deficits in the dorsal stream cause the reading problems found in dyslexics (Amitay et al., 2002; Williams et al., 2003) examined a dyslexic's sensitivity to flicker or high contrast random dot patterns, relative to *no* background pattern or a moving background (Sperling et al., 2006), none of these stimuli being optimal for activating direction-selective cells (Baker, 1990; De Valois et al., 2000). Patterned backgrounds, as opposed to featureless backgrounds, require figure/ground discrimination, suggesting that a core deficit in dyslexia may be figure/ground discrimination analyzed by the dorsal stream, consistent with: (1) the dyslexic's deficits being primarily due to deficits in the spatiotemporal parsing of the letter stream (Vidyasagar, 1999, 2001) that are normally transmitted both by feedforward magnocellular (low-contrast movement) input and feedback at the attended location from LIP to MT (Saalman et al., 2007) and from MT to V1 (Hupe et al., 1998); (2) an impairment in the low gamma frequency oscillations reducing feedback in visual cortical areas (Vidyasagar, 2013); and (3) in excluding noisy backgrounds (Sperling et al., 2006). Training with the stationary background frame of reference provided by multifrequency backgrounds (**Figure 1C**) improved the dyslexic's ability to discriminate the direction of movement (Lawton, 2011), enabling the child to attend to a wider region of space. This study supports the hypothesis (Lawton, 1989) that stationary multifrequency backgrounds confer an advantage when discriminating the direction of motion, providing a wider, more structured frame of reference, most likely by taking advantage of MT's center-surround organization (Allman et al., 1985) to facilitate figure/ground discrimination. Moreover, only with stationary textured backgrounds has motion direction-discrimination training been found to improve reading fluency in all types of dyslexics (Lawton, 2000, 2007, 2011).

This study found that direction-discrimination training, a task that optimally activates the V1-MT network (De Valois et al., 2000), improved: (1) movement direction sensitivity; (2) speed of processing for both motion direction discrimination and reading rates; (3) attention; (4) reading comprehension; (5) phonological processing; and (6) both auditory and visual working-memory, including delayed recall, more than found following phonological training, either by improving auditory timing or word building strategies. These results indicate that direction-discrimination training improves the sensitivity and timing of sluggish magnocellular neurons (improving dorsal stream function), relative to parvocellular neurons early in the dorsal stream, as evidenced by improved motion discrimination sensitivity at higher background contrasts and temporal frequencies. After direction-discrimination training, the highest contrast sensitivities were found for patterns moving from 10–13 Hz, these temporal frequencies being key to improving attention in dyslexics. These results contradict Goswami's temporal sampling framework theory, proposing that the key timing deficits in dyslexia are for movement <10 Hz (Goswami, 2011). This study found that improving visual motion direction-discrimination sensitivity and timing improved processing in the neural networks underlying attention, reading, and working memory in dyslexics. These improvements are found by presumably improving low levels in the dorsal stream, the V1-MT network, which improved functioning at higher levels in the dorsal stream, including the PPC, the dorsal lateral prefrontal cortex (DLPFC), and the attention networks. This study provides additional evidence that *visual* motion processing is fundamental for paying attention, good reading performance, and remediating reading deficits, contrary to common practice based on the assumption that only auditory-based phonological processing can be used to remediate reading deficits (Tallal et al., 1993; Temple et al., 2003; Vellutino et al., 2004; Dehaene, 2009; Olulade et al., 2013).

Initially, the biological basis of dyslexia was assumed to be in the brain regions responsible for the visual perception of text (Hinshelwood, 1917). However presently, the dominant view is that the core deficit underlying reading disabilities is an auditory phonological processing deficit (Bradley and Bryant, 1983; Tallal et al., 1993; Temple et al., 2003; Vellutino et al., 2004; Dehaene, 2009; Olulade et al., 2013). A careful examination of the neuroimaging studies responsible for this paradigm shift reveal that visual word form areas and other visual processing areas were also implicated in many of these studies. For instance, Shaywitz et al. (1998) state "Brain activation patterns differed significantly between the groups with dyslexic readers showing relative underactivation in posterior regions (Wernicke's area, the angular gyrus, and striate cortex) and relative overactivation in an anterior region (inferior frontal gyrus)." Finding the striate (visual) processing area to be hypoactive in persons with dyslexia is widespread in the literature (Eden et al., 1996; Demb et al., 1998; Shaywitz et al., 1998; Shelley-Tremblay et al., 2011) and reliably co-occurs with abnormal patterns of cortical activity in areas more typically associated with auditory analyses. The visual contribution of dorsal stream processing to dyslexia has been dismissed by the American Academy of Pediatrics (2009) based on a version of the magnocellular deficit theory that has been shown to be biologically implausible (Scarborough, 2005).

Proposing that phonological processing deficits are the sole and key abnormal factor in dyslexia is not born out by studies showing visual motion processing deficits are found for all types of dyslexics (Lawton, 2000, 2007, 2011; Ridder et al., 2001). While phonological processing is a reliable and robust predictor of future reading, it cannot fully account for the variance in reading ability and the full range of deficits in dyslexic readers, instead only accounting for approximately 25% of future reading skills (Mann and Liberman, 1984; Wagner, 1997).

Novel Method to Remediate Attention, Reading, and Working Memory in Dyslexics

Movement figure/ground discrimination, a novel method (Lawton, 2000, 2015), is fundamental for detecting and remediating attention, reading, and memory problems for *all* types of dyslexics. This study found that training to improve motion direction-discrimination, most likely by improving the timing and sensitivity of directionally-selective magnocellular neurons relative to parvocellular neurons in the dorsal stream is linked to improved attention skills, enabling the beginning and end of the word, and processing the letters sequentially to be done effortlessly, thereby improving reading performance. Moreover, previous studies (Lawton, 2011) found that the more a student was trained on motion direction-discrimination, the more reading speed improved. Consequently, abnormal visual motion processing is implicated as a fundamental factor underlying the reduced functionality of the attention networks in dyslexics, causing slow reading speeds and poor comprehension. Furthermore, this abnormality can be remediated rapidly by visual training that improves a person's contrast sensitivity for direction-discrimination of dim vertical bars moving relative to a stationary textured background, indicating that visual timing deficits are a cause not a result of dyslexia.

The significant improvements in both phonological processing and auditory working-memory found in this study demonstrate that training to improve visual timing improves auditory skills. Consequently, training early in the visual dorsal stream improved higher levels of processing in the dorsal stream, in particular the PPC, where: (1) there is a supramodal representation of space with convergence of both auditory and visual inputs in the parietal cortex (Farah et al., 1989); and (2) selective endogenous attention activates this area which connects to frontal areas, like the DLPFC (Posner et al., 1984; Posner and Petersen, 1990; Supekar and Menon, 2012). By improving attention, students were able to hear the sequential ordering of sounds more accurately, improving phonological processing and auditory working memory. Students given training aimed at auditory magnocellular function, as embodied by the auditory timing intervention, improved in reading fluency, but the improvements were not significant when compared to the improvements made by controls, as also found in a review of *FFW* studies (Strong et al., 2011).

A major limitation of this study is the small sample size in the group to improve auditory timing. Most of the students in our study were from year-round schools, whose schedules precluded implementing the auditory timing program. Power to detect treatment effects in the auditory timing group was limited, requiring a larger study to determine unequivocally the relative effect of improving auditory timing on reading fluency and attention. Another limitation of this study is the lack of an out of classroom control condition that was comparable in terms of the extent of personal attention from the college students administering the reading interventions. Since half the classroom was pulled to be trained on the timing interventions, the students who stayed in the classroom had much more attention from their classroom teacher. Moreover, there was no evidence of such an effect in the auditory timing group, even though this group experienced the same level of personal interaction with students for 5 days a week compared to only 3 days a week for the visual timing intervention. Hence, it is unlikely that the significant effects observed in the motion direction-discrimination group were driven by effects associated with pulling children from the classroom and personal attention.

This study found that motion direction-discrimination training remediates reading deficits of *both* phonological (requiring accurate temporal sequencing) and visual (requiring accurate spatial sequencing) origin. Moreover, there is evidence that improvements in reading speed after motion direction-discrimination training are sustained over time (Lawton, 2011), whereas improvements in word reading found following auditory interventions to improve phonological processing degrade over time, two years later showing no difference in word reading compared to controls not having the auditory intervention (Wise et al., 2000).

Sluggish Magnocellular Processing Limits Reading Acquisition in Dyslexics

It has been proposed that the visual system exploits the dichotomy of a fast magnocellular channel and a slower parvocellular channel for the purpose of selective attention (Vidyasagar, 2001, 2012, 2013). The faster transmission time of the magnocellular neurons projecting predominantly to the dorsal stream are ideal to provide the input for feedback to intermediate stages in the cortical dorsal and ventral streams, as well as to V1 (Vidyasagar, 1999, 2001, 2013). Feedback from MT has its strongest effects for stimuli of low salience (Hupe et al., 1998), such as the low contrast patterns that maximally activate magnocellular neurons (Kaplan and Shapley, 1986; Sclar et al., 1990) that are being used to train visual movement discrimination in this study. There is parvocellular input to MT from: (1) parvocellular layers in the lateral geniculate nucleus (Nassi et al., 2006); (2) layer 6 V1 cells, having both parvocellular and magnocellular input, projecting to layer 4Cb in V1 which projects to MT (Callaway, 1998); and (3) V4 (Maunsell et al., 1990), enabling parvocellular activity to provide a background frame of reference for discriminating the direction of movement in the dorsal stream. Parvocellular functioning among dyslexics has been found to be equivalent to that in normal controls, whereas magnocellular function is significantly impaired (Lovegrove et al., 1980; Hansen et al., 2001; Kevan and

Pammer, 2009; Gori et al., 2014), being the primary cause for slow reading and attention deficits.

When reading, it has been proposed that the PPC uses the spatial information of the location and overall shape and form of a word it receives through the rapid magnocellular pathway to gate the information going into the temporal stream. The information is gated via attentional feedback to the striate cortex and to other regions in the occipito-temporal cortex (Martinez et al., 1999; Vidyasagar, 1999, 2001), most likely by top-down feedback which uses synchronized neuronal oscillations at the lower end of the gamma frequency range (Vidyasagar, 2013), which can then be used by parvocellular neurons in the ventral stream as a starting point for deciphering the individual letters (Vidyasagar, 2001; see **Figure 4**). Each cycle of gamma oscillation focuses an attentional spotlight on the primary visual cortical representation of just one or two letters before sequential recognition of these letters and their concatenation into word strings. The timing, period, envelope, amplitude, and phase of the synchronized oscillations modulating the incoming signals in the striate cortex have a profound influence on the accuracy and speed of reading (Vidyasagar, 2013). The speed determined by the gamma frequency oscillation is the essential rate-limiting step in dyslexia (Vidyasagar, 2013). Figure/ground movement discrimination training is likely to strengthen coupled: (1) theta/gamma activity for the test patterns moving at 6.7 and 8 Hz; or (2) alpha/gamma activity for the test patterns moving at 10 and 13.3 Hz. Therefore, it is likely that the visual direction-discrimination training paradigm used in this study improves not only magnocellular function and attention, but also magno-parvo integration, figure/ground discrimination, and low gamma frequency oscillation.

Our working hypothesis is that sluggish magnocellular neurons early in the dorsal cortical visual pathway (V1), found in dyslexics (Livingstone et al., 1991), disrupt processing at higher levels of dorsal stream processing, dyslexics having little or no activity in MT (Eden et al., 1996; Demb et al., 1998), including the development of these processes. After 6 weeks of motion direction-discrimination training 3 times/week in dyslexic fourth graders, dorsal stream activity improved as shown by their Visual Evoked Potentials (Shelley-Tremblay et al., 2011), consistent with a recent pilot study using magnetoencephalography (MEG) source imaging (Lawton and Huang, 2015) that found improved function in both the dorsal stream (V1, V3, MT, MST areas) and fronto-parietal attention networks. Magnocellular output from

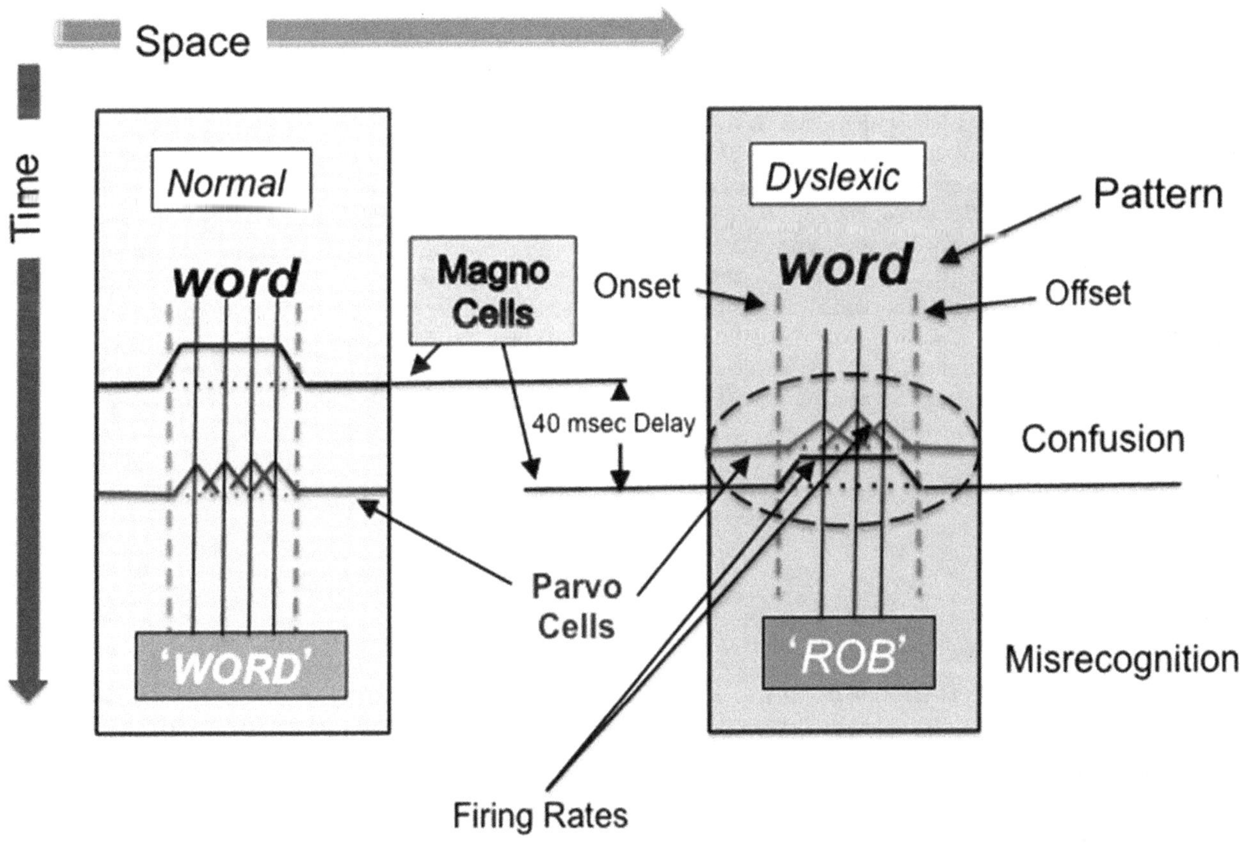

FIGURE 4 | Word distortions resulting from sluggish magnocellular neurons. What happens when the pattern and motion pathways are not working together: dyslexics always go to the middle of word, often not seeing the first letter and flipping the order of the letters. The dorsal stream sets up frame of reference (where is word located) and ventral stream analyses details sequentially. The dyslexic appears to tunnel down to get meaning (individual letters), not knowing where to go next with their eyes since magnocellular neurons are sluggish, being delayed 20–40 ms, causing confusion and misrecognition.

the anterior portion of the dorsal stream, including the PPC, is input to the mid/posterior insula, a hub of the Central Executive Network (CEN), which includes the PPC and the DLPFC (Supekar and Menon, 2012). Magnocellular activity signals the beginning and end of a word, thereby gating the processing of parvocellular activity, as proposed by Vidyasagar (2001, 2013), and illustrated in **Figure 4**. The sluggish magnocellular neurons in dyslexics not only result in attention deficits, an impairment in the low gamma frequencies reducing feedback in visual cortical areas (Vidyasagar, 2013), but also disrupted processing in LIP and FEF, either within a fixation, between fixation sequences, or both (Vidyasagar, 2001; Slaghuis and Ryan, 2006; Fischer, 2012). This study found, for the first time, that direction-discrimination training improved not only reading fluency, but also attention and working memory. Therefore, direction-discrimination training improved CEN functioning, also found using MEG source imaging (Lawton and Huang, 2015), providing more evidence that abnormal visual motion processing is a fundamental cause of attention and subsequent reading problems in dyslexics.

By improving the attention network's functioning, motion direction-discrimination training provides a wider usable field of view so that more objects are perceived in their correct location in a single glance. Motion direction-discrimination training is the key for reading acquisition to happen at an efficient speed for dyslexics, most likely by increasing the ease of magno-parvo integration. When motion direction-discrimination training was followed by guided reading in the classroom, attention, reading fluency, and working memory skills improved significantly more than found after training on linguistic word building or auditory timing interventions. Remediating visual timing deficits in the dorsal stream reveals the causal role of visual motion discrimination and attention in reading acquisition. This study supports the hypothesis that faulty timing in synchronizing the activity of magnocellular (left-right movement discrimination) with parvocellular (stationary background) visual pathways are a fundamental cause of dyslexia and argues against the assumption that reading deficiencies in dyslexia are caused by phonological or language deficits. This study demonstrates that visual movement figure/ground discrimination can be used to not only detect dyslexia early, but also for its successful treatment, so that reading problems do not prevent children from readily learning.

AUTHOR CONTRIBUTIONS

TL designed study, recruited and trained staff, ran daily operations, and wrote article.

ACKNOWLEDGMENTS

I thank Drs. Jack Shelley-Tremblay, Sue Cotter, Norma Graham, Mike Posner, Eric Borsting, Steve Hillyard, Dan Felleman, Jaime Pineda, and Bryan Hansen for many thoughtful and insightful suggestions to help improve this article substantially. I thank Wendy Portnuff, the chief trainer at Scientific Learning, for training and supervising the RAs to administer *FastForWord*, and her vast knowledge of motivational strategies used to improve compliance of all students in this study. I thank Steve Edland, the UCSD biostatistician who designed and analyzed all the statistical analyses for this study using the R statistical package, and helped write earlier versions of this article. I thank Kelly Lawton for helping to automate the computer calibration, training staff using easy to follow written instructions, helping film the video training movies, and help in developing the motivational strategies. I thank Jordan Conway, the Senior Research Assistant, who helped run daily operations, being in charge of the lead assistants at each school, as well as helping to recruit and train the 40 UCSD undergraduates who were in charge of performing these experiments, help in developing the motivational strategies, helping film the video training movies, backing up and calibrating all of the computers, and providing the motivational strategies at each school. I thank the 40 UCSD cognitive science and psychology undergraduates who collected the data. I thank Dr. Doug Stephey for his support, encouragement, and advice, especially recommending we use the CAS Stroop and Number Detection subtests to measure attention, and the TIPS to measure working memory. This work was supported by the Institute of Educational Sciences (IES), US Department of Education (IES Award R305A100389) to UCSD.

REFERENCES

Allman, J., Miezin, F., and McGuiness, E. (1985). Stimulus specific responses from beyond the classical receptive field: neurophysiological mechanisms for local-global comparisons in visual neurons. *Annu. Rev. Neurosci.* 8, 407–430. doi: 10.1146/annurev.ne.08.030185.002203

American Academy of Pediatrics. (2009). Learning disabilities, dyslexia and vision. *Pediatrics* 124, 837–844. Available online at: http://pediatrics.aappublications.org/cgi/reprint/124/2/837

Amitay, S., Ben-Yehudah, G., Banai, K., and Ahissar, M. (2002). Disabled readers suffer from visual and auditory impairments but not from a specific magnocellular deficit. *Brain* 125, 2272–2285. doi: 10.1093/brain/awf231

Atkinson, J. (1991). "Review of human visual development: crowding and dyslexia," in *Vision and Visual Dyslexia*, ed. J. F. Stein (Boston: CRC Press), 44–57.

Baker, C. L. (1990). Spatial and temporal frequency selectivity as a basis for velocity preference in cat striate cortex neurons. *Vis. Neurosci.* 4, 101–113. doi: 10.1017/s0952523800002273

Blakemore, C., and Campbell, F. W. (1969). On the existence of neurones in the human visual system selectively sensitive to the orientation and size of retinal images. *J. Physiol.* 203, 237–260. doi: 10.1113/jphysiol.1969.sp008862

Boden, C., and Giaschi, D. (2007). M-stream deficits and reading-related visual processes in developmental dyslexia. *Psychol. Bull.* 133:346. doi: 10.1037/0033-2909.133.2.346

Boets, B., Vandermosten, M., Cornelissen, P., Wouters, J., and Ghesquiere, P. (2011). Coherent motion sensitivity and reading development in the transition from prereading to reading stage. *Child Dev.* 82, 854–869. doi: 10.1111/j.1467-8624.2010.01527.x

Braddick, O., O'Brien, J. M. D., Wattam-Bell, J., Atkinson, J., Hartley, T., and Turner, R. (2001). Brain areas sensitive to coherent visual motion. *Perception* 30, 61–72. doi: 10.1068/p3048

Bradley, L., and Bryant, P. E. (1983). Categorizing sounds and learning to read: a causal connection. *Nature* 301, 419–421. doi: 10.1038/301419a0

Buchholz, J., and McKone, E. (2004). Adults with dyslexia show deficits on spatial frequency doubling and visual attention tasks. *Dyslexia* 10, 24–43. doi: 10.1002/dys.263

Callaway, E. M. (1998). Local circuits in primary visual cortex of the macaque monkey. *Annu. Rev. Neurosci.* 21, 47–74. doi: 10.1146/annurev.neuro.21.1.47

Chambers, J. M., Freeny, A., and Heiberger, R. M. (1992). "Chapter 5: analysis of variance; designed experiments," in *Statistical Models*, eds J. M. Chambers and T. J. Hastie (Pacific Grove, CA: S. Wadsworth and Brooks/Cole), 853–861.

Cornelissen, P., Richardson, A., Mason, A., Fowler, S., and Stein, J. (1995). Contrast sensitivity and coherent motion detection measured at photopic luminance levels in dyslexics and controls. *Vision Res.* 35, 1483–1494. doi: 10.1016/0042-6989(95)98728-r

Dehaene, S. (Ed.). (2009). "The dyslexic brain," in *Reading in the Brain*, (New York, NY: Penguin Viking), 235–261.

Demb, J. B., Boynton, G. M., and Heeger, D. J. (1998). Functional magnetic resonance imaging of early visual pathways in dyslexia. *J. Neurosci.* 18, 6939–6951.

De Valois, R. L., Cottaris, N. P., Mahon, L. E., Elfar, S. D., and Wilson, J. A. (2000). Spatial and temporal receptive fields of geniculate and cortical cells and directional selectivity. *Vision Res.* 40, 3685–3702. doi: 10.1016/s0042-6989(00)00210-8

Dreher, B., Fukada, Y., and Rodieck, R. W. (1976). Identification, classification and anatomical segregation of cells with X-like and Y-like properties in the lateral geniculate nucleus of old-world primates. *J. Physiol.* 258, 433–452. doi: 10.1113/jphysiol.1976.sp011429

Eden, G. F., VanMeter, J. W., Rumsey, J. M., Maisog, J. M., Woods, R. P., and Zeffiro, T. A. (1996). Abnormal processing of visual motion in dyslexia revealed by functional brain imaging. *Nature* 382, 66–69. doi: 10.1038/382066a0

Facoetti, A., Paganoni, P., Turatto, M., Marzla, V., and Mascetti, G. G. (2000). Visual-spatial attention in developmental dyslexia. *Cortex* 36, 109–123. doi: 10.1016/s0010-9452(08)70840-2

Facoetti, A., Trussardi, A. N., Ruffino, M., Lorusso, M. L., Cattaneo, C., Galli, R., et al. (2010). Multisensory spatial attention deficits are predictive of phonological decoding skills in developmental dyslexia. *J. Cogn. Neurosci.* 22, 1011–1025. doi: 10.1162/jocn.2009.21232

Farah, M. J., Wong, A. B., Monheit, M. A., and Morrow, L. A. (1989). Parietal lobe mechanisms of spatial attention: modality-specific or supramodal? *Neuropsychologia* 27, 461–470. doi: 10.1016/0028-3932(89)90051-1

Felleman, D. J., and Van Essen, D. C. (1991). Distributed hierarchical processing in the primate cerebral cortex. *Cereb. Cortex* 1, 1–47. doi: 10.1093/cercor/1.1.1

Fischer, B. (2012). "Subitizing, dynamic vision, saccade and fixation control in dyslexia, chapter 2," in *Visual Aspects of Dyslexia*, eds J. Stein and Z. Kapoula (New York, NY: Oxford University Press), 15–43.

Georgeson, M. A., and Scott-Samuel, N. E. (1999). Motion contrast: a new metric for direction discrimination. *Vision Res.* 39, 4393–4402. doi: 10.1016/s0042-6989(99)00147-9

Gori, S., Cecchini, P., Bigoni, A., Molteni, M., and Facoetti, A. (2014). Magnocellular-dorsal pathway and sublexical route in developmental dyslexia. *Front. Hum. Neurosci.* 8:460. doi: 10.3389/fnhum.2014.00460

Goswami, U. (2011). A temporal sampling framework for developmental dyslexia. *Trends Cogn. Sci.* 15, 3–10. doi: 10.1016/j.tics.2010.10.001

Guerin, D. W., Griffin, J. R., Gottfried, A. W., and Christenson, G. N. (1993). Concurrent validity and screening efficiency of the dyslexia screener. *Psychol. Assess.* 5, 369–373. doi: 10.1037/1040-3590.5.3.369

Handford, P., and Borsting, E. (2015). Validity of the decoding encoding screener for dyslexia. *Optom. Vis. Sci.* 92, 487–493. doi: 10.1097/opx.0000000000000560

Hansen, P. C., Stein, J. F., Orde, S. R., Winter, J. L., and Talcott, J. B. (2001). Are dyslexics' visual deficits limited to measures of dorsal stream function? *Neuroreport* 12, 1527–1530. doi: 10.1097/00001756-200105250-00045

Higgins, K. E., Jaffe, M. J., Coletta, N. J., Caruso, R. C., and de Monasterio, F. M. (1984). Spatial contrast sensitivity. *Arch. Ophthalmol.* 102, 2067–2074.

Hinshelwood, J. (1917). *Congenital Word-Blindness.* London: H. K. Lewis and Co.

Hupe, J. M., Payne, A. C., Lomer, B. R., Girad, S. G., and Bullier, J. (1998). Cortical feedback improves discrimination between figure and background by V1, V2 and V3 neurons. *Nature* 394, 784–787.

Kaplan, E., and Shapley, R. M. (1986). The primate retina contains two types of ganglion cells, with high- and low-contrast sensitivity. *Proc. Natl. Acad. Sci. U S A* 83, 2755–2757. doi: 10.1073/pnas.83.8.2755

Kevan, A., and Pammer, K. (2009). Predicting early reading skills from pre-reading measures of dorsal stream functioning. *Neuropsychologia* 47, 3174–3181. doi: 10.1016/j.neuropsychologia.2009.07.016

Lawton, T. B. (1989). Outputs of paired Gabor filters summed across background frame of reference predicts direction of movement. *IEEE Trans. Biomed. Eng.* 36, 130–139. doi: 10.1109/10.16458

Lawton, T. B. (2000). *Methods and Apparatus for Diagnosing and Remediating Reading Disorders.* U.S. Patent No. 6,045,515. Washington, DC: U. S. Patent and Trademark Office.

Lawton, T. (2007). Training direction-discrimination sensitivity remediates a wide spectrum of reading skills. *Optom. Vis. Dev.* 38, 37–51.

Lawton, T. (2008). Filtered text and direction discrimination training improved reading fluency for both dyslexic and normal readers. *Optom. Vis. Dev.* 39, 114–126.

Lawton, T. (2011). Improving magnocellular function in the dorsal stream remediates reading deficits. *Optom. Vis. Dev.* 42, 142–154.

Lawton, T. (2015). *Diagnosing and Remediating Cognitive Deficits Involving Attention, Sequential Processing, Reading, Speed of Processing, and Navigation.* U. S. Patent No. 8,979,263 B2. Washington, DC: U. S. Patent and Trademark Office.

Lawton, T., and Huang, M. X. (2015). "Improving visual timing enhances cognitive functioning by altering dorsal stream and attention networks," in *12th Annual World Congress of the Society for Brain Mapping and Therapeutics* (Los Angeles, CA).

Livingstone, M. S., and Hubel, D. H. (1988). Segregation of color, form, movement and depth: anatomy, physiology and perception. *Science* 240, 740–749. doi: 10.1126/science.3283936

Livingstone, M. S., Rosen, G. D., Drislane, F. W., and Galaburda, A. M. (1991). Physiological and anatomical evidence for a magnocellular defect in developmental dyslexia. *Proc. Natl. Acad. Sci. U S A* 88, 7943–7947.

Lovegrove, W. J., Bowling, A., Badcock, D., and Blackwood, M. (1980). Specific reading disability: differences in contrast sensitivity as a function of spatial frequency. *Science* 210, 439–440. doi: 10.1126/science.7433985

Lyon, G. R., Shaywitz, S. E., and Shaywitz, B. A. (2003). Comorbdity, teachers' knowledge of language and reading: a definition of dyslexia. *Ann. Dyslex.* 53, 1–14.

Mann, V. A., and Liberman, I. Y. (1984). Phonological awareness and short-termmemory. *J. Learn. Disabil.* 17, 592–599.

Martinez, A., Anllo-Vento, L., Serono, M. I., Frank, L. R., Buxton, R. B., Dubowitz, D. J., et al. (1999). Involvement of striate and extrastriate cortical areas in spatial attention. *Nat. Neurosci.* 2, 364–369.

Maunsell, J. H., Nealey, T. A., and De Priest, D. D. (1990). Magnocellular and parvocellular contributions to responses in the middle temporal visual area (MT) of the macaque monkey. *J. Neurosci.* 10, 3323–3334.

Merigan, W. H., and Maunsell, J. H. R. (1993). How parallel are the primate visual pathways? *Annu. Rev. Neurosci.* 16, 369–402. doi: 10.1146/annurev.neuro.16.1.369

Nassi, J. J., Lyon, D. C., and Callaway, E. M. (2006). The parvocellular LGN provides a robust disynaptic input to the visual motion area MT. *Neuron* 50, 319–327. doi: 10.1016/j.neuron.2006.03.019

National Center for Educational Statistics. (2013). Available online at: http://nces. ed.gov/nationsreportcard/subject/publications/main2013/pdf/2014451.pdf, page 7.

Nicholson, R. I., and Fawcett, A. J. (2007). Procedural learning difficulties: reuniting the developmental disorders? *Trends Neurosci.* 30, 135–141. doi: 10.1016/j.tins.2007.02.003

Olulade, O. A., Napoliello, E. M., and Eden, G. F. (2013). Abnormal visual motion processing is not a cause of dyslexia. *Neuron* 79, 180–190. doi: 10.1016/j.neuron.2013.05.002

Ostarello, A., and De Ley, L. (2009). *The Effect of Product use Lapses on Student Learning.* Oakland, CA: Scientific Learning Corporation.

Pammer, K., and Wheatley, C. (2001). Isolating the M(y)-cell response in dyslexia using the spatial frequency doubling illusion. *Vision Res.* 41, 2139–2147. doi: 10.1016/s0042-6989(01)00092-x

Pinheiro, J., and Bates, D. (2000). *Mixed-Effects Models in S and S-PLUS.* (US: Springer).

Posner, M. I., and Petersen, S. E. (1990). The attention system of the human brain. *Annu. Rev. Neurosci.* 13, 25–42.

Posner, M. I., Walker, J. A., Friedrich, F. J., and Rafal, R. D. (1984). Effects of parietal injury on covert orienting of attention. *J. Neurosci.* 4, 1863–1874.

Ridder, W. H., Borsting, E., and Banton, T. (2001). All developmental dyslexic subtypes display an elevated motion coherence threshold. *Optom. Vis. Sci.* 78, 510–517. doi: 10.1097/00006324-200107000-00014

Saalman, Y. B., Pigarev, I. N., and Vidyasagar, T. R. (2007). Neural mechanism of visual attention: how top-down feedback highlights relevant locations. *Science* 316, 1612–1615. doi: 10.1126/science.1139140

Scarborough, H. S. (2005). "Developmental relationships between language and reading: reconciling a beautiful hypotheses with some ugly facts," in *The Connections between Language and Reading Disabilities*, eds H. W. Catts and A. G. Kamhi (Mahwah, NJ: Erlbaum), 3–24.

Schatschneider, C., Fletcher, J. M., Francis, D. J., Carlson, C. D., and Foorman, B. R. (2004). Kindergarten prediction of reading skills: a longitudinal comparative analysis. *J. Edu. Psychol.* 96, 265–282. doi: 10.1037/0022-0663.96.2.265

Sclar, G., Maunsell, J. H. R., and Lennie, P. (1990). Coding of image contrast in central visual pathways of the macaque monkey. *Vision Res.* 30, 1–10. doi: 10.1016/0042-6989(90)90123-3

Shaywitz, S. E., Shaywitz, B. A., Pugh, K. R., Fullbright, R. K., Constable, R. T., Mencl, W. E., et al. (1998). Functional disruption in the organization of the brain for reading in dyslexia. *Proc. Natl. Acad. Sci. U S A* 95, 2636–2641. doi: 10.1016/s0006-3223(98)90658-8

Shelley-Tremblay, J. F., Syklawer, S., and Ramkissoon, I. (2011). The effect of magno-parvocellular integration training on fluency and visual evoked potentials in poor readers. *J. Behav. Optom.* 22, 31–37.

Slaghuis, W. L., and Ryan, J. F. (2006). Directional motion contrast sensitivity in developmental dyslexia. *Vision Res.* 46, 3291–3303. doi: 10.1016/j.visres.2006.05.009

Solan, H. A., Larson, S., Shelley-Tremblay, J., Ficarra, A., and Silverman, M. (2001). Role of visual attention on cognitive control of oculomotor readiness in students with reading disabilities. *J. Learn. Disabil.* 34, 107–118. doi: 10.1177/002221940103400202

Solan, H. A., Shelley-Tremblay, J., Hansen, P. C., Silverman, M., Larson, S., and Ficarra, A. (2004). M-cell deficit and reading disability: a preliminary study of the effects of temporal vision-processing therapy. *Optometry* 75, 640–650. doi: 10.1016/s1529-1839(04)70211-0

Sperling, A. J., Lu, Z., Manis, F. R., and Seindemberg, M. S. (2006). Motion-perception deficits and reading impairment: it's the noise, not the motion. *Psychol. Sci.* 17, 1047–1053. doi: 10.1111/j.1467-9280.2006.01825.x

Stanley, G., and Hall, R. (1973). Short-term visual information processing in dyslexics. *Child Dev.* 44, 841–844. doi: 10.2307/1127735

Stein, J. (2001). The magnocellular theory of developmental dyslexia. *Dyslexia* 7, 12–36. doi: 10.1002/dys.186

Stein, J., and Walsh, V. (1997). To see but not to read; the magnocellular theory of dyslexia. *Trends Neurosci.* 20, 147–152.

Strong, G. K., Torgerson, C. J., Torgerson, D., and Hulme, C. (2011). A systematic meta-analytic review of evidence for the effectiveness of the 'FastForWord' language intervention program. *J. Child Psychol. Psychiatry* 52, 224–235. doi: 10.1111/j.1469-7610.2010.02329.x

Stuart, G. W., McAnally, K. I., and Castles, A. (2001). Can contrast sensitivity functions in dyslexia be explained by inattention rather than a magnocellular deficit? *Vision Res.* 41, 3205–3211. doi: 10.1016/s0042-6989(01)00176-6

Supekar, K., and Menon, V. (2012). Developmental maturation of dynamic causal control signals in higher-order cognition: a neurocognitive network model. *PLoS Comput. Biol.* 8:e1002374. doi: 10.1371/journal.pcbi.1002374

Talcott, J. B., Hansen, P. C., Assoku, E. L., and Stein, J. F. (2000). Visual motion sensitivity in dyslexia: evidence for temporal and energy integration deficits. *Neuropsychologia* 38, 935–943. doi: 10.1016/s0028-3932(00)00020-8

Talcott, J. B., Witton, C., and Stein, J. F. (2013). Probing the neurocognitive trajectories of children's reading skills. *Neuropsychologia* 51, 472–481. doi: 10.1016/j.neuropsychologia.2012.11.016

Tallal, P., Miller, S., and Fitch, R. H. (1993). Neurobiological basis of speech: a case for the preeminence of temporal processing. *Ann. N Y Acad. Sci.* 682, 27–47.

Temple, E., Deutsch, G. K., Poldrack, R. A., Miller, S. L., Tallal, P., Merzenich, M. M., et al. (2003). Neural deficits in children with dyslexia ameliorated by behavioral remediation: evidence from functional MRI. *Proc. Natl. Acad. Sci. U S A* 100, 2860–2865. doi: 10.1073/pnas.0030098100

Tyler, C. W. (1974). Observations on spatial-frequency doubling. *Perception* 3, 81–86. doi: 10.1068/p030081

Ungerleider, L. G., and Mishkin, M. (1982). "Two cortical visual systems," in *Analysis of Visual Behavior*, eds D. J. Ingle, M. A. Goodale and R. J. W. Mansfield (Cambridge, UK: MIT Press), 549–586.

Vellutino, F. R., Fletcher, J. M., Snowling, M. J., and Scanlon, D. M. (2004). Specific reading disability (dyslexia): what have we learned in the past four decades? *J. Child Psychol. Psychiatry* 45, 2–40. doi: 10.1046/j.0021-9630.2003.00305.x

Vidyasagar, T. R. (1999). A neuronal model of attentional spotlight: parietal guiding the temporal. *Brain Res. Rev.* 30, 66–76. doi: 10.1016/s0165-0173(99)00005-3

Vidyasagar, T. R. (2001). From attentional gating in macaque primary visual cortex to dyslexia in humans. *Prog. Brain Res.* 134, 297–312. doi: 10.10.1016/S0079-6123(01)34020-7

Vidyasagar, T. R. (2012). "Aetiology of dyslexia: a visual perspective on a phonological marker," in *Visual Aspects of Dyslexia*, eds J. Stein and Z. Kapoula (New York, NY: Oxford University Press), 151–170.

Vidyasagar, T. R. (2013). Reading into neuronal oscillations in the visual system: implications for developmental dyslexia. *Front. Hum. Neurosci.* 7:811. doi: 10.3389/fnhum.2013.00811

Vidyasagar, T. R., and Pammer, K. (2010). Dyslexia: a deficit in visuo-spatial attention, not in phonological processing. *Trends Cogn. Sci.* 14, 57–63. doi: 10.1016/j.tics.2009.12.003

Wagner, R. K. (1997). Changing relations between phonological processing abilities and word-level reading as children develop from beginning to skilled readers: a 5-year longitudinal study. *Dev. Psychol.* 33, 468–479. doi: 10.1037/0012-1649.33.3.468

Wilkins, A. J. (1995). *Experientia.* Oxford: Oxford University Press.

Williams, M. J., Stuart, G. W., Castles, A., and McAnnally, K. I. (2003). Contrast sensitivity in subgroups of developmental dyslexia. *Vision Res.* 43, 467–477. doi: 10.1016/s0042-6989(02)00573-4

Wise, B. W., Ring, J., and Olson, R. K. (2000). Individual differences in gains from computer-assisted remedial reading. *J. Exp. Child Psychol.* 77, 197–235. doi: 10.1006/jecp.1999.2559

Wolf, M., Bowers, P. G., and Biddle, K. (2000). Naming-speed processes, timing and reading: a conceptual review. *J. Learn. Disabil.* 33, 387–407. doi: 10.1177/002221940003300409

Zohary, E. S., Celebrini, S., Britten, K. H., and Newsome, W. T. (1994). Neuronal plasticity that underlies improvement in perceptual performance. *Science* 263, 1289–1292. doi: 10.1126/science.8122114

5

Seven Pervasive Statistical Flaws in Cognitive Training Interventions

David Moreau, Ian J. Kirk and Karen E. Waldie*

Centre for Brain Research and School of Psychology, University of Auckland, Auckland, New Zealand

Edited by:
Claudia Voelcker-Rehage, Technische Universität Chemnitz, Germany

Reviewed by:
Tilo Strobach, Medical School Hamburg, Germany
Florian Schmiedek, German Institute for International Educational Research, Germany

***Correspondence:**
David Moreau
d.moreau@auckland.ac.nz

The prospect of enhancing cognition is undoubtedly among the most exciting research questions currently bridging psychology, neuroscience, and evidence-based medicine. Yet, convincing claims in this line of work stem from designs that are prone to several shortcomings, thus threatening the credibility of training-induced cognitive enhancement. Here, we present seven pervasive statistical flaws in intervention designs: (i) lack of power; (ii) sampling error; (iii) continuous variable splits; (iv) erroneous interpretations of correlated gain scores; (v) single transfer assessments; (vi) multiple comparisons; and (vii) publication bias. Each flaw is illustrated with a Monte Carlo simulation to present its underlying mechanisms, gauge its magnitude, and discuss potential remedies. Although not restricted to training studies, these flaws are typically exacerbated in such designs, due to ubiquitous practices in data collection or data analysis. The article reviews these practices, so as to avoid common pitfalls when designing or analyzing an intervention. More generally, it is also intended as a reference for anyone interested in evaluating claims of cognitive enhancement.

Keywords: brain enhancement, evidence-based interventions, working memory training, intelligence, methods, data analysis, statistics, experimental design

INTRODUCTION

Can cognition be enhanced via training? Designing effective interventions to enhance cognition has proven one of the most promising and difficult challenges of modern cognitive science. Promising, because the potential is enormous, with applications ranging from developmental disorders to cognitive aging, dementia, and traumatic brain injury rehabilitation. Yet difficult, because establishing sound evidence for an intervention is particularly challenging in psychology: the gold standard of double-blind randomized controlled experiments is not always feasible, due to logistic shortcomings or to common difficulties in disguising the underlying hypothesis of an experiment. These limitations have important consequences for the strength of evidence in favor of an intervention. Several of them have been extensively discussed in recent years, resulting in stronger, more valid, designs.

For example, the importance of using active control groups has been underlined in many instances (e.g., Boot et al., 2013), helping conscientious researchers move away from the use of no-contact controls, standard in a not-so-distant past. Equally important is the emphasis on objective measures of cognitive abilities rather than self-report assessments, or on the necessity to use multiple measurements of single abilities to provide better estimates of cognitive constructs and minimize measurement error (Shipstead et al., 2012). Other limitations pertinent to training designs have been illustrated elsewhere with simulations (e.g., fallacious assumptions, Moreau and Conway, 2014; biased samples, Moreau, 2014b), in an attempt to illustrate visually some of the discrepancies observed in the literature. Indeed, much knowledge can be gained by incorporating simulated data to complex research problems (Rubinstein and Kroese, 2011), either because they are difficult to visualize or because the representation of their outcomes is ambiguous. Intervention studies are no exception—they often include multiple extraneous variables, and thus benefit greatly from informed estimates about the respective influence of each predictor variable in a given model. As it stands, the approach typically favored is that good experimental practices (e.g., random assignment, representative samples) control for such problems. In practice, however, numerous designs and subsequent analyses do not adequately allow such inferences, due to single or multiple flaws. We explore here some of the most prevalent of these flaws.

Our objective is three-fold. First, we aim to bring attention to core methodological and statistical issues when designing or analyzing training experiments. Using clear illustrations of how pervasive these problems are, we hope to help design better, more potent interventions. Second, we stress the importance of simulations to improve the understanding of research designs and data analysis methods, and the influence they have on results at all stages of a multifactorial project. Finally, we also intend to stimulate broader discussions by reaching wider audiences, and help individuals or organizations assess the effectiveness of an intervention to make informed decisions in light of all the evidence available, not just the most popular or the most publicized information. We strive, throughout the article, to make every idea as accessible as possible and to favor clear visualizations over mathematical jargon.

A note on the structure of the article. For each flaw we discuss, we include three steps: (1) a brief introduction to the problem and a description of its relation to intervention designs; (2) a Monte Carlo simulation and its visual illustration[1]; and (3) advice on how to circumvent the problem or minimize its impact. Importantly, the article is not intended to be an in-depth analysis of each flaw discussed; rather, our aim is to help visual representations of each problem and provide the tools necessary to assess the consequences of common statistical procedures. However, because the problems we discuss hereafter are complex and deserve further attention, we have referred the interested reader to additional literature throughout the article.

A slightly more technical question pertains to the use of Monte Carlo simulations. Broadly speaking, Monte Carlo methods refer to the use of computational algorithms to simulate repeated random sampling, in order to obtain numerical estimates of a process. The idea that we can refine knowledge by simulating stochastic processes repeatedly rather than via more traditional procedures (e.g., direct integration) might be counterintuitive, yet this method is well suited to the specific examples we are presenting here for a few reasons. Repeated stochastic simulations allow creating mathematical models of ecological processes: the repetition represents research groups, throughout the world, randomly sampling from the population and conducting experiments. Such simulations are also particularly useful in complex problems where a number of variables are unknown or difficult to assess, as they can provide an account of the values a statistic can take when constrained by initial parameters, or a range of parameters. Finally, Monte Carlo simulations can be clearly represented visually. This facilitates the graphical translation of a mathematical simulation, thus allowing a discussion of each flaw with little statistical or mathematical background.

LACK OF POWER

We begin our exploration with a pervasive problem in almost all experimental designs, particularly in training interventions: low statistical power. In a frequentist framework, two types of errors can arise at the decision stage in a statistical analysis: Type I (false positive, probability α) and Type II (false negative, probability β). The former occurs when the null hypothesis (H_0) is true but rejected, whereas the latter occurs when the alternative hypothesis (H_A) is true but the H_0 is retained. That is, in the context of an intervention, the experimental treatment was effective but statistical inference led to the erroneous conclusion that it was not. Accordingly, the power of a statistical test is the probability of rejecting H_0 given that it is false. The more power, the lower the probability of Type II errors, such that power is $(1-\beta)$. Importantly, higher statistical power translates to a better chance of detecting an effect if it is exists, but also a better chance that an effect is genuine if it is significant (Button et al., 2013). Obviously, it is preferable to minimize β, which is akin to maximizing power.

Because α is set arbitrarily by the experimenter, power could be increased by directly increasing α. This simple solution, however, has an important pitfall: since α represents the probability of Type I errors, any increase will produce more false positives (rejections of H_0 when it should be retained) in the long run. Therefore, in practice experimenters need to take into account the tradeoff between Type I and Type II errors when setting α. Typically, $\alpha < \beta$, because missing an existing effect (β) is thought to be less prejudicial than falsely rejecting H_0 (α); however, specific circumstances where the emphasis is on discovering new effects (e.g., exploratory approaches) sometimes justify α increases (for example, see Schubert and Strobach, 2012).

Discussions regarding experimental power are not new. Issues related to power have long been discussed in the behavioral sciences, yet they have drawn heightened attention recently (e.g., Button et al., 2013; Wagenmakers et al., 2015), for good reasons: when power is low, relevant effects might go

[1]Step (2) was implemented in R (R Core Team, 2014) because of its growing popularity among researchers and data scientists (Tippmann, 2015), and because R is free and open-source, thus allowing anyone, anywhere, to reproduce and build upon our analyses. We used R version 3.1.2 (R Core Team, 2014) and the following packages: ggplot2 (Wickham, 2009), gridExtra (Auguie, 2012), MASS (Venables and Ripley, 2002), MBESS (Kelley and Lai, 2012), plyr (Wickham, 2011), psych (Revelle, 2015), pwr (Champely, 2015), and stats (R Core Team, 2014).

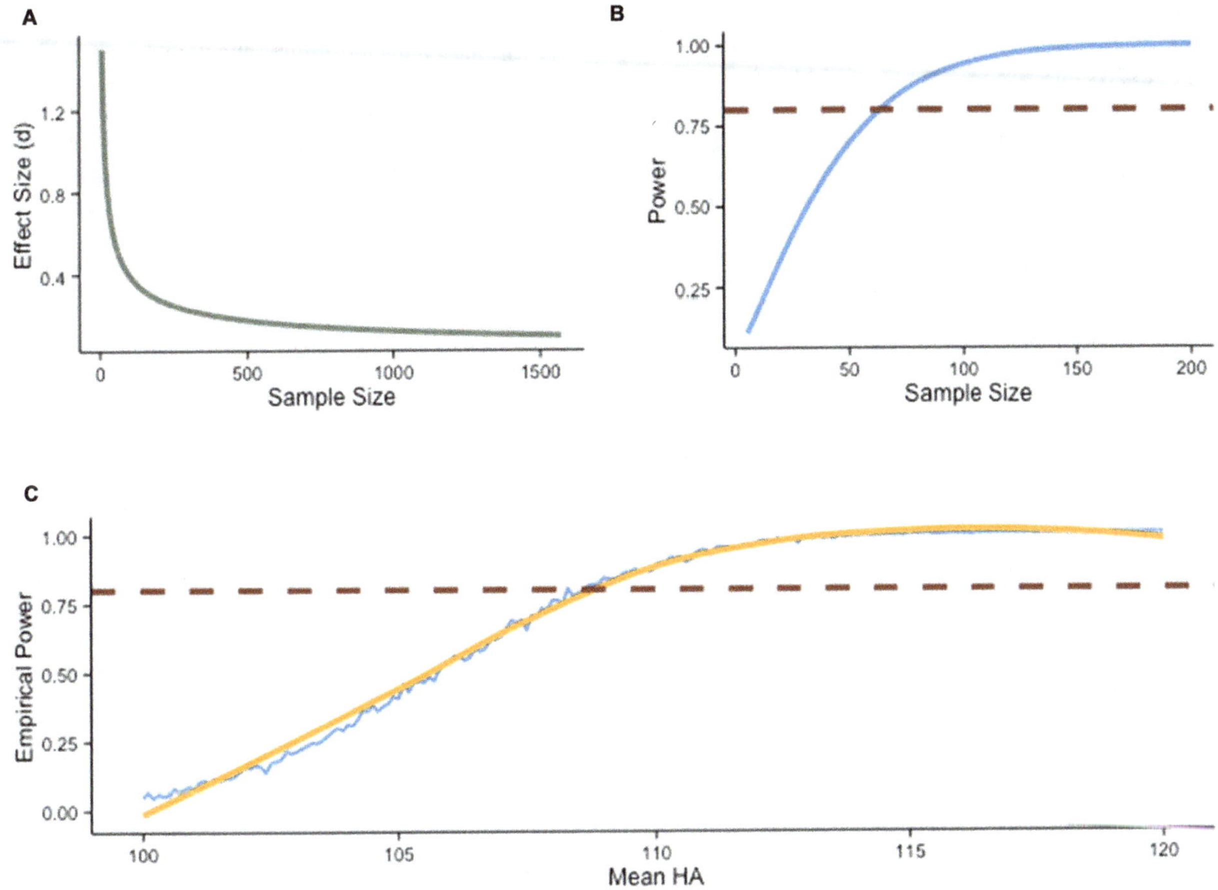

FIGURE 1 | Power analysis. (A) Relationship between effect size (Cohen's *d*) and sample size with power held constant at .80 (two-sample *t*-test, two-sided hypothesis, α = .05). **(B)** Relationship between power and sample size with effect size held constant *d* = 0.5 (two-sample *t* test, two-sided hypothesis, α = .05). **(C)** Empirical power as a function of an alternative mean score (H_A), estimated from a Monte Carlo simulation (*N* = 1000) of two-sample *t*-tests with 20 subjects per group. The distribution of scores under null hypothesis (H_0) is consistent with IQ test score standards (*M* = 100, SD = 15), and H_A varies from 100 to 120 by incremental steps of 0.1. The blue line shows the result of the simulation, with estimated smoothed curve (orange line). The red line denotes power = .80.

undetected, and significant results often turn out to be false positives[2]. Besides α and β levels, power is also influenced by sample size and effect size (**Figure 1A**). The latter depends on the question of interest and the design, with various strategies intended to maximize the effect one wishes to observe (e.g., well-controlled conditions). Noise is often exacerbated in training interventions, because such designs potentially increase sources of non-sampling errors, for example via poor retention rates, failure to randomly assigned participants, use of non-standardized tasks, use of single measures of abilities, or failure to blind participants and experimenters. Furthermore, the influence of multiple variables is typically difficult to estimate (e.g., extraneous factors), and although random assignment is usually thought to control for this limitation, it has been demonstrated repeatedly that such assumption is highly dependent on sample size, with typical designs being rarely satisfactory in this regard (Cohen, 1992b). As a result, the preferred solution to increase power is typically to adjust sample sizes (**Figure 1B**).

Power analyses are especially relevant in the context of interventions because sample size is usually limited by the design and its inherent costs—training protocols require participants to come back to the laboratory multiple times for testing and in some cases for the training regimen itself. Yet despite the importance of precisely determining power before an experiment, power analyses include several degrees of freedom that can radically change outcomes and thus recommended sample sizes (Cohen, 1992b). As informative as it may be, gauging the influence of each factor is difficult using power analyses in the traditional sense, that is, varying factors one at a time. This problem can be circumvented by Monte Carlo methods, where one can visualize the influence of each factor in isolation and in conjunction with one another.

[2]For a given α and effect size, low power results in low Positive Predictive Value (PPV), that is, a low probability that a significant effect observed in a sample reflects a true effect in the population. The PPV is closely related to the False Discovery Rate (FDR) mentioned in the section on multiple comparisons of this article, such that PPV + FDR = 1.

Suppose, for example, that we wish to evaluate the effectiveness of an intervention by comparing gain scores in experimental and control groups. Using a two-sample *t*-test with two groups of 20 subjects, and assuming $\alpha = .05$ and $1-\beta = .80$, an effect size needs to be of about $d = 0.5$ or greater to be detected, on average (**Figure 1C**). Any weaker effect would typically go undetected. This concern is particularly important when considering how conservative our example is: a power of .80 is fairly rare in typical training experiments, and an effect size of $d = 0.5$ is quite substantial—although typically defined as "medium" in the behavioral sciences (Cohen, 1988), an increase of half a standard deviation is particularly consequential in training interventions, given potential applications and the inherent noise of such studies.

We should emphasize that we are not implying that every significant finding with low power should be discarded; however, caution is warranted when underpowered studies coincide with unlikely hypotheses, as this combination can lead to high rates of Type I errors (Krzywinski and Altman, 2013; Nuzzo, 2014). Given the typical lack of power in the behavioral sciences (Cohen, 1992a; Button et al., 2013), the current emphasis on replication (Pashler and Wagenmakers, 2012; Baker, 2015; Open Science Collaboration, 2015) is an encouraging step, as it should allow extracting more signal from noisy, underpowered experiments in the long run. Statistical power directly informs the reader about two elements: if an effect is there, what is the probability to detect it, and if an effect was detected, what is the probability that it was genuine? These are critical questions in the evaluation of scientific evidence, and especially in the field of cognitive training, setting the stage for the central role of power in all the problems discussed henceforth.

SAMPLING ERROR

A pernicious consequence of low statistical power is sampling error. Because a sample is an approximation of the population, a point estimate or statistic calculated for a specific sample may differ from the underlying parameter in the population (**Figures 2A,B**). For this reason, most statistical procedures take into account sampling error, and experimenters try to minimize its impact, for example by controlling confounding factors, using valid and reliable measures, and testing powerful manipulations. Despite these precautions, sampling error can obscure experimental findings in an appreciable number of occurrences (Schmidt, 1992). We provide below an example of its detrimental effect.

Let us consider a typical scenario in intervention designs. Assume we randomly select a sample of 40 individuals from an underlying population and assign each participant either to the experimental or the control group. We now have 20 participants in each group, which we assume are representative of the whole population. This assumption, however, is rarely met in typical designs (e.g., Campbell and Stanley, 1966). In small samples, sampling error can have important consequences, especially when individual characteristics are not homogeneously represented in the population. Differences can be based upon neural plasticity, learning potential, motivational traits, or any other individual characteristic. When sampling from an heterogeneous population, groups might not be matched despite random assignment (e.g., Moreau, 2014b).

In addition, failure to take into account extraneous variables is not the only problem with sampling. Another common weakness relates to differences in pretest scores. As set by α, random sampling will generate significantly different baseline scores on a given task 5% of the time in the long run, despite drawing from the same underlying population (see **Figure 2C**). This is not trivial, especially considering that less sizeable discrepancies can significantly influence the outcome of an intervention, as training or testing effects might exacerbate a difference undetected initially.

There are different ways to circumvent this problem, and one in particular that has been the focus of attention recently in training interventions is to increase power. As we have mentioned in the previous section, this can be accomplished either by using larger samples, or by studying larger effects, or both (**Figure 2D**). But these adjustments are not always feasible. To restrict the influence of sampling error, another potential remedy is to factor pretest performance on the dependent variable into group allocation, via restricted randomization. The idea is to ensure that random assignment has been effective at shuffling predefined characteristics (e.g., scores, demographics, physiological correlates) evenly to the different experimental conditions. If groups are imbalanced, a simple remedy is to perform new iterations of the random assignment procedure until conditions are satisfied. This is sometimes unpractical, however, especially with multiple variables to shuffle. Alternatively, one can then constrain random assignment *a priori* based on pretest scores, via stratified sampling (e.g., Aoyama, 1962). Non-random methods of group assignment are sometimes used in training studies (Spence et al., 2009; Loosli et al., 2012; Redick et al., 2013). An example of such methods, blocking, consists of dividing participants based on pretest scores on a given variable, to create homogenous groups (Addelman, 1969). In second step, random assignment is performed with equal draws from each of the groups, so as to preserve the initial heterogeneity in each experimental group. Other, more advanced approaches can be used (for a review, see Green et al., 2014), yet the rationale remains the same, that is, to reduce the influence of initial discrepancies on the outcome of an intervention. We should point out that these procedures bring problems of their own (Ericson, 2012)—with small samples, no method of assignment is perfect, and one needs to decide on the most suitable approach based on the specific design and hypotheses. In an effort to be transparent, it is therefore important to report how group assignment was performed, particularly in instances where it departed from typical (i.e., simple) randomization.

CONTINUOUS VARIABLE SPLITS

Lack of power and its related issue sampling error are two limitations of experimental designs that often need substantial investment to be remediated. Conversely, splitting

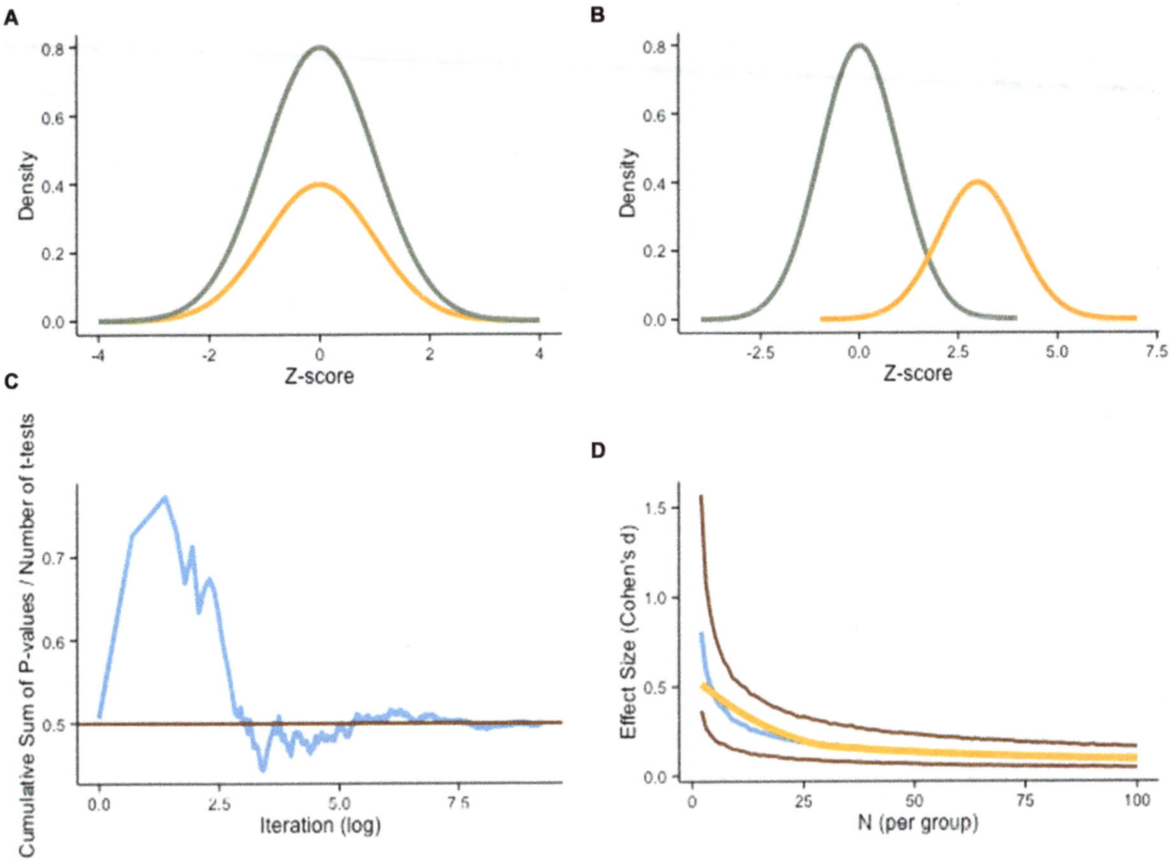

FIGURE 2 | Sampling error. (A) Cognitive training experiments often assume a theoretical ideal where the sample (orange curve) is perfectly representative of the true underlying distribution (green curve). **(B)** However, another possibility is that the sample is not representative of the population of interest due to sampling error, a situation that can lead to dubious claims regarding the effectiveness of a treatment. **(C)** Assuming $\alpha = .05$ in a frequentist framework, the difference between two groups drawn from the same underlying distribution will be unequal 5% of the time, but a more subtle departure from the population is also likely to influence training outcomes meaningfully. The graph shows the cumulative sum of two-sample *t*-test *p*-values divided by the number of tests performed, based on a Monte Carlo simulation ($N = 10{,}000$) of 40 individual IQ scores (normally distributed, $M = 100$, SD = 1) randomly divided in two groups (experimental, control). The red line shows $P = .5$. **(D)** Even when both groups are drawn from a single normal distribution (H_0 is true), small sample sizes will spuriously produce substantial differences (absolute median effect size, blue line), as illustrated here with another Monte Carlo simulation ($N = 10{,}000$). As group samples get larger, effect size estimates get closer to 0. Red lines represent 25th and 75th quartiles, and the orange line is loess smooth on the median.

a continuous variable is a deliberate decision at the analysis stage. Although popular in intervention studies, it is rarely—if ever—justified.

Typically, a continuous variable reflecting performance change throughout training is split into a categorical variable, often dichotomous. Because the idea is to identify individuals who do respond to the training regimen, and those who do not benefit as much, this approach is often called "responder analysis". Most commonly, the dichotomization is achieved via a median split, which refers to the procedure of finding the median score on a continuous variable (e.g., training performance) and split subjects who are below and above this particular score (e.g., low responders vs. high responders).

Median splits are almost always prejudicial (Cohen, 1983), and their use often reflects a lack of understanding of the consequences involved (MacCallum et al., 2002). A full account of the problems associated with this practice is beyond the scope of this article, but the main harms are loss of power and of information, reduction of effect sizes, and inconsistencies in the comparison of results across studies (Allison et al., 1993). Turning a continuous variable into a dichotomy also implies that the original continuum was irrelevant, and that the true nature of the variable is dichotomous. This is seldom the case.

In intervention designs, a detrimental consequence of turning continuous variables into categorical ones and separating low and high performers *post hoc* is the risk of regression toward the mean (Galton, 1886). Regression toward the mean is one of the most well known byproducts of multiple measurements, yet it is possibly one of the least understood (Nesselroade et al., 1980). As for all the notions discussed in this article, regression toward the mean is not exclusive to training experiments; however, estimating its magnitude is made more difficult by potential confounds with testing effects in these types of design.

In short, regression toward the mean is the tendency for a given observation that is extreme, or far from the mean, to be closer to the mean on a second measurement. When a population is normally distributed, extreme scores are not as likely as average scores, therefore making the probability to observe two extreme scores in a row unlikely. Regression toward the mean is the consequence of imperfect correlations between scores from one session to the next—singling out an extreme score on a specific measure therefore increases the likelihood that it will regress to the mean on another measurement.

This phenomenon might be puzzling because it seems to violate the assumption of independent events. Indeed, regression toward the mean can be mistaken as a deterministic linear change from one measurement to the next, whereas it simply reflects the idea that in a bivariate distribution with the correlation between two variables X and Y less that $|1|$, the corresponding value y in Y of a given value x of X is expected to be closer to the mean of Y than x is to the mean of X, provided both are expressed in standard deviation units (Nesselroade et al., 1980). This is easier to visualize graphically—the more a score deviates from the mean on a measurement (**Figure 3A**), the more it will regress to the mean on a second measurement, independently from any training effect (i.e., assuming no improvement from pretest to posttest). This effect is exacerbated after splitting a continuous variable (**Figure 3B**), as absolute gains are influenced by the deviation of pretest scores from the mean, irrespective of genuine improvement (**Figure 3C**).

This is particularly problematic in training interventions because numerous studies are designed to measure the effectiveness of a treatment after an initial selection based on baseline scores. For example, many studies intend to assess the impact of a cognitive intervention in schools after enrolling the lowest-scoring participants on a pretest measure (e.g., Graham et al., 2007; Helland et al., 2011; Stevens et al., 2013). Median- or mean-split designs should always wary the reader, as it does not adequately control for regression toward the mean and other confounds (e.g., sampling bias) - if the groups to be compared are not equal at baseline, any interpretation of improvement is precarious. In addition, such comparison is often obscured by the sole presentation of gains scores, rather than both pretest and posttest scores. Significant gains in one group vs. the other might be due to a true effect of the intervention, but can also arise from unequal baseline scores. The remedy is simple: unless theoretically motivated *a priori*, splitting a continuous variable should be avoided, and unequal performance at baseline should be reported and taken into account when assessing the evidence for an intervention.

Despite the questionable relevance of this practice, countless studies have used median splits on training performance scores in the cognitive training literature (Jaeggi et al., 2011; Rudebeck et al., 2012; Kundu et al., 2013; Redick et al., 2013; Thompson et al., 2013; Novick et al., 2014), following the rationale that transfer effects are moderated by individual differences in gains on the training task (Tidwell et al., 2014). Accordingly, individual differences in response to training and cognitive malleability leads researchers to expect a correlation between training gains and gains on the transfer tasks, a finding that has been commonly reported in the literature (Chein and Morrison, 2010; Jaeggi et al., 2011; Schweizer et al., 2013; Zinke et al., 2014). We explore this idea further in the next section.

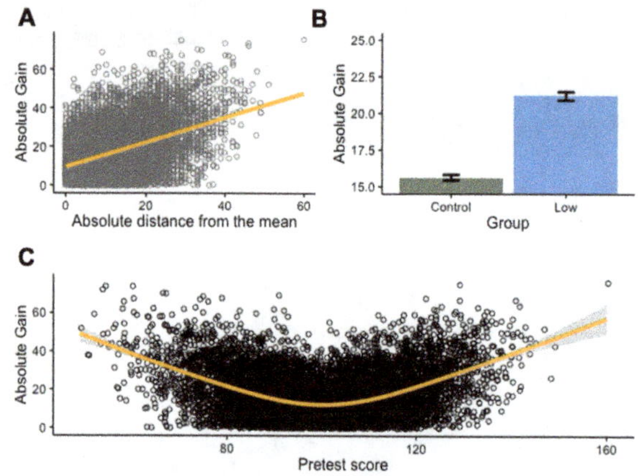

FIGURE 3 | Continuous variable splits and regression toward the mean. Many interventions isolate a low-performing group at pretest and compare the effect of training on this group with a group that includes the remaining participants. This approach is fundamentally flawed, as it capitalizes on regression toward the mean rather than on true training effects. Here, we present a Monte Carlo simulation of 10,000 individual scores drawn from a normally-distributed population (M = 100, SD = 15), before and after a cognitive training intervention (for simplicity purposes, we assume no test-retest effect). **(A)** As can be expected in such a situation, there is a positive relationship between the absolute distance of pretest scores from the mean and the absolute gains from pretest to posttest: the farther a score deviates from the mean (in either direction), the more likely it is to show important changes between the two measurement points. **(B)** This is particularly problematic when one splits a continuous variable (e.g., pretest score) into a categorical variable. In this case, and without assuming any real effect of the intervention, a low-performing group (all scores inferior or equal to the first quartilo) will typically show impressive changes between the two measurement points, compared with a control group (remaining scores). **(C)** This difference is a direct consequence of absolute gains from pretest to posttest being a function of the deviation of pretest scores from the mean, following a curvilinear relationship (U-shaped, orange line).

INTERPRETATION OF CORRELATIONS IN GAINS

The goal in most training interventions is to show that training leads to transfer, that is, gains in tasks that were not part of the training. Decades of research have shown that training on a task results in enhanced performance on this particular task, paving the way for entire programs of research focusing on deliberate practice (e.g., Ericsson et al., 1993). In the field of cognitive training, however, the newsworthy research question is whether or not training is followed by enhanced performance on a *different* task (i.e., transfer). Following this rationale, researchers often look for positive correlations between gains in the training task and in the transfer task, and interpret such effects as evidence supporting the effectiveness of an intervention (Jaeggi et al., 2011; Rudebeck et al., 2012; Kundu et al., 2013; Redick et al., 2013; Thompson et al., 2013; Novick et al., 2014; Zinke et al., 2014).

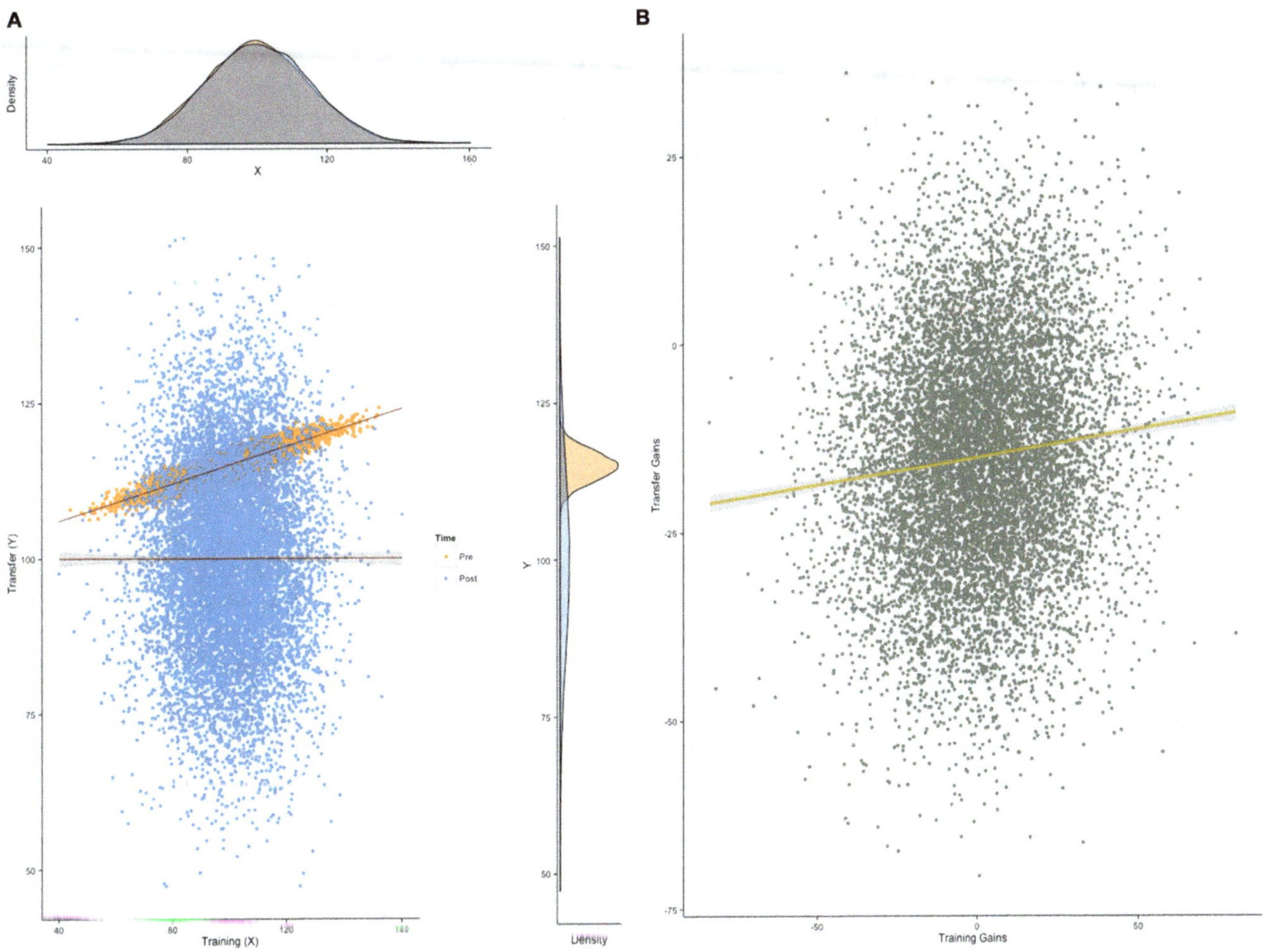

FIGURE 4 | Correlated gain scores. Correlated gain scores between a training variable and a transfer variable can occur regardless of transfer. **(A)** Here, a Monte Carlo simulation (N = 1000) shows normally-distributed individual scores (M = 100, SD = 15) on a training task and a transfer task at two consecutive testing sessions (pretest in orange, posttest in blue). The only constraint on the model is the correlation between the two tasks at pretest (here, r = .92), but not at posttest. **(B)** In this situation, gain scores—defined as the difference between posttest and pretest scores—will be correlated (here, r = .10), regardless of transfer. This pattern can arise irrespective of training effectiveness, due to the initial correlation between training and transfer scores.

Although apparently sound, this line of reasoning is flawed. Correlated gain scores are neither an indication nor a necessity for transfer—transfer can be obtained without any correlation in gain scores, and correlated gain scores do not guarantee transfer (Zelinski et al., 2014).

For the purpose of simplicity, suppose we design a training intervention in which we set out to measure only two dependent variables: the ability directly trained (e.g., working memory capacity, WMC) and the ability we wish to demonstrate transfer to (e.g., intelligence, g). If requirements (a, b, c) are met such that: (a) performance on WMC and g is correlated at pretest, as is often the case due to the positive manifold (Spearman, 1904), (b) this correlation is no longer significant at posttest, and (c) scores at pretest do not correlate well with scores at posttest, both plausible given that one ability is being artificially inflated through training (Moreau and Conway, 2014); then gains in the trained ability and in the transfer ability will be correlated. This correlation will be a consequence of pretest correlations, and cannot be regarded as reflecting evidence for transfer. More strikingly perhaps, performance gains in initially correlated tasks are expected to be correlated even *without* transfer (**Figures 4A,B**). Correlations are unaffected by a linear transformation of the variables they relate to—they are therefore not influenced by variable means. As a result, correlated gain scores is a phenomenon completely independent from transfer. A positive correlation is the consequence of a greater covariance of gain scores within-session than between sessions, but it provides no insight into the behavior of the means we wish to measure—scores could increase, decrease, or remain unchanged, and this information would not be reflected in the correlation of gain scores (Tidwell et al., 2014). Conversely, transfer can happen without correlated gains, although this situation is perhaps less common in training studies, as it often implies that the training task and the transfer task were not initially correlated.

To make things worse, analyses of correlation in gains are often combined with median splits to look for different patterns in a group of responders (i.e., individuals who improved on the training task) and in a group of non-responders (i.e., individuals who did not improve on the training task). The underlying rationale is that if training is effective, only those who improved in the training task should show transfer. This approach, however, combines the flaw we presented herein with the ones discussed in the previous section, therefore increasing the chances to reach erroneous conclusions. Limitations of this approach have been examined before and illustrated via simulations (Tidwell et al., 2014) and structural equation modeling (SEM; Zelinski et al., 2014). To summarize, these articles point out that correlated gain scores do not answer the question they are typically purported to answer, that is, whether improvement was moderated by training conditions.

The remedy to this intuitive but erroneous interpretation of correlated gains lies in alternative statistical techniques. Transfer can be established when the experimental group shows larger gains than controls, demonstrated by a significant interaction on a repeated measures ANOVA (with treatment group as the between-subject factor and session as the within-group factor) or its Bayesian analog. Because this analysis does not correct for group differences at pretest, one should always report *post hoc* comparisons to follow up on significant interactions and provide summary statistics including pretest and posttest scores, not just of gain scores, as is often the case. Due to this limitation, another common approach is to use an ANCOVA, with posttest scores as a dependent variable and pretest scores as a covariate. Although often used interchangeably, the two types of analysis actually answer slightly different research questions. When one wishes to assess the difference in gains between treatment groups, the former approach is most appropriate[3]. Unlike correlated gain scores, this method allows answering the question at hand—does the experimental treatment produce larger cognitive gains than the control?

A different, perhaps more general problem concerns the validity of improvements typically observed in training studies. How should we interpret gains on a specific task or on a cognitive construct? Most experimental tasks used by psychologists to assess cognitive abilities were designed and intended for comparison between individuals or groups, rather than as a means to quantify individual or group improvements. This point may seem trivial, but it hardly is—the underlying mechanisms tapped by training might be task-specific, rather than domain-general. In other words, one might improve via specific strategies that help perform well on a task or set of tasks, without any guarantee of meaningful transfer. In some cases, even diminishment can be viewed as a form of enhancement (Earp et al., 2014). It can therefore be difficult to interpret improvement following a training intervention, as it may reflect different underlying patterns. Hayes et al. (2015, p. 1) emphasize this point in a discussion of training-induced gains in fluid intelligence: "The interpretation of these results is questionable because score *gains* can be dominated by factors that play marginal roles in the scores themselves, and because intelligence gain is not the only possible explanation for the observed control-adjusted far transfer across tasks". Indeed, a possibility that often cannot be discarded is that improvement is driven by strategy refinement rather than general gains. Moreover, it has also been pointed out that gains in a test of intelligence designed to measure between-subject differences do not necessarily imply intelligence gains evaluated within subjects (te Nijenhuis et al., 2007).

Reaching a precise understanding about the nature and meaning of cognitive improvement is a difficult endeavor, but in a field with far-reaching implications for society such as cognitive training, it is worth reflecting upon what training is thought and intended to achieve. Although informed by prior research (e.g., Ellis, 1965; Stankov and Chen, 1988a,b), practicing specific cognitive tasks to elicit transfer is a novel paradigm in its current form, and numerous questions remain regarding the definition and measure of cognitive enhancement (e.g., te Nijenhuis et al., 2007; Moreau, 2014a). Until theoretical models are refined to account for novel evidence, we cannot assume that long-standing knowledge based on more than a century of research in psychometrics applies inevitably to training designs deliberately intended to promote general cognitive improvement.

SINGLE TRANSFER ASSESSMENTS

Beyond matters of analysis and interpretation, the choice of specific tasks used to demonstrate transfer is also critical. Any measurement, no matter how accurate, contains error. More than anywhere else perhaps, this is true in the behavioral sciences—human beings differ from one another on multiple factors that contribute to task performance in any ability. One of the keys to reduce error is to increase the number of measurements. This idea might not be straightforward at first—if measurements are imperfect, why would multiplying them, and therefore the error associated with them, give a better estimate of the ability one wants to probe? The reason multiple measurements are superior to single measurements is because inferring scores from combined sources allows extracting out some, if not most, of the error.

This notion is ubiquitous. Teachers rarely give final grades based on one assessment, but rather average intermediate grades to get better, fairer estimates. Politicians do not rely on single polls to decide on a course of action in a campaign—they combine several of them to increase precision. Whenever precision matters most, we also increase the number of measurements before combining them. In tennis, men play to the best of three sets in most competitions, but to the best of five sets in the most prestigious tournaments, the Grand Slams. The idea is to minimize the noise, or random sources of error, and maximize the signal, or the influence of a true ability, tennis skills in this example.

[3]More advanced statistical techniques (e.g., latent change score models) can help to refine claims of transfer in situations where multiple outcome variables are present (e.g. McArdle and Prindle, 2008; McArdle, 2009; Noack et al., 2014).

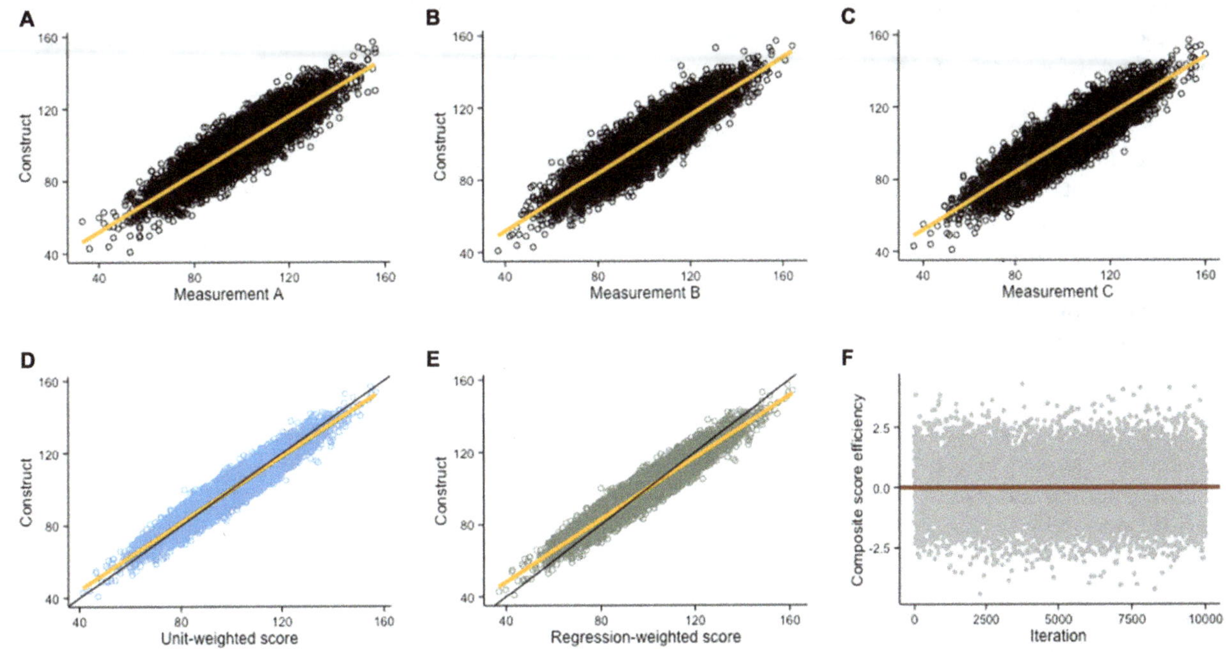

FIGURE 5 | Composite scores. Monte Carlo simulation (N = 10,000) of three imperfect measurements of a hypothetical construct (construct is normally distributed with M = 100 and SD = 15; random error is normally distributed with M = 0 and SD = 7.5). **(A–C)** Scatterplots depicting the relationship between the construct and each of its imperfect measurements (r = .89, in all cases). **(D)** A better estimate of the construct is given by a unit-weighted composite score (r = .96), or by **(E)** a regression-weighted composite score (r = .96) based on factor loadings of each measurement in a factor analysis. **(F)** In this example, the difference between unit-weighted scores and regression-weighted is negligible because the correlations of each measurement with the true ability are roughly equal. Thus, observations above the red line (regression-weighted score is the best estimate) and below the red line (unit-weighted score is the best estimate) approximately average to 0.

This is not the unreasoned caprice of picky scientists—by increasing the number of measurements, we do get better estimates of latent constructs. Nobody says it more eloquently than Randy Engle in *Smarter*, a recent bestseller by Hurley (2014): "Much of the things that psychology talks about, you can't observe. [. . .] They're constructs. We have to come up with various ways of measuring them, or defining them, but we can't specifically observe them. Let's say I'm interested in love. How can I observe love? I can't. I see a boy and a girl rolling around in the grass outside. Is that love? Is it lust? Is it rape? I can't tell. But I define love by various specific behaviors. Nobody thinks any one of those in isolation is love, so we have to use a number of them together. Love is not eye contact over dinner. It's not holding hands. Those are just manifestations of love. And intelligence is the same."

Because constructs are not directly observable (i.e., latent), we rely on combinations of multiple measurements to provide accurate estimates of cognitive abilities. Measurements can be combined into composite scores, that is, scores that minimize measurement error to better reflect the underlying construct of interest. Because they typically improve both reliability and validity in measurements (Carmines and Zeller, 1979), composite scores are key in cognitive training designs (e.g., Shipstead et al., 2012). Relying on multiple converging assessments also allows adequate scopes of measurement, which ensure that constructs reflect an underlying ability rather than task-specific components (Noack et al., 2014). Such precaution in turn allows stronger and more accurate claims of transfer after an intervention. Again, thinking about this idea with an example is helpful. Suppose we simulate an experiment in which we set to measure intelligence (g) in a sample of participants. Defining a construct g and three imperfect measures of g reflecting the true ability plus normally distributed random noise, we obtain single measures that correlate with g such that r = .89 (**Figures 5A–C**). Let us assume three *different* assessments of g rather than three consecutive testing sessions of the same assessment, so that we do not need to take testing effects into account.

Different solutions exist to minimize measurement error, besides ensuring experimental conditions were adequate to guarantee valid measurements. One possibility is to use the median score. Although not ideal, this is an improvement over single testing. Another solution is to average all scores and create a unit-weighted composite score (i.e., mean, **Figure 5D**), which often is a better estimate than the median, unless one or several of the measurements were unusually prone to error. When individual scores are strongly correlated (i.e., collinear), a unit-weighted composite score is often close to the best possible estimate. When individual scores are not or weakly correlated, a regression-weighted composite score is usually a better estimate as it allows minimizing error (**Figure 5E**). Weights for the latter are factor loadings extracted from a factor analysis that includes each measurement, thus minimizing non-systematic error. The power of composite scores is more evident graphically—**Figures 5D,E** show how composite scores are better estimates of a construct than either measure alone (including the median, see in comparison with **Figures 5A–C**). Different methods to generate composite scores can themselves be subsequently compared (see **Figure 5F**). To confidently claim transfer after an intervention, one therefore needs to demonstrate that gains are not exclusive to single tasks, but rather reflect general improvement on latent constructs.

Directly in line with this idea, more advanced statistical techniques such as latent curve models (LCM) and latent change score models (LCSM), typically implemented in a SEM framework, can allow finer assessment of training outcomes (for example, see Ghisletta and McArdle, 2012, for practical implementation). Because of its explicit focus on change across different time points, LCSM is particularly well suited to the analysis of longitudinal data (e.g., Lövdén et al., 2005) and of training studies (e.g., McArdle, 2009), where the emphasis is on cognitive improvement. Other possibilities exist, such as multilevel (Rovine and Molenaar, 2000), random effects (Laird and Ware, 1982) or mixed models (Dean and Nielsen, 2007), all with a common goal: minimizing noise in repeated-measures data, so as to separate out measurement error from predictors or structural components, thus yielding more precise estimates of change.

MULTIPLE COMPARISONS

If including too few dependent variables is problematic, too many can also be prejudicial. At the core of this apparent conundrum lies the multiple comparisons problem, another subtle but pernicious limitation in experimental designs. Following up on one of our previous examples, suppose we are comparing a novel cognitive remediation program targeting learning disorders with traditional feedback learning. Before and after the intervention, participants in the two groups can be compared on measures of reading fluency, reading comprehension, WMC, arithmetic fluency, arithmetic comprehension, processing speed, and a wide array of other cognitive constructs. They can be compared across motivational factors, or in terms of attrition rate. And questionnaires might provide data on extraversion, happiness, quality of life, and so on. For each dependent variable, one could test for differences between the group receiving the traditional intervention and the group enrolled in the new program, with the rationale that differences between groups reflect an inequality of the treatments.

With the multiplication of pairwise comparisons, however, experimenters run the risk of finding differences by chance alone, rather than because of the intervention itself.[4] As we mentioned earlier, mistaking a random fluctuation for a true effect is a false positive, or Type I error. But what exactly is the probability to wrongly conclude that an effect is genuine when it is just random noise? It is easier to solve this problem graphically (**Figure 6A**). When comparing two groups on 10 transfer tasks, the probability to make a wrong judgment because of random fluctuation is about 40%. With 15 tasks, the probability rise to 54%, and with 20 tasks, it reaches 64% (all assuming a $\alpha = .05$ threshold to declare a finding significant).

This problem is well known, and procedures have been developed to account for it. One evident answer is to reduce Type I errors by using a more stringent threshold. With $\alpha = .01$, the percentage of significant differences rising spuriously in our previous scenario drops to 10% (10 tasks), 14% (15 tasks), and 18% (20 tasks). Lowering the significance threshold is exactly what the Bonferroni correction does (**Figure 6B**). Specifically, it requires dividing the significance level required to claim that a difference is significant by the number of comparisons being performed. Therefore, for the example above with 10 transfer tasks, $\alpha = .005$, with 15 tasks, $\alpha = .003$, and with 20 tasks, $\alpha = .0025$. The problem with this approach is that it is often too conservative—it corrects more strictly than necessary. Considering the lack of power inherent to numerous interventions, true effects will often be missed when the Bonferroni procedure is applied; the procedure lowers false discoveries, but by the same token lowers true discoveries as well. This is especially problematic when comparisons are highly dependent (Vul et al., 2009; Fiedler, 2011). For example, in typical fMRI experiments involving the comparisons of thousands of voxels with one another, Bonferroni corrections would systematically prevent yielding any significant correlation. By controlling α levels across all voxels, the method guarantees an error probability of .05 on each single comparison, a level too stringent for discoveries. Although the multiple comparisons problem has been extensively discussed, we should point out that not everyone agrees on its pernicious effects (Gelman et al., 2012).

Provided there is a problem, a potential solution is replication. Obviously, this is not always feasible, can turn out to be expensive, and is not entirely foolproof. Other techniques have been developed to answer this challenge, with good results. For example, the recent rise of Monte Carlo methods or their non-parametric equivalent such as bootstrap and jackknife offers interesting alternatives. In intervention that include brain imaging data, these techniques can be used to calculate cluster-size thresholds, a procedure that relies on the assumption that contiguous signal changes are more likely to reflect true neural activity (Forman et al., 1995), thus allowing more meaningful control over discovery rates.

In line with this idea, one approach that has gained popularity over the years is based on the false discovery rate (FDR). FDR correction is intended to control false discoveries by adjusting α only in the tests that result in a discovery (true or false), thus allowing a reduction of Type I errors while leaving more power to detect truly significant differences. The resulting q-values are corrected for multiple comparisons, but are less stringent than traditional corrections on p-values because they only take into account positive effects. To illustrate this idea, suppose 10% of all cognitive interventions are effective. That is, of all the designs tested by researchers with the intent to improve some aspect of cognition, one in 10 is a successful attempt. This is a deliberately low estimate, consistent with the conflicting evidence

[4]Multiple comparisons introduce additional problems in training designs, such as practice effects from one task to another within a given construct (i.e., hierarchical learning, Bavelier et al., 2012), or cognitive depletion effects (Green et al., 2014).

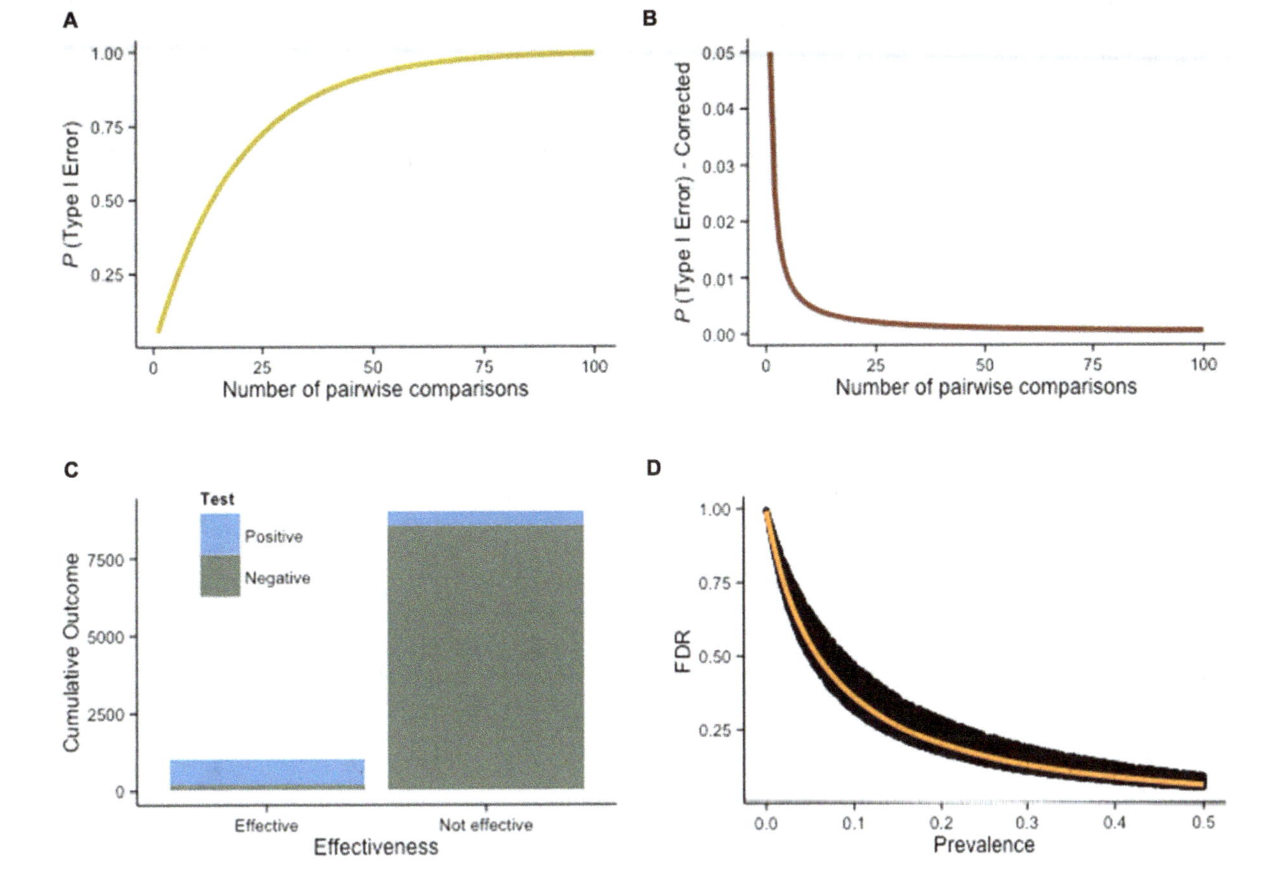

FIGURE 6 | Multiple comparisons problem. (A) True probability of a Type I error as a function of the number of pairwise comparisons (holding $\alpha = .05$ constant for any given comparison). **(B)** A possible solution to the multiple comparisons problem is the Bonferroni correction, a rather conservative procedure—the false discovery rate (FDR) decreases, but so does the true discovery rate, increasing the chance to miss a true difference (β). **(C)** Assuming 10% of training interventions are truly effective (N = 10, 000), with power = .80 and $\alpha = .05$, 450 interventions will yield false positives, while 800 will result in true positives. The FDR in this situation is 36% (more than a third of the positive results are not real), despite high power and standard α criteria. Therefore, this estimate is conservative—assuming 10% of the interventions are effective and $1-\beta = .80$ is rather optimistic. **(D)** As the prevalence of an effect increases (e.g., higher percentage of effective interventions overall), the FDR decreases. This effect is illustrated here with a Monte Carlo simulation of the FDR as a function of prevalence, given $1-\beta$ free to vary such that $.50 \leq 1-\beta \leq 1$ (the orange line shows FDR when $1-\beta = .80$).

surrounding cognitive training (e.g., Melby-Lervåg and Hulme, 2013). Note that we rarely know beforehand the ratio of effective interventions, but let us assume here that we do. Imagine now that we wish to know which interventions will turn out to show a positive effect, and which will not, and that $\alpha = .05$ and power is .80 (both considered standard in psychology). Out of 10,000 interventions, how often will we wrongly conclude that an intervention is effective?

To determine this probability, we first need to determine how many interventions overall will yield a positive result (i.e., the experimental group will be significantly different from the control group at posttest). In our hypothetical scenario, we would detect, with a power of .80, 800 true positives. These are interventions that were effective (N = 1000) and would be correctly detected as such (true positives). However, because our power is *only* .80, we will miss 200 interventions (false negatives). In addition, out of the 9000 interventions that we know are ineffective, 5% (α) will yield false positives. In our example, these amount to 450. The true negatives would be the remaining 8550 (**Figure 6C**).

The FDR is the amount of false positives divided by all the positive results, that is, 36% in this example. More than 1/3 of the positive studies will not reflect a true underlying effect. The positive predictive value (PPV), the probability that a significant effect is genuine, is approximately two thirds in this scenario (64%). This is worth pausing for a moment: more than a third of our positive results, reaching significance with standard frequentist methods, would be misleading. Furthermore, the FDR increases if either power or the percentage of effective training interventions in the population of studies decreases (**Figure 6D**). Because FDR only corrects for positive p-value, the procedure is less conservative than the Bonferroni correction. Many alternatives exist (e.g., Dunnett's test, Fisher's LSD, Newman-Keuls test, Scheffé's method, Tukey's HSD)—ultimately, the preferred method depends on the problem at hand. Is the emphasis on finding new effects, or on the reliability of any discovered effect? Scientific rationale is rarely dichotomized, but thinking about a research question in these terms can help to decide on adequate statistical procedures. In the context of this discussion, one of the best remedies remains to design an intervention with a clear hypothesis about the variables of interest, rather than multiply outcome measures and increase the rate of false positives. Ideally, experiments should explicitly state whereas they are exploratory or confirmatory (Kimmelman et al., 2014), and should always disclose all tasks used in pretest and posttest sessions (Simmons et al., 2011). These measures are part of a broader ongoing effort intended to reduce false positives in psychological research, via more transparency and systematic disclosure of all manipulations, measurements and analyses in experiments, to control for researcher degrees of freedom (Simmons et al., 2011).

PUBLICATION BIAS

Our final stop in this statistical journey is to discuss publication bias, a consequence of research findings being more likely to get published based on the direction of the effects reported or on statistical significance. At the core of the problem lies the overuse of frequentist methods, and particularly H_0 Significance Testing (NHST), in medicine and the behavioral sciences, with an emphasis on the likelihood of the collected data or more extreme data if the H_0 is true—in probabilistic notation, $P(d|H_0)$ - rather than the probability of interest, $P(H_0|d)$, that is, the probability that the H_0 is true given the data collected. In intervention studies, one typically wishes to know the probability that an intervention is effective given the evidence, rather than the less informative likelihood of the evidence if the intervention were ineffective (for an in-depth analysis, see Kirk, 1996). The incongruity between these two approaches has motivated changes in the way findings are reported in leading journals (e.g., Cumming, 2014) punctuated recently by a complete ban of NHST in *Basic and Applied Social Psychology* (Trafimow and Marks, 2015), and is central in the growing popularity of Bayesian inference in the behavioral sciences (e.g., Andrews and Baguley, 2013).

Because of the underlying logic of NHST, only rejecting the H_0 is truly informative—retaining H_0 does not provide evidence to prove that it is true[5]. Perhaps the H_0 is untrue, but it is equally plausible that the strength of evidence is insufficient to reject H_0 (i.e., lack of power). What this means in practice is that null findings (findings that do not allow us to confidently reject H_0) are difficult to interpret, because they can be due to the absence of an effect or to weak experimental designs. Publication of null findings is therefore rare, a phenomenon that contribute to bias the landscape of scientific evidence—only positive findings get published, leading to the false belief that interventions are effective, whereas a more comprehensive assessment might lead to more nuanced conclusions (e.g., Dickersin, 1990).

Single studies are never definitive; rather, researchers rely on meta-analyses pooling together all available studies meeting a set of criteria and of interest to a specific question to get a better estimate of the accumulated evidence. If only studies corroborating the evidence for a particular treatment get published, the resulting literature becomes biased. This is particularly problematic in the field of cognitive training, due to the relative novelty of this line of investigation, which increases the volatility of one's belief, and because of its potential to inform practices and policies (Bossaer et al., 2013; Anguera and Gazzaley, 2015; Porsdam Mann and Sahakian, 2015). Consider for example that different research groups across the world have come to dramatically opposite conclusions about the effectiveness of cognitive training, based on slight differences in meta-analysis inclusion criteria and models (Melby-Lervåg and Hulme, 2013; Karbach and Verhaeghen, 2014; Lampit et al., 2014; Au et al., 2015). The point here is that even a few missing studies in meta-analyses can have important consequences, especially when the accumulated evidence is relatively scarce as is the case in the young field of cognitive training. Again, let us illustrate this idea with an example. Suppose we simulate a pool of study results, each with a given sample size and an observed effect size for the difference between experimental and control gains after a cognitive intervention. The model draws pairs of numbers randomly from a vector of sample size (ranging from $N = 5$ to $N = 100$) and a vector of effect sizes (ranging from $d = 0$ to $d = 2$). We then generate stochastically all kinds of associations, for example large sample sizes with small effect sizes and vice-versa (**Figure 7A**). In science, however, the landscape of published findings is typically different—studies get published when they pass a test of statistical significance, with a threshold given by the p-value. To demonstrate that a difference is significant in this framework, one needs large sample sizes, large effects, or a fairly sizable combination of both. When represented graphically, this produces a funnel plot typically used in meta-analyses (**Figure 7B**); departures from this symmetrical representation often indicate some bias in the literature.

Two directions seem particularly promising to circumvent publication bias. First, researchers often try to make an estimate of the size of publication bias when summarizing the evidence for a particular intervention. This process can be facilitated by examining a representation of all the published studies, with a measure of precision plotted as a function of the intervention effect. In the absence of publication bias, it is expected that studies with larger samples, and therefore better precision, will fall around the average effect size observed, whereas studies with smaller sample size, lacking precision, will be more dispersed. This results in a funnel shape within which most observations fall. Deviations from this shape can raise concerns regarding the objectivity of the published evidence, although it should be noted that other explanations might be equally valid (Lau et al., 2006). These methods can be improved upon, and recent articles have addressed some of the typical concerns of solely relying on funnel plots to estimate publication bias. Interesting alternatives have

[5]David Bakan distinguished between sharp and loose null hypotheses, the former referring to the difference between population means being strictly zero, whereas the latter assumes this difference to be *around* the null. Much of the disagreement with NHST arises from the problem presented by sharp null hypotheses, which, given sufficient sample sizes, are never true (Bakan,

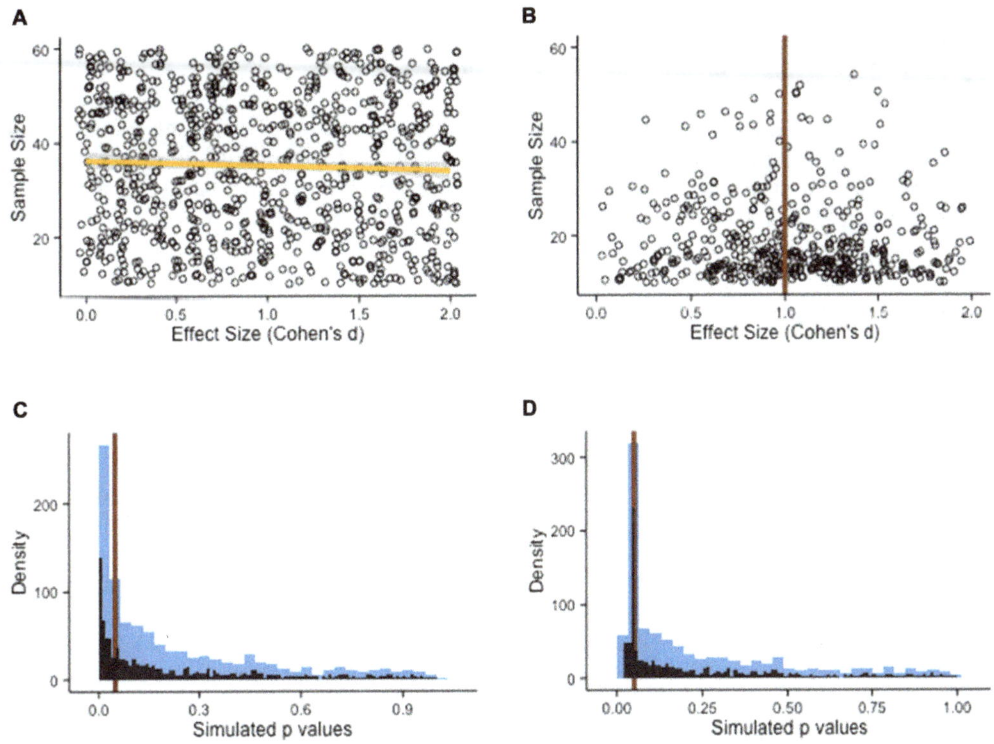

FIGURE 7 | Publication bias. (A) Population of study outcomes, with effect sizes and associated sample sizes. There is no correlation between the two variables, as shown by the slope of the fit line (orange line). **(B)** It is often assumed that in the absence of publication bias, the population of studies should roughly resemble the shape of a funnel, with small sample studies showing important variation and large sample studies clustered around the true effect size (in the example, $d = 1$). **(C)** Alternatives have been proposed (see main text), such as the p-curve. Here, a Monte Carlo simulation of two-sample t-tests with 1000 draws ($N = 20$ per groups, $d = 0.5$, $M = 100$, SD = 20) shows a shape resembling a power-law distribution, with no particular change around the $p = .05$ threshold (red line). The blue bars represent the rough density histogram, while the black bars are more precise estimates. **(D)** When the pool of published studies is biased, a sudden peak can sometimes be observed just below the $p = .05$ threshold (red line). Arguably, this irregularity in the distribution of p-values has no particular justification, if not for bias.

2014a,b) or more direct measures of the plausibility of a set of findings (Francis, 2012). These methods are not infallible (for example, see Bishop and Thompson, 2016), but they represent steps in the right direction.

Second, ongoing initiatives are intended to facilitate the publication of all findings, irrespective of the outcome, on online repositories. Digital storage has become cheap, allowing platforms to archive data for limited cost. Such repositories already exist in other fields (e.g., arXiv), but have not been developed fully in medicine and in the behavioral sciences. Additional incentives to pre-register studies are another step in that direction—for example, allowing researchers to get preliminary publication approval based on study design and intended analyses, rather than on the direction of the findings. Publishing all results would eradicate publication bias (van Assen et al., 2014), and therefore initiatives such as pre-registration should be the favored approach in the future (Goldacre, 2015).

CONCLUSION

Based on Monte Carlo simulations, we have demonstrated that several statistical flaws undermine typical findings in cognitive training interventions. This critique echoes others, which have pointed out the limitations of current research practices (e.g., Ioannidis, 2005), although arguably the flaws we discussed in this article are often a consequence of limited resources—including methodological and statistical guidelines—rather than the result of errors or practices deliberately intended to mislead. These flaws are pervasive, but we believe that clear visual representations can help raise awareness of their pernicious effects among researchers and interested readers of scientific findings. As we mentioned, statistical flaws are not the only kinds of problems in cognitive training interventions. However, the relative opacity of statistics favors situations where one applies methods and techniques popular in a field of study, irrespective of pernicious effects. We hope that our present contribution provides a valuable resource to make training interventions more accessible.

Importantly, not all interventions suffer from these flaws. A number of training experiments are excellent, with strong designs and adequate data analyses. Arguably, these studies have emerged in response to prior methodological concerns and through facilitated communication across scientific fields, such as between evidence-based medicine and psychology, stressing further the importance of discussing good research practices. One example that illustrates the benefits of this dialog is the use of active control groups, which is becoming the norm rather than the exception in the field of cognitive training. When feasible, other important components are being integrated within research procedures, such as random allocation to conditions, standardized data collection and double-blind designs. Following current trends in the cognitive training literature, interventions should be evaluated according to their methodological and statistical strengths—more value, or weight, should be given to flawless studies or interventions with fewer methodological problems, whereas less importance should be conferred to studies that suffer several of the flaws we mentioned (Moher et al., 1998).

Related to this idea, most simulations in this article stress the limit of frequentist inference in its NHST implementation. This idea is not new (e.g., Bakan, 1966), yet discussions of alternatives are recurring and many fields of study are moving away from solely relying on the rejection of null hypotheses that often make little practical sense (Herzog and Ostwald, 2013; but see also Leek and Peng, 2015). In our view, arguing for or against the effectiveness of cognitive training is ill-conceived in a NHST framework, because the overwhelming evidence gathered throughout the last century is in favor of a null-effect. Thus, even well-controlled experiments that fail to reject the H_0 cannot be considered as convincing evidence against the effectiveness of cognitive training, despite the prevalence of this line of reasoning in this literature.

As a result, we believe cognitive interventions are particularly suited to alternatives such as Neyman-Pearson Hypothesis Testing (NPHT) and Bayesian inference. These approaches are not free of caveats, yet they provide interesting alternatives to the prevalent framework. Because NPHT allows non-significant results to be interpreted as evidence for the null-hypothesis (Neyman and Pearson, 1933), the underlying rationale of NPHT favors scientific advances, especially in the context of accumulating evidence against the effectiveness of an intervention. Bayesian inference (Bakan, 1953; Savage, 1954; Jeffreys, 1961; Edwards et al., 1963) also seems particularly appropriate in evaluating training findings, given the relatively limited evidence for novel training paradigms and the variety of extraneous factors involved. Initially, limited data is outweighed by prior beliefs, but more substantial evidence eventually overwhelms the prior and lead to changes in belief (i.e., updated posteriors). Generally, understanding human cognition follows this principle, with each observation refining the ongoing model. In his time, Piaget speaking of children as "little scientists" was hinting on this particular point—we construct, update and refine our model of the world at all times, taking into account the available data and confronting them with prior experience. A full discussion of Bayesian inference applications in the behavioral sciences is outside the scope of this article, but many excellent contributions have been published in recent years, either related to the general advantages of adopting Bayesian statistics (Andrews and Baguley, 2013) or introducing Bayesian equivalents to common frequentist procedures (Wagenmakers, 2007; Rouder et al., 2009; Morey and Rouder, 2011; Wetzels and Wagenmakers, 2012; Wetzels et al., 2012). It follows that evidence should not be dichotomized—some interventions work for some individuals, and what needs to be identified is what particular interventions yield the more sizeable or reliable effects, what individuals benefit from these and why, rather than the elusive question of absolute effectiveness (Moreau and Waldie, 2016).

In closing, we remain optimistic about current directions in evidence-based cognitive interventions—experimental standards have been improved (Shipstead et al., 2012; Boot et al., 2013), in direct response to blooming claims reporting post-intervention cognitive enhancement (Karbach and Verhaeghen, 2014; Au et al., 2015) and their criticisms (Shipstead et al., 2012; Melby-Lervåg and Hulme, 2013). Such inherent skepticism is healthy, yet hurdles should not discourage efforts to discover effective treatments. The benefits of effective interventions to society are enormous, and further research is to be supported and encouraged. In line with this idea, the novelty of cognitive training calls for exploratory designs to discover effective interventions. The present article represents a modest attempt to document and clarify experimental pitfalls so as to encourage significant advances, at a time of intense debates sparking around replication in the behavioral sciences (Pashler and Wagenmakers, 2012; Simons, 2014; Baker, 2015; Open Science Collaboration, 2015; Simonsohn, 2015; Gilbert et al., 2016). By presenting common pitfalls and by reflecting on ways to evaluate typical designs in cognitive training, we hope to provide an accessible reference for researchers conducting experiments in this field, but also a useful resource for neophytes interested in understanding the content and ramifications of cognitive intervention studies. If scientists want training interventions to impact decisions outside research and academia, empirical findings need to be presented in a clear and unbiased manner, especially when the question of interest is complex and the evidence equivocal.

AUTHOR CONTRIBUTIONS

DM designed and programmed the simulations, ran the analyses, and wrote the paper. IJK and KEW provided valuable suggestions. All authors approved the final version of the manuscript.

ACKNOWLEDGMENTS

We are deeply grateful to Michael C. Corballis for providing invaluable suggestions and comments on an earlier version of this manuscript. DM and KEW are supported by philanthropic donations from the Campus Link Foundation, the Kelliher Trust and Perpetual Guardian (as trustee of the Lady Alport Barker Trust).

REFERENCES

Addelman, S. (1969). The generalized randomized block design. *Am. Stat.* 23, 35–36. doi: 10.2307/2681737

Allison, D. B., Gorman, B. S., and Primavera, L. H. (1993). Some of the most common questions asked of statistical consultants: our favorite responses and recommended readings. *Genet. Soc. Gen. Psychol. Monogr.* 119, 155–185.

Andrews, M., and Baguley, T. (2013). Prior approval: the growth of Bayesian methods in psychology. *Br. J. Math. Stat. Psychol.* 66, 1–7. doi: 10.1111/bmsp.12004

Anguera, J. A., and Gazzaley, A. (2015). Video games, cognitive exercises and the enhancement of cognitive abilities. *Curr. Opin. Behav. Sci.* 4, 160–165. doi: 10.1016/j.cobeha.2015.06.002

Aoyama, H. (1962). Stratified random sampling with optimum allocation for multivariate population. *Ann. Inst. Stat. Math.* 14, 251–258. doi: 10.1007/bf02868647

Au, J., Sheehan, E., Tsai, N., Duncan, G. J., Buschkuehl, M., and Jaeggi, S. M. (2015). Improving fluid intelligence with training on working memory: a meta-analysis. *Psychon. Bull. Rev.* 22, 366–377. doi: 10.3758/s13423-014-0699-x

Auguie, B. (2012). *GridExtra: Functions in Grid Graphics.* (R package version 0.9.1).

Bakan, D. (1953). Learning and the principle of inverse probability. *Psychol. Rev.* 60, 360–370. doi: 10.1037/h0055248

Bakan, D. (1966). The test of significance in psychological research. *Psychol. Bull.* 66, 423–437. doi: 10.1037/h0020412

Baker, M. (2015). First results from psychology's largest reproducibility test. *Nature* doi: 10.1038/nature.2015.17433 [Epub ahead of print].

Bavelier, D., Green, C. S., Pouget, A., and Schrater, P. (2012). Brain plasticity through the life span: learning to learn and action video games. *Annu. Rev. Neurosci.* 35, 391–416. doi: 10.1146/annurev-neuro-060909-152832

Bishop, D. V. M., and Thompson, P. A. (2016). Problems in using p -curve analysis and text-mining to detect rate of p -hacking and evidential value. *PeerJ* 4:e1715. doi: 10.7717/peerj.1715

Boot, W. R., Simons, D. J., Stothart, C., and Stutts, C. (2013). The pervasive problem with placebos in psychology: why active control groups are not sufficient to rule out placebo effects. *Perspect. Psychol. Sci.* 8, 445–454. doi: 10.1177/1745691613491271

Bossaer, J. B., Gray, J. A., Miller, S. E., Enck, G., Gaddipati, V. C., and Enck, R. E. (2013). The use and misuse of prescription stimulants as "cognitive enhancers" by students at one academic health sciences center. *Acad. Med.* 88, 967–971. doi: 10.1097/ACM.0b013e318294fc7b

Button, K. S., Ioannidis, J. P. A., Mokrysz, C., Nosek, B. A., Flint, J., Robinson, E. S. J., et al. (2013). Power failure: why small sample size undermines the reliability of neuroscience. *Nat. Rev. Neurosci.* 14, 365–376. doi: 10.1038/nrn3475

Campbell, D. T., and Stanley, J. (1966). *Experimental and Quasiexperimental Designs for Research.* Chicago: Rand McNally.

Carmines, E. G., and Zeller, R. A. (1979). *Reliability and Validity Assessment.* Thousand Oaks, CA: SAGE Publications, Inc.

Champely, S. (2015). *Pwr: Basic Functions for Power Analysis.* (R package version 1.1-2).

Chein, J. M., and Morrison, A. B. (2010). Expanding the mind's workspace: training and transfer effects with a complex working memory span task. *Psychon. Bull. Rev.* 17, 193–199. doi: 10.3758/PBR.17.2.193

Cohen, J. (1983). The cost of dichotomization. *Appl. Psychol. Meas.* 7, 249–253. doi: 10.1177/014662168300700301

Cohen, J. (1988). *Statistical Power Analysis for the Behavioral Sciences.* 2nd Edn. Hillsdale, NJ: Lawrence Earlbaum Associates.

Cohen, J. (1992a). A power primer. *Psychol. Bull.* 112, 155–159. doi: 10.1037/0033-2909.112.1.155

Cohen, J. (1992b). Statistical power analysis. *Curr. Dir. Psychol. Sci.* 1, 98–101. doi: 10.1111/1467-8721.ep10768783

Cumming, G. (2014). The new statistics: why and how. *Psychol. Sci.* 25, 7–29. doi: 10.1177/0956797613504966

Dean, C. B., and Nielsen, J. D. (2007). Generalized linear mixed models: a review and some extensions. *Lifetime Data Anal.* 13, 497–512. doi: 10.1007/s10985-007-9065-x

Dickersin, K. (1990). The existence of publication bias and risk factors for its occurrence. *JAMA* 263, 1385–1389. doi: 10.1001/jama.263.10.1385

Earp, B. D., Sandberg, A., Kahane, G., and Savulescu, J. (2014). When is diminishment a form of enhancement? Rethinking the enhancement debate in biomedical ethics. *Front. Syst. Neurosci.* 8:12. doi: 10.3389/fnsys.2014.00012

Edwards, W., Lindman, H., and Savage, L. J. (1963). Bayesian statistical inference for psychological research. *Psychol. Rev.* 70, 193–242. doi: 10.1037/h0044139

Ellis, H. C. (1965). *The Transfer of Learning.* New York, NY: MacMillian.

Ericson, W. A. (2012). Optimum stratified sampling using prior information. *J. Am. Stat. Assoc.* 60, 311–750. doi: 10.2307/2283243

Ericsson, K. A., Krampe, R. T., and Tesch-Römer, C. (1993). The role of deliberate practice in the acquisition of expert performance. *Psychol. Rev.* 100, 363–406. doi: 10.1037/0033-295x.100.3.363

Fiedler, K. (2011). Voodoo correlations are everywhere-not only in neuroscience. *Perspect. Psychol. Sci.* 6, 163–171. doi: 10.1177/1745691611400237

Forman, S. D., Cohen, J. D., Fitzgerald, M., Eddy, W. F., Mintun, M. A., and Noll, D. C. (1995). Improved assessment of significant activation in functional magnetic resonance imaging (fMRI): use of a cluster-size threshold. *Magn. Reson. Med.* 33, 636–647. doi: 10.1002/mrm.1910330508

Francis, G. (2012). Too good to be true: publication bias in two prominent studies from experimental psychology. *Psychon. Bull. Rev.* 19, 151–156. doi: 10.3758/s13423-012-0227-9

Galton, F. (1886). Regression towards mediocrity in hereditary stature. *J. Anthropol. Inst. Great Br. Irel.* 15, 246–263. doi: 10.2307/2841583

Gelman, A., Hill, J., and Yajima, M. (2012). Why we (usually) don't have to worry about multiple comparisons. *J. Res. Educ. Eff.* 5, 189–211.

Ghisletta, P., and McArdle, J. J. (2012). Teacher's corner: latent curve models and latent change score models estimated in R. *Struct. Equ. Modeling* 19, 651–682. doi: 10.1080/10705511.2012.713275

Gilbert, D. T., King, G., Pettigrew, S., and Wilson, T. D. (2016). Comment on "Estimating the reproducibility of psychological science". *Science* 351:1037. doi: 10.1126/science.aad7243

Goldacre, B. (2015). How to get all trials reported: audit, better data and individual accountability. *PLoS Med.* 12:e1001821. doi: 10.1371/journal.pmed.1001821

Graham, L., Bellert, A., Thomas, J., and Pegg, J. (2007). QuickSmart: a basic academic skills intervention for middle school students with learning difficulties. *J. Learn. Disabil.* 40, 410–419. doi: 10.1177/00222194070400050401

Green, C. S., Strobach, T., and Schubert, T. (2014). On methodological standards in training and transfer experiments. *Psychol. Res.* 78, 756–772. doi: 10.1007/s00426-013-0535-3

Hayes, T. R., Petrov, A. A., and Sederberg, P. B. (2015). Do we really become smarter when our fluid-intelligence test scores improve? *Intelligence* 48, 1–14. doi: 10.1016/j.intell.2014.10.005

Helland, T., Tjus, T., Hovden, M., Ofte, S., and Heimann, M. (2011). Effects of bottom-up and top-down intervention principles in emergent literacy in children at risk of developmental dyslexia: a longitudinal study. *J. Learn. Disabil.* 44, 105–122. doi: 10.1177/0022219410391188

Herzog, S., and Ostwald, D. (2013). Experimental biology: sometimes Bayesian statistics are better. *Nature* 494:35. doi: 10.1038/494035b

Hurley, D. (2014). *Smarter: The New Science of Building Brain Power.* New York, NY: Penguin Group (USA) LLC.

Ioannidis, J. P. A. (2005). Why most published research findings are false. *PLoS Med.* 2:e124. doi: 10.1371/journal.pmed.0020124

Jaeggi, S. M., Buschkuehl, M., Jonides, J., and Shah, P. (2011). Short- and long-term benefits of cognitive training. *Proc. Natl. Acad. Sci. U S A* 108, 10081–10086. doi: 10.1073/pnas.1103228108

Jeffreys, H. (1961). *The Theory of Probability.* 3rd Edn. Oxford, NY: Oxford University Press.

Karbach, J., and Verhaeghen, P. (2014). Making working memory work: a meta-analysis of executive-control and working memory training in older adults. *Psychol. Sci.* 25, 2027–2037. doi: 10.1177/0956797614548725

Kelley, K., and Lai, K. (2012). *MBESS: MBESS.* (R package version 3.3.3).

Kimmelman, J., Mogil, J. S., and Dirnagl, U. (2014). Distinguishing between exploratory and confirmatory preclinical research will improve translation. *PLoS Biol.* 12:e1001863. doi: 10.1371/journal.pbio.1001863

Kirk, R. E. (1996). Practical significance: a concept whose time has come. *Educ. Psychol. Meas.* 56, 746–759. doi: 10.1177/0013164496056005002

Krzywinski, M., and Altman, N. (2013). Points of significance: power and sample size. *Nat. Methods* 10, 1139–1140. doi: 10.1038/nmeth.2738

Kundu, B., Sutterer, D. W., Emrich, S. M., and Postle, B. R. (2013). Strengthened effective connectivity underlies transfer of working memory training to tests of short-term memory and attention. *J. Neurosci.* 33, 8705–8715. doi: 10.1523/JNEUROSCI.2231-13.2013

Laird, N. M., and Ware, J. H. (1982). Random-effects models for longitudinal data. *Biometrics* 38, 963–974. doi: 10.2307/2529876

Lampit, A., Hallock, H., and Valenzuela, M. (2014). Computerized cognitive training in cognitively healthy older adults: a systematic review and meta-analysis of effect modifiers. *PLoS Med.* 11:e1001756. doi: 10.1371/journal.pmed.1001756

Lau, J., Ioannidis, J. P. A., Terrin, N., Schmid, C. H., and Olkin, I. (2006). The case of the misleading funnel plot. *BMJ* 333, 597–600. doi: 10.1136/bmj.333.7568.597

Leek, J. T., and Peng, R. D. (2015). Statistics: P values are just the tip of the iceberg. *Nature* 520:612. doi: 10.1038/520612a

Loosli, S. V., Buschkuehl, M., Perrig, W. J., and Jaeggi, S. M. (2012). Working memory training improves reading processes in typically developing children. *Child Neuropsychol.* 18, 62–78. doi: 10.1080/09297049.2011.575772

Lövdén, M., Ghisletta, P., and Lindenberger, U. (2005). Social participation attenuates decline in perceptual speed in old and very old age. *Psychol. Aging* 20, 423–434. doi: 10.1037/0882-7974.20.3.423

MacCallum, R. C., Zhang, S., Preacher, K. J., and Rucker, D. D. (2002). On the practice of dichotomization of quantitative variables. *Psychol. Methods* 7, 19–40. doi: 10.1037/1082-989x.7.1.19

McArdle, J. J. (2009). Latent variable modeling of differences and changes with longitudinal data. *Annu. Rev. Psychol.* 60, 577–605. doi: 10.1146/annurev.psych.60.110707.163612

McArdle, J. J., and Prindle, J. J. (2008). A latent change score analysis of a randomized clinical trial in reasoning training. *Psychol. Aging* 23, 702–719. doi: 10.1037/a0014349

Melby-Lervåg, M., and Hulme, C. (2013). Is working memory training effective? A meta-analytic review. *Dev. Psychol.* 49, 270–291. doi: 10.1037/a0028228

Moher, D., Pham, B., Jones, A., Cook, D. J., Jadad, A. R., Moher, M., et al. (1998). Does quality of reports of randomised trials affect estimates of intervention efficacy reported in meta-analyses? *Lancet* 352, 609–613. doi: 10.1016/s0140-6736(98)01085-x

Moreau, D. (2014a). Can brain training boost cognition? *Nature* 515:492. doi: 10.1038/515492c

Moreau, D. (2014b). Making sense of discrepancies in working memory training experiments: a Monte Carlo simulation. *Front. Syst. Neurosci.* 8:161. doi: 10.3389/fnsys.2014.00161

Moreau, D., and Conway, A. R. A. (2014). The case for an ecological approach to cognitive training. *Trends Cogn. Sci.* 18, 334–336. doi: 10.1016/j.tics.2014.03.009

Moreau, D., and Waldie, K. E. (2016). Developmental learning disorders: from generic interventions to individualized remediation. *Front. Psychol.* 6:2053. doi: 10.3389/fpsyg.2015.02053

Morey, R. D., and Rouder, J. N. (2011). Bayes factor approaches for testing interval null hypotheses. *Psychol. Methods* 16, 406–419. doi: 10.1037/a0024377

Nesselroade, J. R., Stigler, S. M., and Baltes, P. B. (1980). Regression toward the mean and the study of change. *Psychol. Bull.* 88, 622–637. doi: 10.1037/0033-2909.88.3.622

Neyman, J., and Pearson, E. S. (1933). On the problem of the most efficient tests of statistical hypotheses. *Philos. Trans. R. Soc. A Math. Phys. Eng. Sci.* 231, 289–337. doi: 10.1098/rsta.1933.0009

Noack, H., Lövdén, M., and Schmiedek, F. (2014). On the validity and generality of transfer effects in cognitive training research. *Psychol. Res.* 78, 773–789. doi: 10.1007/s00426-014-0564-6

Novick, J. M., Hussey, E., Teubner-Rhodes, S., Harbison, J. I., and Bunting, M. F. (2014). Clearing the garden-path: improving sentence processing through cognitive control training. *Lang. Cogn. Neurosci.* 29, 186–217. doi: 10.1080/01690965.2012.758297

Nuzzo, R. (2014). Scientific method: statistical errors. *Nature* 506, 150–152. doi: 10.1038/506150a

Open Science Collaboration. (2015). Estimating the reproducibility of psychological science. *Science* 349:aac4716. doi: 10.1126/science.aac4716

Pashler, H., and Wagenmakers, E.-J. (2012). Editors' introduction to the special section on replicability in psychological science: a crisis of confidence? *Perspect. Psychol. Sci.* 7, 528–530. doi: 10.1177/1745691612465253

Porsdam Mann, S., and Sahakian, B. J. (2015). The increasing lifestyle use of modafinil by healthy people: safety and ethical issues. *Curr. Opin. Behav. Sci.* 4, 136–141. doi: 10.1016/j.cobeha.2015.05.004

R Core Team. (2014). *R: A Language and Environment for Statistical Computing.* Vienna, Austria: R Foundation for Statistical Computing.

Redick, T. S., Shipstead, Z., Harrison, T. L., Hicks, K. L., Fried, D. E., Hambrick, D. Z., et al. (2013). No evidence of intelligence improvement after working memory training: a randomized, placebo-controlled study. *J. Exp. Psychol. Gen.* 142, 359–379. doi: 10.1037/a0029082

Revelle, W. (2015). *Psych: Procedures for Personality and Psychological Research.* Evanston, Illinois: Northwestern University.

Rouder, J. N., Speckman, P. L., Sun, D., Morey, R. D., and Iverson, G. (2009). Bayesian *t* tests for accepting and rejecting the null hypothesis. *Psychon. Bull. Rev.* 16, 225–237. doi: 10.3758/pbr.16.2.225

Rovine, M. J., and Molenaar, P. C. (2000). A structural modeling approach to a multilevel random coefficients model. *Multivariate Behav. Res.* 35, 51–88. doi: 10.1207/S15327906MBR3501_3

Rubinstein, R. Y., and Kroese, D. P. (2011). *Simulation and the Monte Carlo Method.* (Vol. 80). New York, NY: John Wiley & Sons.

Rudebeck, S. R., Bor, D., Ormond, A., O'Reilly, J. X., and Lee, A. C. H. (2012). A potential spatial working memory training task to improve both episodic memory and fluid intelligence. *PLoS One* 7:e50431. doi: 10.1371/journal.pone.0050431

Savage, L. J. (1954). *The Foundations of Statistics (Dover Edit.).* New York, NY: Wiley.

Schmidt, F. L. (1992). What do data really mean? Research findings, meta-analysis and cumulative knowledge in psychology. *Am. Psychol.* 47, 1173–1181. doi: 10.1037/0003-066x.47.10.1173

Schubert, T., and Strobach, T. (2012). Video game experience and optimized executive control skills—On false positives and false negatives: reply to Boot and Simons (2012). *Acta Psychol.* 141, 278–280. doi: 10.1016/j.actpsy.2012.06.010

Schweizer, S., Grahn, J., Hampshire, A., Mobbs, D., and Dalgleish, T. (2013). Training the emotional brain: improving affective control through emotional working memory training. *J. Neurosci.* 33, 5301–5311. doi: 10.1523/JNEUROSCI.2593-12.2013

Shipstead, Z., Redick, T. S., and Engle, R. W. (2012). Is working memory training effective? *Psychol. Bull.* 138, 628–654. doi: 10.1037/a0027473

Simmons, J. P., Nelson, L. D., and Simonsohn, U. (2011). False-positive psychology: undisclosed flexibility in data collection and analysis allows presenting anything as significant. *Psychol. Sci.* 22, 1359–1366. doi: 10.1177/0956797611417632

Simons, D. J. (2014). The value of direct replication. *Perspect. Psychol. Sci.* 9, 76–80. doi: 10.1177/1745691613514755

Simonsohn, U. (2015). Small telescopes: detectability and the evaluation of replication results. *Psychol. Sci.* 26, 559–569. doi: 10.1177/0956797614567341

Simonsohn, U., Nelson, L. D., and Simmons, J. P. (2014a). P-curve and effect size: correcting for publication bias using only significant results. *Perspect. Psychol. Sci.* 9, 666–681. doi: 10.1177/1745691614553988

Simonsohn, U., Nelson, L. D., and Simmons, J. P. (2014b). P-curve: a key to the file-drawer. *J. Exp. Psychol. Gen.* 143, 534–547. doi: 10.1037/a0033242

Spearman, C. (1904). "General intelligence" objectively determined and measured. *Am. J. Psychol.* 15, 201–293. doi: 10.2307/1412107

Spence, I., Yu, J. J., Feng, J., and Marshman, J. (2009). Women match men when learning a spatial skill. *J. Exp. Psychol. Learn. Mem. Cogn.* 35, 1097–1103. doi: 10.1037/a0015641

Stankov, L., and Chen, K. (1988a). Can we boost fluid and crystallised intelligence? A structural modelling approach. *Aust. J. Psychol.* 40, 363–376. doi: 10.1080/00049538808260056

Stankov, L., and Chen, K. (1988b). Training and changes in fluid and crystallized intelligence. *Contemp. Educ. Psychol.* 13, 382–397. doi: 10.1016/0361-476x(88)90037-9

Stevens, C., Harn, B., Chard, D. J., Currin, J., Parisi, D., and Neville, H. (2013). Examining the role of attention and instruction in at-risk kindergarteners: electrophysiological measures of selective auditory attention before and after an early literacy intervention. *J. Learn. Disabil.* 46, 73–86. doi: 10.1177/0022219411417877

te Nijenhuis, J., van Vianen, A. E. M., and van der Flier, H. (2007). Score gains on g-loaded tests: no g. *Intelligence* 35, 283–300. doi: 10.1016/j.intell.2006.07.006

Thompson, T. W., Waskom, M. L., Garel, K.-L. A., Cardenas-Iniguez, C., Reynolds, G. O., Winter, R., et al. (2013). Failure of working memory training to enhance cognition or intelligence. *PLoS One* 8:e63614. doi: 10.1371/journal.pone.0063614

Tidwell, J. W., Dougherty, M. R., Chrabaszcz, J. R., Thomas, R. P., and Mendoza, J. L. (2014). What counts as evidence for working memory training? Problems with correlated gains and dichotomization. *Psychon. Bull. Rev.* 21, 620–628. doi: 10.3758/s13423-013-0560-7

Tippmann, S. (2015). Programming tools: adventures with R. *Nature* 517, 109–110. doi: 10.1038/517109a

Trafimow, D., and Marks, M. (2015). Editorial. *Basic Appl. Soc. Psych.* 37, 1–2. doi: 10.1080/01973533.2015.1012991

van Assen, M. A. L. M., van Aert, R. C. M., Nuijten, M. B., and Wicherts, J. M. (2014). Why publishing everything is more effective than selective publishing of statistically significant results. *PLoS One* 9:e84896. doi: 10.1371/journal.pone.0084896

Venables, W. N., and Ripley, B. D. (2002). *Modern Applied Statistics with S.* 4th Edn. New York, NY: Springer.

Vul, E., Harris, C., Winkielman, P., and Pashler, H. (2009). Puzzlingly high correlations in fmri studies of emotion, personality and social cognition. *Perspect. Psychol. Sci.* 4, 274–290. doi: 10.1111/j.1745-6924.2009.01125.x

Wagenmakers, E.-J. (2007). A practical solution to the pervasive problems of p values. *Psychon. Bull. Rev.* 14, 779–804. doi: 10.3758/bf03194105

Wagenmakers, E.-J., Verhagen, J., Ly, A., Bakker, M., Lee, M. D., Matzke, D., et al. (2015). A power fallacy. *Behav. Res. Methods* 47, 913–917. doi: 10.3758/s13428-014-0517-4

Wetzels, R., Grasman, R. P. P. P., and Wagenmakers, E.-J. (2012). A default Bayesian hypothesis test for anova designs. *Am. Stat.* 66, 104–111. doi: 10.1080/00031305.2012.695956

Wetzels, R., and Wagenmakers, E.-J. (2012). A default Bayesian hypothesis test for correlations and partial correlations. *Psychon. Bull. Rev.* 19, 1057–1064. doi: 10.3758/s13423-012-0295-x

Wickham, H. (2009). *ggplot2: Elegant Graphics for Data Analysis.* New York, NY: Springer.

Wickham, H. (2011). The split-apply-combine strategy for data analysis. *J. Stat. Softw.* 40, 1–29. doi: 10.18637/jss.v040.i01

Zelinski, E. M., Peters, K. D., Hindin, S., Petway, K. T., and Kennison, R. F. (2014). Evaluating the relationship between change in performance on training tasks and on untrained outcomes. *Front. Hum. Neurosci.* 8:617. doi: 10.3389/fnhum.2014.00617

Zinke, K., Zeintl, M., Rose, N. S., Putzmann, J., Pydde, A., and Kliegel, M. (2014). Working memory training and transfer in older adults: effects of age, baseline performance and training gains. *Dev. Psychol.* 50, 304–315. doi: 10.1037/a0032982

6

Reading Aloud and Solving Simple Arithmetic Calculation Intervention (Learning Therapy) Improves Inhibition, Verbal Episodic Memory, Focus Attention and Processing Speed in Healthy Elderly People: Evidence from a Randomized Controlled Trial

Rui Nouchi[1,2,3], Yasuyuki Taki[4,5,6], Hikaru Takeuchi[6], Takayuki Nozawa[3,7], Atsushi Sekiguchi[5,8] and Ryuta Kawashima[3,6,7,9]*

[1] Creative Interdisciplinary Research Division, Frontier Research Institute for Interdisciplinary Science (FRIS), Tohoku University, Sendai, Japan, [2] Human and Social Response Research Division, International Research Institute of Disaster Science, Tohoku University, Sendai, Japan, [3] Smart Ageing International Research Centre, Institute of Development, Aging and Cancer, Tohoku University, Sendai, Japan, [4] Department of Nuclear Medicine and Radiology, Institute of Development, Aging and Cancer, Tohoku University, Sendai, Japan, [5] Division of Medical Neuroimage Analysis, Department of Community Medical Supports, Tohoku Medical Megabank Organization, Tohoku University, Sendai, Japan, [6] Division of Developmental Cognitive Neuroscience, Institute of Development, Aging and Cancer, Tohoku University, Sendai, Japan, [7] Department of Ubiquitous Sensing, PreClinical Research Center, Institute of Development, Aging and Cancer, Tohoku University, Sendai, Japan, [8] Department of Adult Mental Health, National Institute of Mental Health, National Center of Neurology and Psychiatry, Tokyo, Japan, [9] Department of Functional Brain Imaging, Institute of Development, Aging and Cancer, Tohoku University, Sendai, Japan

Edited by:
Soledad Ballesteros,
Universidad Nacional de Educación a Distancia (UNED), Spain

Reviewed by:
Hidenao Fukuyama,
Kyoto University, Japan
Eduard Kraft,
University of Munich, Germany

***Correspondence:**
Rui Nouchi
rui.nouchi.a4@tohoku.ac.jp

Background: Previous reports have described that simple cognitive training using reading aloud and solving simple arithmetic calculations, so-called "learning therapy", can improve executive functions and processing speed in the older adults. Nevertheless, it is not well-known whether learning therapy improve a wide range of cognitive functions or not. We investigated the beneficial effects of learning therapy on various cognitive functions in healthy older adults.

Methods: We used a single-blinded intervention with two groups (learning therapy group: LT and waiting list control group: WL). Sixty-four elderly were randomly assigned to LT or WL. In LT, participants performed reading Japanese aloud and solving simple calculations training tasks for 6 months. WL did not participate in the intervention. We measured several cognitive functions before and after 6 months intervention periods.

Results: Compared to WL, results revealed that LT improved inhibition performance in executive functions (Stroop: LT (Mean = 3.88) vs. WL (Mean = 1.22), adjusted $p = 0.013$ and reverse Stroop LT (Mean = 3.22) vs. WL (Mean = 1.59), adjusted $p = 0.015$), verbal episodic memory (Logical Memory (LM): LT (Mean = 4.59) vs. WL (Mean = 2.47), adjusted $p = 0.015$), focus attention (D-CAT: LT (Mean = 2.09) vs. WL

(Mean = −0.59), adjusted $p = 0.010$) and processing speed compared to the WL control group (digit symbol coding: LT (Mean = 5.00) vs. WL (Mean = 1.13), adjusted $p = 0.015$ and Symbol Search (SS): LT (Mean = 3.47) vs. WL (Mean = 1.81), adjusted $p = 0.014$).

Discussion: This randomized controlled trial (RCT) can be showed the benefit of LT on inhibition of executive functions, verbal episodic memory, focus attention and processing speed in healthy elderly people. Our results were discussed under overlapping hypothesis.

Keywords: learning therapy, cognitive training, reading aloud, simple calculation, transfer effect

BACKGROUND

Cognitive function changes during one's lifetime (Hedden and Gabrieli, 2004). Previous reports have described that older adults showed a decline in memory performance (Salthouse, 2003), attentional process (Yakhno et al., 2007), processing speed (Salthouse, 1996) and executive functions (Royall et al., 2004). Defining the term executive function is important. The term "executive function" is used as an umbrella for various complex cognitive processes and sub-processes (Elliott, 2003). Executive function includes the high-level cognitive processes that facilitate new ways of behaving and which optimize one's approach to unfamiliar circumstances (Gilbert and Burgess, 2008). Three main components in executive functions are "updating (constant monitoring and rapid addition/deletion of working-memory contents), shifting (switching flexibly between tasks or mental sets) and inhibition (deliberate overriding of dominant or proponent responses)" (Miyake et al., 2000; Miyake and Friedman, 2012). As described herein, we use executive function as a collective term includes updating, shifting and inhibition.

Previous studies have demonstrated improvements of cognitive functions in older adults (Verhaeghen et al., 1992; Ball et al., 2002; Clare and Woods, 2004; Edwards et al., 2005; Carretti et al., 2007; Green and Bavelier, 2008; Lustig et al., 2009; Jean et al., 2010; Nouchi et al., 2012a; Ballesteros et al., 2014). Cognitive training is an intervention program that provides structured practice on tasks related to aspects of cognitive function. There are many types of cognitive training such as working memory training (Richmond et al., 2011), processing speed training (Edwards et al., 2005, 2009), memory strategic training (Verhaeghen et al., 1992; Mahncke et al., 2006a; Carretti et al., 2007) and brain training game (Nouchi et al., 2012b; Anguera et al., 2013; Lampit et al., 2014; Toril et al., 2014). Developing cognitive training and validating the evidence of cognitive training have been at the forefront of scientific efforts (Nouchi and Kawashima, 2014).

Recently, cognitive training using reading aloud and solving of simple arithmetic calculations, so-called learning therapy (LT), has been developed (Kawashima et al., 2005; Uchida and Kawashima, 2008; Nouchi et al., 2012b). We were motivated to develop the new cognitive training based on following reasons. First, a previous study suggested that cognitive training should be designed in accordance with neuro-scientific evidence (Papp et al., 2009). Consequently, training tasks of learning therapy are created based on recent neuroimaging findings. Learning therapy uses reading text aloud and making simple calculations. Neuroimaging studies show that reading sentences with a voice (Miura et al., 2003, 2005) and simple arithmetic operations (Kawashima et al., 2004; Arsalidou and Taylor, 2011) activated the frontal, temporal and parietal cortices. Second, psychological stress related cognitive training reduced the improvements of cognitive functions after cognitive training (McAvinue et al., 2013). We selected extremely simple and easy tasks to do during intervention periods. Additionally, the training tasks are more familiar activities for older people because reading and calculation are parts of everyday life. Moreover, the training tasks use only papers and pencils. Consequently, elderly people can comprehend and perform training tasks. Third, previous results of studies have suggested that multiple components in training tasks facilitate to improvement of cognitive functions (Stuss et al., 2007; Green and Bavelier, 2008). Reading aloud and solving arithmetic problems are accomplished using a combination of cognitive processes including memory, attention and executive functions (inhibition, shifting and updating; Nouchi et al., 2012b). Therefore, we prepared reading aloud and mathematical calculations tasks as training tasks of learning therapy. Learning therapy is expected to have greater effects than previous cognitive training because it alleviates the difficulties mentioned above.

An earlier report described that learning therapy improves executive functions, episodic memory and processing speed (Kawashima et al., 2005; Uchida and Kawashima, 2008; Yoshida et al., 2014). However, there is no study which investigates the positive effects of learning therapy on various cognitive functions (e.g., memory and attention) in elderly people. Previous studies did not measure any cognitive function except for executive functions and processing speed. It is necessary to test the effectiveness of learning therapy on diverse cognitive functions, because various cognitive functions are necessary to support our actions and behaviors in everyday life.

As we mentioned before, the previous studies using learning therapy showed only improvements of executive functions, episodic memory and processing speed (Kawashima et al., 2005; Uchida and Kawashima, 2008; Yoshida et al., 2014).

It is still unclear whether or not learning therapy can facilitate performance of other cognitive domains such as episodic memory, short term memory, working memory, reading ability and attention. Thus, this study was designed to investigate whether or not learning therapy can improve diverse cognitive functions in elderly people. There were essential differences from previous studies. First, the current study was aimed to validate the previous finding using the different cognitive tests in the same domains such as executive functions and processing speed. For example, previous studies used: (1) Frontal Assessment Battery (FAB) as the executive functional measure (Kawashima et al., 2005; Uchida and Kawashima, 2008); (2) the digit symbol coding as the processing speed measure (Kawashima et al., 2005; Uchida and Kawashima, 2008); and (3) the word list as the episodic memory measure (Yoshida et al., 2014). On the other hand, we newly used Stroop and verbal fluency tests for the executive functional measure, Symbol Search (SS) for the processing speed andLogical Memory (LM) and face-name association memory for the episodic memory measure. Second, we measure other cognitive domains such as focus attention, short-term memory and working memory which did not measure in the previous articles. Thus, we can firstly investigate the beneficial effects of LT on a wide range of cognitive functions in one study.

To elucidate the beneficial effects of learning therapy on a wide range of cognitive function, we conducted single-blinded randomized controlled trials (RCT) using learning therapy. Testers who conducted psychological tests were blinded to the study hypothesis and the group membership (learning therapy group or not). To test the benefits of learning therapy, we assessed a broad range of cognitive functions. We measured inhibition and shifting of executive functions, verbal and facial episodic memory, short-term memory, working memory, reading ability, focus attention and processing speed.

Based on previous studies using cognitive training related to reading and mathematical calculations, we hypothesized that learning therapy would improve the inhibition performance in executive functional domain, verbal episodic memory in episodic memory domain, focus attention and processing speed in the healthy elderly people. Several reasons exist: (1) regarding the inhibition performance, a previous study (Uchida and Kawashima, 2008) found that performance of FAB (Dubois et al., 2000) which measured executive functions improved after learning therapy. Especially, the sub score (sensitivity to an interference task) of FAB was increased after learning therapy. The sensitivity to an interference task requiring behavioral self-regulation under verbal commands conflicts with sensory information. It may be highly correlated with the inhibition ability in executive functions. This task is similar to the Stroop task. Cognitive training using calculation (Takeuchi et al., 2011) and video game training (Nouchi et al., 2013), which included reading aloud and mental calculations, in young adults showed the improvements of the Stroop task. Consequently, we hypothesized that learning therapy can improve the inhibition performance measured by Stroop task performance; (2) for episodic memory, a previous study using working memory training, which included calculation training, demonstrated improvements of episodic memory (McAvinue et al., 2013). An earlier long-term intervention study using reading aloud and calculation revealed improvements of verbal episodic memory as measured by word lists (Yoshida et al., 2014). Consequently, we hypothesized that learning therapy would engender improvements of verbal episodic memory performance measured by LM test; (3) for focus attention, to solve mathematical calculations and reading sentences, it is necessary to examine the present information (focus attention) specifically. We assume that the focus attention ability would be improved by simple calculation and reading aloud tasks; and (4) for processing speed, our report of a previous study described improvements of processing speed measured by digit symbol coding (Uchida and Kawashima, 2008). Additionally, video game training using reading aloud and calculations also showed improvements of processing speed measured by SS (Nouchi et al., 2013). Based on the previous finding, we hypothesized that processing speed measured by SS and digit symbol coding. Therefore, we assumed that learning therapy engenders improvements of inhibition, verbal episodic memory, focus attention and processing speed compared to the control group.

METHODS

Randomized Controlled Trial Design and Setting of this Trial

The following information was the same as our protocol article (Nouchi et al., 2012b). This study was a RCT. This study "conducted in Sendai city, Miyagi prefecture, Japan. Written informed consent to participate in the study was obtained from each participant based on the Declaration of Helsinki before enrolment. Informed consent were approved by the Ethics Committee of the Tohoku University Graduate School of Medicine (ref. 2011-153). This study was registered in the University Hospital Medical Information Network (UMIN) Clinical Trial Registry (UMIN000006998)" (Nouchi et al., 2012b).

To assess the impact of learning therapy on widely diverse cognitive functions in healthy elderly people, we used a single-blinded intervention with two parallel groups: a learning therapy group and a waiting list (WL) control group. Testers were blind to the study's hypothesis and the group membership of participants. The Consolidated Standards of Reporting Trials (CONSORT) statement (http://www.consort-statement.org/home/) was used as a framework for developing the study methodology (see Supplementary Material 1). The trial design is presented in **Figure 1**.

Participants

Seventy-two participants were recruited from Sendai city through advertisements in the local town paper (Kahoku weekly; **Figure 1**). A procedure of recruitment of participants was the same as our previous study (Nouchi et al., 2014). Sample

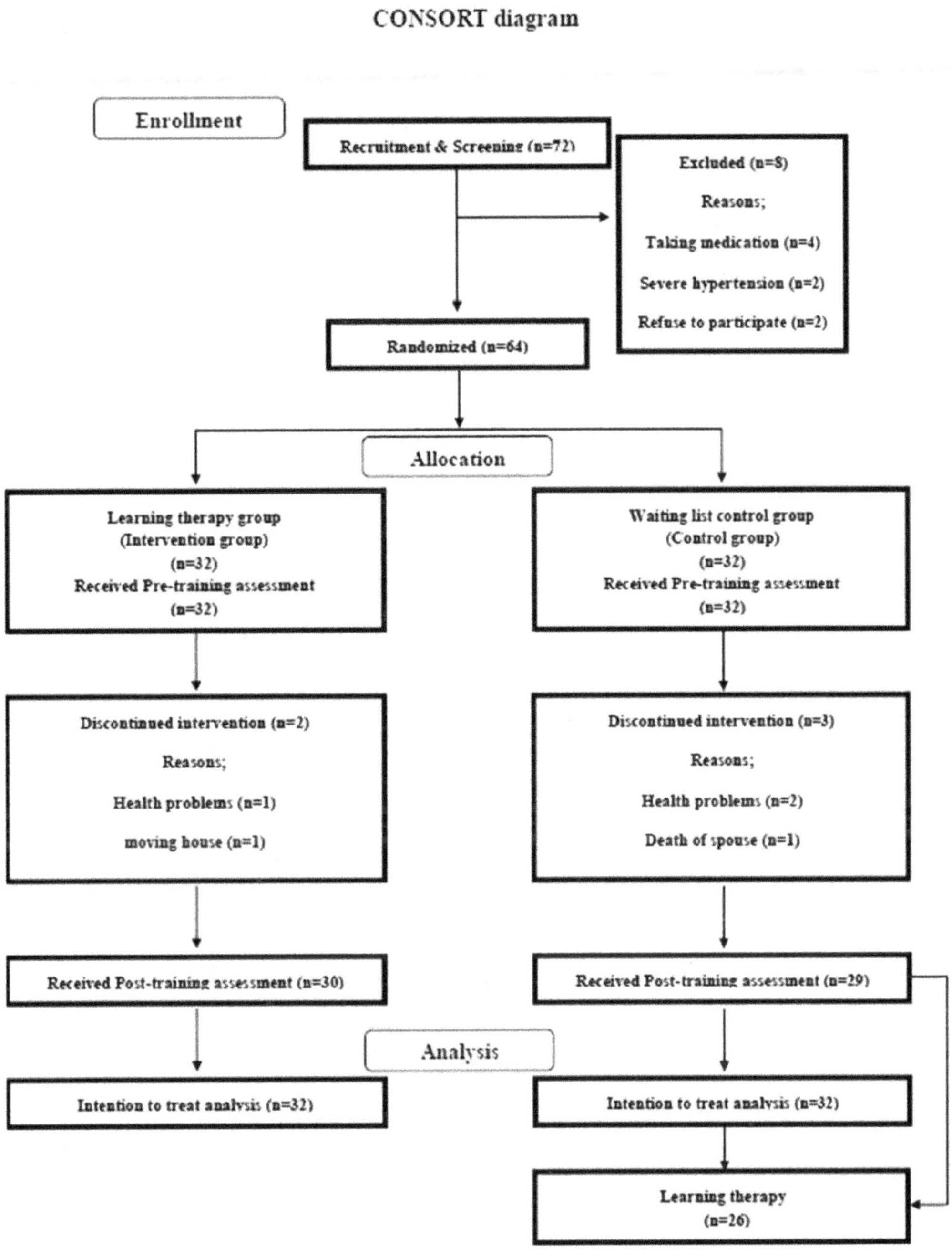

FIGURE 1 | Consolidated standards of reporting trials (CONSORT) flowchart.

size calculation was written in Supplementary Material 2. Interested participants were screened using a semi-structured telephone interview, during which we asked participants for their demographic information (e.g., age and gender) and asked the same questions related to our inclusion and exclusion criteria (e.g., past medical histories of disease known to affect the central nervous system and using medications known to interfere with cognitive functions). "After the telephone interview, four people were excluded because they reported taking medications known to interfere with cognitive function (including benzodiazepines, antidepressants and other central nervous agents)" (Nouchi et al., 2012b). Two people were excluded based on severe hypertension (systolic blood pressure over 180, diastolic blood pressure over 110). Two participants declined to participate before a random assignment. All included participants (n = 64) were invited to visit Tohoku University for more detailed screening assessment (JART) and Mini-Mental State Examination (MMSE;

TABLE 1 | Characteristics of participants in the learning therapy group and the waiting list control groups.

	Learning therapy group		Wait list control group		
	Mean	SD	Mean	SD	*p*-value
Age (years)	72.81	(6.18)	71.38	(4.92)	0.31
Education (years)	13.25	(2.00)	12.69	(1.40)	0.20
MMSE (score)	28.34	(0.86)	28.44	(0.76)	0.65
Arithmetic from WAIS (score)	11.44	(2.42)	11.13	(2.42)	0.61
Vocabulary WAIS (score)	31.19	(4.37)	31.03	(4.65)	0.89
JART (score)	19.97	(3.47)	19.21	(4.30)	0.44
Estimated IQ from JART (score)	109.91	(7.03)	108.50	(8.61)	0.48

No significant difference was found between combination exercise training and the waiting list control groups (two-sample t-test, $p > 0.10$). JART, Japanese Reading test; SD, standard deviation; MMSE, Mini-Mental State Examination; WAIS, Wechsler Adult Intelligence Scale III.

Folstein et al., 1975) and to provide written informed consent. No participant was excluded based on JART scores. Randomization was conducted after receiving the informed consent statement from participants. Before the intervention period, we measured reading abilities using a sub-scale of Wechsler Adult Intelligence Scale (WAIS) such as Vocabulary (Wechsler, 1997) and arithmetic abilities using a sub-scale of WAIS such as Arithmetic (Wechsler, 1997). **Table 1** presents the baseline characteristics. There were no significant differences between the groups in all data (two-sample *t*-test, $p > 0.10$). The scores of MMSE and IQ were within the range of normality.

Details of sample size calculation was described in the protocol of this study (Nouchi et al., 2012b).

Learning Therapy Group (Cognitive Intervention Group)

The cognitive intervention method was the same as that used in our previous study with learning therapy for healthy older adults (Uchida and Kawashima, 2008). Training tasks use two simple tasks (solving arithmetic and Japanese language problems) with systematized basic problems in arithmetic and reading (Uchida and Kawashima, 2008). The example of training tasks showed in **Figures 2, 3.** The lowest level of difficulty in simple calculation was simple addition (e.g., 1 + 3). The highest level of calculation was three figure number division (e.g., 156 ÷ 3). The lowest level of difficulty in reading aloud was reading simple sentences of 17 characters such as Japanese Haiku poems. The highest level was reading fairy tales aloud (about 100–120 characters per page). The difficulties of the Japanese Language problems were based on the number of Japanese characters per page because it takes more time to read aloud sentences with more characters.

Before intervention, we measured the percentages of correct answers and the time it takes to solve the diagnostic tests. The diagnostic tests consisted of 70 simple arithmetic and 16 simple reading tests. Based on the diagnostic tests, the appropriate level and workload in training tasks were set. In these tasks, participant was able to solve the problems with ease and without mental stress within 15 min. The difficulty level of training tasks and workloads did not change during the intervention period.

The cognitive intervention was scheduled to be conducted for 23 weeks. Participants in the cognitive intervention group were asked to go to a classroom at Tohoku University once a week. They were instructed to complete five sheets of each task prepared for each participant for that day. The daily learning time for the two tasks was approximately 15 min. They were required to complete five sheets of each task as homework for 4–6 days a week.

Waiting List Control Group (No Cognitive Intervention Group)

The following texts were the same as our previous protocol article (Nouchi et al., 2012b). "The waiting list control group received no intervention. Those participants were informed by letter that they were scheduled to receive an invitation to participate after a waiting period of 6 months. No placebo was used for the social contact group" (Nouchi et al., 2012b). Results of previous intervention studies (Clark et al., 1997; Mahncke et al., 2006) showed that "a placebo group was unnecessary for study of this type because no difference existed in cognitive or functional improvement between the placebo and no-social-contact groups (control group)" (Nouchi et al., 2012b). After a waiting period of 6 months, 26 elderly people in the waiting list group participated in the learning therapy. Six elderly people declined to receive the learning therapy because three elderly people dropped out during the waiting period and three elderly did not want to receive the learning therapy after the waiting period.

There were several reasons why we used the waiting list control group. To investigate beneficial effects of cognitive training, we should use certain control conditions because of reductions in the influence of practice effects and cognitive declines by aging. Several studies used no-contact or waiting list groups (Levine et al., 2007; Basak et al., 2008; Shatil et al., 2010; McDougall and House, 2012). On the other hand, many activities were selected for active control conditions (Buiza et al., 2008; Peretz et al., 2011; Nouchi et al., 2012a). For instance, there were many types of activities in the active control groups such as selecting letters in the newspaper (Herrera et al., 2012), leaning trivia using web sites (Richmond et al., 2011a) and video games (Nouchi et al., 2012a). From a methodological perspective, it would be better to use an other intervention program as an active

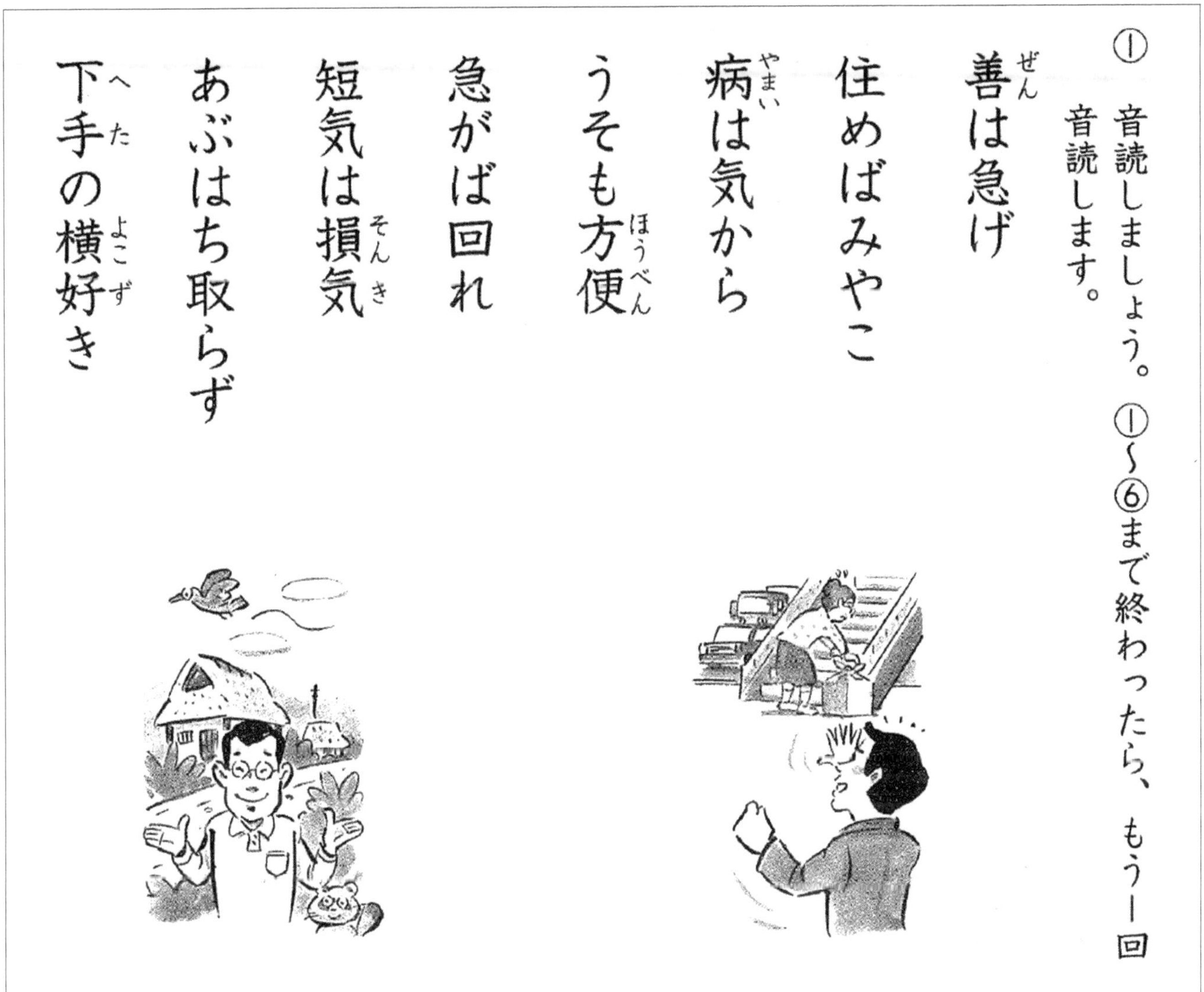
①音読しましょう。①〜⑥まで終わったら、もう一回
音読します。
善は急げ
住めばみやこ
病は気から
うそも方便
急がば回れ
短気は損気
あぶはち取らず
下手の横好き

FIGURE 2 | An example of the training task for reading aloud.

control group in the cognitive training studies compared to use a waiting list control group. However, to use an active control group, we should consider an ethical issue. Using the active control group should be "a reasonable balance of the level of benefit to the time investment required of participants in the treatment group" (Street and Luoma, 2002). An active control group with meaningless and worthless tasks is not suitable. In the cognitive training research field, there is no standard and appropriate task for the active control group. The choice of an active control condition must be considered within costs, research questions and ethical considerations. Additionally, results of previous intervention studies (Clark et al., 1997; Mahncke et al., 2006) reported that a placebo group was unnecessary for study of this type because no difference existed in cognitive or functional improvement between the placebo and no-social-contact groups (control group). Moreover, using the waiting list control group had "the advantage of letting everyone in the study receive the new intervention (sooner or later)" (Nouchi et al., 2014). Therefore, we decided to the waiting list control group.

Cognitive Function Measures

The following texts were the same as our previous article (Nouchi et al., 2012b). To test the positive effects of learning therapy on performance in cognitive functions, we used several cognitive measures (**Table 2**). "Measures of the cognitive functions were divisible into seven categories (executive functions, episodic memory, short-term memory, working memory, reading ability, attention and processing speed)" (Nouchi et al., 2012b). Executive functions were measured by the Stroop Test (ST; Hakoda and Sasaki, 1990; Watanabe et al., 2011) and Verbal fluency task (VFT; Ito et al., 2004). The ST had ST and reverse ST (rST) conditions. For ST, participants were required to select a word corresponding to the ink color in the color–word combination. For rST participants were asked to choose a color

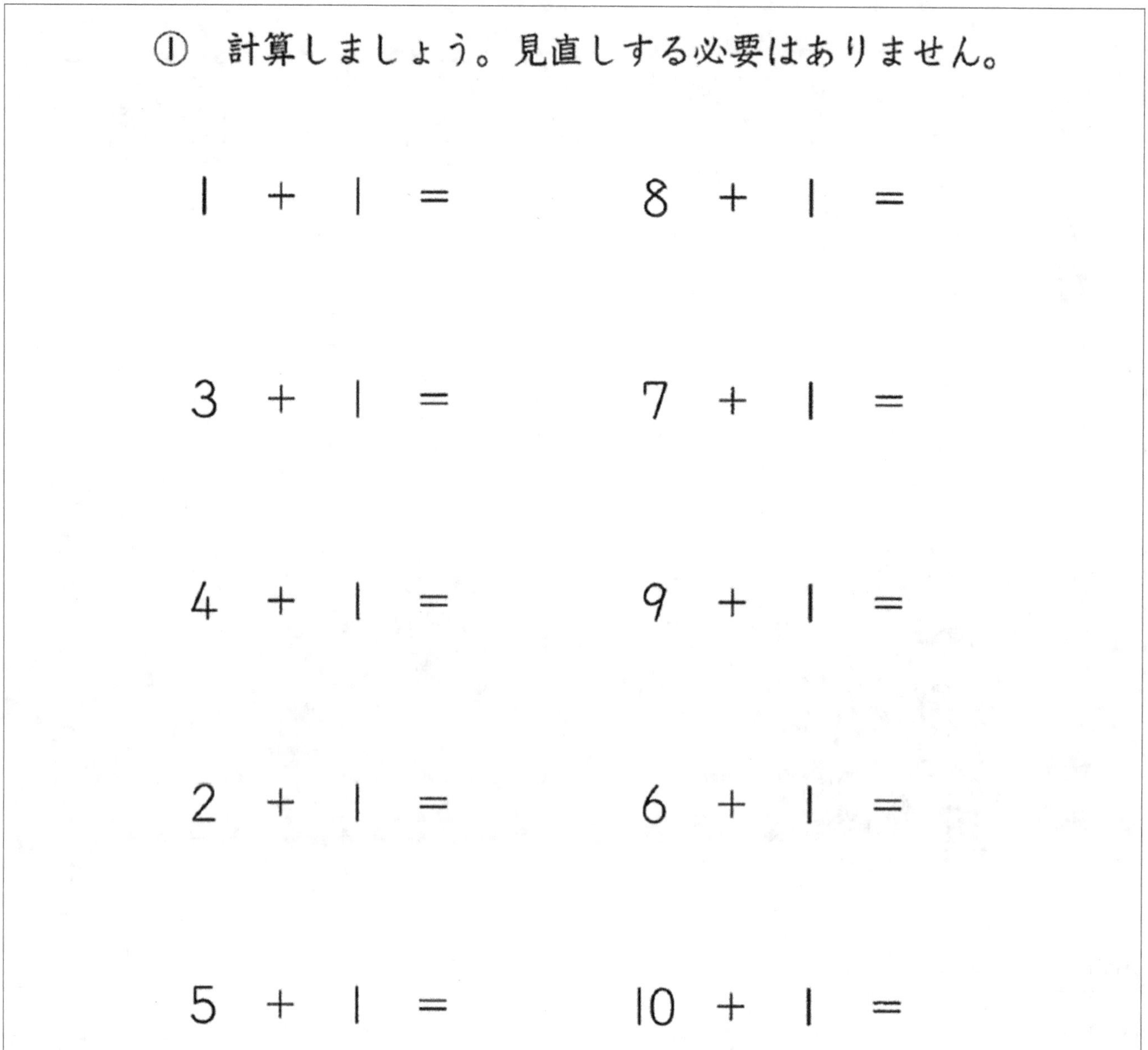

FIGURE 3 | An example of the training task for simple calculation.

item corresponding to a color–word combination's semantic meaning or selection. For VFT, we used Japanese version's letter fluency task (LFT) and category fluency (CFT) task. Participants were asked to generate many words beginning with the specific letter (LFT) or many words of a category (CFT). Episodic memory was measured using LM (Wechsler, 1987) and First and Second Names (FSN; Wilson et al., 1985). For LM, participants were asked to memorize the short story. For FSN, participants were asked to memorize FSN with faces. Verbal short-term memory was measured by Digit Span Forward (DS-F; Wechsler, 1997). For DS-F, participants were asked to memorize numbers and repeat the numbers. Working memory was measured using Digit Span Backward (DS-B; Wechsler, 1997). For DS-B, participants were require to memorize digit numbers and answer the number in reverse order. Reading ability was measured by the Japanese Reading Test (JART; Matsuoka et al., 2006). JART was reading test of 25 Japanese Kanji. The Digit Cancellation Task (D-CAT) was used to measure focus attention (Hatta et al., 2000). For D-CAT, participants were asked to check the target number in 12 rows of 50 digits. Digit Symbol Coding (Cd; Wechsler, 1997) and SS (Wechsler, 1997) were used for processing speed tests. For Cd, participants were required to write the symbol corresponding to the number. For SS, participants were required to search the target symbols in five symbols. Details of all tasks are described in the Supplementary Material 2. We assessed these cognitive function measures before and after the intervention period (6 months).

TABLE 2 | Summary of cognitive function measures.

Cognitive function	Task
Executive functions	Verbal fluency task
	Stroop test
Attention	Digit cancellation task
Episodic memory	Logical memory
	First and second names
Short-term memory	Digit span forward
Working memory	Digit span backward
Reading ability	Japanese reading test
Processing speed	Digit symbol coding
	Symbol Search

Analysis

This study was designed to evaluate the beneficial effect of learning therapy in elderly people. The following analysis method was also presented in our protocol article (Nouchi et al., 2012b). We calculated the change score (post-training score minus pre-training score) in all cognitive function measures. We conducted ANCOVA for the change scores in each cognitive test. The change scores were the dependent variable. Groups (learning therapy, waiting list control) were the independent variable. Pre-training scores in the dependent variable, sex and age were the covariates to exclude the possibility that any pre-existing difference of measure between groups affects the result of each measure and adjust for background characteristics. Significance was inferred for $p < 0.05$. We used Storey's False discovery rate (FDR) correction methods to adjust the p values (Storey, 2002). Moreover, this report describes eta squared (η^2) as an index of effect size (Cohen, 1988). Missing data were imputed using the expectation maximization method, as implemented in the Statistical Package for the Social Sciences (SPSS) Missing Value Analysis. It imputed missing values using maximum likelihood estimation with observed data in an iterative process (Dempster et al., 1977; Nouchi et al., 2012b). All randomized participants were included in the analyses in line with their allocation, irrespective of how many sessions they completed (intention-to-treat principle). All analyses were conducted using software (SPSS ver. 18 or higher; SPSS Inc.).

RESULTS

Sixty-four elderly people participated in this RCT (learning therapy and waiting list control). Thirty of the 32 members of the learning therapy group and 29 of the 32 members of the waiting list control group were completed. We imputed missing values of two participants in the learning therapy group and three participants in the waiting list control group using intention-to-treat principle (see "Analysis" Section). The pre-training and post-training scores in cognitive functions are presented in **Table 3**.

To test the positive effect of the learning therapy on the improvement of cognitive functions, we did ANCOVA for the change scores in each cognitive test (**Table 4**). We found significant group differences in four cognitive domains (executive functions, episodic memory, attention and processing speed). For executive functions, the learning therapy group improved the ST score (learning therapy (Mean = 3.88) vs. waiting list control (Mean = 1.22), $F_{(1,59)}$ = 7.35, η^2 = 0.11, *adjusted p* = 0.013) and the rST score (learning therapy (Mean = 3.22) vs. waiting list control (Mean = 1.59), $F_{(1,59)}$ = 8.72, η^2 = 0.09, *adjusted p* = 0.015). For episodic memory, the learning therapy group improved the LM score (learning therapy (Mean = 4.59) vs. waiting list control (Mean = 2.47), $F_{(1,59)}$ = 9.72, η^2 = 0.12, *adjusted p* = 0.015). For focus attention, learning therapy group improved the D-CAT score (learning therapy (Mean = 2.09) vs. waiting list control (Mean = -0.59), $F_{(1,59)}$ = 12.23, η^2 = 0.14, *adjusted p* = 0.010). For processing speed, learning therapy group improved the Cd score (learning therapy (Mean = 5.00) vs. waiting list control (Mean = 1.13), $F_{(1,59)}$ = 9.85, η^2 = 0.13, *adjusted p* = 0.015) and the SS score (learning therapy (Mean = 3.47) vs. waiting list control (Mean = 1.81), $F_{(1,59)}$ = 7.81, η^2 = 0.10, *adjusted p* = 0.014). These results demonstrate that the learning therapy led to improvements of inhibition performance in executive functions, verbal episodic memory's measures, focus attentional measure and all processing speed's measures.

DISCUSSION

We investigated the positive effects of learning therapy on diverse cognitive functions in healthy elderly people. Results showed clearly that the learning therapy group exhibited improved inhibition performance of executive functions measured by ST and rST, verbal episodic memory measured by LM, focus attention measured by D-CAT and processing speed measured by SS and Cd compared to the waiting list control group. These results supported our hypothesis. The improvements of Cd performance of processing speed after learning therapy are consistent with previous evidence (Kawashima et al., 2005; Uchida and Kawashima, 2008). However, this study extends the previous finding by demonstrating improvements of focus attention and by replicating improvement of inhibition process and processing speed using different cognitive functional measures such as ST, rST and SS after learning therapy.

The overlapping hypothesis can explain the present results (Nouchi et al., 2012a, 2013, 2014). The overlapping hypothesis hypothesizes that improvements of cognitive functions by a certain type of training would occur if the processes during both cognitive training tasks (e.g., reading aloud and calculation simple arithmetic problem) and untrained tasks (e.g., measures of cognitive functions) were overlapped and were involved in similar cognitive processes. In this study, participants were required to undertake learning therapy, which included a reading aloud task and a simple arithmetic calculation problem task. As we described in the background reading aloud and simple arithmetic calculation involve many cognitive components and processes. To perform these tasks, inhibition process related to executive functions, verbal episodic memory,

TABLE 3 | Cognitive function scores before and after training period in both groups.

	Learning therapy group				Wait list control group				
	Pre		Post		Pre		Post		
	Mean	SD	Mean	SD	Mean	SD	Mean	SD	*p*-value
Executive functions									
LFT (number)	8.56	(2.53)	9.38	(2.64)	9.59	(3.35)	10.28	(2.82)	0.17
CFT (number)	11.06	(2.84)	11.72	(2.77)	11.41	(2.08)	11.44	(3.26)	0.58
rST (number)	27.44	(6.87)	31.31	(5.87)	28.63	(6.47)	29.84	(6.66)	0.48
ST (number)	41.41	(9.00)	44.63	(8.29)	40.78	(9.15)	42.38	(8.73)	0.78
Attention									
D-CAT (number)	26.31	(5.87)	28.41	(4.98)	26.84	(5.48)	26.25	(5.47)	0.71
Episodic memory									
LM (score)	7.31	(2.22)	11.91	(2.80)	8.09	(2.84)	10.56	(2.94)	0.23
FSN (score)	2.97	(1.60)	3.34	(1.89)	3.66	(1.79)	4.00	(2.06)	0.11
Short-term memory									
DS-F (score)	5.13	(0.87)	4.97	(1.18)	5.56	(1.37)	5.34	(1.33)	0.16
Working memory									
DS-B (score)	4.09	(0.86)	3.97	(0.82)	4.38	(1.29)	4.13	(1.13)	0.31
Processing speed									
Cd (number)	64.56	(13.15)	69.56	(13.21)	66.84	(11.48)	67.97	(11.37)	0.61
SS (number)	33.00	(6.15)	36.47	(5.51)	32.81	(6.17)	34.63	(6.41)	0.90
Verbal ability									
JART (score)	19.97	(3.47)	20.34	(3.30)	19.25	(4.30)	19.50	(4.15)	0.46

Group comparison (two sample t-tests) of the pre-training scores revealed no significant difference in any measure of cognitive functions between the learning therapy group and the waiting list control group (p > 0.10). Pre, pre-training; post, post-training; SD, standard deviation. Executive functions were measured using the Stroop Test (ST) and Verbal fluency task (VFT). Attention was measured using the Digit Cancellation Task (D-CAT). Episodic Memory was measured using Logical Memory (LM) and First and Second Names (FSN). Short-term memory was measured using Digit Span Forward (DS-F). Working memory was measured using Digit span Backward (DS-B). Processing speed was measured using Digit Symbol Coding (Cd) and Symbol Search (SS). Reading ability was measured using the Japanese Reading Test (JART).

focus attention and processing speed are expected to be recruited. For instance, attentions are necessary to modulate one's own voice during reading sentences aloud and inhibition ability is important to select and use rules of mathematics during calculation. Long-term Memory (semantic and verbal episodic memory) is expected to be necessary to read a sentence and to comprehend the sentence during reading aloud (LaBerge and Samuels, 1974; Myers et al., 2000). When we read a sentence, we construct a mental representation, known as the situation model (Kintsch, 1994; Zwaan and Radvansky, 1998). To facilitate understanding and integration of incoming information from sentence, we use related information from verbal long-term memory (Cook et al., 1998). Both semantic and verbal episodic memories are important to create and elaborate the situation model (Van Dijk and Kintsch, 1983; Kintsch et al., 1999). Some previous studies showed that semantic memory has the most important role in reading and comprehending the sentences (Garrod and Terras, 2000). Especially, the patient with episodic memory dysfunctions has no problem with reading (Tulving et al., 1988). Thus, most theories assume that comprehending and reading a sentence rely on more on semantic rather than on episodic memory. However, for healthy people, verbal episodic memory may influence reading processing as early as general world knowledge (Myers et al., 2000). One previous study reported that the verbal episodic memory for prior text facilitated the reading process (Haviland and Clark, 1974). Verbal episodic memory for prior texts is reactivated automatically when we encounter the related information during reading sentences (Myers and O'Brien, 1998). Consequently, verbal episodic memory is also necessary to read and comprehend texts as well as semantic memory. Focus attention is expected to be necessary to perform each task with concentration. Processing speed has a important role to solve mathematical problems and to read as fast as possible during a training period. The overlapping hypothesis explains the improvements of inhibition in executive functions, verbal episodic memory, focus attention and processing speed after learning therapy that follows. First, it would take the mental processes described above to perform the reading aloud task and the simple arithmetic calculation problem task. Second, both these training tasks and the cognitive tests can share the similar cognitive processes. Third, the cognitive processes described above are expected to be facilitated by these training tasks. Therefore, inhibition performance in executive functions, verbal episodic memory, focus attention and processing speed were improved after these training tasks.

Considering common elements of improved cognitive functional measures, it may be true that learning therapy generally improved the speed of processing related to task performance. Improved cognitive functional measures such as ST, rST, D-CAT, SS and Cd required participants to do the task as quickly as possible during a limited time (please see "Methods" Section). Two training tasks also require that participants complete materials of two training tasks as quickly as possible. Based on the overlapping hypothesis, both cognitive training tasks such as reading aloud and simple calculations and the psychological tests which measured the cognitive

TABLE 4 | Change scores in cognitive functions measures of both groups.

	Learning therapy		Wait list control		Effect size		Adjusted	Results
	Mean	SD	Mean	SD	(η^2)	*p*-value	*p*-value	of ANCOVA
Executive functions								
LFT (number)	0.81	(1.82)	0.69	(2.21)	0.00	0.607	0.759	ns
CFT (number)	0.66	(2.59)	0.03	(2.79)	0.01	0.396	0.566	ns
rST (number)	3.22	(1.90)	1.59	(2.53)	0.09	0.009	0.015	LT > WL
ST (number)	3.88	(3.44)	1.22	(3.90)	0.11	0.005	0.013	LT > WL
Episodic memory								
LM (score)	4.59	(2.75)	2.47	(2.30)	0.12	0.003	0.015	LT > WL
FSN (score)	0.38	(1.79)	0.34	(1.81)	0.00	0.650	0.650	ns
Short-term memory								
DS-F (score)	(0.16)	(1.05)	(0.22)	(0.83)	0.01	0.457	0.784	ns
Working memory								
DS-B (score)	(0.13)	(0.75)	(0.25)	(1.34)	0.00	0.862	0.781	ns
Attention								
D-CAT (number)	2.09	(2.99)	(0.59)	(3.15)	0.14	0.001	0.010	LT > WL
Processing speed								
Cd (number)	5.00	(4.31)	1.13	(4.77)	0.13	0.003	0.015	LT > WL
SS (number)	3.47	(2.98)	1.81	(2.60)	0.10	0.007	0.014	LT > WL
Verbal ability								
JART (score)	0.38	(1.50)	0.25	(1.30)	0.00	0.622	0.691	ns

Change scores were calculated by subtracting the pre-cognitive measure score from the post-cognitive measure score. We conducted analysis of covariance (ANCOVA) for the change scores in each of cognitive tests. In the ANCOVA, pre-training scores in each cognitive test, sex and age were the covariates. Significance was inferred for $p < 0.05$. The p values were adjusted using FDR method. Moreover, this report describes eta square (η^2) as an index of effect size. As a descriptive index of strength of association between an experimental factor (main effect or interaction effect) and a dependent variable, η^2 is defined as the proportion of total variation attributable to the factor, and it ranges in value from 0 to 1. $\eta^2 \geq 0.01$ is regarded as a small effect, $\eta^2 \geq 0.06$ as a medium effect, and $\eta^2 \geq 0.14$ as a large effect. LT, learning therapy; WL, waiting list control group; SD, standard deviation. Executive functions were measured using the Stroop Test (ST) and Verbal fluency task (VFT). Episodic Memory was measured using Logical Memory (LM) and First and Second Names (FSN). Short-term memory was measured using Digit Span Forward (DS-F). Working memory was measured using Digit span Backward (DS-B). Attention was measured using the Digit Cancellation Task (D-CAT). Processing speed was measured using Digit Symbol Coding (Cd) and Symbol Search (SS). Reading ability was measured using the Japanese Reading Test (JART).

functions can share the elements of speed of processing. Therefore, performances of cognitive functional measures that require speed of participants were improved by learning therapy.

It is important to consider dissociations of improvements in executive functions and episodic memory measures. The benefits of learning therapy did not generalize to all tasks in the same functions. In this study, the learning therapy group improved inhibition performance of executive functions (rST and ST) but not other shifting performance of executive functions (LFT and CFT). Additionally, the learning therapy improved verbal episodic memory measure such as LM, but not the facial episodic memory measure such as FSN. According to the overlapping hypothesis, the possibility exists that these training tasks (reading aloud and calculation simple arithmetic problems) and cognitive function measures such as LFT, CFT and FSN might not share the same cognitive processes. For instance, previous studies showed that LFT and CFT require both the generation of words within a subcategory (clustering) and the ability to shift to a new category when a subcategory is exhausted (switching; Troyer et al., 1998). FSN requires a face recognition process and an association between FSN and between faces and names (Wilson et al., 1985). As described earlier herein, these cognitive processes (clustering, switching, face recognition and association) did not include cognitive processes during reading aloud and arithmetic calculation problems. Consequently, the respective levels of performance of LFT, CFT and FSN were not improved by learning therapy.

Dissociation result of episodic memory can also be explained by the following ideas. For episodic memory, participants may become more familiar with the story structure by reading aloud training. Therefore, participants would be able to use the knowledge to encode information better after the reading aloud training. This idea can predict only the improvement of LM, but not the FSN.

From the perspective of definition of executive functions, three main components exist in executive functions. Based on this, learning therapy improved only the inhibition ability in executive functions, but not the shifting ability. The improvement of the inhibition ability after reading aloud and simple calculation training was consistent with our previous results (Uchida and Kawashima, 2008; Nouchi et al., 2013). Our dissociation results of executive functions suggest that it is necessary to prepare multiple cognitive measures in each cognitive domain such as executive functions and episodic memory. Moreover, in future studies, we have to focus on one area of cognitive domain (e.g., working memory) and use varied measures for the specific cognitive domain (operating span, reading span, n-back and digit (spatial) span). It may reveal a great deal about the impact of cognitive intervention on cognitive functions in the elderly people.

In addition, discussion of negative findings of no improvements of verbal ability, short-term memory and working memory is important. For verbal ability measured by JART, participants must read Kanji compound words. The difficulty level of the kanji words in JART is higher than that in the junior high school. However, the difficulty level of kanji in the reading aloud task would be lower than that in JART because our texts for the reading aloud task are based on first-grade to fourth-grade elementary school students (please see "Methods" Section). Thus, the participants did not learn how to read difficult kanji through intervention. Therefore, learning therapy did not show the improvement of JART performance. In addition, we found no significant improvements of short-term and working memory measured by DS-F and DS-B. No improvements of short-term and working memory performance would come from the lack of adaptive elements for the training tasks. Some previous studies demonstrated that intensive adaptive training would facilitate improvements of cognitive functions (Takeuchi et al., 2011; McAvinue et al., 2013). One previous study using mental calculation training in young adults reported that the intensive adaptive training using mental calculation led to improvement of short-term memory performance, but not the no intention adaptive training using mental calculation (Takeuchi et al., 2011). In the present study, we set the appropriate difficulties level of both task based on the diagnostic tests. However, the difficulty level of both training tasks did not change through intervention periods. Thus, learning therapy showed no improvement of short-term and working memory performance. Future studies demand additional detailed studies to ascertain whether learning therapy using the intensive adaptive training would improve short-term and working memory performance.

This study has several strength points compared to earlier studies assessing the effects of cognitive training for elderly people. As we described in our protocol article (Nouchi et al., 2012b), we used easy to learn training tasks such as reading sentence and simple calculation using a paper and pencil. Most training tasks in previous studies were complex tasks using computers (Berry et al., 2010; Li et al., 2010). Using computers might make it easy to record data precisely and to control tasks. Nevertheless, elderly people often have difficulty using computers (Wagner et al., 2010). Recent studies have demonstrated that some barriers to computer use exist, such as lack of interest, lack of knowledge and fear of using computer (Saunders, 2004; Peacock and Künemund, 2007). The difficulty of using computers is one main reason of frustration and other negative emotions, possibly reducing their motivation to continue. On the other hand, our training tasks are easy to do for elderly people. Therefore our training tasks were expected to encourage their willingness.

This study has a limitation. We do not use other cognitive training as an active control group. We used the waiting list control group because previous studies revealed no differences in cognitive or functional improvement between the active control group and the non-training control group (Clark et al., 1997; Mahncke et al., 2006). However, from a study design perspective, it would be suitable to use the active control group to prove the effectiveness of learning therapy. Future intervention studies should be conducted to compare learning therapy to other cognitive training such as working memory training or training programs of other types such as exercise training.

CONCLUSION

In summary, this study was designed to investigate the beneficial effects of learning therapy on diverse cognitive functions in healthy elderly people. This report is the first of a study revealing the beneficial effects of learning therapy on inhibition performance of executive functions, verbal episodic memory, focus attention and processing speed in healthy elderly people. On the other hand, the learning therapy did not improve shifting performance of executive function, facial episodic memory, verbal short-term memory, verbal working memory and reading ability. These positive and negative findings would be important for people who want to use the learning therapy. If people want to improve inhibition performance, verbal episodic memory, focus attention and processing speed, this intervention program would work well. If people want to improve other cognitive domains (e.g., working memory), other cognitive training program such as working memory training would be well for them. This study had some limitations, but produced important and sufficient evidence demonstrating the effectiveness of learning therapy. Given that cognitive functions are important to do daily life activities (Cahn-Weiner et al., 2000, 2002; Lee et al., 2005), our results suggest that cognitive functions in the elderly are enhanced through daily life activities such as reading aloud and calculating simple arithmetic problems.

AUTHOR CONTRIBUTIONS

RN designed, developed the study protocol and calculated the sample size. RN conducted the study. RN wrote the manuscript with YT, HT, TN, AS and RK. RK also provided advice related to the study protocol. All authors read and approved the final manuscript.

ACKNOWLEDGMENTS

This study was an industry–academic collaboration of Tohoku University: Smart Aging Square (http://www2.idac.tohoku.ac.jp/dep/sairc/square.html). This study was supported by the Kumon Institute of Education. This study is also supported by JSPS KAKENHI Grant Number 15H05366 (Grant-in-Aid for Young Scientists (A)) and Research Grant of Frontier Research Institute for Interdisciplinary Science (FRIS), Tohoku University. Funding sources of the trial have no involvement in the study design, collection, analysis, interpretation of data, or writing of articles. We thank A. Kasagi and H. Nouchi for recruiting the participants, testers for performing psychological tests, supporters for conducting learning therapy, the participants and all of our other colleagues in IDAC, Tohoku University for their support.

REFERENCES

Anguera, J. A., Boccanfuso, J., Rintoul, J. L., Al-Hashimi, O., Faraji, F., Janowich, J., et al. (2013). Video game training enhances cognitive control in older adults. *Nature* 501, 97–101. doi: 10.1038/nature12486

Arsalidou, M. and Taylor, M. J. (2011). Is 2+2=4? Meta-analyses of brain areas needed for numbers and calculations. *Neuroimage* 54, 2382–2393. doi: 10.1016/j.neuroimage.2010.10.009

Ball, K., Berch, D. B., Helmers, K. F., Jobe, J. B., Leveck, M. D., Marsiske, M., et al. (2002). Effects of cognitive training interventions with older adults: a randomized controlled trial. *JAMA* 288, 2271–2281. doi: 10.1001/jama.288.18.2271

Ballesteros, S., Prieto, A., Mayas, J., Toril, P., Pita, C., Ponce de León, L., et al. (2014). Brain training with non-action video games enhances aspects of cognition in older adults: a randomized controlled trial. *Front. Aging Neurosci.* 6:277. doi: 10.3389/fnagi.2014.00277

Basak, C., Boot, W. R., Voss, M. W., and Kramer, A. F. (2008). Can training in a real-time strategy video game attenuate cognitive decline in older adults? *Psychol. Aging* 23, 765–777. doi: 10.1037/a0013494

Berry, A. S., Zanto, T. P., Clapp, W. C., Hardy, J. L., Delahunt, P. B., Mahncke, H. W., et al. (2010). The influence of perceptual training on working memory in older adults. *PLoS One* 5:e11537. doi: 10.1371/journal.pone.0011537

Buiza, C., Etxeberria, I., Galdona, N., Gonzalez, M. F., Arriola, E., López de Munain, A., et al. (2008). A randomized, two-year study of the efficacy of cognitive intervention on elderly people: the Donostia Longitudinal Study. *Int. J. Geriatr. Psychiatry* 23, 85–94. doi: 10.1002/gps.1846

Cahn-Weiner, D. A., Boyle, P. A., and Malloy, P. F. (2002). Tests of executive function predict instrumental activities of daily living in community-dwelling older individuals. *Appl. Neuropsychol.* 9, 187–191. doi: 10.1207/s15324826an0903_8

Cahn-Weiner, D. A., Malloy, P. F., Boyle, P. A., Marran, M., and Salloway, S. (2000). Prediction of functional status from neuropsychological tests in community-dwelling elderly individuals. *Clin. Neuropsychol.* 14, 187–195. doi: 10.1076/1385-4046(200005)14:2;1-z;ft187

Carretti, B., Borella, E., and De Beni, R. (2007). Does strategic memory training improve the working memory performance of younger and older adults? *Exp. Psychol.* 54, 311–320. doi: 10.1027/1618-3169.54.4.311

Clark, F., Azen, S. P., Zemke, R., Jackson, J., Carlson, M., Mandel, D., et al. (1997). Occupational therapy for independent-living older adults. A randomized controlled trial. *JAMA* 278, 1321–1326. doi: 10.1001/jama.1997.03550160041036

Clare, L., and Woods, R. T. (2004). Cognitive training and cognitive rehabilitation for people with early-stage Alzheimer's disease: a review. *Neuropsychol. Rehabil.* 14, 385–401. doi: 10.1080/09602010443000074

Cohen, J. (1988). *Statistical Power Analysis for the Behavioral Sciences.* Hillsdale, NJ: L. Erlbaum Associates.

Cook, A. E., Halleran, J. G., and O'Brien, E. J. (1998). What is readily available during reading? A memory-based view of text processing. *Discourse Process.* 26, 109–129. doi: 10.1080/01638539809545041

Dempster, A. P., Laird, N. M., and Rubin, D. B. (1977). Maximum likelihood from incomplete data via the EM algorithm. *J. R. Stat. Soc. Series B Methodol.* 39, 1–38.

Dubois, B., Slachevsky, A., Litvan, I., and Pillon, B. (2000). The FAB: a frontal assessment battery at bedside. *Neurology* 55, 1621–1626. doi: 10.1212/wnl.55.11.1621

Edwards, J. D., Delahunt, P. B., and Mahncke, H. W. (2009). Cognitive speed of processing training delays driving cessation. *J. Gerontol. A Biol. Sci. Med. Sci.* 64, 1262–1267. doi: 10.1093/gerona/glp131

Edwards, J. D., Wadley, V., Vance, D., Wood, K., Roenker, D., and Ball, K. (2005). The impact of speed of processing training on cognitive and everyday performance. *Aging Ment. Health* 9, 262–271. doi: 10.1080/13607860412331336788

Elliott, R. (2003). Executive functions and their disorders. *Br. Med. Bull.* 65, 49–59. doi: 10.1093/bmb/65.1.49

Folstein, M. F., Folstein, S. E., and McHugh, P. R. (1975). "Mini-mental state". A practical method for grading the cognitive state of patients for the clinician. *J. Psychiatr. Res.* 12, 189–198. doi: 10.1016/0022-3956(75)90026-6

Garrod, S., and Terras, M. (2000). The contribution of lexical and situational knowledge to resolving discourse roles: bonding and resolution. *J. Mem. Lang.* 42, 526–544. doi: 10.1006/jmla.1999.2694

Gilbert, S. J., and Burgess, P. W. (2008). Executive function. *Curr. Biol.* 18, R110–R114. doi: 10.1016/j.cub.2007.12.014

Green, C., and Bavelier, D. (2008). Exercising your brain: a review of human brain plasticity and training-induced learning. *Psychol. Aging* 23, 692–701. doi: 10.1037/a0014345

Hakoda, Y., and Sasaki, M. (1990). Group version of the stroop and reverse-stroop test: the effects of reaction mode, order and practice. *Kyoiku Shinrigaku Kenkyu (Jpn. J. Educ. Psychol.)* 38, 389–394.

Hatta, T., Ito, Y., and Yoshizaki, K. (2000). *D-CAT Manual (Screening Test for Attention).* Osaka: Union Press.

Haviland, S. E., and Clark, H. H. (1974). What's new? Acquiring new information as a process in comprehension. *J. Verb. Learn. Verb. Behav.* 13, 512–521. doi: 10.1016/s0022-5371(74)80003-4

Hedden, T., and Gabrieli, J. D. (2004). Insights into the ageing mind: a view from cognitive neuroscience. *Nat. Rev. Neurosci.* 5, 87–96. doi: 10.1038/nrn1323

Herrera, C., Chambon, C., Michel, B. F., Paban, V., and Alescio-Lautier, B. (2012). Positive effects of computer-based cognitive training in adults with mild cognitive impairment. *Neuropsychologia* 50, 1871–1881. doi: 10.1016/j.neuropsychologia.2012.04.012

Ito, E., Hatta, T., Ito, Y., Kogure, T., and Watanabe, H. (2004). Performance of verbal fluency tasks in Japanese healthy adults: effect of gender, age and education on the performance. *Shinkei Shinrigaku Kenkyu (Jpn. J. Neuropsychol.)* 20, 254–263.

Jean, L., Bergeron, M.-È., Thivierge, S., and Simard, M. (2010). Cognitive intervention programs for individuals with mild cognitive impairment: systematic review of the literature. *Am. J. Geriatr. Psychiatry* 18, 281–296. doi: 10.1097/JGP.0b013e3181c37ce9

Kawashima, R., Okita, K., Yamazaki, R., Tajima, N., Yoshida, H., Taira, M., et al. (2005). Reading aloud and arithmetic calculation improve frontal function of people with dementia. *J. Gerontol. A Biol. Sci. Med. Sci.* 60, 380–384. doi: 10.1093/gerona/60.3.380

Kawashima, R., Taira, M., Okita, K., Inoue, K., Tajima, N., Yoshida, H., et al. (2004). A functional MRI study of simple arithmetic–a comparison between children and adults. *Brain Res. Cogn. Brain Res.* 18, 227–233. doi: 10.1016/j.cogbrainres.2003.10.009

Kintsch, W. (1994). Text comprehension, memory and learning. *Am. Psychol.* 49, 294–303. doi: 10.1037/0003-066x.49.4.294

Kintsch, W., Patel, V. L., and Ericsson, K. A. (1999). The role of long-term working memory in text comprehension. *Psychologia* 42, 186–198.

LaBerge, D., and Samuels, S. J. (1974). Toward a theory of automatic information processing in reading. *Cogn. Psychol.* 6, 293–323. doi: 10.1016/0010-0285(74)90015-2

Lampit, A., Hallock, H., and Valenzuela, M. (2014). Computerized cognitive training in cognitively healthy older adults: a systematic review and meta-analysis of effect modifiers. *PLoS Med.* 11:e1001756. doi: 10.1371/journal.pmed.1001756

Lee, Y., Kim, J. H., Lee, K. J., Han, G., and Kim, J. L. (2005). Association of cognitive status with functional limitation and disability in older adults. *Aging Clin. Exp. Res.* 17, 20–28. doi: 10.1007/bf03337716

Levine, B., Stuss, D. T., Winocur, G., Binns, M. A., Fahy, L., Mandic, M., et al. (2007). Cognitive rehabilitation in the elderly: effects on strategic behavior in relation to goal management. *J. Int. Neuropsychol. Soc.* 13, 143–152. doi: 10.1017/s1355617707070178

Li, K. Z., Roudaia, E., Lussier, M., Bherer, L., Leroux, A., and McKinley, P. A. (2010). Benefits of cognitive dual-task training on balance performance in healthy older adults. *J. Gerontol. A Biol. Sci. Med. Sci.* 65, 1344–1352. doi: 10.1093/gerona/glQ161

Lustig, C., Shah, P., Seidler, R., and Reuter-Lorenz, P. A. (2009). Aging, training and the brain: a review and future directions. *Neuropsychol. Rev.* 19, 504–522. doi: 10.1007/s11065-009-9119-9

Mahncke, H. W., Connor, B. B., Appelman, J., Ahsanuddin, O. N., Hardy, J. L., Wood, R. A., et al. (2006). Memory enhancement in healthy older adults using a brain plasticity-based training program: a randomized, controlled study. *Proc. Natl. Acad. Sci. U S A* 103, 12523–12528. doi: 10.1073/pnas.0605194103

Matsuoka, K., Uno, M., Kasai, K., Koyama, K., and Kim, Y. (2006). Estimation of premorbid IQ in individuals with Alzheimer's disease using Japanese ideographic script (Kanji) compound words: Japanese version of National Adult Reading Test. *Psychiatry Clin. Neurosci.* 60, 332–339. doi: 10.1111/j.1440-1819.2006.01510.x

McAvinue, L. P., Golemme, M., Castorina, M., Tatti, E., Pigni, F. M., Salomone, S., et al. (2013). An evaluation of a working memory training scheme in older adults. *Front. Aging Neurosci.* 5:20. doi: 10.3389/fnagi.2013.00020

McDougall, S., and House, B. (2012). Brain training in older adults: evidence of transfer to memory span performance and pseudo-Matthew effects. *Neuropsychol. Dev. Cogn. B Aging Neuropsychol. Cogn.* 19, 195–221. doi: 10.1080/13825585.2011.640656

Miura, N., Iwata, K., Watanabe, J., Sugiura, M., Akitsuki, Y., Sassa, Y., et al. (2003). Cortical activation during reading aloud of long sentences: fMRI study. *Neuroreport* 14, 1563–1566. doi: 10.1097/00001756-200308260-00004

Miura, N., Watanabe, J., Iwata, K., Sassa, Y., Riera, J., Tsuchiya, H., et al. (2005). Cortical activation during reading of ancient versus modern Japanese texts: fMRI study. *Neuroimage* 26, 426–431. doi: 10.1016/j.neuroimage.2005.01.041

Miyake, A., and Friedman, N. P. (2012). The nature and organization of individual differences in executive functions: four general conclusions. *Curr. Dir. Psychol. Sci.* 21, 8–14. doi: 10.1177/0963721411429458

Miyake, A., Friedman, N. P., Emerson, M. J., Witzki, A. H., Howerter, A., and Wager, T. D. (2000). The unity and diversity of executive functions and their contributions to complex "Frontal Lobe" tasks: a latent variable analysis. *Cogn. Psychol.* 41, 49–100. doi: 10.1006/cogp.1999.0734

Myers, J. L., Cook, A. E., Kambe, G., Mason, R. A., and O'Brien, E. J. (2000). Semantic and episodic effects on bridging inferences. *Discourse Process.* 29, 179–199. doi: 10.1207/s15326950dp2903_1

Myers, J. L., and O'Brien, E. J. (1998). Accessing the discourse representation during reading. *Discourse Process.* 26, 131–157. doi: 10.1080/01638539809545042

Nouchi, R. and Kawashima, R. (2014). Improving cognitive function from children to old age: a systematic review of recent smart ageing intervention studies. *Adv. Neurosci.* 2014:235479. doi: 10.1155/2014/235479

Nouchi, R., Taki, Y., Takeuchi, H., Hashizume, H., Akitsuki, Y., Shigemune, Y., et al. (2012a). Brain training game improves executive functions and processing speed in the elderly: a randomized controlled trial. *PLoS One* 7:e29676. doi: 10.1371/journal.pone.0029676

Nouchi, R., Taki, Y., Takeuchi, H., Hashizume, H., Nozawa, T., Kambara, T., et al. (2013). Brain training game boosts executive functions, working memory and processing speed in the young adults: a randomized controlled trial. *PLoS One* 8:e55518. doi: 10.1371/journal.pone.0055518

Nouchi, R., Taki, Y., Takeuchi, H., Hashizume, H., Nozawa, T., Sekiguchi, A., et al. (2012b). Beneficial effects of reading aloud and solving simple arithmetic calculations (learning therapy) on a wide range of cognitive functions in the healthy elderly: study protocol for a randomized controlled trial. *Trials* 13:32. doi: 10.1186/1745-6215-13-32

Nouchi, R., Taki, Y., Takeuchi, H., Sekiguchi, A., Hashizume, H., Nozawa, T., et al. (2014). Four weeks of combination exercise training improved executive functions, episodic memory and processing speed in healthy elderly people: evidence from a randomized controlled trial. *Age (Dordr.)* 36, 787–799. doi: 10.1007/s11357-013-9588-x

Papp, K. V., Walsh, S. J., and Snyder, P. J. (2009). Immediate and delayed effects of cognitive interventions in healthy elderly: a review of current literature and future directions. *Alzheimers Dement.* 5, 50–60. doi: 10.1016/j.jalz.2008.10.008

Peacock, S. E., and Künemund, H. (2007). Senior citizens and Internet technology. *Eur. J. Ageing* 4, 191–200. doi: 10.1007/s10433-007-0067-z

Peretz, C., Korczyn, A. D., Shatil, E., Aharonson, V., Birnboim, S., and Giladi, N. (2011). Computer-based, personalized cognitive training versus classical computer games: a randomized double-blind prospective trial of cognitive stimulation. *Neuroepidemiology* 36, 91–99. doi: 10.1159/000323950

Richmond, L. L., Morrison, A. B., Chein, J. M., and Olson, I. R. (2011). Working memory training and transfer in older adults. *Psychol. Aging* 26, 813–822. doi: 10.1037/a0023631

Royall, D. R., Palmer, R., Chiodo, L. K., and Polk, M. J. (2004). Declining executive control in normal aging predicts change in functional status: the Freedom House Study. *J. Am. Geriatr. Soc.* 52, 346–352. doi: 10.1111/j.1532-5415.2004.52104.x

Salthouse, T. A. (1996). The processing-speed theory of adult age differences in cognition. *Psychol. Rev.* 103, 403–428. doi: 10.1037/0033-295x.103.3.403

Salthouse, T. A. (2003). Memory aging from 18 to 80. *Alzheimer Dis. Assoc. Disord.* 17, 162–167. doi: 10.1097/00002093-200307000-00008

Saunders, E. J. (2004). Maximizing computer use among the elderly in rural senior centers. *Educ. Gerontol.* 30, 573–585. doi: 10.1080/03601270490466967

Shatil, E., Metzer, A., Horvitz, O., and Miller, A. (2010). Home-based personalized cognitive training in MS patients: a study of adherence and cognitive performance. *NeuroRehabilitation* 26, 143–153. doi: 10.3233/NRE-2010-0546

Storey, J. D. (2002). A direct approach to false discovery rates. *J. R. Stat. Soc. Ser. B Stat. Methodol.* 64, 479–498. doi: 10.1111/1467-9868.00346

Street, L. L., and Luoma, J. B. (2002). Control groups in psychosocial intervention research: ethical and methodological issues. *Ethics Behav.* 12, 1–30. doi: 10.1207/s15327019eb1201_1

Stuss, D. T., Robertson, I. H., Craik, F. I., Levine, B., Alexander, M. P., Black, S., et al. (2007). Cognitive rehabilitation in the elderly: a randomized trial to evaluate a new protocol. *J. Int. Neuropsychol. Soc.* 13, 120–131. doi: 10.1017/s1355617707070154

Takeuchi, H., Taki, Y., Sassa, Y., Hashizume, H., Sekiguchi, A., Fukushima, A., et al. (2011). Working memory training using mental calculation impacts regional gray matter of the frontal and parietal regions. *PLoS One* 6:e23175. doi: 10.1371/journal.pone.0023175

Toril, P., Reales, J. M., and Ballesteros, S. (2014). Video game training enhances cognition of older adults: a meta-analytic study. *Psychol. Aging* 29, 706–716. doi: 10.1037/a0037507

Troyer, A. K., Moscovitch, M., Winocur, G., Alexander, M. P., and Stuss, D. (1998). Clustering and switching on verbal fluency: the effects of focal frontal- and temporal-lobe lesions. *Neuropsychologia* 36, 499–504. doi: 10.1016/s0028-3932(97)00152-8

Tulving, E., Schacter, D. L., McLachlan, D. R., and Moscovitch, M. (1988). Priming of semantic autobiographical knowledge: a case study of retrograde amnesia. *Brain Cogn.* 8, 3–20. doi: 10.1016/0278-2626(88)90035-8

Uchida, S., and Kawashima, R. (2008). Reading and solving arithmetic problems improves cognitive functions of normal aged people: a randomized controlled study. *Age (Dordr.)* 30, 21–29. doi: 10.1007/s11357-007-9044-x

Van Dijk, T. A., and Kintsch, W. (1983). *Strategies of Discourse Comprehension.* New York, NY: Academic Press.

Verhaeghen, P., Marcoen, A., and Goossens, L. (1992). Improving memory performance in the aged through mnemonic training: a meta-analytic study. *Psychol. Aging* 7, 242–251. doi: 10.1037/0882-7974.7.2.242

Wagner, N., Hassanein, K., and Head, M. (2010). Computer use by older adults: a multi-disciplinary review. *Comput. Hum. Behav.* 26, 870–882. doi: 10.1016/j.chb.2010.03.029

Watanabe, M., Hakoda, Y., and Matsumoto, A. (2011). Group version of the stroop and reverse-stroop test: an asymmetric developmental trait in two kinds of interference. *Kyusyu Daigaku Shinrigaku Kenkyu (Kyushu Univ. Psychol. Res.)* 12, 41–50. doi: 10.15017/20075

Wechsler, D. A. (1987). *Wechsler Memory Scale Revised.* San Antonio, TX: The Psychological Corporation.

Wechsler, D. A. (1997). *Wechsler Adult Intelligence Scale Third edition.* San Antonio, TX: The Psychological Corporation.

Wilson, B. A., Cockburn, J., and Baddeley, A. D. (1985). *The Rivermead Behavioral Memory Test.* Reading, England: Thamas Valley Test Company.

Yakhno, N. N., Zakharov, V. V., and Lokshina, A. B. (2007). Impairment of memory and attention in the elderly. *Neurosci. Behav. Physiol.* 37, 203–208. doi: 10.1007/s11055-007-0002-y

Yoshida, H., Sun, K., Tsuchida, N., and Ohkawa, I. (2014). Do practices of learning activities improve the cognitive functioning of healthy elderly adults? From the viewpoint of a transfer effect. *Shinrigaku Kenkyu* 85, 130–138. doi: 10.4992/jjpsy.85.13013

Zwaan, R. A., and Radvansky, G. A. (1998). Situation models in language comprehension and memory. *Psychol. Bull.* 123, 162–185. doi: 10.1037/0033-2909.123.2.162

7

Neural Basis of Video Gaming: A Systematic Review

Marc Palaus[1], Elena M. Marron[1], Raquel Viejo-Sobera[1,2] and Diego Redolar-Ripoll[1]*

[1] Cognitive NeuroLab, Faculty of Health Sciences, Universitat Oberta de Catalunya, Barcelona, Spain, [2] Laboratory for Neuropsychiatry and Neuromodulation, Massachusetts General Hospital, Boston, MA, USA

Edited by:
Soledad Ballesteros,
Universidad Nacional de Educación a Distancia, Spain

Reviewed by:
Tao Liu,
Zhejiang University, China
Pierre Mégevand,
Université de Genève, Switzerland
José Manuel Reales,
Universidad Nacional de Educación a Distancia, Spain

***Correspondence:**
Marc Palaus
mpalausg@uoc.edu

Background: Video gaming is an increasingly popular activity in contemporary society, especially among young people, and video games are increasing in popularity not only as a research tool but also as a field of study. Many studies have focused on the neural and behavioral effects of video games, providing a great deal of video game derived brain correlates in recent decades. There is a great amount of information, obtained through a myriad of methods, providing neural correlates of video games.

Objectives: We aim to understand the relationship between the use of video games and their neural correlates, taking into account the whole variety of cognitive factors that they encompass.

Methods: A systematic review was conducted using standardized search operators that included the presence of video games and neuro-imaging techniques or references to structural or functional brain changes. Separate categories were made for studies featuring Internet Gaming Disorder and studies focused on the violent content of video games.

Results: A total of 116 articles were considered for the final selection. One hundred provided functional data and 22 measured structural brain changes. One-third of the studies covered video game addiction, and 14% focused on video game related violence.

Conclusions: Despite the innate heterogeneity of the field of study, it has been possible to establish a series of links between the neural and cognitive aspects, particularly regarding attention, cognitive control, visuospatial skills, cognitive workload, and reward processing. However, many aspects could be improved. The lack of standardization in the different aspects of video game related research, such as the participants' characteristics, the features of each video game genre and the diverse study goals could contribute to discrepancies in many related studies.

Keywords: addiction, cognitive improvement, functional changes, internet gaming disorder, neural correlates, neuroimaging, structural changes, video games

INTRODUCTION

Nowadays, video gaming is a highly popular and prevalent entertainment option, its use is no longer limited to children and adolescents. Demographic data on video gaming shows that the mean age of video game players (VGPs) (31 years old, as of 2014) has been on the rise in recent decades (Entertainment Software Association, 2014), and it is a common activity among young adults. Moreover, the increasing ubiquity of digital technologies, such as smart-phones and tablet computers, has exposed most of the population to entertainment software in the form of casual video games (VGs) or gamified applications. Therefore, an important segment of society, over 30% in tablet computers and 70% in smart phones, has been exposed to these technologies and can be considered now, in some form, casual gamers (Casual Games Association, 2013).

It is not uncommon to hear both positive and negative health claims related to VGs in the mass media. Most of the time, these are unverified and sensationalist statements, based on "expert" opinions, but lacking evidence behind them. On the other side, as VGs become more complex (due to improvements in computer hardware), they cater to audiences other than children, appealing to older audiences, and VGs have gained prevalence as a mainstream entertainment option. Consequently, the number of people who spend hours daily playing these kinds of games is increasing.

There is interest in knowing the possible effects of long-term exposure to VGs, and whether these effects are generally positive (in the shape of cognitive, emotional, motivation, and social benefits) (e.g., Granic et al., 2014) or negative (exposure to graphic violence, contribution to obesity, addiction, cardio-metabolic deficiencies, etc.) (e.g., Ivarsson et al., 2013; Turel et al., 2016). Moreover, VGs possess a series of intrinsic features which make them suitable for use in experimental procedures: they seem to increase participants' motivation better than tasks traditionally used in neuropsychology (e.g., Lohse et al., 2013) and, in the case of purpose-made VGs, they offer a higher degree of control over the in-game variables.

For all the reasons mentioned above, VGs have recently sparked more scientific interest. The number of publications that study or use some form of gaming has been increasing, since 2005, at a constant rate of 20% per year. While during the 90's around 15 VG-related articles were published per year, in 2015 that number was over 350 (see **Figure 1**).

However, the concept of VG is extremely heterogeneous and within the category we find a myriad of hardly comparable genres. The behavioral effects and the neural correlates derived from the use of VGs depend both on the nature of the VG, the exposition to the game (hours of game play, age of onset, etc.) (Kühn and Gallinat, 2014), and, to a large extent, the individual characteristics of each participant (Vo et al., 2011).

Furthermore, due to the popularity of VG genres where graphic violence is prevalent (shooters, survival horror, fantasy), many studies have chosen to focus on this variable. Therefore, there is a reasonable amount of scientific literature devoted to the study of violent behaviors and violence desensitization as a consequence of violence in VGs (e.g., Wang et al., 2009; Engelhardt et al., 2011). Lastly, in particular since the emergence of online VG play, there are concerns about the addictive properties of VGs, akin to gambling and substance abuse, consequently making it another recurrent topic in the literature (e.g., Young, 1998).

For the time being, this whole body of knowledge is a complex combination of techniques, goals and results. On one hand, there are articles which study the effects of VG exposure over the nervous system and over cognition (e.g., Green and Seitz, 2015); it seems that there is solid evidence that exposure to certain kinds of VGs can have an influence on behavioral aspects, and therefore, we should be able to appreciate changes in the neural bases (Bavelier et al., 2012a). Actually, assessing the cognitive and behavioral implications of VG exposure has already been the object of study in recent systematic reviews and meta-analysis that used neuropsychological tasks to measure the influence of these games in healthy individuals. This is highly relevant since they evaluate the possible transfer effects of VG training to wider cognitive domains, providing a global perspective on how experimental and quasi-experimental designs differ in the size of the effect depending on the cognitive function (Powers et al., 2013), and how aging interferes with cognitive training by means of computerized tasks (Lampit et al., 2014) and VGs (Toril et al., 2014; Wang et al., 2016). Knowledge obtained about transfer effects is very important since it allows us to establish a link between VGs and cognition, indirectly helping us understand its neural basis, which in this case acts as a bridge between them. From an applied perspective, this knowledge can be used to design more effective rehabilitation programs, especially those focusing on older populations, keeping the most

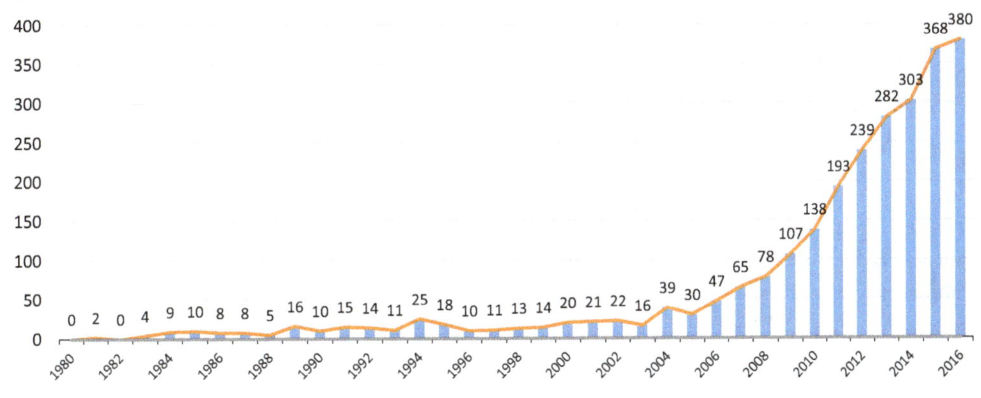

FIGURE 1 | Increasing trend in VG-related articles. Since 2005, the average annual growth is around 20%. (Source: MEDLINE).

useful components and reducing those which are shown to have less benefits.

On the other hand, VGs have been used as a research tool to study the nervous system. In this group of studies, it is common to find exposure to VGs as the independent variable, especially in most studies that use unmodified commercial VGs. However, it is not unusual to employ custom designed VGs, such as the widely used Space Fortress, where in-game variables can be fine-tuned to elicit certain mental processes in consonance with the research hypothesis (e.g., Smith et al., 1999; Anderson et al., 2011; Prakash et al., 2012; Anderson et al., 2015). Nevertheless, in both cases, the study of the VG exposure over the nervous system and the use of VGs as a research tool, VGs are used to obtain information about the underlying neural processes relevant to our research interest.

As yet there is no systematic review on this topic. The aim of this article is to gather all the scientific information referring to neural correlates of VGs and synthesize the most important findings. All articles mentioning functional and structural changes in the brain due to video gaming will be analyzed and information about the most relevant brain regions for each kind of study will be extracted; the main objective of many VG-related articles is not to study their neural correlates directly. Studies focusing on the addictive consequences or the effects of violence will be categorized independently.

Our final goal is to highlight the neural correlates of video gaming by making a comprehensive compilation and reviewing all relevant scientific publications that make reference to the underlying neural substrate related to VG play. This is the first effort in this direction that integrates data regarding VGs, neural correlates and cognitive functions that is not limited to action-VGs or cognitive training programs, the most frequently found research topics.

METHODS

In order to structure reliably the gathered information in this systematic review, the guidelines and recommendations contained in the PRISMA statement (Liberati et al., 2009) have been followed.

Eligibility Criteria

All articles which included neural correlates (both functional and structural) and included VG play in the research protocol or studied the effects of exposure to VGs were included in the review. Both experimental and correlational studies were included. No restrictions regarding publication date were applied.

Healthy participants of any age and gender were considered. Studies include both naive and experienced VG participants. Participants that reported gaming addiction or met criteria for internet gaming disorder (IGD) were also included in the review owing to the interest in observing neural correlates in these extreme cases. Other pathologies were excluded in order to avoid confounding variables.

Articles employing several methodologies were included. These can be organized into three main groups: studies where naive participants were trained in the use of a VG against a control group, studies comparing experienced players vs. non-gamers or low-experience players, and studies comparing differential characteristics of two VG or two VG genres.

The primary outcome measures were any kind of structural and functional data obtained using neuroimaging techniques including computerized tomography (CT) scan, structural magnetic resonance imaging (MRI), functional MRI (fMRI), positron emission tomography (PET), single-photon emission computed tomography (SPECT), magneto encephalography (MEG), transcranial direct current stimulation (tDCS), electroencephalogram (EEG), event-related potentials (ERP), event-related spectral perturbation (ERSP), steady state visually evoked potential (SSVEP), Doppler, and near-infrared spectroscopy (NIRS), following or related to VG use.

Information Sources

Academic articles were located using two electronic databases: MEDLINE and Web of Science, and by scanning reference lists in other studies in the same field. Only the results from these two databases are reported since results from other sources (Scopus, Google Scholar) did not provide any relevant new results. The search was not limited by year of publication and only articles published in English, Spanish, or French were considered for inclusion. The first studies relevant to the topic are from 1992, while the most recent studies included in this review were published in February 2016.

Search

A systematic search was performed using a series of keywords which were expected to appear in the title or abstract of any study containing neural correlates of VGs. These keywords were grouped in two main categories. First of all, a group of keywords trying to identify articles which used VG as a technique or as a study goal. These keywords included search terms related to "video games" proper (in different orthographic variants), types of players (casual, core, and hardcore gamers) and references to serious gaming. In second place, two groups of keywords were used to detect articles which studied the neural basis: (1) keywords related to anatomical features, such as structural or functional changes, gray, or white matter (WM) volumes, cortical features, and connectivity and (2) keywords which mentioned the neuroimaging technique used to obtain that data, such as EEG, MRI, PET, or NIRS. (See Appendix)

Study Selection

Due to the large amount of results obtained by the previous search terms, strict exclusion criteria were applied to limit the final selection of studies. The same criteria were applied in a standardized way by two independent reviewers, and disagreements between reviewers were resolved by consensus. Due to high variability in the terminology and the diversity of keywords used in the search, a large number of false positive studies (65% of items found) appeared during the review process (see **Figure 2**).

By performing a search using standardized terms, a list of studies from the two databases was extracted. A large number of studies (62% of those that met the inclusion criteria) were found

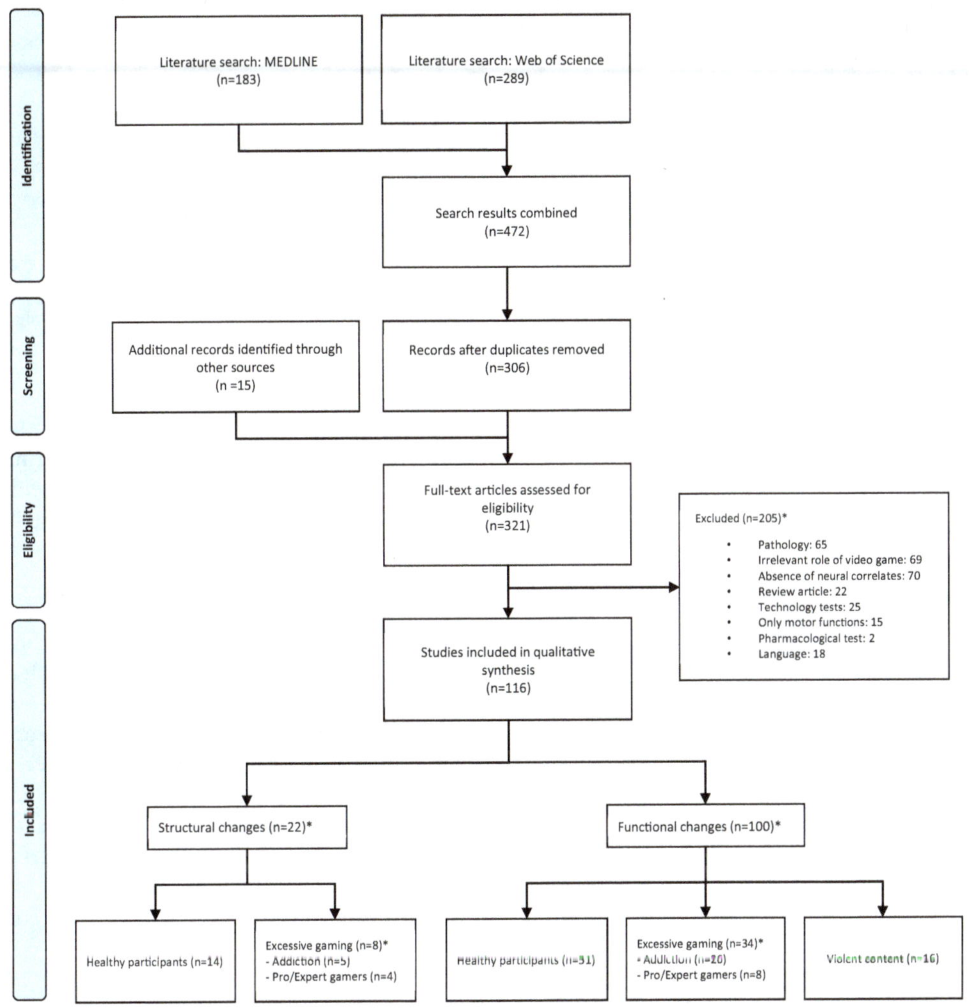

FIGURE 2 | Study selection diagram flow. *Articles in these sections may not be mutually exclusive.

to be duplicates in both databases, so a careful comparison was made in order to merge the references.

No unpublished relevant studies were considered. Studies relevant to the topic but not published in peer-reviewed journals, such as conference posters and abstracts were considered.

Data Collection Process

All the relevant information was classified in a spreadsheet, according to the variables listed below. Variables related to violence and abuse of VGs were also categorized, since a significant portion of the studies focused on these behaviors. A small number of articles ($n = 7$) were found in sources other than the two databases, mainly through references in other articles.

For each study, the following data was extracted: (1) characteristics of the sample, including sample size, average age and range, inclusion and exclusion criteria, and gaming experience; (2) aim of the study, specially noting if it is focused on gaming abuse or exposure to violent content; (3) name and genre of the VG used during the study, if applicable; (4) study design; (5) main neuroimaging technique applied in the study, and whether the technique was applied while participants played; (6) functional and structural neural correlates observed in the study. Studies were then classified in several groups as to whether they provided structural or functional data, and whether they addressed violent or addictive aspects.

Moreover, in order to understand the outcomes derived from the neural correlates, most of the studies establish a connection between these correlates and their cognitive correspondence, either by directly measuring the outcomes using cognitive tasks and questionnaires, or by interpreting their results based on existing literature.

In the discussion section of this review, we attempted to summarize the main findings by associating the neural changes to their cognitive and behavioral correspondences. Whereas, in many cases the original articles provided their own explanation for the phenomena, we also worked on integrating the general trends from a cognitive perspective. We therefore indicate which studies provide and interpret empirical cognitive or/and behavioral data (non-marked), those which discuss cognitive or/and behavioral implications without assessing them (marked with *), and those which did not provide any cognitive nor behavioral information (marked with **).

RESULTS

Study Selection

The combined search of MEDLINE and Web of Science provided a total of 306 unique citations. Of these, 205 studies were discarded because they did not seem to meet the inclusion criteria after reviewing the abstract. The main reasons for exclusion were: being a review article (n = 22), absence of neural correlates (n = 70), presence of pathology in the participants (n = 65), not being related to VGs or using simple computerized tasks which could not be considered VGs (n = 69), testing of new technologies in which the brain correlates were a mere by-product (n = 25), articles focused on motor functions (n = 15), pharmacological studies (n = 2), and finally, articles in languages other than English, Spanish, or French (n = 18). Excluded articles often met more than one exclusion criteria. As mentioned in the eligibility criteria, an exception were those articles in which the pathology consisted of gaming overuse or addiction and articles which featured psychopathology and included groups of healthy participants from whom neural data was provided.

Fifteen extra articles that met the inclusion criteria were found after examining the contents and following the references in the previously selected studies. As expected, articles written in English comprised the vast majority; among the rest (8.9%), 10 of them (4.9%) were discarded from the review solely for language reasons. No unpublished relevant studies were considered. Studies relevant to the topic but not published in peer-reviewed journals, such as conference posters and abstracts were considered. Ultimately, a total of 116 studies were identified for inclusion in the review (see flow diagram in **Figure 2**).

Most studies (n = 100; 86.2%) provided functional data, while only 22 (18.9%) of them studied structural changes in the brain. A few (n = 6; 5.2%) provided both structural and functional data. A significant number of the studies focused their attention on excessive playing or VG addiction. That was the case for 39 (33.6%) of the reviewed articles, so we considered it appropriate to analyze them in their own category. Likewise, 16 studies (13.8%) focusing on the violent component of VGs were also placed in their own category. These categories were not always exclusive, but there was only one case where the two criteria were met. (See **Table 1** for a breakdown by category).

Characteristics of Included Studies

Based on their methodology, studies in this review could be classified as experimental (n = 54; 46.6%), randomly assigning the participant sample to the experimental groups, and quasi-experimental (n = 62; 53.4%), where the groups were usually constructed according to the participants' characteristics. While studies involving excessive gaming almost always followed a quasi-experimental design comparing experienced gamers against low-experience VG players, articles studying normal gaming and the effects of violence exposure used both experimental and quasi-experimental designs. A fraction of the studies (n = 15; 13%), both experimental and quasi-experimental, compared the results to a baseline using a pretest-posttest design. That was the case for most studies involving a training period with VGs.

TABLE 1 | Article breakdown by category.

	Structural	Functional	Both	Total
All	22	100	6	116
Healthy (Non excessive, non-violent)	14	51	3	62
Excessive gaming	8	34	3	39
Excessive gaming, IGD	5	26	2	29
Excessive gaming, Non-IGD	3	8	1	10
Violence	0	16	0	16
Violence + Excessive gaming	0	1	0	1
	Only structural	**Only functional**		
	16	94		

IGD, Internet Gaming Disorder.

The cumulative sample included in this review exceeds 3,880 participants. The exact number cannot be known since participants could have been reused for further experiments and in some cases the sample size was not available. Most studies used adolescents or young adults as the primary experimental group, since that is the main demographic target for video gaming. In many cases, only male participants were accepted. In the cases where VG experience was compared, the criteria varied greatly. For the low video gaming groups, VG usage ranged from <5 h/week to none at all. For the usual to excessive VG groups, it could typically start at 10 h/week. In some cases, where the level of addiction mattered, the score in an addiction scale was used instead.

In more than half of the studies (n = 67; 57.8%) participants actually played a VG as part of the experimental procedure. In the rest, either neural correlates were measured in a resting-state condition or VG related cues were presented to the participants during the image acquisition.

Structural changes in the gray matter (GM) were measured in the form of volumetric changes, whereas WM was assessed using tractography techniques. Functional changes were typically measured comparing activation rates for different brain regions. Nearly half (n = 55; 47.4%) of the assessed studies used fMRI as the neuroimaging technique of choice, while other functional techniques remained in a distant second place. Functional connectivity was assessed in several studies employing resting-state measures. EEG in its multiple forms was also widely used (n = 32; 27.6%) to obtain functional data, either to measure activation differences across regions or in the form of event related potentials. (See **Table 2** for a breakdown by neuroimaging technique).

The high variability in the study designs, participants and objectives meant we focused on describing the studies, their results, their applicability, and their limitations on a qualitative synthesis rather than meta-analysis.

Structural Data

Data regarding structural changes following VG use was available from 22 studies, fourteen of which provided structural data for more than 800 participants that had a normal VG use and included both VGPs and non-VGPs (see **Table 3**). The remaining eight studies examined aspects concerning the excessive or professional use of VG (see **Table 4**).

In studies dealing with healthy, non-addicted participants, eight studies used MRI to provide structural information for the GM, while six focused on the WM using diffusion tension imaging (DTI).

Three studies compared lifetime VG experience prior to the study, while the rest used a training paradigm where participants were exposed to a VG during the experimental sessions prior to the neuroimaging procedure and compared to a baseline. Seven studies provided WM integrity data using the DTI technique while the rest analyzed cortical thickness variations using regular structural MRI.

The most researched areas in studies examining volumetric differences found relevant changes in prefrontal regions, mainly the dorsolateral prefrontal cortex (dlPFC) and surrounding areas, superior and posterior parietal regions, the anterior cingulate cortex (ACC), the cerebellum, the insula, and subcortical nuclei, as well as the striatum and the hippocampus. In addition to this, structural connectivity studies observed changes in virtually all parts of the brain, such as in fibers connecting to the visual, temporal and prefrontal cortices, the corpus callosum, the hippocampus, the thalamus, association fibers like the external capsule, and fibers connecting the basal ganglia.

Functional Data

A 100 articles provided functional data combined with VG use. Of these, around half ($n = 51$) were studies which did not include violence or addiction elements (See **Table 5**). A third ($n = 34$) corresponded to articles aiming at understanding the neural bases of IGD (See **Table 6**), often drawing parallels with other behavioral addictions and trying to find biomarkers for VG addiction. The rest ($n = 16$) were devoted to study the effects of violence exposure in VGs (See **Table 7**). In total, these studies provided functional data for 3,229 experimental subjects, including control groups. Note that there is some overlap with the structural section, since a few ($n = 6$) studies provided both structural and functional data.

The rich diversity of methodologies and research goals means that the study of functional brain correlates covers practically all regions of the brain. The most studied areas are found in frontal and prefrontal regions and are concerned with high-order cognitive processes and motor/premotor functions. Activity changes in parietal regions, like the posterior and superior parietal lobe, relevant for diverse functions such as sensory integration and visual and attentional processing, are also a common find. The anterior and posterior cingulate cortices, together with other limbic areas, such as the amygdala, and the entorhinal cortex, display activity changes possibly as a consequence of learning and emotion processing and memory. Structures in the basal nuclei also have a prominent role, particularly the striatum, in studies related to VG addiction. Finally, we must not overlook a series of brain regions which do not appear as frequently, such as occipital and temporal cortices, the cerebellum, the thalamus, and the hippocampus, where distinctive activity patterns have also been observed as a result of VG play.

TABLE 2 | Neuroimaging techniques used in the reviewed studies.

Technique	N	%
Electrophysiological methods	32	27.6
EEG (standard)	13	11.2
ERP	16	13.8
ERSP	1	0.9
SSVEP	2	1.7
MRI	70	60.3
MRI (structural)	15	12.9
fMRI	55	47.4
NIRS	8	6.9
SPECT	2	1.7
PET	2	1.7
Doppler	1	0.9

EEG, Electroencephalography; ERP, Event-related potentials; ERSP, Event-related spectral Dynamics; fMRI, Functional magnetic resonance imaging; MRI, Magnetic resonance imaging; NIRS, Near-infrared spectroscopy; PET, Positon emission tomography; SPECT, Single-photon emission computed tomography; SSVEP, Steady-state visual evoked potential.

DISCUSSION

Due to the given amount of data provided in the reviewed articles, we decided to categorize all the information based on the cognitive functions which are associated with the neurophysiological correlates, rather than focusing on the main research goal for each study. Thus, the discussion has been grouped into six main sections: attention, visuospatial skills, cognitive workload, cognitive control, skill acquisition, and reward processing. These cognitive processes are not clearly independent since they present some degree of overlap. This is particularly relevant in the cases of cognitive workload, which may be linked to virtually any cognitive function, and attention, which is also closely related to cognitive control, among other functions. Nevertheless, after analyzing the literature, virtually all the articles included in this review focused on one or more of the mentioned cognitive functions in order to explain their findings. Thus, the proposed categories have sufficient presence in the literature to justify their use as separate domains for the study of cognition. While they should not be understood as independent aspects of cognition, the chosen categorization will allow a link between the underlying neural correlates and corresponding behavior to be easily established.

Within each one of the sections, structural and functional correlates are discussed according to their contributions to cognitive functioning, including possible inconsistencies between studies and the presence of transfer effects. Owing to the close link between VG violence, limbic and reward systems, and the possible abnormal reward mechanisms in addicted players, studies previously classified with violence in VGs and VG addiction are predominantly discussed in the reward processing section.

TABLE 3 | Studies providing structural data dealing with healthy, non-expert participants.

Ref.	Year	*N*	Age	Sample	VP experience	VG genre	Technique	Design	Neural correlates
Erickson et al., 2010	2010	39	(18–28)	Healthy young adults	<3 h/week	Action, shooter	MRI	Experimental (randomized)	Predictors of skill acquisition: ▲ DS ▲ VS
Basak et al., 2011	2011	20	70.1 ± 4.81	Healthy older adults	Low VGP (<1 h/week)	Real time strategy	MRI	Quasi-experimental (one group pretest-posttest)	Predictors of skill acquisition: ▲ MFG (left) ▲ PoCG (left) ▲ dlPFC (left) ▲ ACC (right) ▲ Cerebellum
Vo et al., 2011	2011	34	(18–28)	Healthy young adults	Low or Non-VGP	Action, shooter	MRI	Experimental (crossover)	Skill acquisition: ▲ DS
Colom et al., 2012	2012	20	18.95 ± 2.65	Healthy young adults, female	Low or Non-VGP	Puzzle, Brain training	MRI (DTI)	Experimental (randomized with pretest)	After VG training: Gray matter: ▲ PFC (BA9 & BA10) ▲ Small temporal and parietal regions White matter: ▲ HC cingulum ▲ ILF
Kühn et al., 2013	2013	48	24.1 ± 3.8	Healthy young adults	Low or Non-VGP	Action, 3D platforms	MRI	Experimental (randomized with pretest)	After VG training: ▲ HC (right) ▲ dlPFC (right) ▲ Cerebellum
McGarry et al., 2013	2013	7	(60–85)	Healthy older adults	–	Real time strategy	MRI	Quasi-experimental (one group pretest-posttest)	After VG training: ▲ SPG ▲ Lateral IFG ▲ PrCG ▲ FG
Kühn and Gallinat, 2014*	2014	62	28.4 ± 6.07	Healthy young adults, male	Low or Non-VGP ($n = 48$) Excessive ($n = 9$) IGD ($n = 5$)	–	MRI	Quasi-experimental (retrospective)	VG experience: ▲ Entorhinal cortex ▲ HC Game genre: ▲ Entorhinal cortex
Kühn et al., 2014*	2014	152	14.4 ± 0.03	Healthy adolescents	12.6 ± 12.9 h/week	–	MRI	Quasi-experimental (retrospective)	VG experience: ▲ dlPFC (left) ▲ MFG(left) ▲ SFG (left) ▲ FEF (left)
Strenziok et al., 2013	2014	–	(>60)	Healthy older adults	–	Real time strategy Puzzle, Brain training	MRI (DTI)	Experimental (randomized)	After VG training: ▼ Splenium of CC

(Continued)

TABLE 3 | Continued

Ref.	Year	*N*	Age	Sample	VP experience	VG genre	Technique	Design	Neural correlates
Strenziok et al., 2014	2014	42	69.21 ± 4.9	Healthy older adults	–	Action, shooter Real time strategy Puzzle, Brain training	MRI (DTI)	Experimental (randomized with pretest)	After VG training (white matter AD): All 3 groups: ▲ Lingual gyrus (left) ▲ Thalamus (right) Brain training vs. Action shooter: ▲ TO junction (right) Brain training vs. Strategy: ▲ POT junction (right)
Szabó et al., 2014**	2014	56	36.8 ± 10.3	Healthy adults	Low or Non-VGP	Action, 3D platforms	MRI	Experimental (randomized with pretest)	After VG training: ▲ HC (right)
Zhang et al., 2015	2015	45	16.9 ± 2.2 (VGP) 17.1 ± 1.3 (Non-VGP)	Healthy adolescents, male	VGP (19 h/week) Low or Non-VGP (<2 h/week)	Racing Role playing, MMORPG Dance Action, First Person Shooter	MRI (DTI)	Quasi-experimental (retrospective)	VGP vs. Non-VGP (White matter FA): ▲ CST (left) ▲ SLF (left) ▲ ILF ▲ IFOF
Kim Y. H. et al., 2015*	2015	31	29.0 ± 4.1	Healthy young adults	VGP (>3 h/week) Non-VGP (<10 h/year)	Real time strategy	MRI (DTI)	Quasi-experimental (with control group)	VGP vs. Non-VGP: White matter connectivity: ▲ EC (right) & Visual cortex ▲ IFG (right) & ACC
Takeuchi et al., 2016	2016	240	11.1 ± 2.7	Healthy children	0.8 ± 0.75 h/week	–	MRI (DTI)	Quasi-experimental (cross-sectional)	VG experience: ▲ PFC (bilateral) (GM & WM) ▲ ACC ▲ Lateral & Medial temporal cortex ▲ BG ▲ FG ▼ Genu of de CC (Specific areas) ▼ Body of the CC ▼ ACR (bilateral) ▼ SCR (right)
Takeuchi et al., 2016	2016	189	(5.7–16.6)	Healthy children	–	–	MRI (DTI)	Quasi-experimental (longitudinal)	VG experience: ▲ Cluster 1: BG (Gm & WM) (left) Medial temporal lobe (left) Thalamus (bilateral) ▲ Cluster 2: Insula (right) Putamen (right) Thalamus (right) ▲ Cluster 3: MTG & ITC (left) FG Occipital lobe (left)

ACC, Anterior cingulate cortex; ACR, Anterior corona radiata; AD, Axial diffusivity; BA, Brodmann area; BG, Basal ganglia; CC, Corpus callosum; CST, Corticospinal tract; dlPFC, Dorsolateral prefrontal cortex; DS, Dorsal striatum; DTI, Diffusion tensor imaging; EC, External capsule; FA, Fractional anisotropy; FEF, Frontal eye fields; FG, Fusiform gyrus; GM, Gray matter; HC, Hippocampus; IFG, Inferior frontal gyrus; IFOF, Inferior frontooccipital fasciculus; IGD, Internet Gaming Disorder; ILF, Inferior longitudinal fasciculus; ITC, Inferior temporal cortex; MFG, Middle frontal gyrus; MRI, Magnetic resonance imaging; MTG, Middle temporal gyrus; PFC, Prefrontal cortex; PoCG, Post central gyrus; POT, Parieto-occipito-temporal; PrCG, Pre-central gyrus; SCR, Superior corona radiata; SFG, Superior frontal gyrus; SLF, Superior longitudinal fasciculus; SPG, Superior parietal gyrus; TO, Temporo-occipital; VG, Video game; VGP, Video game player; VS, Ventral striatum; WM, White matter. Articles marked with an asterisk (*) discuss cognitive implications without directly assessing this dimension. Articles marked with a double asterisk (**) did not provide either empirical cognitive data nor discuss cognitive implications. The rest of the articles (non-marked) have measured cognitive correlates with specific tasks.

TABLE 4 | Studies providing structural data dealing with VG experts or excessive gaming.

Ref.	Year	*N*	Age	Sample	VG experience	VG genre	Technique	Design	Neural correlates
Han et al., 2012a	2012	55	20.9 ± 2.0 (IGD) 20.8 ± 1.5 (Pro) 20.9 ± 2.1 (Control)	Young adults, male	IGD (9.0 ± 3.7 h/day) Professional VGP (9.4 ± 1.6 h/day) Low or Non-VGP (1.0 ± 0.7 h/day)	Real time strategy	MRI	Quasi-experimental (with control group)	IGD vs. Control: ▲ Thalamus GM (left) ▼ ITG (bilateral) ▼ MOG (right) ▼ IOG (left) Professional vs. Control: ▲ CG (left) ▼ MOG (left) ▼ ITG (right) Professional vs. IGD: ▲ CG (left) ▼ Thalamus (left)
Hou et al., 2012*	2012	14	20.40 ± 2.30 (IGD) 20.44 ± 1.13 (Control)	Young adults	IGD (>8 h/day) Low or Non-VGP (<5 h/day)	–	SPECT	Quasi-experimental (with control group)	IGD vs. Control: ▼ Striatum volume ▼ Striatum weight ▼ Striatum/whole brain ratio
Hyun et al., 2013	2013	23	19.8 ± 1.7	Healthy young adults, male	Professional VGP (9.2 ± 1.6 h/day)	Real time strategy	MRI	Quasi-experimental	Career length: ▲ SFG (right) ▲ SPG (right) ▲ PrCG (right) Winning rates: ▲ PFC
Tanaka et al., 2013	2013	50	24.1 ± 2.9 (Experts) 22.4 ± 3.42 (Control)	Healthy young adults, male	Expert VGP (21.4 ± 10.0 h/week) Low or Non-VGP (<2 h/week)	Action, fighting	MRI	Quasi-experimental (with control group)	Experts vs. Non-experts: ▲ PPC (right)
Yuan et al., 2013a	2013	36	19.4 ± 3.1 (IGD) 19.5 ± 2.8 (Control)	Young adults, male	IGD (10.2 ± 2.6 h/day) Low or Non-VGP (0.8 ± 0.4 h/day)	Role playing, MMORPG	MRI	Quasi-experimental (with control group)	IGD vs. Control: ▲ Precentral cortex (left) ▲ PCu ▲ MFG ▲ ITC ▲ MTG ▼ lOFC (left) (Impaired task performance) ▼ Insula ▼ Lingual gyrus ▼ PoCG (right) ▼ Entorhinal cortex ▼ IPC

(Continued)

TABLE 4 | Continued

Ref.	Year	*N*	Age	Sample	VG experience	VG genre	Technique	Design	Neural correlates
									IGD duration: ▲ Precentral cortex (left) ▲ PCu ▲ Lingual gyrus
Xing et al., 2014	2014	34	19.1 ± 0.7 (IGD) 19.8 ± 1.3 (Control)	Young adults	IGD (9.5 ± 1.3 h/day; 65.7 ± 11.6 IAT) Control (2.2 ± 1.4 h/day; 29.2 ± 4.5 IAT)	Action, Real time strategy	MRI (DTI)	Quasi-experimental (with control group)	IGD vs. Control (FA): ▼ SN tract (right)
Gong et al., 2015*	2015	57	23.26 ± 0.4 (Experts) 22.36 ± 0.38 (Amateurs)	Healthy young adults	Expert VGP (46.67 ± 2.1 h/week) Amateur VGP (14.2 ± 1.1 h/week)	Action, Real time strategy	MRI	Quasi-experimental (with control group)	Experts vs. Amateurs): ▲ Insula (left) ▲ Short insular gyri ▲ Long insular gyrus ▲ Central sulcus
Jin et al., 2016*	2016	46	19.12 ± 1.05 (IGD) 18.76 ± 1.81 (Control)	Adolescents	IGD (5.32 ± 2.10 h/day) Low or Non-VGP (2.07 ± 1.39 h/day)	Action, Real time strategy	MRI	Quasi-experimental (with control group)	IGD vs. Control: ▼ dlPFC ▼ OFC ▼ ACC ▼ SMA (right)

ACC, Anterior cingulate cortex; CG, Cingulate gyrus; dlPFC, Dorsolateral prefrontal cortex; DTI, Diffusion tensor imaging; FA, Fractional anisotropy; GM, Gray matter; IGD, Internet gaming disorder; IOG, Inferior occipital gyrus; IPC, Inferior parietal cortex; ITC, Inferior temporal cortex; lOFC, Lateral orbitofrontal cortex; MFG, Middle frontal gyrus; MMORPG, Massively multiplayer online role-playing game; MOG, Middle occipital gyrus; MRI, Magnetic resonance imaging; MTG, Middle temporal cortex; OFC, Orbitofrontal cortex; PCu, Precuneus; PFC, Prefrontal cortex; PoCG, Post-central gyrus; PPC, Posterior parietal cortex; PrCG, Pre-central gyrus; SFG, Superior frontal gyrus; SMA, Supplementary motor area; SN, Salience network; SPECT, Single-photon emission computed tomography; SPG, Superior parietal gyrus; VGP, Video game player. Articles marked with an asterisk (*) discuss cognitive implications without directly assessing this dimension. Articles marked with a double asterisk (**) did not provide either empirical cognitive data nor discuss cognitive implications. The rest of the articles (non-marked) have measured cognitive correlates with specific tasks.

TABLE 5 | Studies providing functional data dealing with healthy, non-expert participants, without violent content.

Ref.	Year	*N*	Age	Sample	VG experience	VG genre	Technique	Design	Neural correlates
Kelley et al., 1992**	1992	21	31.4 ± 7.8	Healthy adults	–	Breakout	Doppler	Experimental (crossover)	VG play vs. Baseline: ▲ MCA (bilateral) ▲ PCA (left)
Brookings et al., 1996	1996	8	(21–29)	Healthy adults	Air traffic controllers	Simulation	EEG	Experimental (crossover)	Task difficulty (measured in Theta power): High vs. Low difficulty: ▲ F8, C3, Cz, T4, P3, Pz, P4 Medium vs. Low difficulty: ▲ C3, P3, Pz Overload condition vs. Low difficulty: ▲ F3, C3, Pz Overload condition vs. Medium difficulty: ▲ T6, O2 Overload condition vs. High difficulty: ▲ F7, F3, Fz, C3
Koepp et al., 1998**	1998	8	(36–46)	Healthy adults, male	–	Action	PET	Quasi-experimental (with pretest)	VGP vs. baseline: ▼ Striatum (dopamine binding) Performance level: ▼ VS (dopamine binding)
Pellouchoud et al., 1999*	1999	7	(9–15)	Healthy children	–	Puzzle	EEG	Experimental (crossover)	Gameplay vs. resting: ▲ Frontal midline theta (6–7 Hz) ▼ Posterior alpha (9–12 Hz) ▼ Central mu (10–13 Hz)
Smith et al., 1999	1999	6	(22–25)	Healthy young adults	–	Action, shooter	EEG	Quasi-experimental (with pretest)	VG Post vs. Pre: ▼ Central alpha waves ▲ Primary motor cortex alpha waves ▲ Frontal midline theta waves
Izzetoglu et al., 2004*	2004	8	(18–50)	Healthy adults	–	Action, strategy	NIRS	Experimental (crossover)	VG difficulty: ▲ dlPFC (bilateral)
Matsuda and Hiraki, 2004*	2004	6	(23–29)	Healthy young adults	–	Action, First Person Shooter Rhythm Puzzle	NIRS	Experimental (crossover)	VG play vs. rest: ▼ dPFC Viewing VG or non-VG images: ▼ dPFC Fast vs. slow finger tapping: ▲ dPFC Left vs. right finger tapping: ▲ dPFC
Matsuda and Hiraki, 2006*	2006	13	(7–14)	Healthy children	–	Action, fighting Puzzle	NIRS	Experimental (crossover)	Children (VG play vs. rest): ▼ dPFC Children vs. Adults (VG play): = dPFC
Nagamitsu et al., 2006**	2006	12	8 (7–10) (children) 34 (26–44) (adults)	Healthy children Healthy adults	Low and High VGP (>2 h/day) Non-VGP	Action, 2D Platforms	NIRS	Quasi-experimental (with control group)	During VG play: ▲ PFC (bilateral) in 4 adults ▼ PFC (bilateral) in 2 children ▲ PFC & Motor cortex (bilateral) correlation

(Continued)

TABLE 5 | Continued

Ref.	Year	*N*	Age	Sample	VG experience	VG genre	Technique	Design	Neural correlates
Salminen and Ravaja, 2007**	2007	25	23.8	Healthy young adults	VGP (>once a month)	Action, 3D Platforms	EEG	Experimental (crossover)	While playing: Picking up item: ▼ Central theta waves ▼ Frontal high alpha waves ▲ Frontal beta waves Falling: ▼ Central theta ▲ Fronto-central beta waves Reaching goal: ▲ Parietal theta waves ▼ Frontal low alpha waves ▲ Frontal high alpha waves ▼ Central high alpha waves ▲ Parietal high alpha waves ▼ Frontal beta waves ▲ Central beta waves
Sheikholeslami et al., 2007**	2007	2	–	Healthy participants	–	Sports	EEG	Quasi-experimental (with pretest)	Gaming vs. resting: ▲ Frontal midline theta waves ▼ Parietal alpha waves & slow increase
Corradi-Dell'Acqua et al., 2008*	2008	17	–	Healthy young adults	–	Custom VG	fMRI	Experimental (factorial design)	VG character controlled synchronously: Agency vs. Control: ▲ MCG (left) ▲ MFG Agency vs. Control (when changing spatial positions): ▲ POT junction (right)
Russoniello et al., 2009	2009	69	–	–	–	Puzzle	EEG	Experimental (randomized)	VGP vs. Control: ▼ Frontal alpha waves (left)
Bailey et al., 2010	2010	51	(18–33)	Healthy young adults	Low VGP (1.76 ± 4.75 h/week) High VGP (43.4 ± 16.0 h/week)	Action	EEG (ERP)	Quasi-experimental (with control group)	High VGP vs. Low VGP: ▼ Medial frontal negativity amplitude ▼ Frontal slow wave amplitude
Han et al., 2010b*	2010	21	24.1 ± 2.6	Healthy young adults	Low VGP (< 1 h/day) High VGP (>1 h/day)	Action, fighting	fMRI	Quasi-experimental (with control group and pretest)	Excessive VGP vs. Control: ▲ ACC ▲ OFC
Anderson et al., 2011*	2011	20	23.6	Healthy young adults	VGP (low, medium and high)	Action, shooter	fMRI	Experimental (crossover)	During VG play: ▲ Hand motor regions (bilateral) ▲ ACC ▲ PPC ▲ LIPFC ▲ CN ▲ FG
Maclin et al., 2011	2011	39	(19–29)	Healthy young adults	Low or Non-VGP (<3 h/week)	Action, shooter	EEG (ERP)	Experimental (crossover)	Post vs. Pre-training ▼ P300 amplitude (VG "hits") ▼ P300 amplitude (oddball tones) ▲ P300 amplitude (VG "enemies") ▼ Delta power (VG "hits") ▲ Delta power (oddball tones) ▲ Alpha power (VG "hits")

(Continued)

TABLE 5 | Continued

Ref.	Year	*N*	Age	Sample	VG experience	VG genre	Technique	Design	Neural correlates
									▲ Alpha power (oddball tones) ▲ Delta power (VG "enemies") ▲ Alpha power (VG "enemies") ▲ Parietal (Pz) theta power (VG "enemies") ▲ Parietal (Pz) delta power (VG "enemies") Oddball task inside VG vs outside game ▼ P300 amplitude
Mishra et al., 2011	2011	41	21 (VGP) 24 (Non-VGP)	Healthy young adults, male	VGP (9.0 ± 2.7 h/week) Non-VGP (0 h/week)	Action	EEG (SSVEP)	Quasi-experimental (with control group)	VGP vs. Non-VGP: ▲ Suppression SSVEP to unattended peripheral sequences ▲ P300 amplitude
Bavelier et al., 2012a	2012	26	20.50	Healthy young adults	VGP (>5 h/week) Low or Non-VGP (<5 h/week)	Action, First Person Shooter	fMRI	Quasi-experimental (crossover, with control group)	As attentional demands increased: Non-VGP vs. VGP: ▲ FPN
Cole et al., 2012*	2012	57	25.3 ± 9.4	Healthy young adults	–	Action, shooter	fMRI	Experimental (randomized)	VG onset: ▲ CN ▲ NAcc ▲ PHG VG gameplay: ▲ Thalamus ▲ Posterior insula ▲ Putamen ▲ Motor regions ▼ Parietal cortex ▼ Medial PFC VG offset gameplay: ▲ Anterior insula ▲ ACC VG group vs. Control: ▲ CN ▲ NAcc ▲ PHG
Lee H. et al., 2012	2012	75	21.57 ± 2.58	Healthy young adults	Low or Non-VGP (<4 h/week)	Action, shooter	fMRI	Experimental (randomized)	Full emphasis vs. Hybrid variable-priority training (post-training): ▲ PCu (left) ▲ Lateral occipital cortex (left) ▲ Intracalcarine cortex (left) ▲ SFG (right) Post vs. Pre training: ▼ Intracalcarine cortex (bilateral) ▼ Lingual gyrus (bilateral) ▼ Lateral occipital cortex (bilateral) Hybrid variable-priority training vs Control: ▼ dlPFC VG skill improvement: ▼ Intracalcarine cortex (right)
Han et al., 2012a*	2012	19	20.5 ± 1.5	Healthy young adults, male	–	Action, First Person Shooter	fMRI/MRI	Experimental (crossover)	VG vs. Neutral stimuli: ▲ IFG (left) ▲ PHG (left) ▲ Parietal lobe (bilateral) ▲ Thalamus (bilateral) ▲ Cerebellum (right)

(Continued)

TABLE 5 | Continued

Ref.	Year	*N*	Age	Sample	VG experience	VG genre	Technique	Design	Neural correlates
									VG training amount: ▲ Medial frontal lobe (right) ▲ PrCG (bilateral) ▲ PoCG (right) ▲ PHG (right) ▲ PCu (left)
Havranek et al., 2012	2012	20	23.5 ± 3.83	Healthy young adults	VGP (>11.7 h/week) Non-VGP (0.2 h/week)	Role-playing	EEG	Experimental (factorial)	1st person view vs. 3rd person view: ▼ Parietal alpha ▼ Occipital alpha ▼ Limbic cortex alpha Active VGP vs. Passive VGP: ▲ Frontal theta
Klasen et al., 2012*	2012	13	(18–26)	Healthy young adults, male	VGP (15.1 ± 9.0 h/week)	Action, First Person Shooter	fMRI	Experimental (crossover)	Success vs. failure events: ▲ Head of the CN ▲ NAcc ▲ Putamen ▲ Cerebellum ▲ Thalamus ▲ SPG ▲ Motor and premotor areas High vs low focus (presence of enemies): ▲ Cerebellum ▲ Visual areas ▲ PCu ▲ Premotor areas ▼ IPS (bilateral) ▼ OFC ▼ rACC Goal-oriented vs exploratory: ▼ IPS (bilateral) ▲ FFA ▼ dACC ▼ PCu High vs Low control: ▲ Visual areas ▲ Cerebellum ▲ Thalamus ▲ Motor areas ▼ Temporal poles (bilateral) ▼ AG (bilateral)
Liu et al., 2012	2012	68	19.7 ± 2.0	Healthy young adults	–	Racing	NIRS	Experimental (randomized)	Extrinsic orders & Intrinsic orders vs. Control: ▲ Prefrontal activation Extrinsic orders vs. Intrinsic orders: ▲ Prefrontal activation (globally) ▼ Prefrontal activation (in subsequent VG trials)
Mathewson et al., 2012	2012	39	(18–28)	Healthy young adults	Low or Non-VGP (<3 h/week)	Action, shooter	EEG (ERSP)	Experimental (crossover)	Learning rate predicted by: ▲ Frontal alpha power ▲ Alpha ERSPs ▲ Delta ERSPs

(Continued)

TABLE 5 | Continued

Ref.	Year	*N*	Age	Sample	VG experience	VG genre	Technique	Design	Neural correlates
Prakash et al., 2012	2012	66	22 ± 2.90 (Fixed emphasis training) 20.86 ± 2.19 (Hybrid variable-priority training) 21.48 ± 2.71 (Control)	Healthy young adults	Low or Non-VGP (<4 h/week)	Action, shooter	fMRI	Experimental (randomized)	Post vs. Pre (all groups): ▼ MFG (right) ▼ SFG (right) ▼ vmPFC HVT vs. Control: ▼ MFG (right) ▼ SFG (right)
									▼ vmPFC HVT vs. FET: ▼ MFG (right) ▼ SFG (right) ▼ vmPFC ▼ Motor cortices ▼ Sensory cortices ▼ Posteriomedial cortex
Subhani et al., 2012**	2012	10	(19–25)	Healthy young adults	–	Racing	EEG	Quasi-experimental (with pretest)	Gaming vs. rest: ▲ Global theta Fz/alpha Pz ratio
Voss et al., 2012	2012	29	22.24 ± 2.90	Healthy young adults	Low or Non-VGP (<3 h/week)	Action, shooter	fMRI	Experimental (randomized)	Post vs. Pre-training (FC): Changes in the DMN
Wu et al., 2012	2012	16	21.3 (Experimental) 22 (Control)	Healthy young adults	Non-VGP	Action, First Person Shooter	EEG (ERP)	Experimental (randomized with pretest)	FPS vs. Non-action: =N100 amplitude =P100 amplitude ▲ P200 amplitude ▲ P300 amplitude
Anguera et al., 2013	2013	46	67.1 ± 64.2	Healthy older adults	Low or Non-VGP (<2 h/month)	Racing	EEG	Experimental (crossover)	After VG training: ▲ Midline frontal theta power ▲ Frontal-posterior theta coherence
Bailey and West, 2013**	2013	31	20.40 ± 2.01 (Action) 21.77 ± 4.02 (Non-action) 24.22 ± 8.43 (Control)	Healthy adults	Non-VGP (0 h/week)	Action, First Person Shooter Puzzle, Brain Training	EEG (ERP)	Experimental (randomized)	After VG training: Action VG vs. Control: ▲ Frontal amplitude (right) ▲ Posterior amplitude (right) Non-action VG vs. Control: ▲ N200 amplitude ▲ P300 amplitude ▼ Sustained modulation centralparietal region (left) ▲ Sustained modulation frontal region Post vs Pre: Action & Non-action VG vs. Control: ▲ P300 amplitude
Berta et al., 2013	2013	22	26.3 ± 5.5	Healthy young adults	VGP and Non-VGP	Action, shooter	EEG	Experimental (crossover)	VG difficulty differences in: Alpha frequency Low-beta frequency Mid beta frequency
Khairuddin et al., 2013*	2013	29	21.73 ± 1.59	Healthy young adults	–	Racing	EEG	Experimental (crossover)	3D vs. 2D VG play: ▲ Occipital CPEI complexity ▲ Occipital Hjorth complexity ▲ Temporal Hjorth complexity

(Continued)

TABLE 5 | Continued

Ref.	Year	*N*	Age	Sample	VG experience	VG genre	Technique	Design	Neural correlates
Krishnan et al., 2013	2013	24	–	–	Action VGP (9 h/week) Non-action VGP (15 h/week)	Action, First Person Shooter Role-playing	EEG (SSVEP)	Quasi-experimental (with control group)	Non-action VGP: (Hit rate at attended 8.6 Hz flicker) ▲ Parietal activation (task difficulty at attended 8.6 flicker) ▲ Frontal activation Action VGP: (Hit rate at ignored 3 Hz flicker) ▲ Parietal activation (task difficulty at ignored 3 Hz flicker) ▲ Frontal activation
Mathiak et al., 2013	2013	13	(18–26)	Healthy young adults, male	VGP (>5 h/week)	Action, First Person Shooter	fMRI	Quasi-experimental (crossover)	Decrease of positive affect: ▲ Insula (bilateral) ▲ Amygdala (bilateral) Increase of negative affect: ▼ vmPFC (bilateral) ▼ PCu ▼ HC
Martínez et al., 2013	2013	20	18.95 ± 2.65	Healthy young adults, female	Low or Non-VGP	Puzzle, Brain training	fMRI	Experimental (randomized, with pretest)	Post vs. pre-training (resting state): ▲ Parietofrontal correlated activity VG training vs. control group (resting state): ▲ PCu (bilateral) ▲ PCC ▲ Retrosplenial cortex ▲ Inferior parietal/supramarginal (B40) ▲ TPJ ▲ TO junction ▲ PTC (BA21, 22) ▲ Temporal pole (left) ▲ IFG (left) ▲ dlPFC & vmPFC (BA10, 11) (bilateral) ▲ MFG (BA9) (left) ▲ ACC (BA24, 32) ▲ Cuneus (BA18, 19) (bilateral) ▲ Cerebellum (bilateral) ▲ Thalamus
McGarry et al., 2013	2013	7	(60–85)	Healthy older adults	–	Strategy	fMRI	Quasi-experimental (with pretest)	After VG training (FC): ▲ PPC & AG
Tachtsidis and Papaioannou, 2013**	2013	30	24.00	Healthy young adults	≪Some≫ experience in VG	Action, fighting Puzzle	NIRS	Experimental (randomized with pretest)	VG playing vs. baseline: ▲ PFC Fighting vs. puzzle game: ▲ PFC (1st third of gameplay) ▼ PFC (3rd third of gameplay)
Hahn et al., 2014	2014	27	25.5 ± 4.18 (VGP) 24.5 ± 2.85 (Non-VGP)	Healthy young adults	VGP (>4 h/week) Non-VGP (0 h/week)	Role-playing, MMORPG	fMRI	Quasi-experimental (with control group)	VGP vs. Non-VGP (reward anticipation): ▼ VS VGP vs. Non-VGP (resting-state): ▲ VS regional homogeneity (right)
Nikolaidis et al., 2014	2014	45	21.74 ± 5.09	Healthy young adults	Low or Non-VGP (<4 h/week)	Action, shooter	fMRI	Experimental (crossover)	Post vs. Pre-training (predictors of working memory performance): ▲ Superior parietal lobule ▲ PoCG ▲ PCu
Strenziok et al., 2014	2014	46	69.21 ± 4.9	Healthy older adults	–	Action, Shooter real time strategy puzzle, Brain training	fMRI	Experimental (randomized with pretest)	Puzzle & Shooter vs. Strategy (FC): ▼ SPG & ITG

(Continued)

TABLE 5 | Continued

Ref.	Year	*N*	Age	Sample	VG experience	VG genre	Technique	Design	Neural correlates
Yoshida et al., 2014*	2014	20	22.3 ± 1.2	Healthy young adults	–	Puzzle	NIRS	Experimental (crossover)	Flow vs. boredom condition: ▲ vlPFC (bilateral) ▲ dlPFC (bilateral) ▲ Frontal pole areas (bilateral)
Anderson et al., 2015	2015	40	24.0	Healthy young adults	–	Action, shooter	fMRI	Experimental (crossover)	Predictor of VG skill: ▲ DS (right) ▲ Sequential structure of whole brain activation
Hsu et al., 2015	2015	41	26.3	Healthy young adults	–	Racing	tDCS	Experimental (crossover)	Anodal tDCS vs. Sham: ▲ dlPFC (left) enhanced multitasking performance 2nd session vs. 1st session: ▲ dlPFC (left) decreased multitasking cost
Kim Y. H. et al., 2015*	2015	31	29.0 ± 4.1	Healthy young adults	VGP (>3 h/week) Non-VGP (<10 h/year)	Strategy	fMRI	Quasi-experimental (with control group and pretest)	VGP vs. Non-VGP: ▲ IFG (right) ▲ ACC ▲ Striatum
Liu T. et al., 2015	2015	51	21.0 ± 2.2	Healthy young adults	Low and High VGP	Racing	NIRS	Experimental (factorial)	Single vs. Paired (low VGP group) ▲ PFC Low vs. High VGP (paired group) ▼ PFC
Lorenz et al., 2015	2015	50	23.8 ± 3.9 (Experimental) 23.4 ± 3.7 (Control)	Healthy young adults	Low or Non-VGP (0.7 ± 1.97 h/month)	Action, 3D Platforms	fMRI	Experimental (randomized)	Post vs. Pre-test (reward anticipation, VG training & control group): ▼ VS Post vs. Pre-test (VG training group): =VS Post vs. Pre-test (control group) ▼ VS
McMahan et al., 2015	2015	30	20.87 (18–43)	Healthy adults	Low and High VGP (20% >20 h/week)	Action, 2D Platforms	EEG	Experimental (crossover)	High vs. Low intensity VG events: ▲ Betta power ▲ Gamma power
Patten et al., 2015	2015	–	–	–	Low or Non-VGP VGP	–	EEG (ERP)	Quasi-experimental (with control group)	VGP vs. Non-VGP: ▼ Latency Pd component
West et al., 2015	2015	59	23.88 ± 3.94 (Action) 24.36 ± 3.68 (Non-action)	Healthy young adults	Action VGP (17.9 ± 10.44 h/week) Non-Action VGP (0 h/week)	Action, First Person Shooter, Adventure	EEG (ERP)	Quasi-experimental (with control group)	Action vs. Non-VGP: ▼ Visual cortex amplitude (N2pc) in near condition. ▲ Visual cortex amplitude (N2pc) in far condition ▲ P3 component amplitude in targets.

ACC, Anterior cingulate cortex; AG, Angular gyrus; CN, Caudate nucleus; CPEI, Composite permutation entropy index; dACC, Dorsal anterior cingulate cortex; dlPFC, Dorsolateral prefrontal cortex; DS, Dorsal striatum; EEG, Electroencephalography; ERP, Event-related potentials; ERSP, Event-related spectral dynamics; FFA, Fusiform face area; FC, Functional connectivity; FG, Fusiform gyrus; fMRI, Functional magnetic resonance imaging; FPN, Frontoparietal network; HC, Hippocampus; IFG, Inferior frontal gyrus; ITG, Inferior temporal gyrus; IPS, Intraparietal sulcus; liPFC, Lateral inferior prefrontal cortex; MCA, Middle cerebral artery; MCG, Middle cingulate gyrus; MFG, Middle frontal gyrus; MRI, Magnetic resonance imaging; NAcc, Nucleus accumbens; NIRS, Near-infrarred spectroscopy; OFC, Orbitofrontal cortex; PCA, Posterior cerebral artery; PPC, Posterior cingulate cortex; PCu, Precuneus; PFC: Prefrontal cortex; PHG, Parahippocampal gyrus; PoCG, Post central gyrus; POT, Parieto-occipito-temporal; PPC, Posterior parietal cortex; PrCG, Pre-central gyrus; PTC, Posterior temporal cortex; rACC, Rostral anterior cingulate cortex; SFG, Superior frontal gyrus; SPG, Superior parietal gyrus; SSVEP, Steady state visually evoked potential; tDCS, Transcranial direct current stimulation; TO, Temporo-occipital; TPJ, Temporo-parietal junction; VG, Video game; VGP, Video game player; vmPFC, Ventromedial prefrontal cortex; VS, Ventral striatum. Articles marked with an asterisk (*) discuss cognitive implications without directly assessing this dimension. Articles marked with a double asterisk (**) did not provide either empirical cognitive data nor discuss cognitive implications. The rest of the articles (non-marked) have measured cognitive correlates with specific tasks.

TABLE 6 | Studies providing functional data dealing with VG experts or excessive gaming

Ref.	Year	*N*	Mean age (range)	Sample	VG experience/Addiction	VG genre	Technique	Design	Neural correlates
Thalemann et al., 2007*	2007	30	Young adults, male	28.75 ± 6.11 (Excessive VGP) 25.73 ± 8.14 (Control)	Excessive VGP (4.31 ± 2.17 h/day) Casual VGP (0.25 ± 0.46 h/day	–	EEG (ERP)	Quasi-experimental (with control group)	Excessive vs. Casual VGP (exposition to gaming cues): ▲ Pz ▲ P4
Allison and Polich, 2008**	2008	14	23.5 ± 5.1	Healthy young adults	Expert VGP (>10 h/week)	Action, First Person Shooter	EEG (ERP)	Experimental (crossover)	Correlated with gaming workload: ▼ N100 amplitudes (largest in Cz, smallest in Pz) ▼ P200 amplitudes (largest in Cz) ▼ N200 amplitudes (largest in Cz) ▼ sP300 amplitudes (largest in Pz, smallest on Fz)
Ko et al., 2009*	2009	20	(21–25)	Young adults, male	IGD (>30 h/week) Control (<2 h/day)	Role playing, MMORPG	fMRI	Quasi-experimental (with control group)	IGD vs. Control (exposition to gaming pictures): ▲ OFC (right) ▲ NAcc (right) ▲ ACC & Medial frontal cortex (bilateral) ▲ dlPFC (right) ▲ CN (right)
Granek et al., 2010*	2010	26	24 ± 3.1 and 26 ± 4.6	Healthy young adults, male	Expert VGP (12.8 ± 8.6 h/week) Non-VGP	–	fMRI	Quasi-experimental	Expert VGP vs. Non-VGP: ▲ SFG ▲ dlPFC (including MFG (BA 46) & IFG) ▲ vlPFC (including IFG (BA 45), ventro-orbital frontal gyrus (BA 47) and rostral lateral sulcus (BA 45) ▲ PPC (including parietooccipital sulcus (BA 7, 19), PCu (BA 7), IPS (BA 7) and IPC (BA 7)
Liu et al., 2010*	2010	38	Young adults	21.0 ± 1.3 (IAD) 20.0 ± 1.8 (Control)	IAD (=6 h/day) Non-IAD	–	fMRI	Quasi-experimental (with control group)	IAD vs. Control (Regional homogeneity): ▲ Cerebellum ▲ Brainstem ▲ CG (right) ▲ PHG (bilateral) ▲ Frontal lobe (rectal gyrus, IFG & MFG) (right) ▲ SFG (left) ▲ PCu (left) ▲ PoCG (right)

(Continued)

TABLE 6 | Continued

Ref.	Year	*N*	Mean age (range)	Sample	VG experience/Addiction	VG genre	Technique	Design	Neural correlates
						–			▲ MOG (right) ▲ ITG (right) ▲ STG (left) ▲ MTG
Doty et al., 2011*	2011	14	–	–	VG Dependent VG Non-dependent	Action, First Person Shooter	EEG (ERP)	Quasi-experimental (with control group)	Dependent vs. Non-dependent group: ▼ PFC (Pre-event) ▼ PFC Theta waves (Post-event) ▼ Prefrontal and frontal regions (general activation)
Dong et al., 2012*	2012	29	24.2 ± 3.5 (IAD) 24.6 ± 3.8 (Control)	Young adults, male	IAD (>80% time playing VG) Control (16.3 ± 4.3 Young's scale score)	–	fMRI	Quasi-experimental (with control group)	IGD vs. Control (Regional Homogeneity): ▲ Brainstem ▲ IPC ▲ Posterior cerebellum (left) ▲ MFG (left) ▼ ITG (left) ▼ Occipital lobe (left) ▼ PoCG (left) ▼ MCG (left)
Ding et al., 2013*	2013	41	16.94 ± 2.73 (Internet addiction group) 15.87 ± 2.69 (Control group)	Adolescents	Internet Addiction (26.44 ± 21.47 h/week; CIAS 64.59 ± 6.43) Control (10.50 ± 11.60 h/week; CIAS 45.70 ± 7.81)	–	fMRI	Quasi-experimental (with control group)	IGD vs. Control (FC): ▲ Bilateral cerebellum posterior lobe & MTG ▼ IPC (bilateral) & ITG (right)
Feng et al., 2013*	2013	33	16.93 ± 2.34 (IGD) 16.33 ± 2.61 (Control)	Adolescents	IGD (25.47 ± 17.89 h/week; 66.73 ± 3.01 Chen Internet Addiction Scale) Control (9.28 ± 12.90 h/week; 40.50 ± 8.42 Chen Internet Addiction Scale)	–	fMRI	Quasi-experimental (with control group)	IGD vs. Control: ▲ ITC/FG (left) ▲ PHG/Amygdala (left) ▲ Medial frontal lobe /ACC (right) ▲ Insula (bilateral) ▲ MTG (right) ▲ PrCG (right) ▲ SMA (left) ▲ CG (left) ▲ IPC (right) ▼ MTG (left) ▼ MOG (left) ▼ CG (right)

(Continued)

TABLE 6 | Continued

Ref.	Year	*N*	Mean age (range)	Sample	VG experience/Addiction	VG genre	Technique	Design	Neural correlates
Kätsyri et al., 2013a*	2013	11	25.6 (22–33)	Healthy young adults, male	VG Experts (>10 h/week)	Action, First Person Shooter	fMRI	Experimental (crossover)	Winning vs. Losing: ▲ omPFC Active vs. Vicarious playing: ▼ Midbrain ▼ Striatum (especially anterior putamen, in loss events)
Kätsyri et al., 2013b*	2013	17	24.8 (20–33)	Healthy young adults, male	VG Experts (>10 h/week)	Action, First Person Shooter	fMRi	Experimental (crossover)	Winning vs. Losing: ▲ vmPFC ▲ VS ▲ DS Winning condition (FC): ▲ VS & ▲ Insula (right) ▲ VS & ▲ DS ▲ VS & ▲ PrCG & PoCG ▲ VS & ▲ Visual association cortices Human vs. Computer opponent: ▲ vmPFC ▲ DS
Ko et al., 2013*	2013	45	24.67 ± 3.11 (IGD) 24.80 ± 2.68 (Remission) 24.47 ± 2.83 (Control)	Young adults, male	IGD IGD in remission Control (Non-IGD)	Role playing, MMORPG	fMRI	Quasi-experimental (with control group)	IGD vs. Control (exposition to gaming cues): ▲ dlPFC (bilateral) ▲ PCu ▲ PHG (left) ▲ PCC ▲ ACC (right)
Kim et al., 2013	2013	5	18 ± 0	Adolescents, male	IGD (>4 h/day) Control (0 h/day)	–	EEG (ERP)	Quasi-experimental (with control group and pretest)	Pre vs. Post course: ▲ P300 fronto-central areas (bilateral) IGD vs. Control (current density, post-course): ▼ Midline paracentral lobule ▼ PCu
Latham et al., 2013	2013	31	23.27 ± 0.88 (VGP) 25.69 ± 1.19 (Non-VGP)	Healthy young adults, male	Expert VGP (34.67 ± 5.01 h/week) Non-VGP	Action, shooter; Strategy or Role Playing, MMORPG	EEG (ERP)	Quasi-experimental	Expert VPG vs. Low VPG: Earlier Visual N1

(Continued)

TABLE 6 | Continued

Ref.	Year	*N*	Mean age (range)	Sample	VG experience/Addiction	VG genre	Technique	Design	Neural correlates
Song et al., 2013*	2013	39	Healthy young adults, male	20.5 ± 1.6 (2D) 20.4 ± 2.1 (3D)	Professional VGP (2D strategy VG) Professional VGP (3D strategy VG)	Real time strategy	fMRI	Quasi-experimental (with control group)	2D vs. 3D strategy game: ▲ SFG (right) ▲ Medial frontal gyrus (bilateral) ▲ Occipital lobe (right) ▼ MFG (left) ▼ FG (left) ▼ Cerebellum (left)
Yuan et al., 2013b	2013	36	Adolescents and young adults	19.4 ± 3.1 (IGD) 19.5 ± 2.8 (Control)		Role playing, MMORPG	fMRI	Quasi-experimental (with control group)	IGD vs. Control: ▲ medial OFC (left) ▲ PCu (left) ▲ SMA (left) ▲ PHG (right) ▲ MCG (bilateral)
Chen et al., 2014	2014	30	24.67 ± 3.12 (IGD) 24.47 ± 2.83 (Control)	Young adults, male	IGD (>4 h/day; 76.00 ± 12.09 Chen Internet Addiction Scale) Control (26.0 ± 0.0 Chen Internet Addiction Scale)	Role playing, MMORPG	fMRI	Quasi-experimental (with control group)	IGD vs. Control: ▼ SMA (right) ▼ preSMA (right)
Tian et al., 2014*	2014	12	Young adults, male	23.5 ± 2.58 (IGD) 22.7 ± 1.27 (Control)	IGD (77.6 ± 6.8 Young's scale score) Control (28.7 ± 3.7 Young's scale score)	Role playing, MMORPG	PET	Quasi-experimental (with control group and pretest)	IGD vs. Control (glucose metabolism): ▲ Cuneus (right) ▲ Calcarine (right) ▼ Medial temporal cortex (left) Within group (monoamine receptors): ▲ Correlation with IGD severity ▼ Putamen ▼ OFC/cerebellum ratio Glucose vs. monoamine: ▲ Striatum/cerebellum ratio ▲ OFC/cerebellum ratio
Wee et al., 2014*	2014	33	Adolescents	17.3 ± 2.6 (IAD) 17.7 ± 2.5 (Control)	IAD (4.8 ± 22 h/day; 62.4 ± 17.1 Young's Internet Addiction Scale) Control (1.3 ± 0.6 h/day; 37.0 ± 10.6 Young's Internet Addiction Scale)	–	fMRI	Quasi-experimental (with control group)	IAD vs. Control (FC): Frontal, occipital, and parietal lobes

(Continued)

TABLE 6 | Continued

Ref.	Year	*N*	Mean age (range)	Sample	VG experience/Addiction	VG genre	Technique	Design	Neural correlates
Xing et al., 2014	2014	34	Young adults	19.1 ± 0.7 (IGD) 19.8 ± 1.3 (Control)	IGD (9.5 ± 1.3 h/day; 65.7 ± 11.6 IAT) Control (2.2 ± 1.4 h/day; 29.2 ± 4.5 IAT)	Action, Real time strategy	fMRI	Quasi-experimental (with control group)	IGD vs. Control (FC): =FC
Gong et al., 2015*	2015	57	23.26 ± 0.4 (Experts) 22.36 ± 0.38 (Amateurs)	Healthy young adults	Expert VGF (46.67 ± 2.1 h/week) Amateur VGP (14.2 ± 1.1 h/week)	Action, Real time strategy	fMRI	Quasi-experimental (with control group)	Experts vs. Amateurs (FC): ▲ Between insular regions (especially left) VG experience (FC): ▲ Insular functional integration (left)
Han et al., 2015	2015	47	15.2 ± 1.9 (IGD) 14.9 ± 1.9 (Control)	Adolescents, male	IGD (>30 h/week) Non-IGD	Role playing Real time strategy First Person Shooter Others	fMRI	Quasi-experimental (with control group)	IGD vs. Control: ▲ FEF (left) to dACC ▲ FEF (left) to anterior insula (right) ▲ dlPFC (left) to TPJ (left) ▲ dlPFC (right) to TPJ (right) ▲ Auditory cortex (right) to motor cortex (right) ▲ Auditory cortex (right) to SMA ▲ Auditory cortex (right) to dACC
Hong et al., 2015*	2015	23	13.4 ± 2.31(IGD) 14.81 ± 0.87(Control)	Adolescents, male	IGD (14.25 ±1 2.12 h/week; 57.00 ± 17.39 Young Internet Addiction Test) Controls (16.86 ± 6.51 h/week; 38.36 ± 7.31 Young Internet Addiction Test)	–	fMRI	Quasi-experimental (with control-group)	IGD vs. Control (FC): ▼ Dorsal putamen & (Posterior insula, parietal operculum) Internet addiction scores (FC): ▲ Dorsal putamen & PoCG (bilateral)
Kim H. et al., 2015*	2015	31	21.63 ± 5.92 (IGD) 25.4 ± 5.29 (Control)	Young adults, male	IGD (5.95 ± 2.27 h/day; 75.81 ± 4.72 Young's Internet Addiction Test) Control (<2 h/day; 23.80 ± 14.81 Young's Internet Addiction Test)	–	fMRI	Quasi-experimental (with control group)	IGD vs. Control (Regional Homogeneity): ▲ PCC ▼ STG (right) Internet addiction scores correlated in (Regional Homogeneity): ▲ Medial frontal cortex ▲ PCu/PCC ▲ ITC (left)

(Continued)

TABLE 6 | Continued

Ref.	Year	*N*	Mean age (range)	Sample	VG experience/Addiction	VG genre	Technique	Design	Neural correlates
Lee et al., 2015	2015	38	Adolescents, male	13.6 ± 0.9 (IGD) 13.4 ± 1.0 (Control)	IGD Control (Non-IGD)	–	fMRI	Quasi-experimental (with control group)	IGD vs. Control (Angry facial stimuli): ▼ dACC ▲ Insula ▼ PPC ▲ FG IGD vs. Control (FC): ▲ (Insula & ▼ dlPFC, ▼ MTG, ▼ cerebellum, PPC)
Liu J. et al., 2015*	2015	40	Young adults	21.4 ± 1.0 (IGD) 20.8 ± 1.1 (Control)	IGD (=6 h/day in internet) Control (<3 h/day in internet)	Role playing, MMORPG	fMRI	Quasi-experimental (with control group)	IGD vs. Control: ▲ SPG (right) ▲ Insular lobe (right) ▲ PCu (right) ▲ CG (right) ▲ STG (right) ▲ Brainstem (left) ▲ Frontal cortex
Luijten et al., 2015	2015	45	Young adults, male	20.83 ± 3.05 (IGD) 21.38 ± 3.03 (Control)	IGD (Video game Addiction Test score = 2.5) Control (Video game Addiction Test score = 1.5)	–	fMRI	Quasi-experimental (with control group)	IGD vs. Control: ▼ IFG (left) ▼ IPC (right)
Wang et al., 2015*	2015	31	Adolescents	16.94 ± 2.73 (IGD) 15.87 ± 2.69 (Control)	IGD (64.59 ± 6.43 Chen Internet Addiction Scale) Control (45.70 ± 7.81 Chen Internet Addiction Scale)	–	fMRI	Quasi-experimental (with control group)	IGD vs. Control (FC): ▼ SFG (orbital part) (bilateral) ▼ IFG (orbital part) ▼ MFG ▼ SFG
Dong and Potenza, 2016	2016	36	21.33 ± 2.18 (IGD) 21.90 ± 2.33 (Control)	Young adults, male	IGD (>80% online time) Low or Non-VGP	–	fMRI	Quasi-experimental (with control group)	IGD vs. Control: ▼ ACC ▼ PCC ▼ MTG ▼ IFG (RT) ▼ STG (RT)

(Continued)

TABLE 6 | Continued

Ref.	Year	*N*	Mean age (range)	Sample	VG experience/Addiction	VG genre	Technique	Design	Neural correlates
Gong et al., 2016	2016	45	23.3 ± 4.3 (Experts) 22.3 ± 3.46 (Amateurs)	Healthy young adults, male	Experts (ELO > 1,800) Amateurs (ELO < 1,200)	Action, Real time strategy	fMRI	Quasi-experimental (with control group)	Action VG Experts vs. Amateurs: ▲ SN & CEN (global characteristics) ▲ Local regions of SN & CEN (nodal characteristics) ▲ SN & CEN (FC)
Han et al., 2016	2016	102	20.2 ± 3.2 (IGD) 20.2 ± 2.9 (Control)	Adolescent or young adults, male	IGD (>30 h/week) Low or Non-VGP	Role playing Real time strategy First Person Shooter Others	fMRI	Quasi-experimental (with control group)	IGD vs. Control (During executive task): ▲ Lateral occipital cortex (right) ▲ PCu
Jin et al., 2016*	2016	46	19.12 ± 1.05 (IGD) 18.76 ± 1.81 (Control)	Adolescents	IGD (5.32 ± 2.10 h/day) Low or Non-VGP (2.07 ± 1.39 h/day)	Action, Real time strategy	fMRI/MRI	Quasi-experimental (with control group)	IGD vs. Control (FC): ▼ (dlPFC, OFC, ACC & SMA) & (Insula, temporal cortices, occipital cortices) ▼ (dlPFC, OFC, ACC & SMA) & (DS, pallidum, thalamus)
Park et al., 2016	2016	36	Young adults, male	24.2 ± 3.2 (OGA-CBT) 23.6 ± 2.7 (OGA-VRT) 23.3 ± 2.9 (Control)	IGD (>30 h/week) Control (<3 h/week)	–	fMRI	Quasi-experimental (with control group)	IGD vs. Control (baseline, ALFF): ▼ MFG (right) IGD vs. Control (baseline, FC) ▼ Cortico-striatal limbic circuit
Zhang et al., 2016	2016	115	Young adults	22.28 ± 1.98 (IGD) 23.02 ± 2.09 (Control)	IGD (78.36 ± 8.43 Chen Internet Addiction Scale) Control (43.49 ± 9.64 Chen Internet Addiction Scale)	–	fMRI	Quasi-experimental (with control group)	IGD vs. Control (FC): ▲ (Anterior insula & ACC, Putamen, Angular gyrus, PCu) ▲ (Posterior insula & PoCG, PrCG, SMA, STG) IGD severity (FC): ▲ (Anterior insula & Angular gyrus, STG) ▲ (Posterior insula & STG)

ACC, Anterior cingulate cortex; CEN, Central executive network; CG, Cingulate gyrus; CIAS, Chen's Internet addiction scale; CN, Caudate nucleus; dACC, Dorsal anterior cingulate cortex; dlPFC, Dorsolateral prefrontal cortex; DS, Dorsal striatum; FC, Functional connectivity; FEF, Frontal eye fields; FG, Fusiform gyrus; IFG, Inferior frontal gyrus; IGD, Internet gaming disorder; IPC, Inferior parietal cortex; IPS, Intraparietal sulcus; ITC, Inferior temporal cortex; ITG, Inferior temporal gyrus; MCG, Middle cingulate gyrus; MFG, Middle frontal gyrus; MOG, Middle occipital gyrus; MTG, Middle temporal gyrus; NAcc, Nucleus accumbens; OFC, Orbitofrontal cortex; omPFC, Orbitomedial prefrontal cortex; PCC, Posterior cingulate cortex; PCu, Precuneus; PFC, Prefrontal cortex; PHG, Parahippocampal gyrus; PoCG, Post-central gyrus; PrCG, Pre-central gyrus; preSMA, Pre-supplementary motor area; SFG, Superior frontal gyrus; SMA, Supplementary motor area; SN, Salience network; SPG, Superior temporal gyrus; STG, Superior temporal gyrus; TPJ, Temporo-parietal junction; vlPFC, Ventrolateral prefrontal cortex; VS, Ventral striatum. Articles marked with an asterisk (*) discuss cognitive implications without directly assessing this dimension. Articles marked with a double asterisk (**) did not provide either empirical cognitive data nor discuss cognitive implications. The rest of the articles (non-marked) have measured cognitive correlates with specific tasks.

TABLE 7 | Studies providing functional data focused on the violent contents of VG.

Ref.	Year	*N*	Sample	Age	VG experience	VG genre	Technique	Design	Neural correlates
Bartholow et al., 2006	2006	39	Healthy young adults	19.50	Violent VGP Non-violent VGP	"Violent" VG "Non-violent" VG	EEG (ERP)	Quasi experimental (with control group)	Violent vs. Non-violent: ▼ P300 amplitudes
Mathiak and Weber, 2006*	2006	13	Healthy young adults, male	(18–26)	VGP (15.1 ± 9.0 h/week)	Action, First Person Shooter	fMRI	Quasi-experimental	During violent scenes: ▲ dACC ▼ rACC ▼ Amygdala
Weber et al., 2006*	2006	13	Healthy young adults	23.00 (18–26)	VGP (15.1 h/week)	Action, First Person Shooter	fMRI	Experimental (crossover)	During virtual violence exposure: ▼ Amygdala ▼ ACC
Wang et al., 2009	2009	44	Healthy adolescents	14.8 ± 1.2 (Violent group) 15.0 ± 1.1 (Non-violent group)	–	Sports, Racing Action, First person shooter	fMRI	Experimental (randomized)	Violent vs. Non-violent (Counting Stroop task): ▼ PFC Violent vs. Non-violent (Counting Stroop task, FC): ▼ dlPFC & ACC (left) Violent vs. Non-violent (Emotional Stroop task): ▲ Amygdala (right) ▼ Medial PFC Violent vs. Non-violent (Emotional Stroop task, FC): ▼ Amygdala & Medial PFC (non-violent group) =FC (violent group)
Hummer et al., 2010	2010	45	Healthy adolescents	14.9 ± 0.3 (Non-violent) 14.5 ± 0.3 (Violent)	–	Sports, Racing Action, First Person Shooter	fMRI	Experimental (randomized)	Violent vs. Non-violent (Go/No-go): ▼ dlPFC (right) Non-violent VG (FC): ▼ dlPFC & ▲ PCu
Regenbogen et al., 2010*	2010	22	Healthy young adults, male	25.9 ± 2.9	VGP (131 h/year violent VG) Low or Non-VGP (6 h/year violent VG)	Violent VG	fMRI	Quasi-experimental (with control group)	Real vs. Non-violent content (VGP): ▲ IFG (right) ▲ Lingual gyrus (left) ▲ STG Virtual vs. Non-violent content (VGP): ▲ IFG (bilateral) ▲ Occipital cortex ▲ PoCG ▲ MTG (right) ▲ FG (left) Real vs. Non-violent content (Control): ▲ Frontal regions (left) ▲ Insula ▲ SFG Virtual vs. Non-violent content (Control): ▲ Posterior regions

(Continued)

TABLE 7 | Continued

Ref.	Year	*N*	Sample	Age	VG experience	VG genre	Technique	Design	Neural correlates
Bailey et al., 2011*	2011	48	Healthy young adults, male	19.73 ± 1.28 (low VGP) 19.87 ± 3.52 (high VGP)	Low VGP (3 h/week) High VGP (33 h/week)	"Violent" VG	EEG (ERP)	Quasi-experimental (with control group)	High vs. Low VGP: (Negative & violent) vs. (neutral and positive) stimuli: ▼ FCz (@125 ms) ▼ Oz (@280 ms) Early posterior negativity (EPN) ▲ PO4 & F9 (500-1000 ms) Late positive potential (LPP) High (positive & violent vs. neutral stimuli) vs. Low VGP (Positive vs. neutral stimuli): ▼ Fpz (@100 ms) ▲ C3, CP3 (400–900 ms) ▼ Iz (400–900 ms) Low vs. High VGP (negative vs. violent stimuli): ▲ F9 (sustained) ▲ TP8 (sustained) ▲ PO9 (@300 ms)
Engelhardt et al., 2011	2011	70	Healthy young adults	(18–22)	Violent VGP Non-violent VGP	Action, First Person Shooter, Adventure Action, Adventure, Sports, Platforms	EEG (ERP)	Quasi-experimental (with control group)	Violent vs. Non-violent: ▼ P3 component at parietal (P3, Pz, and P4) regions
Mathiak et al., 2011*	2011	13	Healthy young adults, male	22.7 ± 2.0	VGP (15.1 ± 9.0 h/week)	Action, First Person Shooter	fMRI	Quasi-experimental	(Failure & success events) vs. Baseline: ▲ Visual cortex Failure vs. Success events: ▼ OFC ▼ CN Negative vs. Positive affect (only failure events): ▼ Temporal pole (right)
Montag et al., 2012*	2012	40	Healthy young adults, male	23.33 ± 4.45	Experienced VGP in First person Shooters (18.83 ± 9.12 h/week) Low or Non-VGP (2.00 ± 3.82 h/week)	Action First Person Shooter	fMRI	Quasi-experimental (with control group)	VGP vs. Control (during negative emotional stimuli): ▼ Lateral medial frontal lobe (left) VGP vs. Control (during VG cues): ▲ Frontal regions ▲ Temporal regions
Chou et al., 2013*	2013	30	Healthy young adults	24.67 ± 4.7	VGP (3.1 h/week)	Action, Fighting Action, 3D platforms	SPECT	Experimental (crossover)	Post vs. Pre-training: ▼ PFC ▲ Temporal cortex ▲ Occipital cortex Violent vs. Non-violent VG: ▼ dACC (in males)

(Continued)

TABLE 7 | Continued

Ref.	Year	*N*	Sample	Age	VG experience	VG genre	Technique	Design	Neural correlates
Lianekhammy and Werner-Wilson, 2015*	2015	45	Healthy adolescents	14.3 ± 1.5	Brain training VG group (4.8 ± 10.6 h/week) Violent VG group (17.7 ± 17.4 h/week) Non-violent VG (9.3 ± 8.4 h/week)	Puzzle Action, First Person Shooter Action, 3D platforms	EEG	Experimental (randomized)	High empathy vs. Low empathy: ▲ Right hemisphere frontal EEG asymmetry scores (violent and non-violent) ▲ Right hemisphere High vs. Low helpfulness: ▲ Left hemisphere (non-violent group)
Liu Y. et al., 2015	2015	49	Healthy young adults	20.76 ± 1.76	–	Strategy Sports, Racing	EEG (ERP)	Experimental (randomized)	Prosocial vs. Neutral VG: ▼ P300 amplitudes
Petras et al., 2015	2015	30	Healthy adults	25.96 (18–44)	21 Non habitual VGP (<once a week) 9 Habitual VGP (≥once a week)	Action, Shooter	EEG (ERP)	Experimental (randomized, factorial)	Egocentric vs. Bird-view perspective: ▲ N1 amplitudes (shoot task) ▼ Pre-stimulus alpha power (shoot task)
Zvyagintsev et al., 2016*	2016	18	Healthy young adults, male	25.1 ± 2.7	VGP (>5 h/week)	Sports, Racing (Violent)	fMRI	Experimental (crossover)	Violent vs. Non-violent (FC): ▼ Sensory-motor networks ▼ Reward network ▼ DMN ▼ FPN (right)

3D, Three-dimensional; ACC, Anterior cingulate cortex; CN, Caudate nucleus; dACC, Dorsal anterior cingulate cortex; dlPFC, Dorsolateral prefrontal cortex; DMN, Default mode network; EEG, Electroencephalography; ERP, Event-related potentials; FC, Functional connectivity; FG, Fusiform gyrus; fMRI, Functional Magnetic Resonance Imaging; FPN, Frontoparietal network; IFG, Inferior frontal gyrus; MTG, Middle temporal gyrus; OFC, Orbitofrontal cortex; Pcu, Precuneus; PFC, Prefrontal cortex; PoCG, Post-central gyrus; rACC, Rostral anterior cingulate cortex; SFG, Superior frontal gyrus; SPECT, Single-photon emission computed tomography; STG, Superior temporal gyrus; VG, Video game; VGP, Video game player. Articles marked with an asterisk (*) discuss cognitive implications without directly assessing this dimension. Articles marked with a double asterisk (**) did not provide either empirical cognitive data nor discuss cognitive implications. The rest of the articles (non-marked) have measured cognitive correlates with specific tasks.

Attention

Attentional resources are one of the main cognitive domains in which VGs are involved and one of the most researched. The involvement of attentional networks during gameplay is closely related with other brain regions responsible for cognitive control, especially when more complex operations toward a specific goal are required. Many brain regions are involved in attention, particularly nodes in the dorsal frontoparietal system, mediating top-down attentional processes in goal-oriented behavior, but also nodes in the ventral network, responsible for bottom-up sensory stimulation (e.g., Vossel et al., 2014) dealing with those salient stimuli to which the player must pay attention.

There is evidence that VGPs display enhanced performance in a range of top-down attentional control areas, such as selective attention, divided attention, and sustained attention (Bavelier et al., 2012b). The ACC is an area that consistently shows functional activity during VG play due to its involvement as the main hub in top-down attentional processes (selective or focused attention) and goal-oriented behavior (e.g., Anderson et al., 2011*; Bavelier et al., 2012b).

Non-VGPs, compared to VGPs, showed greater frontoparietal recruitment, a source of selective attention, as task demands increased, showing that habitual gamers have more efficient top-down resource allocation during attentional demanding tasks (Bavelier et al., 2012a). That resource optimization effect can also be observed in attentional control areas, such as the right middle frontal gyrus (MFG), right superior frontal gyrus (SFG), and the ventromedial prefrontal cortex (vmPFC) (Prakash et al., 2012*). Functional connectivity changes in the attentional ventral stream, particularly in occipitotemporal WM, responsible for bottom-up reorienting toward novel stimuli, have also been observed as a result of VG training and were linked to cognitive improvement (Strenziok et al., 2014*). Integration between attentional and sensoriomotor functions has been observed in expert VGPs in the form of increased structural GM and functional connectivity in anterior and posterior insular sub regions where long-term exposure to attentional VG demands coordinated with the fine skills involved in using the VG controller may have resulted in plastic changes in these two regions that are respectively involved in attentional and sensoriomotor networks (Gong et al., 2015*).

Using electrophysiological techniques, it seems that VG play correlates with an increment of the frontal midline theta rhythm, associated with focused attention (Pellouchoud et al., 1999*), and increases with VG practice (Sheikholeslami et al., 2007**; Smith et al., 1999), both in an action and a puzzle VG, attributable to ACC activity. Likewise, amplitudes in the P200 (Wu et al., 2012), an early visual stimuli perceptual component, and P300 components (Mishra et al., 2011; Wu et al., 2012), which involved in early stages of decision-making, were also linked to top-down spatial selective attention improvements after training and lifetime exposure to action VG. Action VGPs and non-action VGPs seem to respond differently in the way they deploy attention to central and peripheral targets in visual attention tasks, as measured by the N2pc component (West et al., 2015), which is also linked to selective attention.

If we consider different VG genres, it seems that action VGs are better at improving selective attention than other slow-paced VGs such as role-playing games (RPG) (Krishnan et al., 2013), puzzle (Green and Bavelier, 2003), or strategy VGs (Tsai et al., 2013) which require high planning skills and other forms of proactive cognitive control. This is probably due to the extensive use of attentional systems, paired with precise timings that action VGs require. While these improved attentional skills are typically observed in habitual VGPs, it is possible to achieve long-lasting improvements as a result of a single VG training procedure (Anguera et al., 2013).

Visuospatial Skills

Visuospatial skills encompass processes that allow us to perceive, recognize, and manipulate visual stimuli, including visuomotor coordination and navigational skills, and VGs are predominantly interactive visual tasks.

The areas implicated in visuospatial processing have traditionally been classified along a visual ventral stream (responsible for object recognition) and a visual dorsal stream (responsible for spatial location). Both depart from the visual cortex, in the occipital lobe, and reach the posterior parietal cortex (dorsal stream) and the inferior temporal cortex (ventral stream). More recent proposals have refined that model, broadening the traditional conceptualization of the two-stream model (for further details see Kravitz et al., 2011). Among other nodes, the role of the hippocampus stands out for its function in higher order visual processing and memory (Kravitz et al., 2011; Lee A. C. H. et al., 2012).

Neural correlates related to visuospatial skills have been detected in relationship with structural volume enlargements of the right hippocampus (HC), both in long-term gamers and experimentally after a VG training period (Kühn et al., 2013; Kühn and Gallinat, 2014*). Increased hippocampal volumes were also found by Szabó et al. (2014**), although the authors do not attribute that effect to the VG training. The entorhinal cortex, associated with navigational skills (Schmidt-Hieber and Häusser, 2013), which together with the HC is involved in spatial memory (Miller et al., 2015), was also correlated with lifetime experience in logic/puzzle and platform VG (Kühn and Gallinat, 2014*).

Decreased activation in occipitoparietal regions, associated with the dorsal visuospatial stream (Goodale and Milner, 1992), has also been linked to improved visuomotor task performance, suggesting a reduction of the cognitive costs as a consequence of the VG training, dependent on the training strategy used in the VG (Lee H. et al., 2012). Earlier N100 latencies in the visual pathways are another feature found in long-term VGPs, which may contribute to faster response times in visual tasks after years of practice (Latham et al., 2013).

Reduced WM integrity in interhemispheric parietal networks for spatially-guided behavior could be another symptom for a decreased reliance on specific visuospatial networks after VG training as performance improved (Strenziok et al., 2013*). However, other studies found that increased WM integrity in visual and motor pathways was directly responsible for better visuomotor performance in long term VGPs (Zhang et al., 2015*). Despite these connectivity changes, brain functional differences between VGPs and non-VGPs do not always reflect performance in visuospatial skills, which were best predicted by non-visual areas (Kim Y. H. et al., 2015*).

Cognitive Workload

Brain activation patterns depend on the cognitive demands of the environment and also on the associated level of workload (Vogan et al., 2016), which is directly related to the allocation of resources to the working memory and its associated attentional processes (Barrouillet et al., 2007). When we manipulate this variable and observe its neural correlates, it is likely that we are seeing the result of neural recruitment mechanisms as the cognitive demands increase (Bavelier et al., 2012a). VGs have often been employed to obtain cerebral measures of cognitive workload, given the ability to adjust many of their features, particularly in a purpose-made VG, such as the popular Space Fortress. Due to the nature of this task, it is likely that functional changes related to the manipulation of cognitive load appear along the attentional networks and in specific key nodes related to executive functions, mainly in prefrontal and parietal cortices.

Cognitive workload is not a unitary concept; some studies have been able to identify different activation patterns by manipulating the difficulty of a task (e.g., Anderson et al., 2011*). Namely, the number of stimuli appearing simultaneously on the screen and the complexity of each stimulus seem to elicit different responses from the brain. For instance, in the context of an air traffic control simulator, when directly manipulating the task difficulty by increasing the number of planes that a participant had to attend, the theta band power increased (Brookings et al., 1996). Theta band power also displayed higher power compared to a resting condition, and gradually increased during gameplay (Sheikholeslami et al., 2007**). The theta band seems to be directly related to the level of cognitive demand in a wide range of cognitive abilities, such as attention, memory, and visuospatial processes, although this finding is not universal and decreased theta band power has been observed as a feature of sustained attention. So it appears that it is both related to task complexity and levels of arousal and fatigue. On the other hand, beta band power seemed to be more associated with the complexity of the task, especially in frontal and central areas, likely indicating a qualitative change in the cognitive strategy followed by the participant or the type of processing done by the brain (Brookings et al., 1996).

Assessing cognitive workload with ERP shows that during VG play, amplitudes tend to correlate negatively with game difficulty in expert VGPs, with most ERP (P200, N200) having its maximum amplitude in frontoparietal locations, with the exception of the P300, being larger in parietal regions (Allison and Polich, 2008). This is consistent with previous literature about cognitive workload related to attention and working memory demands and ERP peak amplitude decrements (Watter et al., 2001).

Frontoparietal activity, linked to attentional processes, also exhibits recruitment effects as game difficulty increases, which also affects reaction times, making them slower (Bavelier et al., 2012a). As mentioned above, comparing habitual VGPs with non-VGPs, it appears that the former show less recruitment of frontoparietal networks when compared to the non-gamers, which could be attributed to their VG experience and the optimization of their attentional resources (Bavelier et al., 2012a). Increased blood flow in prefrontal areas like dlPFC was also associated with increasing cognitive demands related to attention, verbal and spatial working memory and decision making (Izzetoglu et al., 2004*).

The intensity of the events displayed in the VG was also linked with certain electrophysiological correlates. High intensity events, such as the death of the VG character, were associated with increased beta and gamma power when compared with general gameplay (McMahan et al., 2015).

Cognitive Control

During the course of a VG, the player can encounter many situations in which he has to use one of several possible actions. For instance, while playing a game, the player might be required to interrupt and quickly implement an alternate strategy, or manipulate a number of elements in a certain way in order to solve a puzzle and progress in the storyline. All these abilities can be characterized under the "umbrella" of cognitive control, which includes reactive and proactive inhibition, task switching and working memory (Obeso et al., 2013). These cognitive control aspects are key to overcoming the obstacles found the VG. In fact, they are frequently used in parallel (Nachev et al., 2008) in order to engage in goal-directed behavior. These processes have their neural substrate in the prefrontal cortex, supported by posterior parietal areas and the basal ganglia (Alvarez and Emory, 2006). Therefore, most changes regarding cognitive control observed after VG play will likely be detected in these regions.

Indeed, prefrontal regions are one of the brain areas in which GM volumetric changes have been observed as a result of a cognitive training with a VG, which is remarkable if we consider that the common VG training period spans from a few weeks to a couple of months. These regions, such as the dlPFC, determinant for cognitive control (Smith and Jonides, 1999), show volumetric changes that seem to correlate with VG performance and experience, likely as a result of the continuous executive demands found in a VG, such as attentional control and working memory (Basak et al., 2011). These volumetric changes even result in correlations with transfer effects in cognitive control tasks (Hyun et al., 2013). Volumetric-behavioral correlations work both ways, since individuals with decreased orbitofrontal cortex (OFC) volumes as a consequence of VG addiction show poorer performance in similar tasks (Yuan et al., 2013a).

During VG play, these prefrontal regions increase their activation in response to the cognitive demands (game difficulty) and display a positive correlation with performance measures (Izzetoglu et al., 2004*). Still, prefrontal activity is not only affected by the complexity of the task, but also by the nature of the task and the individual differences of the participants (Biswal et al., 2010). Some research groups have found deactivation of dorsal prefrontal regions during gameplay. A possible explanation for this phenomenon could be the interference effect of attentional resources during visual stimuli, since activity in the dlPFC remained stable while passively watching a VG, but not while actively playing it (Matsuda and Hiraki, 2004*). Likewise, the same team also found that finger movement while handling the game controller did not seem to contribute as a source of prefrontal deactivation. Further studies also noted that the observed prefrontal deactivation was not affected by age or performance level (Matsuda and Hiraki, 2006*), although some authors have challenged that finding, claiming that prefrontal activation during video gaming was age-dependent, where most adults tended to show increased prefrontal activity while it was attenuated in some of the children. So prefrontal activation could be a result of age, game performance, level of interest and attention dedicated to the VG (Nagamitsu et al., 2006**).

It has been possible to establish a causal relationship between dlPFC activation and cognitive control using non-invasive stimulation methods. Stimulating the left dlPFC using tDCS results in a perceptible improvement in multitasking performance in a three-dimensional VG (Hsu et al., 2015).

Changes in functional activity after a training period in other executive-related nodes, such as the superior parietal lobe (SPL) have also been associated with working memory improvements (Nikolaidis et al., 2014).

Connectivity-wise, Martínez et al. (2013) found resting-state functional connectivity changes in widespread regions (frontal, parietal, and temporal areas) as a result of a VG training program, which were attributed to the interaction of cognitive control and memory retrieval and encoding.

Despite the observed structural and functional changes in prefrontal areas, executive functions trained in a VG show poor transfer effects as measured with cognitive tasks (Colom et al., 2012; Kühn et al., 2013). Others, showing neural correlates related to executive functions, visuospatial navigation and fine motor skills, failed to observe far transfer effects even after a 50 h training period, as measured by neuropsychological tests (Kühn et al., 2013). By studying lifelong experts or professional gamers, some studies have detected structural GM changes that correlated with improved executive performance, involving posterior parietal (Tanaka et al., 2013), and prefrontal (Hyun et al., 2013) regions. Regarding structural connectivity, WM integrity changes in thalamic areas correlated with improved working memory, but integrity of occipitotemporal fibers had the opposite effect (Strenziok et al., 2014). VG experience also seems to consolidate the connectivity between executive regions (dlPFC and the posterior parietal cortex -PPC-) and the salience network, composed by the anterior insula and the ACC, and responsible for bottom-up attentional processes (Gong et al., 2016).

Different VG genres seem to affect which cognitive skills will be trained. Training older adults in a strategy VG seemed to improve verbal memory span (McGarry et al., 2013), but not problem solving or working memory, while using a 2D action VG improved everyday problem solving and reasoning. Transfer effects were even more relevant in the case of a brain training/puzzle VG, where working memory improvements were also observed (Strenziok et al., 2014). Using a younger sample, working memory improvements were detected after training with a 2D action VG (Space Fortress, Nikolaidis et al., 2014). Nevertheless, training periods found in scientific literature vary greatly and it is difficult to ascertain if a lack of transferred skills cannot be due to a short training period.

Regarding electrophysiological methods, electroencephalography studies have shown functional correlations with alpha oscillations in the frontal cortex that could reflect cognitive control engagement in the training VG (Mathewson et al., 2012).

Skill Acquisition

Several studies have attempted to determine which regions could act as predictors for skill acquisition. Since this is a domain in which multiple cognitive functions are involved, volumetric and functional changes will appear in a wide range of cortical regions. Most of the learning in VGs is non-declarative, including visuospatial processing, visuomotor integration, and motor planning and execution. Improvements in these areas will generally lead to decreased cortical activation in the involved areas due to the optimization of resources, whereas this is not the case for striatal and medial prefrontal areas, which display a distinctive pattern of activation and typically increase their activity due to skill acquisition (Gobel et al., 2011).

Striatal volumes were determined as predictors for skill acquisition, although structural changes in the hippocampal formation were not (Erickson et al., 2010). Particularly, the anterior half of the dorsal striatum was the region which more accurately predicted skill acquisition in a complex VG (Vo et al., 2011). Other areas identified as predictors were the medial portion of the Brodmann area 6, located in the frontal cortex and associated with motor control in cognitive operations and response inhibition and the cerebellum, likely associated with motor skill acquisition (Basak et al., 2011). The same authors also considered the post-central gyrus, a somatosensory area that could be related to a feedback mechanism between prefrontal and motor regions, while the volume of the right central portion of the ACC also correlated with skill acquisition and is responsible for monitoring conflict. Finally, dlPFC volumes, with a central role on the executive functions, also showed correlation with VG performance over time (Basak et al., 2011).

On a functional level, Koepp et al. (1998**) was the first team to identify a relationship between striatum activity, associated with learning and the reward system, and performance level in a VG. The study by Anderson et al. (2015) also support the notion that the striatum, particularly the right dorsal striatum, composed of the caudate nucleus and the claustrum, is a key area in skill acquisition. However, the same team was able to predict learning rates more accurately by comparing whole sequential brain activation patterns to an artificial intelligence model.

Learning gains seemed to be best predicted by individual differences in phasic activation in those regions which had the highest tonic activation (Anderson et al., 2011*). Differences related to learning rates were also observed in the activation of the default mode network, especially when different training strategies were employed by the participants. Using electrophysiological methods, the best predictors were the alpha rhythms (Smith et al., 1999), particularly frontal regions, and alpha and delta ERSP, which are associated with cognitive control (task switching and inhibition) and attentional control networks (Mathewson et al., 2012). Frontal midline theta rhythms, linked with focused concentration and conscious control over attention, seemed to increase over the course of the training sessions with a VG (Smith et al., 1999).

Reward Processing

Addiction

VG addiction is understood as an impulse-control disorder with psychological consequences, not unlike other addictive disorders, especially non-substance addictions such as pathological gambling (Young, 1998). Internet Gaming Disorder (IGD) has been recently proposed for inclusion as a psychiatric diagnosis under the non-substance addiction category in the Diagnostic and Statistical Manual for Mental Disorders 5th ed. (DSM-5) (American Psychiatric Association, 2013), with its diagnostic criteria being adapted from those of pathological gambling. Efforts in order to find a consensus regarding its assessment are still ongoing (Petry et al., 2014). In some cases, VG addiction is included as a subset within the broader definition of Internet addiction, although this categorization is not always consistent, since many VGs in which addiction is studied do not have an online component. Several instruments have been developed to assess gaming addictions: the Internet Addiction Test (IAT) by Young (1998) and the Chen Internet Addiction Scale (CIAS) (Chen et al., 2004) being the most used in research and clinical practice.

Within the VG literature, there is a great deal of interest in knowing the neurobiological basis of VG addiction and whether it can be related to other behavioral addictions by observing abnormal reward processing patterns. This seems to be the case, since many regions involved in the reward system have been found affected in people with VG addiction (e.g., Liu et al., 2010*; Hou et al., 2012*; Hahn et al., 2014). Among the complex set of structures that are involved in the reward system, the cortico-ventral basal ganglia circuit is the center of the network responsible for assessing the possible outcomes of a given behavior, especially in those situations where, during a goal-oriented behavior, complex choices must be made and the value and risk of secondary rewards must be weighed (Haber, 2011).

Differential structural and functional changes in addicted individuals can be found throughout the reward system. The main components of this circuit are the OFC, the ACC, the ventral striatum, ventral pallidum, and midbrain dopaminergic neurons (Haber, 2011), but many other regions seem to be involved in the wider context of addiction.

By exposing the participants to gaming cues, it is possible to elicit a craving response and study which regions show stronger correlation in IGD patients compared to controls. The model proposed by Volkow et al. (2010) involves several regions, which are mentioned consistently across studies, to explain the complexity of the craving. First, the precuneus, which showed higher activation in addicted individuals (Ko et al., 2013*), is an area associated with attention, visual processes, and memory retrieval and integrates these components, linking visual information (the gaming cues) to internal information. Regions commonly associated with memory and emotional functions are also involved: the HC, the parahippocampus and the amygdala seem responsible for providing emotional memories and contextual information for the cues (Ding et al., 2013*), regions where subjects showed higher activation (O'Brien et al., 1998). Central key regions of the reward system, like the limbic system and the posterior cingulate have a role in integrating the motivational information and provide expectation and reward significance for gaming behaviors (O'Doherty, 2004). The OFC and the ACC are responsible for the desire for gaming and providing a motivational value of the cue-inducing stimuli (Heinz et al., 2009), contributing to the activation and intensity of the reward-seeking behavior (Kalivas and Volkow, 2005; Brody et al., 2007; Feng et al., 2013*). In the last step, prefrontal executive areas such as the dlPFC have also shown involvement during craving responses (Han et al., 2010a*; Ko et al., 2013*), and are linked to the formation of behavioral plans as a conscious anticipation of VG play. All these frontal regions[dlPFC, OFC, ACC, and the supplementary motor area (SMA)] tend to show reduced GM volumes in participants with IGD (Jin et al., 2016*).

Striatal volumes, particularly the ventral striatum, responsible for a key role in reward prediction, were reduced in people with excessive internet gaming compared to healthy controls (Hou et al., 2012*) and in the insula, with its role in conscious urges to abuse drugs (Naqvi and Bechara, 2009).

Overall, these features are characteristic of reward deficiencies that entail dysfunctions in the dopaminergic system, a shared neurobiological abnormality with other addictive disorders (Ko et al., 2009*, 2013*; Cilia et al., 2010; Park et al., 2010; Kim et al., 2011).

Several regions seem to be related to the intensity of the addiction. In a resting state paradigm, connectivity between the left SPL, including the posterior cingulate cortex (PCC), and the right precuneus, thalamus, caudate nucleus, nucleus accumbens (NAcc), SMA and lingual gyrus (regions largely associated with the reward system) correlated with the CIAS score, while at the same time, functional connectivity with the cerebellum and the superior parietal cortex (SPC) correlated negatively with that score (Ding et al., 2013*). The distinctive activation and connectivity patterns related to the PCC (Liu et al., 2010*), an important node in the DMN and reward system (Kim H. et al., 2015), could be used as a biomarker for addiction severity, both in behavioral and substance dependence. As the addiction severity increases, changing from a voluntary to a compulsive substance use, there is a transition from prefrontal to striatal control, and also from a ventral to a dorsal striatal control over behavior (Everitt and Robbins, 2005), Matching evidence in the form of weaker functional connectivity involving the dorsal-caudal putamen has been found in IGD patients (Hong et al., 2015*).

It is important to note that, even controlling the amount of time playing VGs, professional and expert gamers display very different neural patterns compared to addicted VGPs. Gamers falling into the addiction category show increased impulsiveness and perseverative errors that are not present in professional gamers and, on a neural level, they differ in GM volumes in the left cingulate gyrus (increased in pro-gamers) and thalamus (decreased in pro-gamers), which together may be indicative of an unbalanced reward system (Sánchez-González et al., 2005; Han et al., 2012b).

Exposure to Violent Content

Many articles use violent VGs in their designs as a way to study the effects of violence exposure, emotional regulation and long-term desensitization. Exposure to violent content has been associated with reduced dlPFC activity and interference in executive tasks (inhibition, go/no-go task) (Hummer et al., 2010), which cannot be interpreted without studying the link with the limbic and reward systems. It is likely that repeated exposure to violent content will trigger desensitization processes that affect regions linked to emotional and attentional processing, particularly a frontoparietal network encompassing the left OFC, right precuneus and bilateral inferior parietal lobes (Strenziok et al., 2011). It is hypothesized that this desensitization may result in diminished emotional responses toward violent situations, preventing empathy and lowering the threshold for non-adaptive behaviors linked to aggressiveness (Montag et al., 2012).

Limbic areas are associated with violence interactions, shown by the activation changes detected in the ACC and the amygdala in the presence of violent content (Mathiak and Weber, 2006*; Weber et al., 2006*). Lateral (especially left) prefrontal regions might be involved as well, integrating emotion and cognition and therefore working as a defense mechanism against negative emotions by down-regulating limbic activity (Montag et al., 2012). Wang et al. (2009) also provided evidence of that regulation mechanism by observing differing functional correlations between the left dlPFC and the ACC, and medial prefrontal regions & the amygdala during an executive task after a short-term exposure to a violent VG.

The reward circuit also seems to be implicated in the presence of violent content. Activation decreases in the OFC and caudate appeared in the absence of an expected reward. However, it does not seem that violence events were intrinsically rewarding (Mathiak et al. (2011*). Zvyagintsev et al. (2016*) found that resting-state functional connectivity was reduced within sensory-motor, reward, default mode and right frontotemporal networks after playing a violent VG, which could be linked to short-term effects on aggressiveness.

Gender differences in neural correlates were observed in one study (Chou et al., 2013*) after being exposed to violent content, with reduced blood flow in the dorsal ACC after playing a violent VG in males, but not females, possibly as a result of the role of the ACC in regulating aggressive behavior in males.

The effect of certain personality traits, particularly empathy, have been assessed using violent VG exposure (Lianekhammy and Werner-Wilson, 2015*). However, while empathy scores correlated with neural activity (frontal asymmetry during EEG), they were not affected by the presence of violent content. Markey and Markey (2010) found that some personality profiles, especially those with high neuroticism and low conscientiousness and agreeableness, are more prone to be affected by the exposure to violent VGs.

VG player's perspective may also be determinant to the level of moral engagement; while ERP N100 amplitudes were greater during a first person violent event, if the player was using a distant perspective, general alpha power was greater, which is indicative of lower arousal levels (Petras et al., 2015).

Montag et al. (2012), observed that regular gamers have been habituated to violence exposure and show less lateral prefrontal activation, linked to limbic down-regulation, compared to non-gamers. However, gamers have not lost the ability to distinguish real from virtual violence, as Regenbogen et al. (2010*) found, although that also depended on each person's learning history.

While attenuated P300 amplitudes have been linked to violence desensitization, both in short and long term exposure (Bartholow et al., 2006), these amplitudes did not increase using a pro-social VG (Liu Y. et al., 2015). Engelhardt et al. (2011), experimentally linked the lower P300 amplitudes to violence desensitization and their effects on aggression. Bailey et al. (2010) also supported the link between violent VG exposure and desensitization to violent stimuli, associating it with early processing differences in attentional orienting.

Flow

Flow and boredom states during VG play have also been the subject of research using neural correlates. The concept of flow, described by Csikszentmihalyi (1990), is understood as a mind state of being completely focused on a task that is intrinsically motivating. Among other characteristics, the state of flow implies a balance between the task difficulty and the person's skills, the absence of ambiguity in the goals of the task, and is commonly accompanied by a loss of awareness of time. Considering that the concept of flow is a complex construct which itself cannot be directly measured, it is necessary to operationalize its components. Some authors have identified some of these components as sustained attention (focus), direct feedback, balance between skill and difficulty, clear goals and control over the activity (Klasen et al., 2012*) and it has been theorized to be firmly linked to attentional and reward processes (Weber et al., 2009).

VGs provide the appropriate context in which flow states are encouraged to occur, since feedback is offered continuously and the level of difficulty is programmed to raise progressively, in order to match the improving skills of the player (Hunicke, 2005; Byrne, 2006). Therefore, VGs are perfect candidates to operationalize the components involved in the flow theory.

During gameplay in an action VG, Klasen et al. (2012*) could not relate the feedback component to any meaningful neural activity, but the four remaining flow-contributing factors showed joint activation of somatosensory networks. Furthermore, motor regions were implicated in the difficulty, sustained attention and control components. Together, the authors identify this sensorimotor activity as a reflection of the simulated physical activity present in the VG, which can contribute to the state of flow. The rest of the components elicited activity in several different regions. The reward system was involved in the skill-difficulty balance factor, observed by activation in the ventral striatum and other basal nuclei, rewarding the player in successful in-game events. In addition to activity in reward regions, this factor also correlated with simultaneous activity in a motor network comprised of the cerebellum and premotor areas. The factor comprising concentration and focusing during the VG was associated with changes in attentional networks and the visual system, as players switched away from spatial orientation to processing the numerous elements of the VG in high focus settings. Goal-oriented behavior showed decreased activity in the precuneus and regions of the ACC, while activity in bilateral intraparietal sulcus and right fusiform face area (associated with face processing) increased, which the authors explain as a result of a shift from navigation in a known environment to seeking new game content (Klasen et al., 2012*).

When manipulating the VG settings to elicit states or boredom, operationalized as the absence of goal-oriented behavior, one of the main aspects of flow, affective states appear. While the lack of goal-directed behavior resulted in an increase of positive affect, the neural correlates were characterized by lower activation in the amygdala and the insula (Mathiak et al., 2013). However, a different neural circuit was responsible when negative affect increased, characterized by activation in the ventromedial prefrontal cortex and deactivation of the HC and the precuneus, that seemed to counteract the state of boredom, possibly by planning future actions during inactive periods (Mathiak et al., 2013). Involvement of frontal regions was also observed by Yoshida et al. (2014) related to flow and boredom states. During the state of flow, activity in bilateral ventrolateral prefrontal cortex (vlPFC) [comprising the inferior frontal gyrus (IFG) and lateral OFC] increased, and it decreased when participants were subject to a boredom state. The OFC is linked to reward and emotion processing (Carrington and Bailey, 2009), and monitoring punishment (Kringelbach and Rolls, 2004). However, this study employed boredom differently, using a low difficulty level in the VG instead of the suppressing goal-directed behavior.

Brain-computer interfaces, using electrophysiological methods to measure brain activity, have been able to differentiate states of flow and boredom, created by adjusting the level of difficulty of a VG. The EEG frequencies that were able to discern between flow states were in the alpha, low-beta and mid-beta bands, measured in frontal (F7 and F8) and temporal (T5 and T6) locations (Berta et al., 2013).

Gender Differences

Although some studies have already discussed the presence of gender differences in cognitive processes related to VG playing, the lack of studies dealing with this topic and providing neural data are notable. The most relevant study of gender differences (Feng et al., 2007*) found that a 10-h training in an action VG (but not in a non-action VG) was enough to compensate for baseline gender differences in spatial attention, and to reduce the gap in mental rotation skills. Whether the initial difference was innate or a product of lesser exposure to this kind of activities in women is a matter of debate (Dye and Bavelier, 2010). Actually, one of the reasons men do not improve as much as women could be explained by a ceiling effect due to previous exposure to VGs. On the other hand, women with less experience in these activities are able to achieve equal performances in visuospatial skills that reach the same ceiling effect with a short training period. In this respect, Dye and Bavelier comment on the possible effects of lifetime VG exposure since the gender gap in attentional and non-attentional skills is smaller or non-existent during childhood compared to adult life, and the greater development of these skills in male individuals is partially due to games targeting a male audience.

Other authors (Ko et al., 2005) have focused on other psychosocial factors to explain gender differences in online VG addictions. Considering most online VGPs are men and this difference is also observed in addiction cases, they studied the possible factors and observed that lower self-esteem and lower daily life satisfaction are determinant in men, but not women. They attribute these differences to the reasons on why they play VGs: while men declared to play to pursue feelings of achievement and social-bonding, it was not the case for women. This aspect is not new to VG addiction and is shared aspect with other addictions. It is likely that VGs are used as a way to cope with these problems, leading up to the development of the addiction.

LIMITATIONS

The study of neural correlates of VGs entails a number of inherent difficulties. The main limitation encountered during the development of this review was the dual nature of studies with regard to VGs as a research tool or as an object of study. The lack of standardization in study objectives is another limitation that should be addressed. Despite the recent popularity of VG-related studies, there are a multitude of similar research lines that offer hardly comparable results, making it difficult to draw general conclusions. We aimed to unify all sorts of studies in order to interpret and generalize the results.

First of all, we compared a large number of studies that not only used completely different techniques, but also had very heterogeneous research goals. We grouped them together with the aim of extracting all the available neuroimaging information, but it is likely that some information that would have been relevant for us was missed in the studies because their research objectives differed greatly from our own. In fact, in certain cases, VGs were almost irrelevant to the aim of the study and were only used as a substitute for a cognitive task, so the provided results may not directly reflect the VG neural correlates. Similarly, VGs were sometimes used as tools to provide violence exposure or to study the effects of behavioral addictions without the VG being the central object of study.

Another issue was the lack of a proper classification for VG genres. While the most common division is between action and non-action VGs, it would be interesting to establish which variables determine this classification. For instance, both first person shooters and fighting games could be considered action VGs. Both demand quick response times and high attentional resources, but first person shooter games require much higher visuospatial skills while fighting games do not. Consequently, efforts should be made to determine which aspects of each VG genre are related with each cognitive process and its associated neural correlates.

Apart from these aspects, comparisons between gamers and non-gamers are common in VG literature. Nevertheless, there is no consensus on the inclusion requirements for each group and it seems that no scientific criterion has been used to establish a cut-off line. Current dedication to VGs, measured in hours per week, seems to be the most common classification method. Non-gamer groups sometimes are so strict as to exclude any gaming experience, but on other occasions, for the same category, several weekly VG hours are tolerated. This is problematic since, in some cases, cognitive changes have been found after just a few weeks of VG training. However, in most cases, the onset age of active VG play, which is a particularly relevant aspect (Hartanto et al., 2016), is not taken into account. Another relevant variable, which tends to be forgotten, is lifetime VG experience, usually measured in hours. Moreover, despite the clearly different outcomes caused by different VG genres, this variable is not included when describing a participant's VG experience. Therefore, VG experience should be measured taking into account all the variables mentioned above: onset age, lifetime VG experience (in hours), current VG dedication (hours per week) and VG genres.

With regard to this review, it was really difficult to extract all the relevant information because of the limitations of the existing literature about the topic. But we did our best to clarify the results and to extract valuable conclusions.

Another limitation was the link between neural changes and cognitive functions. The neural correlates of VGs are the focus of this review, and we found it essential to complement this data by discussing their cognitive implications. In most cases these implications were directly assessed by the individual studies, but in some cases they were extrapolated based on previous literature. Furthermore, even when functional or structural changes are detected, they do not always reflect cognitive changes. This may be due to a lack of sensitivity in the cognitive and behavioral tasks employed. In order to detect both neural and cognitive changes, specific research designs, with sufficiently sensitive measurements of the three dimensions (functional, structural, and cognitive) are needed. Ideally, to determine when each change starts to appear as a result of VG exposure, an experimental design, including a VG training period, should be used. In this design, the neural and cognitive data would be assessed along a series of time points until the three types of changes were detected. An exhaustive discussion of the cognitive implications of VGs is beyond our scope since there are already other works that deal with this particular issue (Powers et al., 2013; Lampit et al., 2014; Toril et al., 2014; Wang et al., 2016).

Efforts should be made to systematize VG-related research, establishing VG training protocols and determining the effects of lifetime VG exposure, in order that more comparable results can be obtained and to improve the generalizability of results.

CONCLUSIONS

The current work has allowed us to integrate the great deal of data that has been generated during recent years about a topic that has not stopped growing, making it easier to compare the results of multiple research groups. VG use has an effect in a variety of brain functions and, ultimately, in behavioral changes and in cognitive performance.

The attentional benefits resulting from the use of VG seem to be the most evidence-supported aspect, as many studies by Bavelier and Green have shown (Green and Bavelier, 2003, 2004, 2006, 2007, 2012; Dye et al., 2009; Hubert-Wallander et al., 2011; Bavelier et al., 2012b). Improvements in bottom-up and top-down attention, optimization of attentional resources, integration between attentional and sensorimotor areas, and improvements in selective and peripheral visual attention have been featured in a large number of studies.

Visuospatial skills are also an important topic of study in VG research, where optimization of cognitive costs in visuomotor task performance is commonly observed. Some regions show volumetric increases as a result of VG experience, particularly the HC and the entorhinal cortex, which are thought to be directly related to visuospatial and navigational skills. Optimization of these abilities, just like in attention and overall skill acquisition, is usually detected in functional neuroimaging studies as decreased activation in their associated pathways (in this case, in regions linked to the dorsal visual stream). It is likely that the exposure to a task first leads to an increase of activity in the associated regions, but ultimately, as the performance improves after repeated exposures, less cortical resources are needed for the same task.

Likewise, although not always consistent, even short VG training paradigms showed improvements in cognitive control related functions, particularly working memory, linked to changes in prefrontal areas like the dlPFC and the OFC. How to achieve far transfer in these functions remains one of the most interesting questions regarding cognitive control. Despite VGs being good candidates for cognitive training, it is still not well-known what the optimum training parameters for observing the first effects are. It seems intuitive that longer training periods will have a greater chance of inducing far transfer, but how long should they be? We also commented on how VG genre can have differential effects on cognitive control, so we cannot expect to observe these effects without first controlling this variable, since different VG genres often have little in common with each other.

Cognitive workload studies have offered the possibility of observing neural recruitment phenomena to compensate for the difficulty and complexity of a cognitive task and a number of studies have pointed to the importance of frontoparietal activity for this purpose.

It has been also possible to link skill acquisition rates with certain cerebral structures. Several brain regions are key in this regard, mainly the dlPFC, striatum, SMA, premotor area, and cerebellum. Moreover, as suggested by Anderson et al. (2015), models of whole-brain activation patterns can also be used as an efficient tool for predicting skill acquisition.

The role of the reward system is always present when we talk about VGs, due to the way they are designed. Addiction has a heavy impact throughout the neural reward system, including components like the OFC, the ACC, the ventral striatum, ventral pallidum, and midbrain dopaminergic neurons, together with diverse regions that have support roles in addiction. The role of structures that link addiction to its emotional components, such as the amygdala and the HC should not be underestimated.

Limbic regions work together with the PCC to integrate the motivational information with the expectation of reward.

Exposure to violent content has implications regarding the reward circuits and also emotional and executive processing. Reduced functional connectivity within sensory-motor, reward, default mode and right frontotemporal networks are displayed after playing a violent VG. The limbic system, interacting with the lateral prefrontal cortex, has a role in down-regulating the reaction to negative emotions, like those found in violent contexts, which may lead to short-term violence desensitization.

Despite the difficulties in locating the main components of flow in the brain, it seems that several networks are involved in this experience. General activation of somatosensory networks is observed while being in this state, whereas activation in motor regions is only linked to three components of flow: skill-difficulty balance, sustained attention and control over the activity. The reward system has key implications in the experience of flow, showing that the ventral striatum and other basal ganglia are directly linked to the skill-difficulty balance in a task. When seeking new content in order to avoid boredom, the bilateral intraparietal sulcus and the right fusiform face area seem to be the most implicated regions. During a flow-evoking task, the absence of boredom is shown by activity in the IFC, the OFC, and the vmPFC. Flow is also linked to emotional responses, and both positive and negative affect during a VG have shown changes in the amygdala, insula, vmPFC and the HC.

It is also worth commenting on the negative effects of VGs. While much has been written about the possible benefits of VG playing, finding articles highlighting the negative outcomes in non-addicted or expert VGPs is much less common. To our knowledge, only four studies pointed out neural correlates which predicted hindered performance in a range of cognitive domains. VG use has been linked with reduced recruitment in the ACC, associated with proactive cognitive control and possibly related to reduced attentional skills (Bailey et al., 2010). Likewise, exposure to violent content in VG is associated with lower activity in the dlPFC, interfering with inhibitory control. The same team (Bailey and West, 2013) observed how VG play had beneficial effects on visuospatial cognition, but in turn had negative effects on social information processing. Lastly, VG exposition has been linked to delayed microstructure development in extensive brain regions and lower verbal IQ (Takeuchi et al., 2016).

Finally, although this review is focused on the neural correlates of VG, not their cognitive or behavioral effects, we believe in the importance of integrating all these aspects, since raw neuroimaging data often offer little information without linking it to its underlying cognitive processes. Despite the fact that this integration is increasingly common in the literature, this is not always the case and it is an aspect that could be addressed in future studies.

AUTHOR CONTRIBUTIONS

All authors had an equal involvement during the process of making this review article. The article's design, data acquisition, and analysis of its content has been made by consensus among all the authors.

ACKNOWLEDGMENTS

We would like to sincerely thank our colleague Cristina García Palma for her assistance during the whole process of extracting and processing information from the scientific databases and for her valuable contributions during the course of this work. We would also like to express our gratitude to Nicholas Lumsden, who assisted in the proof-reading and English-language correction of the manuscript.

REFERENCES

Allison, B. Z., and Polich, J. (2008). Workload assessment of computer gaming using a single-stimulus event-related potential paradigm. *Biol. Psychol.* 77, 277–283. doi: 10.1016/j.biopsycho.2007.10.014

Alvarez, J. A., and Emory, E. (2006). Executive function and the frontal lobes: a meta-analytic review. *Neuropsychol. Rev.* 16, 17–42. doi: 10.1007/s11065-006-9002-x

American Psychiatric Association (2013). *Diagnostic and Statistical Manual of Mental Disorders, 5th Edn.* Washington, DC.

Anderson, J. R., Bothell, D., Fincham, J. M., and Moon, J. (2015). The Sequential structure of brain activation predicts skill. *Neuropsychologia* 81, 94–106. doi: 10.1016/j.neuropsychologia.2015.12.014

Anderson, J. R., Bothell, D., Fincham, J. M., Anderson, A. R., Poole, B., and Qin, Y. (2011). Brain regions engaged by part- and whole-task performance in a video game: a model-based test of the decomposition hypothesis. *J. Cogn. Neurosci.* 23, 3983–3997. doi: 10.1162/jocn_a_00033

Anguera, J. A., Boccanfuso, J., Rintoul, J. L., Al-Hashimi, O., Faraji, F., Janowich, J., et al. (2013). Video game training enhances cognitive control in older adults. *Nature* 501, 97–101. doi: 10.1038/nature12486

Bailey, K., and West, R. (2013). The effects of an action video game on visual and affective information processing. *Brain Res.* 1504, 35–46. doi: 10.1016/j.brainres.2013.02.019

Bailey, K., West, R., and Anderson, C. A. (2010). A negative association between video game experience and proactive cognitive control. *Psychophysiology* 47, 34–42. doi: 10.1111/j.1469-8986.2009.00925.x

Bailey, K., West, R., and Anderson, C. A. (2011). The association between chronic exposure to video game violence and affective picture processing: an ERP study. *Cogn. Affect. Behav. Neurosci.* 11, 259–276. doi: 10.3758/s13415-011-0029-y.

Barrouillet, P., Bernardin, S., Portrat, S., Vergauwe, E., and Camos, V. (2007). Time and cognitive load in working memory. *J. Exp. Psychol. Learn. Mem. Cogn.* 33, 570–585. doi: 10.1037/0278-7393.33.3.570

Bartholow, B. D., Bushman, B. J., and Sestir, M. A. (2006). Chronic violent video game exposure and desensitization to violence: behavioral and event-related brain potential data. *J. Exp. Soc. Psychol.* 42, 532–539. doi: 10.1016/j.jesp.2005.08.006

Basak, C., Voss, M. W., Erickson, K. I., Boot, W. R., and Kramer, A. F. (2011). Regional differences in brain volume predict the acquisition of skill in a complex real-time strategy videogame. *Brain Cogn.* 76, 407–414. doi: 10.1016/j.bandc.2011.03.017

Bavelier, D., Achtman, R. L., Mani, M., and Föcker, J. (2012a). Neural bases of selective attention in action video game players. *Vision Res.* 61, 132–143. doi: 10.1016/j.visres.2011.08.007

Bavelier, D., Green, C. S., Pouget, A., and Schrater, P. (2012b). Brain plasticity through the life span: learning to learn and action video games. *Annu. Rev. Neurosci.* 35, 391–416. doi: 10.1146/annurev-neuro-060909-152832

Berta, R., Bellotti, F., De Gloria, A., Pranantha, D., and Schatten, C. (2013). Electroencephalogram and physiological signal analysis for assessing flow in games. *IEEE Trans. Comput. Intell. AI Games* 5, 164–175. doi: 10.1109/TCIAIG.2013.2260340

Biswal, B. B., Eldreth, D. A., Motes, M. A., and Rypma, B. (2010). Task-dependent individual differences in prefrontal connectivity. *Cereb. Cortex* 20, 2188–2197. doi: 10.1093/cercor/bhp284

Brody, A. L., Mandelkern, M. A., Olmstead, R. E., Jou, J., Tiongson, E., Allen, V., et al. (2007). Neural substrates of resisting craving during cigarette cue exposure. *Biol. Psychiatry* 62, 642–651. doi: 10.1016/j.biopsych.2006.10.026

Brookings, J. B., Wilson, G. F., and Swain, C. R. (1996). Psychophysiological responses to changes in workload during simulated air traffic control. *Biol. Psychol.* 42, 361–377. doi: 10.1016/0301-0511(95)05167-8

Byrne, E. (2006). *Game Level Design, 1st Edn.* Newton Center, MA: Charles River Media Inc.

Carrington, S. J., and Bailey, A. J. (2009). Are there theory of mind regions in the brain? A review of the neuroimaging literature. *Hum. Brain Mapp.* 30, 2313–2335. doi: 10.1002/hbm.20671

Casual Games Association (2013). *Games Market Sector Report: Smartphone & Tablet Gaming 2013*. Smithfield, UT.

Chen, C. Y., Huang, M. F., Yen, J. Y., Chen, C. S., Liu, G. C., Yen, C. F., et al. (2014). Brain correlates of response inhibition in Internet gaming disorder. *Psychiatry Clin. Neurosci.* 69, 201–209. doi: 10.1111/pcn.12224

Chen, S. H., Weng, L. J., Su, Y. J., Wu, H. M., and Yang, P. F. (2004). Development of Chinese Internet Addiction Scale and its psychometric study. *Chinese J. Psychol.* 45, 279–294.

Chou, Y.-H., Yang, B.-H., Hsu, J.-W., Wang, S.-J., Lin, C.-L., Huang, K.-L., et al. (2013). Effects of video game playing on cerebral blood flow in young adults: a SPECT study. *Psychiatry Res.* 212, 65–72. doi: 10.1016/j.pscychresns.2012.10.002

Cilia, R., Ko, J. H., Cho, S. S., van Eimeren, T., Marotta, G., Pellecchia, G., et al. (2010). Reduced dopamine transporter density in the ventral striatum of patients with Parkinson's disease and pathological gambling. *Neurobiol. Dis.* 39, 98–104. doi: 10.1016/j.nbd.2010.03.013

Cole, S. W., Yoo, D. J., and Knutson, B. (2012). Interactivity and reward-related neural activation during a serious videogame. *PLoS ONE* 7:e33909. doi: 10.1371/journal.pone.0033909

Colom, R., Quiroga, M. Á., Solana, A. B., Burgaleta, M., Román, F. J., Privado, J., et al. (2012). Structural changes after videogame practice related to a brain network associated with intelligence. *Intelligence* 40, 479–489. doi: 10.1016/j.intell.2012.05.004

Corradi-Dell'Acqua, C., Ueno, K., Ogawa, A., Cheng, K., Rumiati, R. I., and Iriki, A. (2008). Effects of shifting perspective of the self: an fMRI study. *Neuroimage* 40, 1902–1911. doi: 10.1016/j.neuroimage.2007.12.062

Csikszentmihalyi, M. (1990). *Flow: The Psychology of Optimal Experience.* New York, NY: Harper and Row.

Ding, W., Sun, J., Sun, Y., Zhou, Y., Li, L., Xu, J., et al. (2013). Altered default network resting-state functional connectivity in adolescents with Internet gaming addiction. *PLoS ONE* 8:e59902. doi: 10.1371/journal.pone.0059902

Dong, G., and Potenza, M. N. (2016). Risk-taking and risky decision-making in Internet gaming disorder: implications regarding online gaming in the setting of negative consequences. *J. Psychiatr. Res.* 73, 1–8. doi: 10.1016/j.jpsychires.2015.11.011

Dong, G., Huang, J., and Du, X. (2012). Alterations in regional homogeneity of resting-state brain activity in internet gaming addicts. *Behav. Brain Funct.* 8:41. doi: 10.1186/1744-9081-8-41

Doty, R., Rosenthal, S., McDonald, D., O'Leary, C., and Donnelly, M. (2011). *EEG Prefrontal Activity During Video Game Reward Events.* Boston, MA: Society for Psychophysiological Research.

Dye, M. W. G., and Bavelier, D. (2010). Differential development of visual attention skills in school-age children. *Vision Res.* 50, 452–459. doi: 10.1016/j.visres.2009.10.010

Dye, M. W. G., Green, C. S., and Bavelier, D. (2009). The development of attention skills in action video game players. *Neuropsychologia* 47, 1780–1789. doi: 10.1016/j.neuropsychologia.2009.02.002

Engelhardt, C. R., Bartholow, B. D., Kerr, G. T., and Bushman, B. J. (2011). This is your brain on violent video games: neural desensitization to violence predicts increased aggression following violent video game exposure. *J. Exp. Soc. Psychol.* 47, 1033–1036. doi: 10.1016/j.jesp.2011.03.027

Entertainment Software Association (2014). *2014 Sales, Demographic, and Usage Data Essential Facts about the Computer and Video Game Industry.* Washington, DC.

Erickson, K. I., Boot, W. R., Basak, C., Neider, M. B., Prakash, R. S., Voss, M. W., et al. (2010). Striatal volume predicts level of video game skill acquisition. *Cereb. Cortex* 20, 2522–2530. doi: 10.1093/cercor/bhp293

Everitt, B. J., and Robbins, T. W. (2005). Neural systems of reinforcement for drug addiction: from actions to habits to compulsion. *Nat. Neurosci.* 8, 1481–1489. doi: 10.1038/nn1579

Feng, J., Spence, I., and Pratt, J. (2007). Playing an action video game reduces gender differences in spatial cognition. *Psychol. Sci.* 18, 850–855. doi: 10.1111/j.1467-9280.2007.01990.x

Feng, Q., Chen, X., Sun, J., Zhou, Y., Sun, Y., Ding, W., et al. (2013). Voxel-level comparison of arterial spin-labeled perfusion magnetic resonance imaging in adolescents with internet gaming addiction. *Behav. Brain Funct.* 9:33. doi: 10.1186/1744-9081-9-33

Gobel, E. W., Parrish, T. B., and Reber, P. J. (2011). Neural correlates of skill acquisition: decreased cortical activity during a serial interception sequence learning task. *Neuroimage* 58, 1150–1157. doi: 10.1016/j.neuroimage.2011.06.090

Gong, D., He, H., Liu, D., Ma, W., Dong, L., Luo, C., et al. (2015). Enhanced functional connectivity and increased gray matter volume of insula related to action video game playing. *Sci. Rep.* 5:9763. doi: 10.1038/srep09763

Gong, D., He, H., Ma, W., Liu, D., Huang, M., Dong, L., et al. (2016). Functional integration between salience and central executive networks: a role for action video game experience. *Neural Plast.* 2016:9803165. doi: 10.1155/2016/9803165

Goodale, M. A., and Milner, A. D. (1992). Separate visual pathways for perception and action. *Trends Neurosci.* 15, 20–25. doi: 10.1016/0166-2236(92)90344-8

Granek, J. A., Gorbet, D. J., and Sergio, L. E. (2010). Extensive video-game experience alters cortical networks for complex visuomotor transformations. *Cortex* 46, 1165–1177. doi: 10.1016/j.cortex.2009.10.009

Granic, I., Lobel, A., and Engels, R. C. M. E. (2014). The benefits of playing video games. *Am. Psychol.* 69, 66–78. doi: 10.1037/a0034857

Green, C. S., and Bavelier, D. (2003). Action video game modifies visual selective attention. *Nature* 423, 534–537. doi: 10.1038/nature01647

Green, C. S., and Bavelier, D. (2004). "The cognitive neuroscience of video games," in *Digital Media: Transformation in Human Communication*, eds P. Messaris and L. Humphreys (New York, NY: Peter Lang), 211–224.

Green, C. S., and Bavelier, D. (2006). Effect of action video games on the spatial distribution of visuospatial attention. *J. Exp. Psychol. Hum. Percept. Perform.* 32, 1465–1478. doi: 10.1037/0096-1523.32.6.1465

Green, C. S., and Bavelier, D. (2007). Action-video-game experience alters the spatial resolution of vision. *Psychol. Sci.* 18, 88–94. doi: 10.1111/j.1467-9280.2007.01853.x

Green, C. S., and Bavelier, D. (2012). Learning, attentional control, and action video games. *Curr. Biol.* 22, R197–R206. doi: 10.1016/j.cub.2012.02.012

Green, C. S., and Seitz, A. R. (2015). The impacts of video games on cognition (and how the government can guide the industry). *Behav. Brain Sci.* 2, 101–110. doi: 10.1177/2372732215601121

Haber, S. N. (2011). "Neuroanatomy of reward: a view from the ventral striatum," in *Neurobiology of Sensation and Reward*, ed J. Gottfried (Boca Raton, FL: CRC Press/Taylor & Francis), 235–261. doi: 10.1201/b10776-15

Hahn, T., Notebaert, K. H., Dresler, T., Kowarsch, L., Reif, A., and Fallgatter, A. J. (2014). Linking online gaming and addictive behavior: converging evidence for a general reward deficiency in frequent online gamers. *Front. Behav. Neurosci.* 8:385. doi: 10.3389/fnbeh.2014.00385

Han, D. H., Bolo, N., Daniels, M. A., Arenella, L., Lyoo, I. K., and Renshaw, P. F. (2012a). Brain activity and desire for Internet video game play. *Compr. Psychiatry* 52, 88–95. doi: 10.1016/j.comppsych.2010.04.004

Han, D. H., Hwang, J. W., and Renshaw, P. F. (2010a). Bupropion sustained release treatment decreases craving for video games and cue-induced brain activity in patients with Internet video game addiction. *Exp. Clin. Psychopharmacol.* 18, 297–304. doi: 10.1037/a0020023

Han, D. H., Kim, S. M., Bae, S., Renshaw, P. F., and Anderson, J. S. (2015). Brain connectivity and psychiatric comorbidity in adolescents with Internet gaming disorder. *Addict. Biol.* 22, 802–812. doi: 10.1111/adb.12347

Han, D. H., Kim, S. M., Bae, S., Renshaw, P. F., and Anderson, J. S. (2016). A failure of suppression within the default mode network in depressed adolescents with compulsive internet game play. *J. Affect. Disord.* 194, 57–64. doi: 10.1016/j.jad.2016.01.013

Han, D. H., Kim, Y. S., Lee, Y. S., Min, K. J., and Renshaw, P. F. (2010b). Changes in cue-induced, prefrontal cortex activity with video-game play. *Cyberpsychol. Behav. Soc. Netw.* 13, 655–661. doi: 10.1089/cyber.2009.0327

Han, D. H., Lyoo, I. K., and Renshaw, P. F. (2012b). Differential regional gray matter volumes in patients with on-line game addiction and professional gamers. *J. Psychiatr. Res.* 46, 507–515. doi: 10.1016/j.jpsychires.2012.01.004

Hartanto, A., Toh, W. X., and Yang, H. (2016). Age matters: the effect of onset age of video game play on task-switching abilities. *Attent. Percept. Psychophys.* 78, 1125–1136. doi: 10.3758/s13414-016-1068-9

Havranek, M., Langer, N., Cheetham, M., and Jäncke, L. (2012). Perspective and agency during video gaming influences spatial presence experience and brain activation patterns. *Behav. Brain Funct.* 8:34. doi: 10.1186/1744-9081-8-34

Heinz, A., Beck, A., Grüsser, S. M., Grace, A. A., and Wrase, J. (2009). Identifying the neural circuitry of alcohol craving and relapse vulnerability. *Addict. Biol.* 14, 108–118. doi: 10.1111/j.1369-1600.2008.00136.x

Hong, S.-B., Harrison, B. J., Dandash, O., Choi, E.-J., Kim, S.-C., Kim, H.-H., et al. (2015). A selective involvement of putamen functional connectivity in youth with internet gaming disorder. *Brain Res.* 1602, 85–95. doi: 10.1016/j.brainres.2014.12.042

Hou, H., Jia, S., Hu, S., Fan, R., Sun, W., Sun, T., et al. (2012). Reduced striatal dopamine transporters in people with internet addiction disorder. *J. Biomed. Biotechnol.* 2012:854524. doi: 10.1155/2012/854524

Hsu, W.-Y., Zanto, T. P., Anguera, J. A., Lin, Y.-Y., and Gazzaley, A. (2015). Delayed enhancement of multitasking performance: effects of anodal transcranial direct current stimulation on the prefrontal cortex. *Cortex* 69, 175–185. doi: 10.1016/j.cortex.2015.05.014

Hubert-Wallander, B., Green, C. S., Sugarman, M., and Bavelier, D. (2011). Changes in search rate but not in the dynamics of exogenous attention in action videogame players. *Atten. Percept. Psychophys.* 73, 2399–2412. doi: 10.3758/s13414-011-0194-7

Hummer, T. A., Wang, Y., Kronenberger, W. G., Mosier, K. M., Kalnin, A. J., Dunn, D. W., et al. (2010). Short-term violent video game play by adolescents alters prefrontal activity during cognitive inhibition. *Media Psychol.* 13, 136–154. doi: 10.1080/15213261003799854

Hunicke, R. (2005). "The case for dynamic difficulty adjustment in games," in *Proceedings of the 2005 ACM SIGCHI International Conference on Advances in Computer Entertainment Technology—ACE'05* (New York, NY: ACM Press), 429–433.

Hyun, G. J., Shin, Y. W., Kim, B.-N. N., Cheong, J. H., Jin, S. N., and Han, D. H. (2013). Increased cortical thickness in professional on-line gamers. *Psychiatry Investig.* 10, 388–392. doi: 10.4306/pi.2013.10.4.388

Ivarsson, M., Anderson, M., Åkerstedt, T., and Lindblad, F. (2013). The effect of violent and nonviolent video games on heart rate variability, sleep, and emotions in adolescents with different violent gaming habits. *Psychosom. Med.* 75, 390–396. doi: 10.1097/PSY.0b013e3182906a4c

Izzetoglu, K., Bunce, S., Onaral, B., Pourrezaei, K., and Chance, B. (2004). Functional optical brain imaging using near-infrared during cognitive tasks. *Int. J. Hum. Comput. Interact.* 17, 211–227. doi: 10.1207/s15327590ijhc1702_6

Jin, C., Zhang, T., Cai, C., Bi, Y., Li, Y., Yu, D., et al. (2016). Abnormal prefrontal cortex resting state functional connectivity and severity of internet gaming disorder. *Brain Imaging Behav.* 10, 719–729. doi: 10.1007/s11682-015-9439-8

Kalivas, P. W., and Volkow, N. D. (2005). The neural basis of addiction: a pathology of motivation and choice. *Am. J. Psychiatry* 162, 1403–1413. doi: 10.1176/appi.ajp.162.8.1403

Kätsyri, J., Hari, R., Ravaja, N., and Nummenmaa, L. (2013a). Just watching the game ain't enough: striatal fMRI reward responses to successes and failures in a video game during active and vicarious playing. *Front. Hum. Neurosci.* 7:278. doi: 10.3389/fnhum.2013.00278

Kätsyri, J., Hari, R., Ravaja, N., and Nummenmaa, L. (2013b). The opponent matters: elevated FMRI reward responses to winning against a human versus a computer opponent during interactive video game playing. *Cereb. Cortex* 23, 2829–2839. doi: 10.1093/cercor/bhs259

Kelley, R. E., Chang, J. Y., Scheinman, N. J., Levin, B. E., Duncan, R. C., and Lee, S. C. (1992). Transcranial Doppler assessment of cerebral flow velocity during cognitive tasks. *Stroke.* 23, 9–14.

Khairuddin, H. R., Malik, A. S., Mumtaz, W., Kamel, N., and Xia, L. (2013). Analysis of EEG signals regularity in adults during video game play in 2D and 3D. *Conf. Proc. IEEE Eng. Med. Biol. Soc.* 2013, 2064–2067. doi: 10.1109/EMBC.2013.6609938

Kim, H., Kim, Y. K., Gwak, A. R., Lim, J.-A. A., Lee, J.-Y. Y., Jung, H. Y., et al. (2015). Resting-state regional homogeneity as a biological marker for patients with Internet gaming disorder: a comparison with patients with alcohol use disorder and healthy controls. *Prog. Neuro Psychopharmacol. Biol. Psychiatry* 60, 104–111. doi: 10.1016/j.pnpbp.2015.02.004

Kim, P. W., Kim, S. Y., Shim, M., Im, C.-H. H., and Shon, Y.-M. M. (2013). The influence of an educational course on language expression and treatment of gaming addiction for massive multiplayer online role-playing game (MMORPG) players. *Comput. Educ.* 63, 208–217. doi: 10.1016/j.compedu.2012.12.008

Kim, S. H., Baik, S.-H., Park, C. S., Kim, S. J., Choi, S. W., and Kim, S. E. (2011). Reduced striatal dopamine D2 receptors in people with Internet addiction. *Neuroreport* 22, 407–411. doi: 10.1097/WNR.0b013e328346e16e

Kim, Y.-H., Kang, D.-W., Kim, D., Kim, H.-J., Sasaki, Y., and Watanabe, T. (2015). Real-time strategy video game experience and visual perceptual learning. *J. Neurosci.* 35, 10485–10492. doi: 10.1523/JNEUROSCI.3340-14.2015

Klasen, M., Weber, R., Kircher, T. T. J., Mathiak, K. A., and Mathiak, K. (2012). Neural contributions to flow experience during video game playing. *Soc. Cogn. Affect. Neurosci.* 7, 485–495. doi: 10.1093/scan/nsr021

Ko, C. H., Liu, G. C., Hsiao, S., Yen, J. Y., Yang, M. J., Lin, W. C., et al. (2009). Brain activities associated with gaming urge of online gaming addiction. *J. Psychiatr. Res.* 43, 739–747. doi: 10.1016/j.jpsychires.2008.09.012

Ko, C. H., Liu, G. C., Yen, J. Y., Chen, C. Y., Yen, C. F., and Chen, C. S. (2013). Brain correlates of craving for online gaming under cue exposure in subjects with Internet gaming addiction and in remitted subjects. *Addict. Biol.* 18, 559–569. doi: 10.1111/j.1369-1600.2011.00405.x

Ko, C.-H., Yen, J.-Y., Chen, C.-C., Chen, S.-H., and Yen, C.-F. (2005). Gender differences and related factors affecting online gaming addiction among Taiwanese adolescents. *J. Nerv. Ment. Dis.* 193, 273–277. doi: 10.1097/01.nmd.0000158373.85150.57

Koepp, M. J., Gunn, R. N., Lawrence, A. D., Cunningham, V. J., Dagher, A., Jones, T., et al. (1998). Evidence for striatal dopamine release during a video game. *Nature* 393, 266–268. doi: 10.1038/30498

Kravitz, D. J., Saleem, K. S., Baker, C. I., and Mishkin, M. (2011). A new neural framework for visuospatial processing. *Nat. Rev. Neurosci.* 12, 217–230. doi: 10.1038/nrn3008

Kringelbach, M. L., and Rolls, E. T. (2004). The functional neuroanatomy of the human orbitofrontal cortex: evidence from neuroimaging and neuropsychology. *Prog. Neurobiol.* 72, 341–372. doi: 10.1016/j.pneurobio.2004.03.006

Krishnan, L., Kang, A., Sperling, G., and Srinivasan, R. (2013). Neural strategies for selective attention distinguish fast-action video game players. *Brain Topogr.* 26, 83–97. doi: 10.1007/s10548-012-0232-3

Kühn, S., and Gallinat, J. (2014). Amount of lifetime video gaming is positively associated with entorhinal, hippocampal and occipital volume. *Mol. Psychiatry* 19, 842–847. doi: 10.1038/mp.2013.100

Kühn, S., Gleich, T., Lorenz, R. C., Lindenberger, U., and Gallinat, J. (2013). Playing Super Mario induces structural brain plasticity: gray matter changes resulting from training with a commercial video game. *Mol. Psychiatry* 19, 265–271. doi: 10.1038/mp.2013.120

Kühn, S., Lorenz, R. C., Banaschewski, T., Barker, G. J., Büchel, C., Conrod, P. J., et al. (2014). Positive association of video game playing with left frontal cortical thickness in adolescents. *PLoS ONE* 9:e91506. doi: 10.1371/journal.pone.0091506

Lampit, A., Hallock, H., and Valenzuela, M. (2014). Computerized cognitive training in cognitively healthy older adults: a systematic review and meta-analysis of effect modifiers. *PLoS Med.* 11:e1001756. doi: 10.1371/journal.pmed.1001756

Latham, A. J., Patston, L. L. M., Westermann, C., Kirk, I. J., and Tippett, L. J. (2013). Earlier visual N1 latencies in expert video-game players: a temporal basis of enhanced visuospatial performance? *PLoS ONE* 8:e75231. doi: 10.1371/journal.pone.0075231

Lee, A. C. H., Yeung, L.-K., and Barense, M. D. (2012). The hippocampus and visual perception. *Front. Hum. Neurosci.* 6:91. doi: 10.3389/fnhum.2012.00091

Lee, H., Voss, M. W., Prakash, R. S., Boot, W. R., Vo, L. T. K., Basak, C., et al. (2012). Videogame training strategy-induced change in brain function during a complex visuomotor task. *Behav. Brain Res.* 232, 348–357. doi: 10.1016/j.bbr.2012.03.043

Lee, J., Lee, S., Chun, J. W., Cho, H., Kim, D., and Jung, Y.-C. (2015). Compromised prefrontal cognitive control over emotional interference in adolescents with internet gaming disorder. *Cyberpsychol. Behav. Soc. Netw.* 18, 661–668. doi: 10.1089/cyber.2015.0231

Lianekhammy, J., and Werner-Wilson, R. (2015). Links to prosocial factors and alpha asymmetry in adolescents during violent and non-violent video game play. *Child Stud. Asia Pac. Context* 5, 63–81. doi: 10.5723/csac.2015.5.2.063

Liberati, A., Altman, D. G., Tetzlaff, J., Mulrow, C., Gøtzsche, P. C., Ioannidis, J. P. A., et al. (2009). The PRISMA Statement for Reporting Systematic Reviews and Meta-Analyses of Studies That Evaluate Health Care Interventions: explanation and Elaboration. *PLoS Med.* 6:e1000100. doi: 10.1371/journal.pmed.1000100

Liu, J., Gao, X.-P. P., Osunde, I., Li, X., Zhou, S.-K. K., Zheng, H.-R., et al. (2010). Increased regional homogeneity in internet addiction disorder: a resting state functional magnetic resonance imaging study. *Chin. Med. J.* 123, 1904–1908. doi: 10.3760/cma.j.issn.0366-6999.2010.14.014

Liu, J., Li, W., Zhou, S., Zhang, L., Wang, Z., Zhang, Y., et al. (2015). Functional characteristics of the brain in college students with internet gaming disorder. *Brain Imaging Behav.* 10, 60–67. doi: 10.1007/s11682-015-9364-x

Liu, T., Saito, H., and Oi, M. (2012). Distinctive activation patterns under intrinsically versus extrinsically driven cognitive loads in prefrontal cortex: a near-infrared spectroscopy study using a driving video game. *Neurosci. Lett.* 506, 220–224. doi: 10.1016/j.neulet.2011.11.009

Liu, T., Saito, H., and Oi, M. (2015). Online monitoring of the social presence effects in a two-person-like driving video game using near-infrared spectroscopy. *Jpn. Psychol. Res.* 57, 242–253. doi: 10.1111/jpr.12080

Liu, Y., Teng, Z., Lan, H., Zhang, X., and Yao, D. (2015). Short-term effects of prosocial video games on aggression: an event-related potential study. *Front. Behav. Neurosci.* 9:193. doi: 10.3389/fnbeh.2015.00193

Lohse, K., Shirzad, N., Verster, A., Hodges, N., and Van der Loos, H. F. M. (2013). Video games and rehabilitation: using design principles to enhance engagement in physical therapy. *J. Neurol. Phys. Ther.* 37, 166–175. doi: 10.1097/NPT.0000000000000017

Lorenz, R. C., Gleich, T., Gallinat, J., and Kühn, S. (2015). Video game training and the reward system. *Front. Hum. Neurosci.* 9:40. doi: 10.3389/fnhum.2015.00040

Luijten, M., Meerkerk, G.-J., Franken, I. H. A., van de Wetering, B. J. M., and Schoenmakers, T. M. (2015). An fMRI study of cognitive control in problem gamers. *Psychiatry Res. Neuroimaging* 231, 262–268. doi: 10.1016/j.pscychresns.2015.01.004

Maclin, E. L., Mathewson, K. E., Low, K. A., Boot, W. R., Kramer, A. F., Fabiani, M., et al. (2011). Learning to multitask: effects of video game practice on electrophysiological indices of attention and resource allocation. *Psychophysiology* 48, 1173–1183. doi: 10.1111/j.1469-8986.2011.01189.x

Markey, P. M., and Markey, C. N. (2010). Vulnerability to violent video games: a review and integration of personality research. *Rev. Gen. Psychol.* 14, 82–91. doi: 10.1037/a0019000

Martínez, K., Solana, A. B., Burgaleta, M., Hernández-Tamames, J. A., Alvarez-Linera, J., Román, F. J., et al. (2013). Changes in resting-state functionally connected parietofrontal networks after videogame practice. *Hum. Brain Mapp.* 34, 3143–3157. doi: 10.1002/hbm.22129

Mathewson, K. E., Basak, C., Maclin, E. L., Low, K. A., Boot, W. R., Kramer, A. F., et al. (2012). Different slopes for different folks: alpha and delta EEG power predict subsequent video game learning rate and improvements in cognitive control tasks. *Psychophysiology* 49, 1558–1570. doi: 10.1111/j.1469-8986.2012.01474.x

Mathiak, K. A., Klasen, M., Weber, R., Ackermann, H., Shergill, S. S., and Mathiak, K. (2011). Reward system and temporal pole contributions to affective evaluation during a first person shooter video game. *BMC Neurosci.* 12:66. doi: 10.1186/1471-2202-12-66

Mathiak, K. A., Klasen, M., Zvyagintsev, M., Weber, R., and Mathiak, K. (2013). Neural networks underlying affective states in a multimodal virtual environment: contributions to boredom. *Front. Hum. Neurosci.* 7:820. doi: 10.3389/fnhum.2013.00820

Mathiak, K., and Weber, R. (2006). Toward brain correlates of natural behavior: fMRI during violent video games. *Hum. Brain Mapp.* 27, 948–956. doi: 10.1002/hbm.20234

Matsuda, G., and Hiraki, K. (2004). "Prefrontal cortex deactivation during video game play," in *Gaming, Simulations, and Society,* eds R. Shiratori, K. Arai, and F. Kato (Tokyo: Springer-Verlag), 101–109. doi: 10.1007/4-431-26797-2_11

Matsuda, G., and Hiraki, K. (2006). Sustained decrease in oxygenated hemoglobin during video games in the dorsal prefrontal cortex: a NIRS study of children. *Neuroimage* 29, 706–711. doi: 10.1016/j.neuroimage.2005.08.019

McGarry, W., Strenziok, M., Cisler, D. S., Clarke, E., Santa Cruz, S. A., Thompson, J. C., et al. (2013). "Real-time strategy video game training increases fronto-parietal cortical thickness, default mode network connectivity, and reasoning ability in healthy older adults," in *20th Annual Meeting of the Cognitive-Neuroscience-Society* (San Francisco, CA), 132–132.

McMahan, T., Parberry, I., and Parsons, T. D. (2015). Modality specific assessment of video game player's experience using the Emotiv. *Entertain. Comput.* 7, 1–6. doi: 10.1016/j.entcom.2015.03.001

Miller, J. F., Fried, I., Suthana, N., and Jacobs, J. (2015). Repeating spatial activations in human entorhinal cortex. *Curr. Biol.* 25, 1080–1085. doi: 10.1016/j.cub.2015.02.045

Mishra, J., Zinni, M., Bavelier, D., and Hillyard, S. A. (2011). Neural basis of superior performance of action videogame players in an attention-demanding task. *J. Neurosci.* 31, 992–998. doi: 10.1523/JNEUROSCI.4834-10.2011

Montag, C., Weber, B., Trautner, P., Newport, B., Markett, S., Walter, N. T., et al. (2012). Does excessive play of violent first-person-shooter-video-games dampen brain activity in response to emotional stimuli? *Biol. Psychol.* 89, 107–111. doi: 10.1016/j.biopsycho.2011.09.014

Nachev, P., Kennard, C., and Husain, M. (2008). Functional role of the supplementary and pre-supplementary motor areas. *Nat. Rev. Neurosci.* 9, 856–869. doi: 10.1038/nrn2478

Nagamitsu, S., Nagano, M., Yamashita, Y., Takashima, S., and Matsuishi, T. (2006). Prefrontal cerebral blood volume patterns while playing video games-A near-infrared spectroscopy study. *Brain Dev.* 28, 315–321. doi: 10.1016/j.braindev.2005.11.008

Naqvi, N. H., and Bechara, A. (2009). The hidden island of addiction: the insula. *Trends Neurosci.* 32, 56–67. doi: 10.1016/j.tins.2008.09.009

Nikolaidis, A., Voss, M. W., Lee, H., Vo, L. T. K., and Kramer, A. F. (2014). Parietal plasticity after training with a complex video game is associated with individual differences in improvements in an untrained working memory task. *Front. Hum. Neurosci.* 8:169. doi: 10.3389/fnhum.2014.00169

Obeso, I., Robles, N., Marrón, E. M., and Redolar-Ripoll, D. (2013). Dissociating the role of the pre-SMA in response Inhibition and switching: a combined online and offline TMS approach. *Front. Hum. Neurosci.* 7:150. doi: 10.3389/fnhum.2013.00150

O'Brien, C. P., Childress, A. R., Ehrman, R., and Robbins, S. J. (1998). Conditioning factors in drug abuse: can they explain compulsion? *J. Psychopharmacol.* 12, 15–22.

O'Doherty, J. P. (2004). Reward representations and reward-related learning in the human brain: insights from neuroimaging. *Curr. Opin. Neurobiol.* 14, 769–776. doi: 10.1016/j.conb.2004.10.016

Park, H. S., Kim, S. H., Bang, S. A., Yoon, E. J., Cho, S. S., and Kim, S. E. (2010). Altered regional cerebral glucose metabolism in internet game overusers: a ^{18}F-fluorodeoxyglucose positron emission tomography study. *CNS Spectr.* 15, 159–166. doi: 10.1017/S1092852900027437

Park, S. Y., Kim, S. M., Roh, S., Soh, M.-A., Lee, S. H., Kim, H., et al. (2016). The effects of a virtual reality treatment program for online gaming addiction. *Comput. Methods Programs Biomed.* 129, 99–108. doi: 10.1016/j.cmpb.2016.01.015

Patten, J., Gaspar, J., McDonald, J., and Spalek, T. (2015). Active Suppression in video-game players: an ERP study. *J. Vis.* 15:872. doi: 10.1167/15.12.872

Pellouchoud, E., Smith, M. E., McEvoy, L. K., and Gevins, A. (1999). Mental effort-related EEG modulation during video-game play: comparison between juvenile subjects with epilepsy and normal control subjects. *Epilepsia* 40 (Suppl. 4), 38–43. doi: 10.1111/j.1528-1157.1999.tb00905.x

Petras, K., Ten Oever, S., and Jansma, B. M. (2015). The effect of distance on moral engagement: event related potentials and alpha power are sensitive to perspective in a virtual shooting task. *Front. Psychol.* 6:2008. doi: 10.3389/fpsyg.2015.02008

Petry, N. M., Rehbein, F., Gentile, D. A., Lemmens, J. S., Rumpf, H.-J., Mößle, T., et al. (2014). An international consensus for assessing internet gaming disorder using the new DSM-5 approach. *Addiction* 109, 1399–1406. doi: 10.1111/add.12457

Powers, K. L., Brooks, P. J., Aldrich, N. J., Palladino, M. A., and Alfieri, L. (2013). Effects of video-game play on information processing: a meta-analytic investigation. *Psychon. Bull. Rev.* 20, 1055–1079. doi: 10.3758/s13423-013-0418-z

Prakash, R. S., De Leon, A. A., Mourany, L., Lee, H., Voss, M. W., Boot, W. R., et al. (2012). Examining neural correlates of skill acquisition in a complex videogame training program. *Front. Hum. Neurosci.* 6:115. doi: 10.3389/fnhum.2012.00115

Regenbogen, C., Herrmann, M., and Fehr, T. (2010). The neural processing of voluntary completed, real and virtual violent and nonviolent computer game scenarios displaying predefined actions in gamers and nongamers. *Soc. Neurosci.* 5, 221–240. doi: 10.1080/17470910903315989

Russoniello, C. V., O'brien, K., and Parks, J. M. (2009). EEG, HRV and psychological correlates while playing Bejeweled II: a randomized controlled study. *Annu. Rev. CyberTherapy Telemed.* 7, 189–192. doi: 10.3233/978-1-60750-017-9-189

Salminen, M., and Ravaja, N. (2007). Oscillatory brain responses evoked by video game events: the case of super monkey ball 2. *Cyberpsychol. Behav.* 10, 330–338. doi: 10.1089/cpb.2006.9947

Sánchez-González, M. A., García-Cabezas, M. A., Rico, B., and Cavada, C. (2005). The primate thalamus is a key target for brain dopamine. *J. Neurosci.* 25, 6076–6083. doi: 10.1523/JNEUROSCI.0968-05.2005

Schmidt-Hieber, C., and Häusser, M. (2013). Cellular mechanisms of spatial navigation in the medial entorhinal cortex. *Nat. Neurosci.* 16, 325–331. doi: 10.1038/nn.3340

Sheikholeslami, C., Yuan, H., He, E. J., Bai, X., Yang, L., and He, B. (2007). A high resolution EEG study of dynamic brain activity during video game play. *Conf. Proc. IEEE Eng. Med. Biol. Soc.* 2007, 2489–2491. doi: 10.1109/IEMBS.2007.4352833

Smith, E. E., and Jonides, J. (1999). Storage and executive processes in the frontal lobes. *Science* 283, 1657–1661. doi: 10.1126/science.283.5408.1657

Smith, M. E., McEvoy, L. K., and Gevins, A. (1999). Neurophysiological indices of strategy development and skill acquisition. *Cogn. Brain Res.* 7, 389–404. doi: 10.1016/S0926-6410(98)00043-3

Song, W. H., Han, D. H., and Shim, H. J. (2013). Comparison of brain activation in response to two dimensional and three dimensional on-line games. *Psychiatry Investig.* 10, 115–120. doi: 10.4306/pi.2013.10.2.115

Strenziok, M., Clarke, E., Santa Cruz, S. A., Thompson, J. C., Parasuraman, R., and Greenwood, P. M. (2013). "Effects of real-time strategy video game training on white matter integrity in interhemispheric posterior callosal connections of the precuneus in healthy aging," in *20th Annu. Meet. Cogn.* (San Francisco, CA), 190.

Strenziok, M., Krueger, F., Deshpande, G., Lenroot, R. K., Van der meer, E., and Grafman, J. (2011). Fronto-parietal regulation of media violence exposure in adolescents: a multi-method study. *Soc. Cogn. Affect. Neurosci.* 6, 537–547. doi: 10.1093/scan/nsq079

Strenziok, M., Parasuraman, R., Clarke, E., Cisler, D. S., Thompson, J. C., and Greenwood, P. M. (2014). Neurocognitive enhancement in older adults: comparison of three cognitive training tasks to test a hypothesis of training transfer in brain connectivity. *Neuroimage* 85(Pt 3), 1027–1039. doi: 10.1016/j.neuroimage.2013.07.069

Subhani, A. R., Likun, X., and Saeed Malik, A. (2012). Association of autonomic nervous system and EEG scalp potential during playing 2D grand turismo 5. *Conf. Proc. IEEE Eng. Med. Biol. Soc.* 2012, 3420–3423. doi: 10.1109/EMBC.2012.6346700

Szabó, C., Kelemen, O., and Kéri, S. (2014). Low-grade inflammation disrupts structural plasticity in the human brain. *Neuroscience* 275, 81–88. doi: 10.1016/j.neuroscience.2014.06.002

Tsai, M.-H., Cherng, R.-J., and Chen, J.-Y. (2013). "Visuospatial attention abilities in the action and real time strategy video game players as compared with nonplayers," in *2013 1st International Conference on Orange Technologies (ICOT)* (Tainan: IEEE), 264–265.

Tachtsidis, I., and Papaioannou, A. (2013). Investigation of frontal lobe activation with fNIRS and systemic changes during video gaming. *Adv. Exp. Med. Biol.* 789, 89–95. doi: 10.1007/978-1-4614-7411-1_13

Takeuchi, H., Taki, Y., Hashizume, H., Asano, K., Asano, M., Sassa, Y., et al. (2016). Impact of videogame play on the brain's microstructural properties: cross-sectional and longitudinal analyses. *Mol. Psychiatry* 21, 1781–1789. doi: 10.1038/mp.2015.193

Tanaka, S., Ikeda, H., Kasahara, K., Kato, R., Tsubomi, H., Sugawara, S. K., et al. (2013). Larger right posterior parietal volume in action video game experts: a behavioral and voxel-based morphometry (VBM) study. *PLoS ONE* 8:e66998. doi: 10.1371/journal.pone.0066998

Thalemann, R., Wölfling, K., and Grüsser, S. M. (2007). Specific cue reactivity on computer game-related cues in excessive gamers. *Behav. Neurosci.* 121, 614–618. doi: 10.1037/0735-7044.121.3.614

Tian, M., Chen, Q., Zhang, Y., Du, F., Hou, H., Chao, F., et al. (2014). PET imaging reveals brain functional changes in internet gaming disorder. *Eur. J. Nucl. Med. Mol. Imaging* 41, 1388–1397. doi: 10.1007/s00259-014-2708-8

Toril, P., Reales, J. M., and Ballesteros, S. (2014). Video game training enhances cognition of older adults: a meta-analytic study. *Psychol. Aging* 29, 706–716. doi: 10.1037/a0037507

Turel, O., Romashkin, A., and Morrison, K. M. (2016). Health outcomes of information system use lifestyles among adolescents: videogame addiction, sleep curtailment and cardio-metabolic deficiencies. *PLoS ONE* 11:e0154764. doi: 10.1371/journal.pone.0154764

Vo, L. T. K., Walther, D. B., Kramer, A. F., Erickson, K. I., Boot, W. R., Voss, M. W., et al. (2011). Predicting individuals' learning success from patterns of pre-learning MRI activity. *PLoS ONE* 6:e16093. doi: 10.1371/journal.pone.0016093

Vogan, V. M. M., Morgan, B. R. R., Powell, T. L. L., Smith, M. L. L., and Taylor, M. J. J. (2016). The neurodevelopmental differences of increasing verbal working memory demand in children and adults. *Dev. Cogn. Neurosci.* 17, 19–27. doi: 10.1016/j.dcn.2015.10.008

Volkow, N. D., Wang, G.-J., Fowler, J. S., Tomasi, D., Telang, F., and Baler, R. (2010). Addiction: decreased reward sensitivity and increased expectation sensitivity conspire to overwhelm the brain's control circuit. *Bioessays* 32, 748–755. doi: 10.1002/bies.201000042

Voss, M. W., Prakash, R. S., Erickson, K. I., Boot, W. R., Basak, C., Neider, M. B., et al. (2012). Effects of training strategies implemented in a complex videogame on functional connectivity of attentional networks. *Neuroimage* 59, 138–148. doi: 10.1016/j.neuroimage.2011.03.052

Vossel, S., Geng, J. J., and Fink, G. R. (2014). Dorsal and ventral attention systems: distinct neural circuits but collaborative roles. *Neuroscientist* 20, 150–159. doi: 10.1177/1073858413494269

Wang, P., Liu, H.-H., Zhu, X.-T., Meng, T., Li, H.-J., and Zuo, X.-N. (2016). Action video game training for healthy adults: a meta-analytic study. *Front. Psychol.* 7:907. doi: 10.3389/fpsyg.2016.00907

Wang, Y., Mathews, V. P., Kalnin, A. J., Mosier, K. M., Dunn, D. W., Saykin, A. J., et al. (2009). Short term exposure to a violent video game induces changes in frontolimbic circuitry in adolescents. *Brain Imaging Behav.* 3, 38–50. doi: 10.1007/s11682-008-9058-8

Wang, Y., Yin, Y., Sun, Y., Zhou, Y., Chen, X., Ding, W., et al. (2015). Decreased prefrontal lobe interhemispheric functional connectivity in adolescents with internet gaming disorder: a primary study using resting-state fMRI. *PLoS ONE* 10:e0118733. doi: 10.1371/journal.pone.0118733

Watter, S., Geffen, G. M., and Geffen, L. B. (2001). The n-back as a dual-task: P300 morphology under divided attention. *Psychophysiology* 38, 998–1003. doi: 10.1111/1469-8986.3860998

Weber, R., Ritterfeld, U., and Mathiak, K. (2006). Does playing violent video games induce aggression? Empirical evidence of a functional magnetic resonance imaging study. *Media Psychol.* 8, 39–60. doi: 10.1207/S1532785XMEP0801_4

Weber, R., Tamborini, R., Westcott-Baker, A., and Kantor, B. (2009). Theorizing flow and media enjoyment as cognitive synchronization of attentional and reward networks. *Commun. Theor.* 19, 397–422. doi: 10.1111/j.1468-2885.2009.01352.x

Wee, C.-Y., Zhao, Z., Yap, P.-T., Wu, G., Shi, F., Price, T., et al. (2014). Disrupted brain functional network in internet addiction disorder: a resting-state functional magnetic resonance imaging study. *PLoS ONE* 9:e107306. doi: 10.1371/journal.pone.0107306

West, G. L., Drisdelle, B. L., Konishi, K., Jackson, J., Jolicoeur, P., and Bohbot, V. D. (2015). Habitual action video game playing is associated with caudate nucleus- dependent navigational strategies. *Proc. R. Soc. London B Biol. Sci.* 282:20142952. doi: 10.1098/rspb.2014.2952

Wu, S., Cheng, C. K., Feng, J., D'Angelo, L., Alain, C., and Spence, I. (2012). Playing a first-person shooter video game induces neuroplastic change. *J. Cogn. Neurosci.* 24, 1286–1293. doi: 10.1162/jocn_a_00192

Xing, L., Yuan, K., Bi, Y., Yin, J., Cai, C., Feng, D., et al. (2014). Reduced fiber integrity and cognitive control in adolescents with internet gaming disorder. *Brain Res.* 1586, 109–117. doi: 10.1016/j.brainres.2014.08.044

Yoshida, K., Sawamura, D., Inagaki, Y., Ogawa, K., Ikoma, K., and Sakai, S. (2014). Brain activity during the flow experience: a functional near-infrared spectroscopy study. *Neurosci. Lett.* 573, 30–34. doi: 10.1016/j.neulet.2014.05.011

Young, K. S. (1998). Internet addiction: the emergence of a new clinical disorder. *CyberPsychol. Behav.* 1, 237–244. doi: 10.1089/cpb.1998.1.237

Yuan, K., Cheng, P., Dong, T., Bi, Y., Xing, L., Yu, D., et al. (2013a). Cortical thickness abnormalities in late adolescence with online gaming addiction. *PLoS ONE* 8:e53055. doi: 10.1371/journal.pone.0053055

Yuan, K., Jin, C., Cheng, P., Yang, X., Dong, T., Bi, Y., et al. (2013b). Amplitude of low frequency fluctuation abnormalities in adolescents with online gaming addiction. *PLoS ONE* 8:e78708. doi: 10.1371/journal.pone.0078708

Zhang, J.-T., Yao, Y.-W., Li, C.-S. R., Zang, Y.-F., Shen, Z.-J., Liu, L., et al. (2016). Altered resting-state functional connectivity of the insula in young adults with Internet gaming disorder. *Addict. Biol.* 21, 743–751. doi: 10.1111/adb.12247

Zhang, Y., Du, G., Yang, Y., Qin, W., Li, X., and Zhang, Q. (2015). Higher integrity of the motor and visual pathways in long-term video game players. *Front. Hum. Neurosci.* 9:98. doi: 10.3389/fnhum.2015.00098

Zvyagintsev, M., Klasen, M., Weber, R., Sarkheil, P., Esposito, F., Mathiak, K. A., et al. (2016). Violence-related content in video game may lead to functional connectivity changes in brain networks as revealed by fMRI-ICA in young men. *Neuroscience* 320, 247–258. doi: 10.1016/j.neuroscience.2016.01.056

8

Working Memory Training for Healthy Older Adults: The Role of Individual Characteristics in Explaining Short- and Long-Term Gains

Erika Borella[1], Elena Carbone[1], Massimiliano Pastore[2], Rossana De Beni[1] and Barbara Carretti[1]**

[1] Department of General Psychology, University of Padova, Padova, Italy, [2] Department of Developmental and Social Psychology, University of Padova, Padova, Italy

Edited by:
Soledad Ballesteros,
Universidad Nacional de Educación a Distancia, Spain

Reviewed by:
José Manuel Reales,
Universidad Nacional de Educación a Distancia, Spain
Tiina Salminen,
Synaptikon GmbH (NeuroNation), Germany

***Correspondence:**
Erika Borella
erika.borella@unipd.it
Barbara Carretti
barbara.carretti@unipd.it

Objective: The aim of the present study was to explore whether individual characteristics such as age, education, vocabulary, and baseline performance in a working memory (WM) task—similar to the one used in the training (criterion task)—predict the short- and long-term specific gains and transfer effects of a verbal WM training for older adults.

Method: Four studies that adopted the Borella et al. (2010) verbal WM training procedure were found eligible for our analysis as they included: healthy older adults who attended either the training sessions (WM training group), or alternative activities (active control group); the same measures for assessing specific gains (on the criterion WM task), and transfer effects (nearest on a visuo-spatial WM task, near on short-term memory tasks and far on a measure of fluid intelligence, a measure of processing speed and two inhibitory measures); and a follow-up session.

Results: Linear mixed models confirmed the overall efficacy of the training, in the short-term at least, and some maintenance effects. In the trained group, the individual characteristics considered were found to contribute (albeit only modestly in some cases) to explaining the effects of the training.

Conclusions: Overall, our findings suggest the importance of taking individual characteristics and individual differences into account when examining WM training gains in older adults.

Keywords: working memory training, older adults, age, working memory baseline performance, general cognitive ability, training benefits, individual differences, individual characteristics

INTRODUCTION

Working memory (WM), i.e., the ability to retain and manipulate information for use in complex cognitive tasks, is one of the core mechanisms involved in higher-order cognitive abilities (e.g., fluid intelligence, problem-solving, and reading comprehension; de Ribaupierre, 2001; Borella et al., 2011). Though characterized by a limited capacity, WM is a crucial mechanism in cognition. It is also one of the cognitive processes that suffer a clear and linear decline with aging (e.g., Borella et al., 2008; Mammarella et al., 2013). WM is consequently one of the general processes targeted by the new generation of process-based cognitive training. The assumption that WM is trainable is based on evidence of the plasticity of our cognitive system across the whole life span (i.e., Hertzog et al., 2008). Further, according to some WM models, such as the continuity model (see Cornoldi and Vecchi, 2003; Cornoldi, 2010), WM is characterized by different processes that depend on the type of content processed (verbal vs. spatial) and also on the involvement of executive control. Therefore, by improving WM, its related processes can also theoretically be enhanced. The Cornoldi and Vecchi WM model distinguished between a "basic structure" (a sort of personal biological equipment), and a "used ability" determined by the way in which individuals use their WM. On this basis, the benefits of training may presumably concern not only the basic structure of WM, but also its usage.

The aim of WM training in aging is thus to improve older adults' information processing system (e.g., Zinke et al., 2012; Bürki et al., 2014), in order to sustain their cognitive functioning for an active aging. WM training was shown to improve performance not only in the trained tasks (or in tasks similar to the one used in the training), but also in untrained tasks (transfer effects). Training changes the way in which individuals process information, enabling them to make more flexible use of their own resources.

The recent meta-analysis by Karbach and Verhaeghen (2014), focusing on aging, showed that WM training for older people could promote significant gains both in the trained tasks and in other similar tasks (near transfer effects). There also seemed to be some improvements in untrained tasks that shared some cognitive processes with the task used in the training (far transfer effects), though they were usually small in terms of effect size (see Karbach and Verhaeghen, 2014). There have been mixed reports on the matter of the efficacy of WM training in aging (see **Table 1**), however, making it necessary to identify which factors are involved in giving rise to training benefits. Among the numerous factors to consider, individual characteristics—such as age, general cognitive ability, and baseline cognitive resources—believed to predict the benefits of memory training (e.g., Verhaeghen and Marcoen, 1996) may also have a role as modulators of WM training outcomes (Bürki et al., 2014). Surprisingly, their role has not been the focus of WM training studies as yet.

Age is one of the crucial factors that may explain whether and to what extent individuals may gain more or less in terms of both specific training gains (in a given trained task) and transfer effects (e.g., von Bastian and Oberauer, 2014). Some WM training studies examined the role of age in explaining the benefits of training by comparing young and older adults, or considering older adults in different age brackets (see also Borella et al., 2014 for a review). Some of the studies that included both young and older adults analyzed how performance changed over the course of the training sessions (Dahlin et al., 2008; Li et al., 2008; Richmond et al., 2011; Brehmer et al., 2012; von Bastian et al., 2013; Bürki et al., 2014). Brehmer et al. (2012), for instance, considered weekly WM performance scores, pooling participants' daily performance in 7 WM training tasks into a single t-standardized WM performance score. They found that young adults gained more than older adults from week 1 to 2, but then the two age groups showed comparable improvements from the second week to the end of training, from week 2 to 4. Bürki et al. (2014) found that age-related differences in the performance of young and older adults persisted over 10 training sessions (with greater improvements in the former). Li et al. (2008) found significant improvements for both young and older adults in two trained spatial n-back tasks (though the best performance reached by the older adults was still not as good as that of the younger adults). Other studies reported mixed results, however: age-related differences in favor of young adults were found in some of the trained tasks, while improvements were comparable between the two age groups in others.

As concerns specific training gains (i.e., in the criterion tasks), as shown in **Table 1**, mixed results were found: comparable benefits in young and older adults in tasks strictly similar to those used in the training were obtained in five studies (Li et al., 2008; Richmond et al., 2011; von Bastian et al., 2013; Bürki et al., 2014; Zając-Lamparska and Trempała, 2016); three studies showed greater improvements in young than in older adults (Dahlin et al., 2008; Heinzel et al., 2014; Salminem et al., 2015); one study obtained mixed results with age-related differences for some criterion tasks but not for others (Brehmer et al., 2012); two studies showed that older adults reached the young adults' baseline performance level on the WM criterion tasks immediately after the training-i.e., at the post-test assessment-(Li et al., 2008; Salminem et al., 2015), and one study found that older adults exceeded the young participants' baseline performance in the criterion task.

Similarly, for near as well as far transfer effects (when found), studies found either no differences between the two age groups, or larger effects in young adults than in older adults, or again mixed results (see **Table 1**). As for any long-term effects, if they were examined, Brehmer et al. (2012), and Dahlin et al. (2008) found a comparable maintenance of specific training gains between young and older adults. Brehmer et al. (2012) also identified the maintenance of both near and far transfer effects in both age groups. Partially in contrast, Li et al. (2008) found larger long-term specific training gains for young adults than for older ones, while the long-term near transfer effects were comparable between the two age groups (see **Table 1**).

Among the studies focusing only on older adults (see **Table 1**), the ones that found significant specific training gains and transfer effects, along with their maintenance were those involving young-old participants (from 60 to 74 years old). Studies that included old-old participants (from 75 to 87 years old), and those considering a broad age range (i.e., from 60 to 82) reported mixed findings in terms of specific and transfer training gains in the short term (see **Table 1**). As for the maintenance effects, some found limited transfer benefits (Borella et al., 2010, 2013, 2017; Zinke et al., 2013), and others found none (Buschkuehl et al., 2008). In one of these studies, older age also emerged as a negative predictor of training gains and at least some transfer effects (Zinke et al., 2013); it is worth noting that the effect sizes for transfer effects in this case were medium to large for tasks assessing near effects, but only small for far transfer effects (see **Table 1**).

Taken together, the above studies seem to support a negative role of age in determining the benefits of WM training.

TABLE 1 | Peer-reviewed studies of the effects of WM training studies involving older adults and the sample's characteristics (i.e., age).

	Age	Short-term gains			Long-term gains			
		Specific	Near	Far	Follow-up	Specific	Near	Far
YOUNG ADULTS VS. OLDER ADULTS								
Li et al., 2008	Young: 20–30 Old: 70–80	Yes (Y = O)	Yes (Y = O)	No	3 months	Yes (Y > O)	Yes (Y = O)	No
Dahlin et al., 2008	Young: 23.88 ± 2.52 Old: 68.31 ± 1.69	Yes (Y > O)	Yes (Y > O but in general restricted to young adults)	No	18 months	Yes (Y = O)	No	No
Richmond et al., 2011	Young: 20 Old: 60–80	Yes (Y = O)	NE	NE	NE			
Brehmer et al., 2012	Young: 20–30 Old: 60–70	Yes (Mixed*)	Yes (Mixed*)	Yes (Mixed*)	3 months	Yes (Y = O)	Yes (Y = O)	Yes (Y = O)
von Bastian et al., 2013	Young: 19–36 Old: 62–77	Yes (Y = O)	Yes (Y = O but minimal for both age groups)	No	NE			
Bürki et al., 2014	Young: 18–38 Old: 67.98 ± 5.41	Yes (Y = O)	Yes (Y = O but mixed**)	No	NE			
Heinzel et al., 2014	Young: 24–30 Old: 61–75	Yes (Y > O)	Yes (Y > O)	Yes (Y > O)	NE			
Salminem et al., 2015	Young: 20–31 Old: 57–77	Yes (Y > O)	Yes (Y = O)	No	NE			
Zając-Lamparska and Trempała, 2016	Young: 20–33 Old: 60–85	Yes (Y = O)	Yes (Y = O)	Yes (Y = O)	NE			
OLDER ADULTS FROM DIFFERENT AGE BRACKETS								
Buschkuehl et al., 2008	80.00 ± 3.3	Yes	Yes	Yes (Mixed**)	12 months	No	No	No
Borella et al., 2010	65–75	Yes	Yes	Yes	8 months	Yes	No	Yes (Mixed**)
Richmond et al., 2011	60–80	Yes	Yes (Mixed**)	Yes (Mixed**)	NE			
Brehmer et al., 2011	60–70	Yes	Yes	Yes (only in a measure of sustained attention)	NE			
Zinke et al., 2012	77–96	Yes	No	No	NE			
Borella et al., 2013	75–87	Yes	No	No	8 months	Yes	No	Yes (only in a measure of inhibition)
Carretti et al., 2013b	65–75	Yes	Yes	Yes	6 months	Yes	Yes	Yes
Zinke et al., 2013	65–95	Yes	Yes (Mixed**)	Yes (Mixed**)	9 months	Yes	Yes (only in a verbal WM task)	No
Borella et al., 2014	65–84	Yes	Yes (only for young-adults)	Yes (only for young-adults)	8 months	Yes	No	No
Stepankova et al., 2014	65–74	Yes	Yes	Yes	NE			
Xin et al., 2014	60–82	Yes	Yes	Yes	NE			
Cantarella et al., 2017	65–75	Yes	NE	Yes	NE			
Borella et al., 2017	65–75	Yes	No	Yes (only in the processing speed measure)	6 months	Yes	Yes (Mixed**)	Yes (only in the processing speed measure)

*Y, younger adults; O, older adults; Y > O, greater improvements in young adults than in older adults; Y = O, comparable benefits in young adults and older adults; NE, not examined; WM, working memory; STM, short term memory; *Mixed, greater improvements in young adults than in older adults in some tasks, but comparable benefits in young and older adults in other tasks; **Mixed, significant results only in some of the measures considered.*

Another variable that may influence the efficacy of cognitive training is general cognitive ability, operationalized in some studies with crystallized intelligence, i.e., performance in a vocabulary test (Zinke et al., 2013). This can be considered an index of general cognitive ability (e.g., Baltes, 1987), and a possible moderator of WM training benefits. The only WM training study that considered this variable found, however, that it did not contribute to explaining WM training gains and transfer effects (Zinke et al., 2013).

Individual differences in cognitive resources, such as WM baseline performance, are another factor that may predict training outcomes (see Jaeggi et al., 2014 for evidence in young adults), but only two WM training studies that focused on older adults (aged 77 to 96, Zinke et al., 2012; aged 65 to 80 and over: Zinke et al., 2013) have considered this variable. One study found a negative correlation between specific gains and participants' baseline WM performance, i.e., those with a weaker baseline WM performance gained more in the trained tasks than those whose WM performance was better (Zinke et al., 2012). The other confirmed this association, i.e., the lower the baseline WM performance, the larger the specific gains in the trained tasks (Zinke et al., 2013). In another study by Bürki et al. (2014), the pre-test score obtained in a reasoning measure was considered instead, and the results indicated that the effects of the training were predicted not by this reasoning score, but by age group.

Overall, the pattern of results concerning the role of individual characteristics and individual differences in training-related performance gains and transfer effects is rather mixed. It is also worth noting that, despite the importance of analyzing individual factors when assessing the benefits of WM training, only three studies have so far addressed this issue directly in relation to aging (Zinke et al., 2012, 2013; Bürki et al., 2014).

Hence the present study, the aim of which was to examine the role of individual differences (or individual characteristics) by jointly considering different factors to identify those capable of influencing short- and longer-term training-induced plasticity, measured in terms of both specific training gains and transfer effects. The factors considered as potential mediators of the efficacy of training (e.g., von Bastian and Oberauer, 2014) were demographic characteristics (i.e., age), baseline WM performance (Zinke et al., 2012) and general cognitive ability (i.e., crystallized intelligence measured with a vocabulary test; Zinke et al., 2013). The role of education was also examined because education is considered an index of cognitive efficiency that can preserve cognitive functioning, and because it is also used as a proxy of cognitive reserve (e.g., Stern, 2002; Staff et al., 2004), although no studies have examined whether it interacts with the trainability of WM.

We investigated the role of these variables by analyzing data emerging from studies that adopted the same WM training procedure, developed by Borella et al. (2010). This is one of the few procedures to have been used across different studies, generating consistent and promising results in terms of short- and long-term benefits (Borella et al., 2010, 2017)—also in tasks related to everyday abilities (Carretti et al., 2013b; Cantarella et al., 2017)—in normal and pathological aging (in healthy young-old and old-old, Borella et al., 2013, 2014; in amnestic Mild Cognitive Impairment, Carretti et al., 2013a). The effectiveness of the training has been attributed to the fact that it involves participants practicing with a complex WM span task, combining an adaptive procedure with a systematic variation of the demands of the task, so that it remains constantly novel and challenging, keeping participants interested and motivated during the proposed activities. According to the authors, the training also engages numerous different processes that include encoding, maintaining and inhibiting information, simultaneously managing two tasks, sustaining and shifting attention. Together, these aspects are believed to promote learning and particularly to enable the training to favor transfer effects (see Borella et al., 2010). To date, seven studies have adopted this procedure (see **Table 2** for a summary), and four were selected for the present analysis because: (i) the same verbal procedure was adopted; (ii) the same measures were used to assess training gains and transfer effects; (iii) a follow-up session was included; and (iv) a sample of healthy older adults was considered (see **Tables 2, 3**).

Specific training gains and transfer effects were categorized along a conceptually-based continuum of nearest to far transfer tasks (i.e., Noack et al., 2009). The complex WM task (the Categorization Working Memory Span task, CWMS) was used to assess specific training gains because it is similar to the task administered to participants during the training sessions. Another complex WM task measuring the same narrow ability (WM), and also involving active processes (see Cornoldi and Vecchi, 2003), but with a different type of material (visuo-spatial, the Dot Matrix Task) was administered to assess what we describe here as *nearest transfer effects*. Measures of the same broad ability (memory), but with different demands from those of the other complex WM tasks (the Forward and Backward Digit Span tests; see meta-analyses by Bopp and Verhaeghen, 2005) were used to assess near transfer effects. Finally, tasks assessing fluid intelligence (the Cattell test), processing speed (the Pattern Comparison task), and inhibitory mechanisms (Stroop Color test and intrusion errors in the CWMS), i.e., mechanisms differing from WM but known to correlate with WM and to help explaining the age-related decline in WM (e.g., de Ribaupierre and Lecerf, 2006), were used to measure far transfer effects.

Linear mixed effects (LME) models were used to examine the role of individual characteristics (demographic variables) and individual differences in predicting improvements in the measures used to assess the effects of the training (in terms of training gains and transfer effects). These models afford a more robust analytical approach for addressing problems associated with hierarchical and correlated data than the traditional analyses generally conducted in training studies (e.g., ANOVA, *t*-test). In particular, LME models allow for a more flexible approach in dealing with individual changes over time when repeated measures are considered (e.g., Gueorguieva and Krystal, 2004; Wainwright et al., 2007; Baayen et al., 2008).

In general, we expected to confirm the beneficial effect of the WM training in terms of short- and long-term gains in the criterion task, and at least short-term transfer effects for all the measures considered. The advantage of performing such an analysis on all four studies sharing the same procedure lay in enabling us to establish the strength of the effects (i.e., effect sizes) on a larger sample.

TABLE 2 | Summary of the characteristics and results of the seven studies that employed the Borella et al. (2010) training program.

Study	Training task	Months since training: follow-up	Older adults' characteristics	Specific effects	Nearest/near transfer effects	Far transfer effects	Maintenance effects
Borella et al., 2010	Verbal WM task (CWMS)	8 months	Healthy 65–75 ($M = 69 \pm 3.18$)	Yes	Yes (verbal STM)	Yes (processing speed, inhibition, fluid intelligence)	Yes (verbal WM, processing speed, fluid intelligence)
Carretti et al., 2013b	Verbal WM task (CWMS)	6 months	Healthy 65–75 ($M = 69 \pm 3.30$)	Yes	Yes (WM updating)	Yes (comprehension, fluid intelligence)	Yes (all short-term effects)
Borella et al., 2013	Verbal WM task (CWMS)	8 months	Healthy 75–87 ($M = 79 \pm 3.22$)	Yes	No	No	Yes (verbal WM, inhibition)
Borella et al., 2017	Verbal WM task (CWMS) ± mental imagery strategy	6 months	Healthy ($M = 69 \pm 4.33$)	Yes (all trained groups)	No	Yes (processing speed, more consistent for WM trained group)	Yes (verbal WM, verbal STM, processing speed more consistent for WM trained group)
Carretti et al., 2013a	Verbal WM task (CWMS)	NE	Amnestic MCI 65–75 ($M = 70 \pm 2.40$)	Yes	Yes (visuo-spatial WM)	Yes (fluid intelligence)	NE
Borella et al., 2014	Visuo-spatial WM task (The Matrix Task)	8 months	Healthy 65–75 ($M = 69 \pm 2.84$), 76–84 ($M = 80 = 2.29$)	Yes (all age groups)	Yes (verbal WM, visuo-spatial STM, only young-old)	Yes (processing speed, only young-old)	Yes (visuo-spatial WM, verbal WM, all age groups)
Cantarella et al., 2017	Verbal WM task (CWMS)	NE	Healthy 65–75 ($M = 69 \pm 3.08$)	Yes	NE	Yes (everyday problems solving, reasoning)	NE

WM, working memory; STM, short-term memory; MCI, mild cognitive impairment; NE, not examined.

TABLE 3 | Summary of the sample sizes and outcome measures considered in the four studies conducted using the Borella et al. (2010) training program and analyzed in the present study.

Study	Specific effects						Nearest transfer effects			Near transfer effects		Far transfer effects				
	N	Trained group	Control Group	Ed	Voc	VWM	Working memory			Short-term memory		Comprehension	Fluid intelligence		Processing speed	Inhib.
						CWMS	Listening span test	Dot matrix task	Jigsaw puzzle test	Updating task	Forward and backward digit span task	Listening and reading comprehension	Cattell test	Letter sets	Pattern comparison task	Stroop color task
Borella et al., 2010	40	20	20	+	+	+		+			+		+		+	+
Carretti et al., 2013b	36	17	19	+	+	+				+		+	+			
Borella et al., 2013	36	18	18	+	+	+		+			+		+		+	+
Borella et al., 2017^	36	18	18	+	+	+	+		+		+			+	+	
Total Sample	148	73	75	148	148	148	36	76	36	36	112	36	112	36	112	76
Common measures				*	*	*		*			*		*		*	*

The measures that the studies had in common are identified in the bottom row of the table with an asterisk. Ed, Education; Voc, Vocabulary Score; VWM, verbal Working Memory; Inhib., inhibition; CWMS, Categorization Working Memory Span Task (De Beni et al., 2008); Listening Span Test (De Beni et al., 2008); Dot Matrix Task (adapted from Miyake et al., 2001); Jigsaw Puzzle Test (De Beni et al., 2008); Updating Task, Working Memory Updating Word Span (Carretti et al., 2010); Forward and Backward Digit Span Task (De Beni et al., 2008); Listening and Reading Comprehension, Listening Comprehension of Spatial Description (Pazzaglia et al., 2007) and Reading Comprehension of Expository Tests (see Borella et al., 2011); Cattell Test, Culture Fair Test, Scale 3 (Cattell and Cattell, 1963); Letter Sets (Ekstrom et al., 1976); Pattern Comparison Test (adapted from Salthouse and Babcock, 1991); Stroop Color Task (adapted from Trenerry et al., 1989).

^Only the group that attended the Verbal WM training without the use of the imagery strategy was considered here.

Concerning the main objective of the study, we used LME models to analyze participants' individual characteristics and differences vis-à-vis the short- and long-term effects of their training. Analyzing these potential predictors will enable us to test the two proposed theoretical explanations for individual differences in training-related performance gains, i.e., a compensation or a magnification effect of process-based training on cognition in older adults (see for example Titz and Karbach, 2014; see also Lövdén et al., 2012). If there is a magnification effect, then individuals who already perform well will benefit the most from the WM training. In other words, high-performing participants may have more efficient cognitive resources and therefore be in a better position to learn and implement new abilities. The WM training should therefore result in a magnification of age-related (in older adults) and individual differences; baseline cognitive performance should also be positively associated with training-related gains and transfer effects. If there is a compensation effect, on the other hand, then high-performing individuals will benefit less from the training because they are already functioning at their optimal level, and thus have less room for improvement. In this case, age-related and individual differences should be reduced after the training, and baseline cognitive performance should be negatively associated with training-induced gains.

The magnification and compensation effects would thus lead in opposite directions. Among the older adults, the younger participants with a good cognitive status, as represented by a measure of crystallized intelligence (vocabulary), a good WM (revealed by their baseline CWMS performance), and a good education might profit more from an adaptive training on a complex aspect of cognition—WM—because a relatively high level of functioning is required to actively engage in and benefit from the activities proposed in the training (Bissig and Lustig, 2007; Lustig et al., 2009), which would, in turns, magnify their abilities. On the other hand, older participants with a worse cognitive status might benefit more from the WM training (Zinke et al., 2012, 2013) because it could counteract the suboptimal use of resources typical of aging by prompting a more flexible use of these resources, more reliant on controlled than on automatic processes, that would re-activate the older participants' potential, having a compensatory effect.

There is also the possibility, as emerges from the results obtained by Zinke et al. (2013), that the factors thought to predict training-related gains might depend on the measures considered, because these factors may also take effect independently. In fact, the individual characteristics examined may explain the training gains differently, as the transfer tasks vary in several aspects—not only in terms of their relationship with WM, but also in terms of the processes involved, such as the type of control (passive as in the short-term memory tasks vs. active as in the reasoning task), or the more or less strong involvement of fluid abilities (stronger in reasoning and in processing speed than in short-term memory tasks) and/or those related to knowledge.

METHOD

Table 1 lists the characteristics and the main results of the seven studies that used the verbal WM training procedure developed by Borella et al. (2010). As mentioned in the Introduction, three studies (in the last rows of **Table 2**) were not considered because: one involved a sample of older adults with mild cognitive impairment (Carretti et al., 2013a); one used a visuo-spatial version of the training program (Borella et al., 2014); and one did not include a follow-up assessment (Cantarella et al., 2017).

The four studies considered eligible for the present analysis had in common: (i) the same verbal procedure; (ii) the same measures for assessing training gains and transfer effects (see **Table 3**); and (iii) a follow-up assessment.

Participants

All the four studies considered here included a sample of healthy older adults (all native Italian speakers) recruited from the University of the Third Age, at social clubs in north-eastern Italy, or by word of mouth, who all volunteered for the study.

They were told, either individually (Borella et al., 2010, 2017) or at a plenary session (Borella et al., 2013; Carretti et al., 2013b), that they would be involved in one of two different programs each consisting of five individual sessions, plus a final one at a later date (follow-up). They were also told that the activities proposed in one program would concern their cognitive functioning (i.e., practicing with memory tasks), while in the other one they would be asked to reflect on aspects of memory (e.g., autobiographical recall) and complete some questionnaires.

Depending on the study, participants had to meet the following inclusion criteria: (i) good physical and mental health, assessed by means of a questionnaire and a semi-structured interview, respectively (as in Borella et al., 2010; Carretti et al., 2013b); (ii) none of the exclusion criteria proposed by Crook et al. (1986) as in Borella et al. (2010, 2013); (iii) a Mini-Mental State Score (Folstein et al., 1975) higher than 27 (as in Borella et al., 2013); (iv) a maximum score on the Italian Checklist for Multidimensional Assessments (SVAMA; Gallina et al., 2006), i.e., no signs of incipient dementia (as in Borella et al., 2017). In all four studies, participants were randomly assigned to either the trained group or the active control group.

Overall, 148 participants were involved in the four studies considered, with 73 forming the trained groups, and 75 the active control groups. The pooled trained and control groups were comparable in terms of age (age range: 61–87; trained group: $M = 71.63$, $SD = 5.53$; control group: $M = 71.61$ $SD = 5.67$), $F_{(1, 146)} < 1$, years of formal education (from 8 to 24 years; trained group: $M = 9.42$ $SD = 4.54$; control group: $M = 9.97$ $SD = 4.72$), $F_{(1, 146)} < 1$, and vocabulary score in the Wechsler Adult Intelligence Scale—Revised (WAIS–R; Wechsler, 1981; max 70; trained group: $M = 49.21$ $SD = 10.89$; control group: $M = 47.04$ $SD = 11.87$), $F_{(1, 146)} = 1.33, p = 0.25$.

As common outcome measures used to assess transfer effects varied within the four studies considered, pooled trained and control groups were compared with respect to demographic characteristics and vocabulary score. The pooled trained and control groups were not statistically different in terms of age, years of formal education, and vocabulary score[1].

[1]As for the Forward and the Backward Digit Span tasks and the Pattern Comparison task, these measures were used in three

MATERIALS

Criterion Task

Categorization Working Memory Span (CWMS) task (De Beni et al., 2008)

The task consisted of 10 sets of word lists, each including 20 lists of words (divided into groups containing from 2 to 6 lists). Participants listened to a set of word lists audio-recorded at a rate of 1 word per second and they had to tap with their hand on the table whenever an animal noun was heard (processing phase). The interval between word lists was 2 s. At the end of a set, participants recalled the last word on each list (maintenance phase)—i.e., they needed to remember from 2 to 6 words altogether, depending on the difficulty of the set.

The total number of words recalled was used as the measure of WM performance (maximum 20).

Nearest Transfer Effects

Visuo-Spatial WM Task

Dot Matrix task (adapted from Miyake et al., 2001)

In this task participants had to check a matrix equation consisting of an addition or a subtraction presented as lines drawn on a 3 × 3 matrix, and to memorize sequences of dots presented on a 5 × 5 grid. They were given a maximum of 4.5 s to check each equation and say "True" or "False." Immediately after they gave their answer, they were shown a 5 × 5 grid containing a dot in one of the squares for 3 s. After seeing sets of two to six pairs of equations and grids, they had to indicate the positions of the dots on a blank 5 × 5 grid. There was one practice trial with two equations, each with one dot. The number of dot locations to recall increased from two to six. A total of 28 equations and 28 matrices were presented. The total number of dot positions correctly recalled was considered as the dependent variable (maximum score 14).

(Borella et al., 2010, 2013, 2017) of the four studies considered. The pooled trained ($n = 56$) and control ($n = 56$) groups from these three studies did not differ in terms of age (trained group: $M = 72.43$ $SD = 5.81$; control group: $M = 72.04$, $SD = 6.16$), $F_{(1, 110)} < 1$, years of formal education (trained group: $M = 9.482$ $SD = 4.72$; control group: $M = 10.30$ $SD = 4.65$), $F_{(1, 110)} < 1$, or vocabulary score on the Wechsler Adult Intelligence Scale - Revised (WAIS-R; Wechsler, 1981; trained group: $M = 50.23$ $SD = 11.27$; control group: $M = 49.07$ $SD = 11.45$), $F_{(1, 110)} < 1$.

As for the Cattell test, this was used in three (Borella et al., 2010, 2013; Carretti et al., 2013b) of the four studies considered. The pooled trained ($n = 55$) and control ($n = 57$) groups from these two studies did not differ in terms of age (trained group: $M = 72.35$, $SD = 5.86$; control group: $M = 72.72$ $SD = 5.47$), $F_{(1, 110)} < 1$, years of formal education (trained group: $M = 7.80$ $SD = 3.73$; control group: $M = 8.49$ $SD = 4.07$), $F_{(1, 110)} < 1$, or vocabulary score on the Wechsler Adult Intelligence Scale—Revised (WAIS-R; Wechsler, 1981; trained group: $M = 45.11$ $SD = 8.89$; control group: $M = 43.16$ $SD = 10.25$), $F_{(1, 110)} = 1.15$, $p = 0.28$.

The Dot Matrix task and the Stroop Color task were used in two (Borella et al., 2010, 2013) of the four studies considered. The pooled trained ($n = 38$) and control ($n = 38$) groups from these two studies did not differ in terms of age (trained group: $M = 73.84$, $SD = 6.12$; control group: $M = 73.89$ $SD = 5.85$), $F_{(1, 74)} < 1$, years of formal education (trained group: $M = 7.66$ $SD = 3.79$; control group: $M = 8.24$ $SD = 3.62$), $F_{(1, 74)} < 1$, or vocabulary score on the Wechsler Adult Intelligence Scale—Revised (WAIS-R; Wechsler, 1981; trained group: $M = 44.79$ $SD = 8.93$; control group: $M = 44.21$ $SD = 9.65$), $F_{(1, 74)} < 1$.

Near Transfer Effects

Short-Term Memory Tasks

Forward and Backward Digit Span tasks (De Beni et al., 2008)

Participants had to repeat series of digits in the same (forward) or reverse (backward) order. Each level (from 3 to 9 digits for the forward task, from 2 to 8 digits for the backward task) contained two series of digits. After two consecutive recall errors, the task was discontinued. One point was awarded for each correctly recalled series. The final score corresponded to the total number of series recalled correctly (maximum score of 14 for both tasks).

Far Transfer Effects

Fluid Intelligence

Culture Fair test (Cattell test; Cattell and Cattell, 1963)

This task consisted of 4 subtests (to be completed in 2.5–4 min., depending on the subtest) in which participants were asked to: (1) choose from among six different options which ones correctly completed a series of figures; (2) identify figures or shapes that did not belong in a sequence; (3) choose items that correctly completed matrices of abstract figures; (4) assess relationships between sets of items. The dependent variable was the number of correct answers across the four subtests (maximum score 50).

Processing Speed

Pattern comparison task (adpated from Salthouse and Babcock, 1991)

In this task, participants had to decide whether arrangements of line segments were identical or not. The items to be compared were set out on two pages each containing 30 items. Responses consisted of writing *S* (for *Si* [*Yes*], for identical items) or *N* (for *No*, for different items) on the line between the two items in each pair. The experimenter used a stopwatch to record the time taken to complete each page. Three practice trials were run before the experiment started. The dependent variable was the total time taken to complete the task.

Inhibition

Stroop Color task (adapted from Trenerry et al., 1989)

In this task participants were shown six cards. The first two contained names of colors printed in an incongruent ink color (Incongruent condition); the third and fourth contained names of colors printed in a congruous ink color (Congruent condition); and the last two contained color patches (Control condition). Participants had to name the ink color of each stimulus and were asked to process the stimuli as quickly and accurately as possible. The experimenter recorded response latencies for all conditions by using a stopwatch to time the interval between naming the first and last stimuli—as typically done in other studies using the paper version (e.g., West and Alain, 2000; Van der Elst et al., 2006; Troyer et al., 2006)—and noted the respondents' accuracy by hand on a prepared form. The dependent variable—in order to control for individual differences at the baseline (e.g., Borella et al., 2009)—was the interference index computed in terms of relative difference between the time taken to complete the task in the incongruent and control conditions, that is [(incongruent condition − control condition)/control condition]. A higher score thus implied a greater difficulty in controlling the prepotent response in the incongruent condition.

Intrusion errors in the CWMS -CWMS intrusion errors- (De Beni et al., 2008)

The total intrusion errors made in the CWMS, i.e., words that were not actually the last in of each string of words presented, were also considered as a measure of inhibition, representing a participant's ability to inhibit no longer relevant information (Borella et al., 2007).

For each task, two parallel versions were devised and administered in a counterbalanced order across the testing sessions.

Procedure

Participants attended six individual sessions: the first and fifth were the pre-test and the post-test sessions, and the sixth was for the follow-up (held 6–8 months later). For the other three sessions, the trained participants attended the training program, while the active controls were involved in alternative activities. For both groups, all activities were completed within a 2-week time frame, with a fixed 2-day break between sessions. The duration of the sessions and the amount of interaction with the experimenter were much the same for the two groups.

The three sessions of WM training (sessions 2-3-4) lasted about 30–40 min. Participants were presented with lists of words audio-recorded and organized in the same way as for the CWMS task, and asked to recall target words, and to tap with their hand on the table when they heard an animal noun. The maintenance demand of the CWMS task was manipulated by increasing the number of words that successful participants were asked to recall, and by presenting the lowest memory load to participants who were unsuccessful (session 2). The demands of the task also varied and, depending on the session, they could involve having to recall: (i) the last or first word in each list; (ii) words preceded by a beep sound. The processing demand (tapping on the table when an animal noun occurred) was also manipulated by varying the frequency of the animal words in the lists (session 3). Participants in the active control group were asked to complete questionnaires on memory (session 1: Autobiographical Memory questionnaire; session 2: Memory Sensitivity questionnaire—De Beni et al., 2008), and on psychological well-being (De Beni et al., 2008; see Borella et al., 2010 for more details of the training program and the active control group's activities).

The procedure was completed in accordance with the Declaration of Helsinki (2008).

RESULTS

Linear Mixed Models

Linear mixed effects (LME) models were used to analyze the data because, unlike the more classical and frequently-used methods, they enable estimates to be adjusted for repeat sampling (when more than one observation arises from the same individual), and for sampling imbalance (when some individuals are sampled more than others), and because they allow for variation among individuals within the data (McElreath, 2016). Adopting the Bayesian approach when estimating parameters enabled us to exploit all the advantages of LME modeling, focus directly on the probability of an effect, given the observed data (posterior probability), and compute the evidence of our results.

Analytical Plan

For each of the eight measures of interest (i.e., the total number of words recalled in the CWMS, the total number of dots recalled in the Dot Matrix task, the total number of series correctly recalled in the Forward and in the Backward Span tasks, the total number of correctly answered items in the Cattell test, the total time taken to complete the task in the Pattern Comparison test, the interference index in the Stroop Color task, and the total number of intrusion errors in the CWMS), we tested several mixed effects models including all combinations of predictors, i.e., group (trained vs. control), age, education, vocabulary, baseline performance in the verbal WM task (the CWMS), and subjects as random effects. More precisely, we started from the null model (i.e., the model with no predictors), considering only the longitudinal effect (pre-test, post-test, follow-up) and subsequently introduced all the predictors and the interactions of all the predictors with the sessions.

For data analysis, we proceeded as follows:

(i) A first graphical inspection of the univariate and bivariate distributions of all the outcome variables considered, then their summarizing with descriptive statistics (see **Table 4**). This step was done to: (i) check the data distributions and identify any errors/anomalies (e.g., wrong label codes or potential outliers); and to (ii) ascertain which model to adopt for a better fit of our data and choose appropriate priors for the parameters.

(ii) Model fitting and parameter estimation: each model was fitted (separately for each measure of interest) using the Bayesian MCMC estimation method implemented in the STAN probabilistic programming language (Stan Development Team, 2015) with the R packages rstanarm (Gabry and Goodrich, 2016) and brms (Buerkner, 2016).

For the regression parameters (β) we used normal priors ($M = 0$ and $SD = 10$), and for standard deviation parameters we used half-Student t ($df = 3$, $M = 0$, $SD = 10$); convergences were assessed by examining the potential scale reduction factor (PSRF; Gelman and Rubin, 1992).

(iii) Comparison between the models (separately for each measure of interest) to identify the best one. We considered the Widely Applicable Information Criterion (WAIC; Watanabe, 2010), where lower values indicate a better fit, and the Akaike Weight, i.e., an estimate of the likelihood of a model making the best prediction on new data, conditional on the set of models considered (Burnham et al., 2011; McElreath, 2016).

(iv) Analysis of the best model using posterior distributions of parameters. Parameter estimates were summarized by using posterior means and 95% Credibility Intervals (CI; Kruschke, 2011).

TABLE 4 | Descriptive statistics for the outcome measures by group (trained vs. controls) and by assessment session (pre-test, post-test, follow-up).

	Trained group										Active control group										
	Pre-test				Post-test			Follow-up			Pre-test				Post-test			Follow-up		
	N	*M*	*SD*	Min–Max	*M*	*SD*	Min–Max	*M*	*SD*	Min–Max	*N*	*M*	*SD*	Min–Max	*M*	*SD*	Min–Max	*M*	*SD*	Min–Max
CWMS	73	10.23	3.82	4–19	14.68	3.32	6–20	14.05	3.34	6–20	75	10.04	4.30	3–20	10.41	4.18	3–20	10.17	4.20	1–19
Dot Matrix Task	38	5.13	2.18	1–10	7.45	2.84	2–12	5.47	2.02	2–11	38	4.92	2.54	1–12	5.16	2.26	1–12	5.00	2.63	0–10
Forward Span	56	6.21	1.75	2–11	7.18	1.64	3–11	6.46	1.53	3–13	56	6.04	1.63	3–11	5.84	1.45	2–9	5.82	1.40	3–10
Backward Span	56	5.43	1.61	2–10	6.45	1.72	3–10	5.66	1.45	3–11	56	5.02	1.67	2–10	4.84	1.39	2–8	5.12	1.28	2–8
Cattell Test	55	15.13	4.71	6–24	18.87	5.14	7–28	17.9	5.03	7–32	57	15.60	5.46	5–29	16.23	5.32	7–27	15.91	5.49	5–28
Pattern Comparison Test	56	155.15	50.53	59.43–270	127.12	35.67	56.50–229	135.98	33.54	70.12–251	56	165.48	45.87	66.28–261	162.64	46.49	67.40–289	161.28	46.85	59.32–267
Stroop Color index on RTs	38	0.92	0.45	0.08–2.35	0.86	0.44	0.13–1.83	0.94	0.37	0.28–2.03	38	0.95	0.50	0.20–1.89	0.95	0.39	0.40–2.01	0.87	0.47	−0.03 to 1.75
CWMS intrusions	73	1.95	1.88	0–8	1.14	1.65	0–7	0.97	1.28	0–7	75	1.77	2.15	0–8	1.59	1.73	0–8	1.84	2.09	0–9

CWMS, Categorization Working Memory Span Task; RTs, response times; CWMS intrusions, intrusion errors in the CWMS.

Data Inspection

Table 3 contains the descriptive statistics for each of the measures of interest by group (trained and control), and by assessment session (pre-test, post-test, and follow-up).

Model Fitting and Parameter Estimation

In all, 1,026 models, 58 for the CWMS, and 121 for each of the other measures of interest, were fitted. The fit indices of the 5 best models for each measure of interest are given in **Table 5**.

Model Comparison and Best Model Analysis

For each outcome measure we compared the fit indices of the 5 best models. Then, focusing on the best one (the one with the lowest WAIC), we proceeded with a graphical inspection of the Group (trained vs. control) X Session (pre-test vs. post-test vs. follow-up) interaction to assess the effectiveness of the training (see **Figure 1**).

To gain a better understanding of the extent of the benefits of training on the trained group's performance, the effect size was computed on the differences between the two groups (trained and control) at pre-test, post-test, and follow-up (see **Table 6**). In addition, to ascertain the dimension of the immediate (pre- vs. post-test) and long-term (pre-test vs. follow-up) gains obtained in the trained group, Cohen's d was computed using the following formula: {(Post-test or follow-up for the trained group − Pre-test for the trained group) − (Post-test or follow-up for the controls − Pre-test for the controls)}/(Pooled *SD* of the difference; see Weisz and Hawley, 2001). This enabled us to adjust the gains shown by the trained group in relation to the gain obtained by the active control group (see **Table 6**).

Then, for the trained group, we conducted a graphical inspection (separately for each session) of the values fitted for the significant effects of the best model (see **Figure 2**), supported by the evidence ratio for the hypothesis involving the *ß* coefficients considered (see **Table 7**).

The evidence ratio represents the evidence of the targeted hypothesis (e.g., $ß > 0$) with respect to the opposite hypothesis (e.g., $ß < 0$). If the evidence ratio equals 1, then the two hypotheses are equally plausible. An evidence ratio larger than 1 indicates that the target hypothesis is more plausible than the opposite one, and an evidence ratio of <1 means that the opposite hypothesis is more plausible than the targeted one. In the present study, the evidence ratio was used to assess the differences between the pre- and post-test slopes, and between the post-test and follow-up slopes.

Criterion Task

CWMS

For the CWMS we considered a total of 58 models[2]. The best model was the one with the Session X Group X Vocabulary interaction, with a probability of 59.1% (see **Table 5**).

Figure 1A shows the Group (trained vs. control) X Session (pre-test vs. post-test vs. follow-up) interaction from the best model: the trained group performed better at post-test than at pre-test, and maintained its better performance from post-test

[2]For the CWMS, the baseline performance in the CWMS was not entered as a predictor because of multicollinearity problems.

TABLE 5 | Fit indices of the five best models for each variable of interest.

Measure of interest		Model	Formula	WAIC	δ_{WAIC}	weight
CWMS	1	M236	ss × group × vocab	1912.49	0.00	0.59
	2	M313	ss × age + ss × group + ss × vocab	1914.53	2.03	0.21
	3	M216	ss × group + ss × vocab	1916.38	3.88	0.08
	4	M333	ss × age × group × vocab	1917.19	4.69	0.05
	5	M311	ss × age + ss × educ + ss × group	1920.38	7.89	0.01
Dot Matrix task	1	M336	ss × age × group × vocab	879.12	0.00	0.84
	2	M316	ss × age + ss × group + ss × vocab	884.74	5.62	0.05
	3	M233	ss × age × group	885.14	6.02	0.04
	4	M413	ss × age + ss × CWMS baseline + ss × group + ss × vocab	886.33	7.21	0.02
	5	M213	ss × age + ss × group	887.01	7.89	0.01
Forward Span task	1	M340	ss × educ × group × vocab	985.33	0.00	0.27
	2	M339	ss × CWMS baseline × group × vocab	985.63	0.29	0.23
	3	M336	ss × age × group × vocab	986.19	0.85	0.17
	4	M220	ss × group + ss × vocab	988.06	2.72	0.06
	5	M316	ss × age + ss × group + ss × vocab	988.13	2.79	0.06
Backward Span task	1	M334	ss × age × educ × group	1023.03	0.00	0.48
	2	M531	ss × age × educ × vocab × group × CWMS baseline	1024.05	1.01	0.29
	3	M336	ss × age × group × vocab	1025.06	2.02	0.17
	4	M431	ss × age × CWMS baseline × educ × group	1028.94	5.90	0.02
	5	M433	ss × age × CWMS baseline × group × vocab	1029.49	6.45	0.01
Cattell Test	1	M332	ss × age × CWMS baseline × group	1747.97	0.00	0.43
	2	M233	ss × age × group	1749.88	1.90	0.16
	3	M334	ss × age × educ × group	1750.31	2.33	0.13
	4	M434	ss × age × educ × group × vocab	1751.08	3.10	0.09
	5	M314	ss × age + ss × educ + ss × group	1751.45	3.47	0.07
Pattern Comp. Task	1	M339	ss × CWMS baseline × group × vocab	3132.28	0.00	0.38
	2	M233	ss × age × group	3133.55	1.26	0.20
	3	M114	ss × group	3135.60	3.31	0.07
	4	M433	ss × age × CWMS baseline × group × vocab	3135.65	3.36	0.07
	5	M332	ss × age × CWMS baseline × group	3136.00	3.71	0.05
Stroop color index on RTs	1	M233	ss × age × group	174.18	0.00	0.22
	2	M020	Age	176.69	2.51	0.06
	3	M111	ss × age	176.89	2.71	0.05
	4	M060	CWMS baseline	177.35	3.17	0.04
	5	M000	(1 | subject)	177.37	3.18	0.04
CWMS intrusions	1	M332	ss × age × CWMS baseline × group	1481.79	0.00	0.93
	2	M431	ss × age × CWMS baseline × educ × group	1487.59	5.79	0.05
	3	M337	ss × CWMS baseline × educ × group	1491.27	9.48	0.01
	4	M433	ss × age × CWMS baseline × group × vocab	1492.32	10.53	0.00
	5	M531	ss × age × educ × vocab × group × CWMS baseline	1493.49	11.70	0.00

CWMS, Categorization Working Memory Span Task; ss, session; vocab, vocabulary; educ, education; CWMS baseline, baseline performance level; in the Categorization Working Memory Span Task; CWMS intrusions, intrusion errors in the CWMS; WAIC, Widely Applicable Information Criterion (lower values indicate better fit; Watanabe, 2010); δ_{WAIC}, Widely Applicable Information Criterion difference between the best model and the others; weigth, Akaike Weight, i.e., an estimate of the probability that the model will make the best prediction on new data conditional on the set of models considered (Burnham et al., 2011; McElreath, 2016).

to follow-up. The effect sizes for group differences were large at both post-test and follow-up (see **Table 6**). No differences were found for the active control group. The trained group outperformed the control group at post-test and follow-up (see **Figure 1A**). The net effect size index for the trained group, adjusted on the control group's performance, was large for

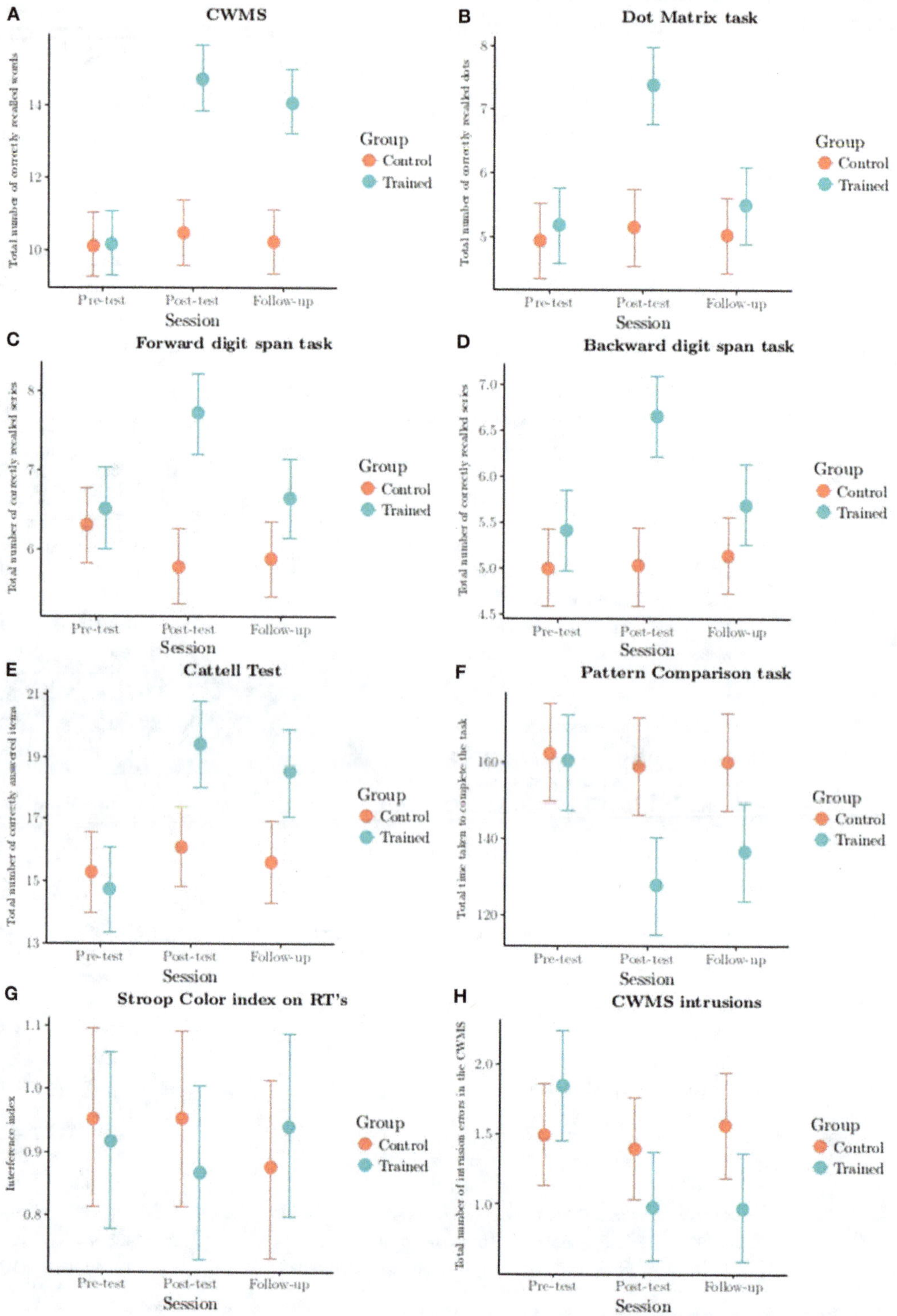

FIGURE 1 | Group (trained vs. control) X Session (pre-test vs. post-test vs. follow-up) interaction from the best model for each measure of interest. Categorization Working Memory Span task **(A)**, Dot Matrix task **(B)**, Forward **(C)** and Backward **(D)** digit span tasks, Cattell test **(E)**, Pattern Comparison task **(F)**, Stroop Color task **(G)** and intrusion errors in the Categorization Working Memory Span task **(H)**. CWMS, Categorization Working Memory Span Task; CWMS intrusions, intrusion errors in the Categorization Working Memory Span Task; RTs, Response Times. Segments represent the 95% credibility intervals.

TABLE 6 | Effect sizes.

	d of Cohen			Net effect sizes	
	Trained group—Active control group			Trained group vs. Active control group	
	Pre-test	Post-test	Follow-up	Short-term gains*	Long-term gains**
CWMS	0.05	1.13	1.02	1.48	1.54
Dot Matrix Task	0.09	0.89	0.20	0.95	0.16
Forward Digit Span	0.10	0.87	0.43	0.91	0.39
Backward Digit Span	0.25	1.03	0.39	0.80	0.10
Cattell Test	−0.09	0.50	0.39	0.67	0.78
Pattern Comparison Test	−0.21	−0.86	−0.62	−0.72	−0.47
Stroop Color index on RTs	−0.07	−0.22	0.15	−0.12	0.23
CWMS intrusions	0.09	−0.27	−0.50	−0.36	−0.66

*Cohen's d of the difference between the trained and control groups at pre-test, post-test, and follow-up, for each measure of interest (first three columns); and net effect sizes computed immediately after the training (pre-test vs. post-test; short-term gains), then 6/8 months later (pre-test vs. follow-up; long-term gains) for all measures of interest (last two columns). CWMS, Categorization Working Memory Span Task; CWMS intrusions, intrusion errors in the CWMS; RTs, Response Times. *For short-term gains, the net effect size was computed with the formula {(Post-test for the training groups − Pre-test for the training groups) − (Post-test for the controls − Pre-test for the controls)}/(Pooled SD of the difference). **For the long-term gains, the net effect size was computed with the formula {(Follow-up for the training groups − Pre-test for the training groups) − (Follow-up for the controls − Pre-test for the controls)}/(Pooled SD of the difference).*

immediate gains (pre- vs. post-test) and for long-terms gains (see **Table 6**).

Figure 2A shows the fitted values from the best model for the trained group alone, as a function of vocabulary score at the three assessment sessions, with the relative estimated linear trend. The regression slope decreased from session 0 (pre-test) to session 1 (post-test), with an evidence ratio of 89.91 (see **Table 7**), and it became flat at follow-up, as shown by the evidence ratio (see **Table 7**). These results indicate that participants with low vocabulary scores were the ones who showed an improvement in performance in the criterion WM task from pre-test to post-test, and maintained this gain at follow-up.

Nearest Transfer Effects

Visuo-Spatial Working Memory

Dot Matrix task

For the Dot Matrix task we considered a total of 121 models. The best model was given by the Session X Age X Group X Vocabulary interaction with a probability of 84.7%. This model was about 17 times more evident than the next one, which achieved a probability of around 5.1% (see **Table 5**).

As for the Group (trained vs. control) X Session (pre-test vs. post-test vs. follow-up) interaction, the two groups did not differ at pre-test. The trained group performed better at post-test than at pre-test, but this gain was not maintained at follow-up, when performance was not as good as at post-test (see **Figure 1B**). Effect sizes for group differences were large at post-test and became small at follow-up (see **Table 6**). No differences were found for the control group. The trained group only outperformed the control group at post-test (see **Figure 1B**). The net effect size for the trained group, adjusted on the control group's performance, was large for the immediate gains (pre- vs. post-test), but became small for the long-terms gains (see **Table 6**).

Figure 2B shows the values fitted from the best model for the trained group alone, as a function of age, and of vocabulary score at the three assessment sessions, with the corresponding estimated linear trend. For age, the regression slope suggests a change—with an evidence ratio of 32.06 (see **Table 7**)—from session 0 (pre-test) to session 1 (post test), and a slight deterioration from post-test to follow-up (evidence ratio of 7.05; see **Table 7**): it was the younger participants whose performance improved from pre-test to post-test, and then dropped back at follow-up to much the same as their pre-test performance.

As for vocabulary, the regression slope rose from session 0 (pre-test) to session 1 (post-test), with an evidence ratio of 5.02 (see **Table 7**), and clearly dropped again, becoming flat at follow up (see evidence ratio): it was the participants with high vocabulary scores whose performance improved in terms of the number of dots correctly recalled from pre-test to post-test, but not at follow-up when their performance clearly deteriorated.

Near Transfer Effects

Short-Term Memory

Forward Digit Span task

A total of 121 models, one of which did not converge, were considered for the Forward Digit Span task. The best model was represented by the Session X Education X Group X Vocabulary interaction with a probability of 27.3%. This model did not seem much more evident than the next two, for which the probability was around 23.5 and 17.7%, respectively (see **Table 4**).

As for the Group (trained vs. control) X Session (pre-test vs. post-test vs. follow-up) interaction, the two groups did not differ at pre-test. The trained group performed better at post-test than at pre-test, but this gain was not maintained at follow-up, when performance was worse than at post-test (see **Figure 1C**). The effect sizes for group differences were large at post-test and became small at follow-up (see **Table 6**). No differences were seen

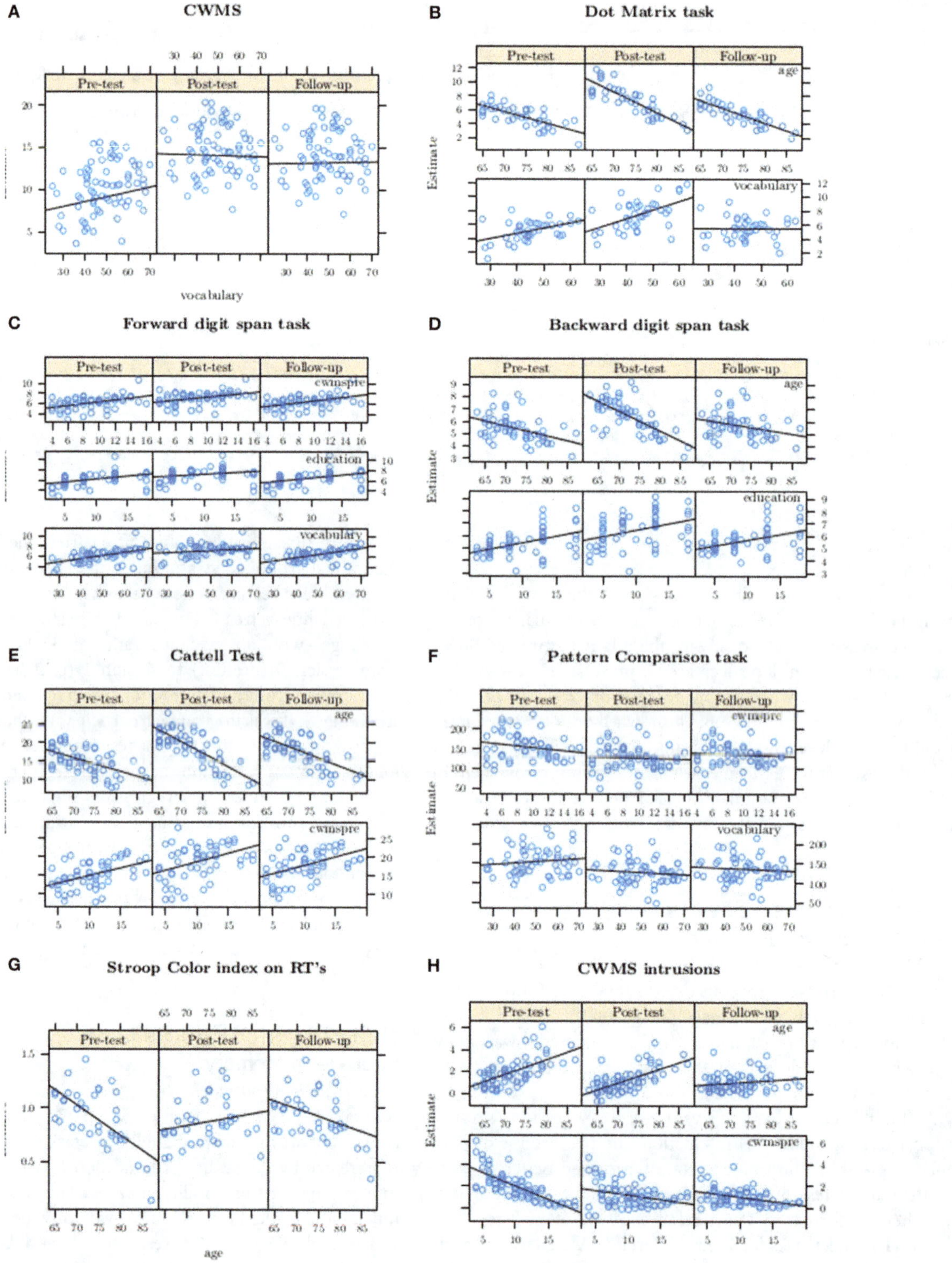

FIGURE 2 | Fitted values from the best model for the trained group alone for each variable of interest. Categorization Working Memory Span task **(A)**, Dot Matrix task **(B)**, Forward **(C)** and Backward **(D)** digit span tasks, Cattell test **(E)**, Pattern Comparison task **(F)**, Stroop Color task **(G)** and intrusion errors in the Categorization Working Memory Span task **(H)**. CWMS, Categorization Working Memory Span Task; CWMS intrusions, intrusion errors in the Categorization Working Memory Span Task; RTs, Response Times; cwmspre, CWMS baseline performance level.

TABLE 7 | Evidence ratio of the differences between pre- and post-test slopes, and between post-test and follow-up slopes, for each variable of interest, by fit index.

Measure of interest	Fitted value	Targeted hypothesis	Alternative hypothesis	Estimate	Estimate error	Evidence ratio
CWMS	Vocabulary	$\beta_0 > \beta_1$	$\beta_0 < \beta_1$	0.08	0.04	89.91
		$\beta_1 < \beta_2$	$\beta_1 > \beta_2$	−0.02	0.04	2.86
Dot Matrix task	Age	$\beta_0 > \beta_1$	$\beta_0 < \beta_1$	0.13	0.07	32.06
		$\beta_1 < \beta_2$	$\beta_1 > \beta_2$	−0.08	0.07	7.05
	Vocabulary	$\beta_0 < \beta_1$	$\beta_0 > \beta_1$	−0.04	0.05	5.02
		$\beta_1 > \beta_2$	$\beta_1 < \beta_2$	0.12	0.05	306.69
Forward Span task	Education	$\beta_0 > \beta_1$	$\beta_0 < \beta_1$	0.05	0.04	7.39
		$\beta_1 < \beta_2$	$\beta_1 > \beta_2$	−0.05	0.04	8.83
	Vocabulary	$\beta_0 > \beta_1$	$\beta_0 < \beta_1$	0.04	0.02	199
		$\beta_1 < \beta_2$	$\beta_1 > \beta_2$	−0.04	0.02	199
	CWMS baseline	$\beta_0 > \beta_1$	$\beta_0 < \beta_1$	−0.02	0.06	0.63
		$\beta_1 > \beta_2$	$\beta_1 < \beta_2$	−0.02	0.06	0.67
Backward Span task	Education	$\beta_0 > \beta_1$	$\beta_0 < \beta_1$	0.00	0.05	0.97
		$\beta_1 < \beta_2$	$\beta_1 > \beta_2$	0.01	0.05	0.67
	Age	$\beta_0 > \beta_1$	$\beta_0 < \beta_1$	0.08	0.04	77.43
		$\beta_1 < \beta_2$	$\beta_1 > \beta_2$	−0.11	0.03	665.67
Cattell Test	Age	$\beta_0 > \beta_1$	$\beta_0 < \beta_1$	0.28	0.10	433.44
		$\beta_1 < \beta_2$	$\beta_1 > \beta_2$	−0.18	0.09	41.11
	CWMS baseline	$\beta_0 > \beta_1$	$\beta_0 < \beta_1$	−0.04	0.14	0.61
		$\beta_1 < \beta_2$	$\beta_1 > \beta_2$	0.00	0.15	0.99
Pattern Comparison Task	Vocabulary	$\beta_0 > \beta_1$	$\beta_0 < \beta_1$	0.65	0.45	13.13
		$\beta_1 < \beta_2$	$\beta_1 > \beta_2$	−0.07	0.45	1.25
	CWMS baseline	$\beta_0 < \beta_1$	$\beta_0 > \beta_1$	−1.63	1.58	5.77
		$\beta_1 > \beta_2$	$\beta_1 < \beta_2$	0.19	1.00	1.21
Stroop color index on RTs	Age	$\beta_0 < \beta_1$	$\beta_0 > \beta_1$	−0.04	0.01	665.67
		$\beta_1 > \beta_2$	$\beta_1 < \beta_2$	0.02	0.01	27.99
CWMS intrusions	Age	$\beta_0 > \beta_1$	$\beta_0 < \beta_1$	0.01	−0.05	1.49
		$\beta_1 > \beta_2$	$\beta_1 < \beta_2$	0.1	0.04	189.48
	CWMS baseline	$\beta_0 < \beta_1$	$\beta_0 > \beta_1$	−0.16	0.06	799
		$\beta_1 < \beta_2$	$\beta_1 > \beta_2$	0	0.06	1.14

CWMS, Categorization Working Memory Span Task; RTs, Response Times; CWMS intrusions, intrusion errors in the CWMS.

for the control group. The trained group only outperformed the control group at post-test (see **Figure 1C**). The net effect size for the trained group, adjusted on the control group's performance, was large for immediate gains (pre- vs. post-test), but became small for long-terms gains (see **Table 6**).

Figure 2C shows the values fitted from the best model for the trained group alone as a function of education, vocabulary, and pre-test performance in the WM criterion task, at the three assessment sessions, with the corresponding estimated linear trend. A minimal change from pre-test to post-test emerged for all the variables: the evidence ratio between session 0 (pre-test) and session 1 (post-test) was 7.39 for education, 199 for vocabulary, and 0.63 for pre-test performance in the WM criterion task (see **Table 7**). At follow-up, there was a change from post-test (see evidence ratio), with performance dropping back to pre-test levels. In particular, it was the participants who had a limited education, low vocabulary scores, and a poor pre-test performance in the WM criterion task who experienced a slight improvement in their performance, but only at post-test.

Backward digit span task

For the Backward Digit Span task we considered a total of 121 models, one of which did not converge. The best model emerged for the Session X Age X Education X Group interaction, with a probability of 48.3%. This model was about two times more evident than the next one, for which the probability was around 29% (see **Table 5**).

For the Group (trained vs. control) X Session (pre-test vs. post-test vs. follow-up) interaction, the two groups did not differ at pre-test. The trained group performed better at post-test than at pre-test, and then its performance deteriorated from post-test to follow-up (see **Figure 1D**). The effect sizes for group differences were large at post-test and became small at follow-up (see **Table 6**). No differences were identified in the control group. The trained group only outperformed the control group at post-test (see **Figure 1D**). The net effect size for the trained group, adjusted on the control group's performance, was large for immediate gains (pre- vs. post-test), but became small for long-terms gains (see **Table 6**).

Figure 2D shows the values fitted from the best model for the trained group alone as a function of education, and of age at the three assessment sessions, with the corresponding estimated linear trend. For education, there was no change in the slope. For age, the younger the participants, the greater the improvement in performance from pre-test to post-test, with an evidence ratio of 77.43 (see **Table 7**). From post-test to follow-up, there was a decline in the slope, with an evidence ratio of 665.67 (see **Table 7**), meaning that performance returned to the levels seen at pre-test.

Far Transfer Effects

Fluid Intelligence

Cattell test

For the Cattell test we considered a total of 121 models. The best model was obtained with the Session X Age X CWMS baseline X Group interaction, with a probability of 43.1%. This model was about three times more evident than the next, for which the probability was around 16.6% (see **Table 5**).

For the Group (trained vs. control) X Session (pre-test vs. post-test vs. follow-up) interaction, the two groups did not differ at pre-test. The trained group performed better at post-test than at pre-test, and then its performance declined from post-test to follow-up (see **Figure 1E**). The effect sizes for group differences were medium at post-test and became small at follow-up (see **Table 6**). No differences came to light for the control group. The trained group outperformed the control group at both post-test and follow-up (see **Figure 1E**). The net effect size for the trained group, adjusted on the control group's performance, was medium for both immediate gains (pre- vs. post-test) and long-term gains (see **Table 6**).

Figure 2E shows the values fitted from the best model for the trained group alone as a function of age, and of pre-test performance in the WM criterion task at the three assessment sessions, with the corresponding estimated linear trend. For age, it was the younger participants whose performance was better at post-test than at pre-test, with an evidence ratio of 443.44 (see **Table 7**), and they also maintained their better level of performance at follow-up, with an evidence ratio of 41.11 (see **Table 7**).

There was no differences in the slopes for pre-test performance in the WM criterion task, as confirmed by the evidence ratio. It is worth noting that there was a slightly higher variability in the Cattell test at post-test for participants with low scores for pre-test performance in the WM criterion task.

Processing Speed

Pattern Comparison task

We considered a total of 121 models for the Pattern Comparison task. The best model was the one with the Session X CWMS baseline X Group X Vocabulary interaction, reaching a probability of 38.5%. This model was about two times more evident than the next, which reached a probability of around 20.5% (see **Table 5**).

For the Group (trained vs. control) X Session (pre-test vs. post-test vs. follow-up) interaction, the two groups did not differ at pre-test. The trained group performed better (taking less time to complete the task) at post-test than at pre-test, and maintained this improvement from post-test to follow-up (see **Figure 1F**). The effect sizes for group differences were large at post-test and became medium at follow-up (see **Table 6**). No differences were found for the control group. The trained group outperformed the control group at post-test and, to a certain extent at, at follow-up too (see **Figure 1F**). The net effect size for the trained group, adjusted on the control group's performance, was medium for both immediate gains (pre- vs. post-test) and long-term gains (see **Table 6**).

Figure 2F shows the values fitted from the best model for the trained group alone, as a function of vocabulary, and pre-test performance in the WM criterion task at the three assessment sessions, with the corresponding estimated linear trend. There was a very weak effect for vocabulary—the evidence ratio was 13.13 (see **Table 7**)—and it was the participants who had a higher pre-test vocabulary score who improved in the processing speed measure from pre- to post-test. No differences were found in the slope when the WM criterion task at pre-test was considered; a high individual variability also emerged (see **Figure 2**).

Inhibition

Stroop color task

We considered a total of 121 models for the Stroop color index on response times (RTs). The best model coincided with the Session X Age X Group interaction, with a probability of 22%, which is rather low, though this model was about 4 times more evident than the next one, which reached a probability of around 6.3% (see **Table 5**). As shown in **Figure 1G**, no Group (trained vs. control) X Session (pre-test vs. post-test vs. follow-up) interaction was found. This is in line with the null effect size identified on the differences between the groups, both immediately after the training and at follow-up (see **Table 6**), and also on the effect size computed for the immediate and long-term training gains obtained by the trained group (see **Table 6**).

The best model was only examined for the trained group. **Figure 2G** shows the values fitted from the best model as a function of age at the three assessment sessions, with the corresponding estimated linear trend. The results suggest that younger participants were more sensitive to interference, and that it decreased from pre-test to post-test, with an evidence ratio of 665.67 (see **Table 7**), but then rose again to the pre-test level at follow-up.

CWMS intrusions

We considered a total of 121 models for the CWMS intrusion errors. The best model was the one with the Session X Age X CWMS baseline X Group interaction, with a probability of 93%. This model showed a higher evidence than the others, since the associated probability was 18 times higher than that of the next model (see **Table 5**).

The differences were not very large for the Group (trained vs. control) X Session (pre-test vs. post-test vs. follow-up) interaction. Performance seemed to deteriorate from pre-test to post-test in the trained group, but not in the control group, while the number of errors increased at follow-up (see **Figure 1H**). The effect sizes for group differences were small at post-test and became medium at follow-up (see **Table 6**), but the two groups did not differ. The net effect size for the trained group, adjusted on the control group's performance, was small for immediate gains (pre- vs. post-test), but became medium for long-term gains (see **Table 6**).

Figure 2H the values fitted from the best model for the trained group alone as a function of age, and of pre-test performance in the WM criterion task, at the three assessment sessions, with the corresponding estimated linear trend. The regression slope for age decreased from post-test to follow-up, but not from pre-test to post-test, as supported by the evidence ratio, indicating that it was the older individuals who made more mistakes at pre-test, and it was only at follow-up that they were likely to experience fewer intrusion errors. The regression slopes for baseline performance in the WM criterion task decreased from session 0 (pre-test) to session 1 (post-test), with an evidence ratio of 799 (see **Table 7**), and then became flat, as supported by the evidence ratio (see **Table 7**): all the participants with a poor WM performance made more mistakes, in terms of intrusion errors, at pre-test, and fewer mistakes at post-test, and this improvement was maintained at follow-up.

DISCUSSION AND CONCLUSIONS

Our aim in the present study was to delineate how certain individual characteristics contribute to explaining WM training gains and transfer effects. Despite the importance of individual characteristics in cognition, only three studies in the aging literature have considered this issue. Here, age, formal education, general cognitive ability (operationalized with the vocabulary score), and WM baseline performance level were considered as a predictor of the short- and long-term specific training gains and transfer effects of a verbal WM training in a sample of healthy older adults.

To elucidate this issue, an analysis was conducted using linear generalized mixed effects models on data from four previous studies on healthy older adults that adopted the verbal WM training program developed by Borella et al. (2010). Part of the interest of such an analysis lies in that—for the first time, to our knowledge at least—all the studies examined were based on the same procedure and the same assessment measures, and they all included a follow-up session. The Borella et al. (2010) training program seems to be the only WM procedure to have been applied repeatedly in older adults with consistent results across studies. It is worth adding that another advantage of the studies selected for the present analysis is the inclusion of an active control group, and parallel versions of the tasks were presented (as recommended, but rarely done, in the literature; Zinke et al., 2012). The effects identified therefore cannot be attributed to the influence of item-specific practice.

Overall, our findings confirmed the efficacy of the verbal WM training procedure proposed by Borella et al. (2010): the trained group showed specific gains, performing better in the criterion task than the active control group immediately after the training, and maintaining this benefit at follow-up. Positive effects of the WM training were also generally apparent in terms of transfer effects, in the short term at least (at post-test), since the trained group outperformed the active controls in all the near transfer measures considered. As for the far transfer measures, the trained group again outperformed the active controls in all tasks, but not in terms of the Stroop Color index on RTs or CWMS intrusion errors.

This pattern of results was confirmed by the generally large post-test effect sizes (over 0.80) computed on the differences between the trained and active control groups, with the exception of the reasoning task -the Cattell test- (medium effect sizes) and intrusion errors in the CWMS (small effect sizes). At follow-up, the differences remained large for the criterion task, but became medium in the processing speed task—the Pattern Comparison task—and for intrusion errors in the CWMS, and small in the other tasks (Forward Digit and Backward Digit Span tasks, Dot Matrix task, and Cattell test). There were no changes in the effect size of the Stroop Color index on RTs, which confirms the absence of an effect of the training—the fact that there were no group differences—between the trained and control groups. Also by considering the net effect size of the training activities on participants' performance, that is changes in the trained group across sessions—pre-test, post-test and follow-up—(see **Table 6**) after adjusting the value for any change in the control group, the training benefits were confirmed. It is consequently reasonable to say that the training produced some maintenance effects on the trained group's performance.

These overall findings are consistent with the previously-published results obtained with the same WM training program. Although the present training regimen is quite short (only three training sessions) near and far training gains were found, confirming that this WM training procedure is effective. As also suggested by the meta-analysis conducted by Karbach and Verhaeghen (2014), the length of a training does not seem a crucial factor in determining its efficacy: in fact, most of the WM training procedures for older adults failed to document any benefits although they were much longer than the one considered here (see Borella et al., 2017; see also **Table 1**). The adaptive regimen adopted may well have favored training gains by: (i) ensuring that the tasks were always challenging, cognitively demanding and novel, consequently inducing participants to adhere to the task; (ii) producing a change in participants' allocation of attentional resources because the training engages several processes (including encoding, retaining information, inhibiting no longer relevant information, managing two tasks simultaneously, shifting attention, and attentional control) for an efficient handling of the different demands of the tasks. On the other hand, the lack of any short-term transfer effects for the two inhibitory measures may mean that inhibitory mechanisms are less amenable to training (see Zavagnin and Riboldi, 2012). Some degree of caution is required in interpreting the findings obtained with the Stroop Color task because they were based on RTs, which are not a very reliable indicator (e.g., de Ribaupierre et al., 2003; see Ludwig et al., 2010; Borella et al., 2017), and the sample was reduced for this particular measure (see **Table 3**). It is also possible, as discussed below, that it would take longer to prompt any detectable change for the inhibitory measures, or some of them at least.

Concerning long-term effects of the training, there was evidence of the maintenance of the specific training gain (in the criterion WM task), in line with all the WM training studies in the aging literature. In the transfer tasks, the training gains were only maintained for the Cattell test and the Pattern Comparison task, as seen in other studies using the same training procedure: the advantage of the trained group over the controls lay in the range of a medium effect size (or near-medium for the Pattern Comparison task). Such a selective maintenance of the training gains may be attributable to the well-documented strong relationship between WM and (i) processing speed (measured with the Pattern Comparison task), and (ii) reasoning ability (for a comprehensive discussion see Borella et al., 2010).

Improving WM performance makes cognitive operations more efficient, thus fostering the ability to move among the basic information processes. The other tasks may call upon more task-specific processes and abilities instead, leading to only transient (immediate) transfer effects (for a discussion, see Borella et al., 2010). One of the inhibitory measures examined, intrusion errors in the CWMS, seems particularly intriguing in that it only showed a clear improvement (fewer intrusion errors in the criterion task) at follow-up. This may mean that it would take longer to see a benefit of the training for some measures (inhibitory mechanisms in the present case). This phenomenon (i.e., clear transfer effects only at follow-up) has been found in other training studies in aging too (e.g., Borella et al., 2017), and has been called the "sleeper" effect. Although its nature needs to be further investigated (see Jaeggi et al., 2014), it may indicate that certain abilities take longer to show a significant improvement in performance. Future studies should make an effort to examine this issue.

Such a result on the intrusion errors and not in the Stroop Color task (leaving aside the problems associated with measuring RTs and the reduced sample size) may even indicate that WM training is more beneficial for some inhibitory functions than for others. In fact, intrusion errors in the CWMS and the Stroop Color task do belong to two different inhibitory functions. CWMS intrusion errors—an internal measure of the WM task and therefore closely related thereto (see Robert et al., 2009)—represent the resistance to proactive interference function of inhibition, which helps attention to be focused on relevant items and simultaneously-presented irrelevant items to be ignored; the Stroop Color task measures the resistance to prepotent response function of inhibition, which blocks dominant and prepotent cognitive responses automatically activated by the stimulus presented (e.g., Borella et al., in press). Resistance to proactive interference is also considered the only inhibitory function related to the control of information coming from memory content (Friedman and Miyake, 2004).

In light of the present findings, the questions following are: 1. Do any individual characteristics have a part to play in these findings? Are the effects of training supported by magnification or compensation effects, or both? Of course, there could be several aspects, such as methodological issues, but also participants' individual characteristics, capable of explaining the training gains and supporting the results. Here, we particularly analyzed the role of certain demographic variables (age and educational level), cognitive abilities in WM (i.e., pre-test performance in the criterion task), and a vocabulary test score as an indicator of crystallized intelligence.

Our findings showed that the role of the individual characteristics considered depended on the type of measure examined, and the effect of these variables was very modest for some tasks. The most interesting aspect seems to be that the factors considered would support either a compensation or a magnification effect immediately after the training, depending on which measure was analyzed. In particular, irrespective of the near or far transfer effects, the more the tasks demanded active information processing (i.e., the Dot Matrix, Backward Digit Span and Pattern Comparison tasks, the Cattell test, and the Stroop Color task), the more the factors examined seemed to support a magnification effect (of variable robustness). In other words, participants who had a higher initial performance in the crystallized measure used here and/or were younger, were more likely to improve after the training. For more passive tasks, on the other hand (i.e., the Forward Digit Span task, which is a short-term memory task), our results supported a compensation effect: participants with lower baseline vocabulary scores, an older age, and a weaker WM performance benefited more from the training. A particular pattern emerged for the criterion task (i.e., the task similar to the one used in the training) and for a closely related measure (CWMS intrusion errors): although the criterion task is complex, participants with a lower performance in a task of crystallized intelligence, as assessed with the vocabulary test, gained more from the training than those with higher vocabulary scores. That vocabulary should have such a role suggests that knowledge can counteract age-related decline (e.g., Baltes, 1987). Further, the role of vocabulary in explaining specific training gains may also suggest that participants exhibiting transfer effects were those who acquired new knowledge, rather than a greater processing efficiency. A finely-graded analysis at individual level may be able to clarify this issue.

As for intrusion errors there was evidence of a compensation effect related to age and baseline WM performance, with older participants and those with a lower baseline WM performance improving the most. These results may mean that the exercises used in the training enabled individuals with a lower crystallized ability to adapt to the demands of the tasks, engage better-controlled processes, and make more efficient use of their resources. It is hardly surprising that such a pattern of results should emerge with a training task that involves an adaptive procedure, which may have enabled progress to be made during the training, leading to a better performance and fewer intrusion errors at post-test and its maintenance at follow-up. Similarly, participants with a low baseline WM performance also became better able to manage no longer relevant information (CWMS intrusion errors).

One way to interpret these results could be by referring to the supply-demand mismatch conceptualized by Lövdén et al. (2010). According to these authors, changes in cognitive performance are induced by a mismatch between available resources and task demands: to cope with this mismatch, individuals engage in activities that promote flexibility, and consequently also plasticity. This hypothesis enables us to predict how individual differences might affect the benefits gained from a training regimen, depending on a task's complexity. The compensation effect seen for the criterion task (which closely resembled the task used in the training) may be due to the fact that using an adaptive procedure while practicing with the training task favored the "right amount" of supply-demand mismatch (i.e., demands exceeding than the available capacity) for individuals with a weaker profile in terms of their general cognitive abilities to re-activate their potential, and thus benefit from the training in terms of a better performance in the criterion task. It might have been easier to support this interpretation if our training procedure had been designed to enable us to test how performance changed from one training session to the next. Such an analysis would also shed light on what happens to individuals with the opposite profile (good general cognitive abilities—high vocabulary scores in the present study), who would only experience the mismatch if the WM tasks used in the training were more difficult, so instead of benefiting in terms of performance in the trained task they would gain in terms of plasticity in the transfer tasks.

According to the mismatch concept, the magnification effect found for the more demanding transfer tasks may indicate that in participants with a higher profile, in terms of age (i.e., younger individuals), or crystallized intelligence (i.e., those with higher vocabulary scores) the training induced a supply-demand mismatch that gave an impetus to change, thus engendering a flexible behavior. In participants with a lower profile, on the other hand, the high demands of the tasks used in the training might prevent any supply-demand mismatch because these individuals might abandon any attempt or be unable to apply resources and processes suited to the task.

The mixed results emerging from the present analysis as concerns the role of individual characteristics in explaining the compensation or magnification effects are consistent with a report from Zinke et al. (2013): the authors found that participants with weaker transfer effects were older (magnification), and that those with smaller training gains had stronger transfer effects (compensation). The role of age and WM performance varied, however, depending on the transfer tasks considered. The role of the predictors was examined too, but the effect size was small for some of the transfer tasks, and this limits the value of the results obtained.

It has to be said that the results found in the present study were modest too, so some degree of caution is warranted in interpreting them. Further, such a pattern of findings was found at post-test and, except for the criterion task and the intrusion errors, the role of the predictors was not maintained at follow-up for the other measures. Such a result could be interpreted in two different ways: one stems from on the idea that, because of the training, the individual characteristics are no longer significant because something beyond them has been modified during the training, such as the way in which participants process information; the other simply attributes the result to the fact that the effects of the training were not maintained. It therefore seems important to analyze the influence of other individual characteristics on the effects of WM training. This has been done, for the first time, at least to our knowledge, in both the short and the long term; the other three studies that approached such an issue did not consider the role of the predictors in the long term.

Our findings also suggest that compensatory and magnification effects are not mutually exclusive in explaining training gains; they may both contribute to characterizing and explaining the outcome of training. It would therefore be important for future WM training studies in general (and in aging, in particular) to make the effort to examine the role of individual factors. We are aware that large samples are needed for such analyses, but it is only by trying to overcome such practical problems that research can advance and enable us to ascertain the real usefulness of intervention to promote an active aging.

A number of limitations of the present study have to be acknowledged. First, single measures were used to represent the constructs of interest, whereas using multiple indicators of the same process (e.g., Shipstead et al., 2010) in training studies would enable us to draw stronger conclusions. Second, we were unable to consider training gains *per-se*, i.e., the role of individual differences in improvements induced by training across the sessions, the rate of learning, in predicting the outcome of the training, because the particular procedure used did not allow for these aspects to be analyzed. Examining what progress a given individual makes, and how it relates to the effects of the training could shed further light on the value of the present training program (Zinke et al., 2013; Bürki et al., 2014). A third limitation lies in that we analyzed the role of a limited number of factors potentially influencing training gains. In future studies we plant to conduct a more complete assessment of general cognitive ability, and assessing them with tasks not used to test transfer effects (to avoid multi-collinearity problems). Since we acknowledge the exploratory nature of our results, we have discussed overall trends for the transfer tasks, rather than the influence of each of the specific predictors on each task. There are also other factors, of course, that may have influenced the training gains, and that have yet to be considered, such as metacognitive (motivational) variables, mood, and psychological well-being (e.g., von Bastian and Oberauer, 2014; Könen and Karbach, 2015). It might also be of interest to analyze the influence of genetics (such as dopamine availability) on training gains (von Bastian and Oberauer, 2014). Future studies should therefore strive to include a broad array of factors, with larger and more homogeneous samples (i.e., with same size) than the one used here, in an effort to delineate all the conditions capable of shaping the effects of WM training in older adults.

To conclude, the present study provides further evidence of the elderly gaining in cognitive flexibility and plasticity from a verbal WM training. It also highlights the importance of analyzing the factors influencing WM training gains in aging. Also, although we showed that older people's WM can be improved thanks to a plasticity that persists with aging, we found that the role of individual characteristics depended on the transfer measure examined. It is consequently important to ascertain "who" gains from the training, but also "who gains in which tasks," in order to be able to design the most effective WM training to suit an individual's cognitive profile. This study could thus be considered as one of the first promising steps toward clarifying the impact of individual characteristics on the short- and long-term efficacy of WM training.

AUTHOR CONTRIBUTIONS

EB designed the study, assisted in carrying out the analyses, and wrote the paper. EC wrote the paper and assisted in carrying out the analyses. MP carried out the statistical analyses. RD assisted in writing the paper. BC designed the study, assisted in carrying out the analyses, and wrote the paper.

REFERENCES

Baayen, R. H., Davidson, D. J., and Bates, D. M. (2008). Mixed-effects modeling with crossed random effects for subjects and items. *J. Mem. Lang.* 59, 390–412. doi: 10.1016/j.jml.2007.12.005

Baltes, P. B. (1987). Theoretical propositions of life-span developmental psychology: on the dynamics between growth and decline. *Dev. Psychol.* 23, 611–626. doi: 10.1037/0012-1649.23.5.611

Bissig, D., and Lustig, C. (2007). Training memory: who benefits from memory training? *Psychol. Sci.* 8, 720–726. doi: 10.1111/j.1467-9280.2007.01966.x

Bopp, K. L., and Verhaeghen, P. (2005). Aging and verbal memory span: a meta-analysis. *J. Gerontol. B Psychol. Sci. Soc. Sci.* 60, 223–233. doi: 10.1093/geronb/60.5.P223

Borella, E., Carretti, B., and De Beni, R. (2008). Working memory and inhibition across the adult life span. *Acta Psychol.* 128, 33–44. doi: 10.1016/j.actpsy.2007.09.008

Borella, E., Carretti, B., Cantarella, A., Riboldi, F., Zavagnin, M., and De Beni, R. (2014). Benefits of training visuospatial working memory in young-old and old-old. *Dev. Psychol.* 50, 714–727. doi: 10.1037/a0034293

Borella, E., Carretti, B., Cornoldi, C., and De Beni, R. (2007). Working memory, control of interference and everyday experience of thought interference: when age makes the difference. *Aging Clin. Exp. Res.* 19, 200–206. doi: 10.1007/BF03324690

Borella, E., Carretti, B., Mitolo, M., Zavagning, M., Caffarra, P., Mammarella, N., et al. (2017). Characterizing cognitive inhibitory deficits in mild cognitive impairment. *Psychiatry Res.* 251, 342–348. doi: 10.1016/j.psychres.2016.12.037

Borella, E., Carretti, B., Riboldi, F., and De Beni, R. (2010). Working memory training in older adults: of transfer and maintenance effects. *Psychol. Aging* 25, 767–778. doi: 10.1037/a0020683

Borella, E., Carretti, B., Sciore, R., Capotosto, E., Tacownat, L., Cornoldi, C., et al. (in press). Training working memory in older adults: is there an advantage when strategies are used? *Psychol. Aging.*

Borella, E., Carretti, B., Zanoni, G., Zavagnin, M., and De Beni, R. (2013). Working memory training in old age: an examination of transfer and maintenance effects. *Arch. Clin. Neuropsychol.* 28, 331–347. doi: 10.1093/arclin/act020

Borella, E., Delaloye, C., Lecerf, T., Renaud, O., and de Ribaupierre, A. (2009). Do age differences between young and older adults in inhibitory tasks depend on the degree of activation of information? *Eur. J. Cogn. Psychol.* 21, 445–472. doi: 10.1080/09541440802613997

Borella, E., Ghisletta, P., and de Ribaupierre, A. (2011). Age differences in text processing: the role of working memory, inhibition and processing speed. *J. Gerontol. B Psychol. Sci. Soc. Sci.* 66, 311–320. doi: 10.1093/geronb/gbr002

Brehmer, Y., Rieckmann, A., Bellander, M., Westerberg, H., Fischer, H., and Bäckman, L. (2011). Neural correlates of training-related working-memory gains in old age. *Neuroimage* 4, 1110–1120. doi: 10.1016/j.neuroimage.2011.06.079

Brehmer, Y., Westerberg, H., and Backman, L. (2012). Working-memory training in younger and older adults: training gains, transfer and maintenance. *Front. Hum. Neurosci.* 6:63. doi: 10.3389/fnhum.2012.00063

Buerkner, P.-C. (2016). *brms: Bayesian Regression Models using Stan. R Package Version 0.10.10.* Available online at: https://CRAN.R-project.org/package=brms

Bürki, C., Ludwig, C., Chicherio, C., and de Ribaupierre, A. (2014). Individual differences in cognitive plasticity: an investigation of training curves in younger and older adults. *Psychol. Res.* 78, 821–835. doi: 10.1007/s00426-014-0559-3

Burnham, K. P., Anderson, D. R., and Huyvaert, K. P. (2011). AIC model selection and multimodel inference in behavioral ecology: some background, observations, and comparisons. *Behav. Ecol. Sociobiol.* 65, 23–35. doi: 10.1007/s00265-010-1029-6

Buschkuehl, M., Jaeggi, S. M., Hutchison, S., Perrig-Chiello, P., Däpp, C., Müller, M., et al. (2008). Impact of working memory training on memory performance in old-old adults. *Psychol. Aging* 23, 743–753. doi: 10.1037/a0014342

Cantarella, A., Borella, E., Carretti, B., Kliegel, M., and de Beni, R. (2017). Benefits in tasks related to everyday life competences after a working memory training in older adults. *Int. J. Geriatr. Psychiatry.* 32, 86–93. doi: 10.1002/gps.4448

Carretti, B., Belacchi, C., and Cornoldi, C. (2010). Difficulties in working memory updating in individuals with intellectual disability. *J. Intellect. Disabil. Res.* 54, 337–345. doi: 10.1111/j.1365-2788.2010.01267.x

Carretti, B., Borella, E., Fostinelli, S., and Zavagnin, M. (2013a). Benefits of training working memory in amnestic mild cognitive impairment: specific and transfer effects. *Int. J. Geriatr. Psychiatry* 25, 617–626. doi: 10.1017/S1041610212002177

Carretti, B., Borella, E., Zavagnin, M., and De Beni, R. (2013b). Gains in language comprehension relating to working memory training in healthy older adults. *Int. J. Geriatr. Psychiatry* 28, 539–546. doi: 10.1002/gps.3859

Cattell, R. B., and Cattell, A. (1963). *Measuring Intelligence with the Culture Fair Tests.* Champaign, IL: Institute for Personality and Ability Testing.

Cornoldi, C. (2010). "Metacognition, intelligence, and academic performance," in *Metacognition, Strategy Use, and Instruction,* eds H. S. Waters and W. Schneider (New York, NY: Guilford Press), 257–277.

Cornoldi, C., and Vecchi, T. E. (2003). *Visuo-Spatial Working Memory and Individual Differences.* Hove: Psychology Press.

Crook, T., Bartus, R. T., Ferris, S. H., Whitehouse, P., Cohen, G. D., and Gershon, S. (1986). Age-associated memory impairment: proposed diagnostic criteria and measures of clinical change—report of a National Institute of Mental Health work group. *Dev. Neuropsychol.* 2, 261–276. doi: 10.1080/87565648609540348

Dahlin, E., Nyberg, L., Bäckman, L., and Stigsdotter Neely, A. (2008). Plasticity of executive functioning in young and older adults: immediate gains, transfer, and long-term maintenance. *Psychol. Aging* 23, 720–730. doi: 10.1037/a00114296

De Beni, R., Borella, E., Carretti, B., Marigo, C., and Nava, L. (2008). *BAC. Portfolio per la Valutazione del Benessere e delle Abilità Cognitive nell'età adulta e Avanzata [The Assessment of Well-being and Cognitive Abilities in Adulthood and Aging].* Firenze: Giunti, OS.

de Ribaupierre, A. (2001). "Working memory and attentional processes across the life span," in *Life Span Development of Human Memory,* eds P. Graf and N. Otha (Cambridge, MA: MIT Press), 59–80.

de Ribaupierre, A., and Lecerf, T. (2006). Relationships between working memory and intelligence from a developmental perspective: convergent evidence from a neo-Piagetian and a psychometric approach. *Eur. J. Cogn. Psychol.* 18, 109–137. doi: 10.1080/09541440500216127

de Ribaupierre, A., Borella, E., and Delaloye, C. (2003). "Inhibition et variabilite' individuelle: ge'ne' ralite' ou spe'cificite' des processus inhibiteurs [Inhibition and individual variability: generality or specificity of inhibitory processes]," in *Inhibition Neurale et Cognitive*, ed S. Moutier (Paris: Herme's), 103–124.

Ekstrom, R. B., French, J. W., Harman, H. H., and Dermen, D. (1976). *Manual for Kit of Factor-Referenced Cognitive Tests.* Princeton, NJ: Educational Testing Service.

Folstein, M., Folstein, S. E., and McHugh, P. R. (1975). "Mini-Mental State": a practical method for grading the cognitive state of patients for the clinician. *J. Psychiatr. Res.* 12, 189–198. doi: 10.1016/0022-3956(75)90026-6

Friedman, N. P., and Miyake, A. (2004). The relations among inhibition and interference control functions: a latent-variable analysis. *J. Exp. Psychol. Gen.* 133, 101–135. doi: 10.1037/0096-3445.133.1.101

Gabry, J., and Goodrich, B. (2016). *rstanarm: Bayesian Applied Regression Modeling via Stan. R Package Version 2.10.11.* Available online at: https://cran.rstudio.com/web/packages/rstanarm/

Gallina, P., Saugo, M., Antoniazzi, M., Fortuna, P., Toffanin, R., Maggi, S., et al. (2006). Validazione della scheda per la Valutazione Multidimensionale dell'Anziano (SVAMA) [Validation of the checklist for the assessment multidimensional of the elderly]. *Tendenze Nuove* 3, 229–264.

Gelman, A., and Rubin, D. B. (1992). Inference from iterative simulation using multiple sequences (with discussion). *Stat. Sci.* 7, 457–511. doi: 10.1214/ss/1177011136

Gueorguieva, R., and Krystal, J. H. (2004). Move over ANOVA: progress in analyzing repeated-measures data and its reflection in papers published in the archives of general psychiatry. *Arch. Gen. Psychiatr.* 61, 310–317. doi: 10.1001/archpsyc.61.3.310

Heinzel, S., Schulte, S., Onken, J., Duong, Q.-L., Riemer, T. G., Heinz, A., et al. (2014). Working memory training improvements and gains in non-trained cognitive tasks in young and older adults. *Neuropsychol. Dev. Cogn. B Aging Neuropsychol. Cogn.* 21, 146–173. doi: 10.1080/13825585.2013.790338

Hertzog, C., Kramer, A. F., Wilson, R. S., and Lindenberger, U. (2008). Enrichment effects on adult cognitive development. *Psychol. Sci. Public Interest* 9, 1–65. doi: 10.1111/j.1539-6053.2009.01034.x

Jaeggi, S. M., Buschkuehl, M., Shah, P., and Jonides, J. (2014). The role of individual differences in cognitive training and transfer. *Mem. Cogn.* 42, 464–480. doi: 10.3758/s13421-013-0364-z

Karbach, J., and Verhaeghen, P. (2014). Making working memory work: a meta-analysis of executive-control and working memory training in older adults. *Psychol. Sci.* 25, 2027–2037. doi: 10.1177/0956797614548725

Könen, T., and Karbach, J. (2015). The benefit of looking at intraindividual dynamics in cognitive training data. *Front. Psychol.* 6:615. doi: 10.3389/fpsyg.2015.00615

Kruschke, J. K. (2011). *Doing Bayesian Data Analysis.* Burlington, MA: Academic Press.

Li, S.-C., Schmiedeck, F., Huxhold, O., Röcke, C., Smith, J., and Lindenberger, U. (2008). Working memory plasticity in old age: practice gain, transfer, and maintenance. *Psychol. Aging* 23, 731–742. doi: 10.1037/a0014343

Lövdén, M., Bäckman, L., Lindenberger, U., Schaefer, S., and Schmiedek, F. (2010). A theoretical framework for the study of adult cognitive plasticity. *Psychol. Bull.* 136, 659–676. doi: 10.1037/a0020080

Lövdén, M., Brehmer, Y., Li, S.-C., and Lindenberger, U. (2012). Training-induced compensation versus magnification of individual differences in memory performance. *Front. Hum. Neurosci.* 6:141. doi: 10.3389/fnhum.2012.00141

Ludwig, C., Borella, E., Tettamanti, M., and de Ribaupierre, A. (2010). Adult age differences in the Stroop color test: a comparison between an item-by-item and a blocked version. *Arch. Gerontol. Geriat.* 51, 35–142. doi: 10.1016/j.archger.2009.09.040

Lustig, C., Shah, P., Seidler, R., and Reuter-Lorenz, P. A. (2009). Aging, training, and the brain: a review and future directions. *Neuropsychol. Rev.* 19, 504–522. doi: 10.1007/s11065-009-9119-9

Mammarella, I. C., Borella, E., Pastore, M., and Pazzaglia, F. (2013). The structure of visuospatial memory in adulthood. *Learn. Individ. Diff.* 25, 99–110. doi: 10.1016/j.lindif.2013.01.014

McElreath, R. (2016). *Statistical Rethinking: A Bayesian Course with Examples in R and Stan.* Boca Raton, FL: Chapman and Hall/CRC.

Miyake, A., Friedman, N. P., Rettinger, D. A., Shah, P., and Hegarty, M. (2001). How are visuospatial working memory, executive functioning, and spatial abilities related? A latent-variable analysis. *J. Exp. Psychol. Gen.* 130, 621–640. doi: 10.1037/0096-3445.130.4.621

Noack, H., Lövdén, M., Schmiedek, F., and Lindenberger, U. (2009). Cognitive plasticity in adulthood and old age: gauging the generality of cognitive intervention effects. *Restor. Neurol. Neurosci.* 27, 435–453. doi: 10.3233/RNN-2009-0496

Pazzaglia, F., De Beni, R., Meneghetti, C. (2007). The effects of verbal and spatial interference in the encoding and retrieval of spatial and non spatial texts. *Psychol. Res.* 71, 484–494. doi: 10.1007/s00426-006-0045-7

Richmond, L. L., Morrison, A. B., Chein, J. M., and Olson, I. R. (2011). Working memory training and transfer in older adults. *Psychol. Aging* 26, 813–822. doi: 10.1037/a0023631

Robert, C., Borella, E., Fagot, D., Lecerf, T., and De Ribaupierre, A. (2009). Working memory and inhibitory control across the life span: intrusion errors in the Reading Span Test. *Mem. Cog.* 37, 336–345. doi: 10.3758/MC.37.3.336

Salminem, T., Frensch, P., Storbach, T., and Schubert, T. (2015). Age-specific differences of dual n-back training. *Aging Neuropsychol. Cogn.* 23, 18–39. doi: 10.1080/13825585.2015.1031723

Salthouse, T. A., and Babcock, R. L. (1991). Decomposing adult age differences in working memory. *Dev. Psychol.* 27, 763–776. doi: 10.1037/0012-1649.27.5.763

Shipstead, Z., Redick, T., and Engle, R. (2010). Does working memory training generalize? *Psychol. Belg.* 50, 245–276. doi: 10.5334/pb-50-3-4-245

Staff, R. T., Murray, A. D., Deary, I. J., and Whalley, L. J. (2004). What provides cerebral reserve? *Brain* 127, 1191–1199. doi: 10.1093/brain/awh144

Stan Development Team (2015). *Stan Modeling Language User's Guide and Reference Manual. Version 2.10.10.* Available online at: http://mc-stan.org

Stepankova, H., Lukavsky, J., Buschkuehl, M., Kopecek, M., Ripova, D., and Jaeggi, S. M. (2014). The malleability of working memory and visuospatial skills: a randomized controlled study in older adults. *Dev. Psychol.* 50, 1049–1059. doi: 10.1037/a0034913

Stern, Y. (2002). What is cognitive reserve? Theory and research application of the reserve concept. *J. Int. Neuropsychol. Soc.* 8, 448–460. doi: 10.1017/S1355617702813248

Titz, C., and Karbach, J. (2014). Working memory and executive functions: effects of training on academic achievement. *Psychol. Res.* 78, 852–868. doi: 10.1007/s00426-013-0537-1

Trenerry, M. R., Crosson, B., De Boe, J., and Lever, W. R. (1989). *Stroop Neuropsychological Screening Test.* Lutz, FL: Psychological Assessment Resources.

Troyer, A. K., Leach, L., and Strauss, E. (2006). Aging and response inhibition: normative data for the Victoria Stroop test. *Aging Neuropsychol. Cogn.* 13, 20–35. doi: 10.1080/138255890968187

Van der Elst, W., Van Boxtel, M. P. J., Van Breukelen, G. J. P., and Jolles, J. (2006). The Stroop color–word test: influence of age, sex, and education, and normative data for a large sample across the adult age range. *Assessment* 13, 62–79. doi: 10.1177/1073191105283427

Verhaeghen, P., and Marcoen, A. (1996). On the mechanisms of plasticity in young and older adults after instruction in the method of loci: evidence for an amplification model. *Psychol. Aging* 11, 164–178. doi: 10.1037/0882-7974.11.1.164

von Bastian, C. C., and Oberauer, K. (2014). Effects and mechanisms of working memory training: a review. *Psychol. Res.* 6, 803–820. doi: 10.1007/s00426-013-0524-6

von Bastian, C. C., Langer, N., Jäncke, L., and Oberauer, K. (2013). Effects of working memory training in young and old adults. *Mem. Cogn.* 41, 611–624. doi: 10.3758/s13421-012-0280-7

Wainwright, P. E., Leatherdale, S. T., and Dubin, J. A. (2007). Advantages of mixed effects models over traditional ANOVA models in developmental studies: a worked example in a mouse model of fetal alcohol syndrome. *Dev. Psychobiol.* 49, 664–674. doi: 10.1002/dev.20245

Watanabe, S. (2010). Asymptotic equivalence of Bayes cross validation and widely applicable information criterion in singular learning theory. *J. Mach. Learn. Res.* 11, 3571–3594.

Wechsler, D. (1981). *Wechsler Adult Intelligence Scale—Revised (WAIS-R).* New York, NY: Psychological Corporation.

Weisz, J. R., and Hawley, K. M. (2001). *Procedural and Coding Manual for Identification of Evidence-Based Treatments.* Los Angeles, CA: University of California.

West, R. L., and Alain, C. (2000). Age-related decline in inhibitory control contributes to the increased Stroop effect observed in older adults. *Psychophysiology* 37, 179–189. doi: 10.1017/S0048577200981460

Xin, Z., Lai, Z. R., Li, F., and Maes, J. H. (2014). Near- and far-transfer effects of working memory updating training in elderly adults. *Appl. Cogn. Psychol.* 28, 403–408. doi: 10.1002/acp.3011

Zając-Lamparska, L., and Trempała, J. (2016). Effects of working memory and attentional control training and their transfer onto fluid intelligence in early and late adulthood. *Health Psychol. Rep.* 4, 41–53. doi: 10.5114/hpr.2016.56846

Zavagnin, M., and Riboldi, F. (2012). Training di potenziamento della memoria di lavoro e delle funzioni esecutive nella popolazione anziana: una rassegna. [Training of working memory and executive functions in elderly people: A review]. *Giornale Italiano di Psicologia* 4, 745–770. doi: 10.1421/73141

Zinke, K., Zeintl, M., Eschen, A., Herzog, C., and Kliegel, M. (2012). Potentials and limits of plasticity induced by working memory training in old-old age. *Gerontology* 58, 79–87. doi: 10.1159/000324240

Zinke, K., Zeintl, M., Rose, N. S., Putzmann, J., Pydde, A., and Kliegel, M. (2013). Working memory training and transfer in old age: effects of age, baseline performance and training gains. *Dev. Psychol.* 50, 304–315. doi: 10.1037/a0032982

9

Spatial Frequency Training Modulates Neural Face Processing: Learning Transfers from Low- to High-Level Visual Features

Judith C. Peters[1,2]*, *Carlijn van den Boomen*[3,4] and *Chantal Kemner*[3,4]

[1]Department of Cognitive Neuroscience, Faculty of Psychology and Neuroscience, Maastricht University, Maastricht, Netherlands, [2]Department of Neuroimaging and Neuromodeling, Netherlands Institute for Neuroscience, Institute of the Royal Netherlands Academy of Arts and Sciences (KNAW), Amsterdam, Netherlands, [3]Department of Experimental Psychology, Helmholtz Institute, Utrecht, Netherlands, [4]Department of Developmental Psychology, Utrecht University, Utrecht, Netherlands

Edited by:
Soledad Ballesteros,
National University of Distance
Education, Spain

Reviewed by:
Elvire Vaucher,
Université de Montréal, Canada
Joseph Allen Harris,
Otto von Guericke University
Magdeburg, Germany

***Correspondence:**
Judith C. Peters
j.peters@maastrichtuniversity.nl

Perception of visual stimuli improves with training, but improvements are specific for trained stimuli rendering the development of generic training programs challenging. It remains unknown to which extent training of low-level visual features transfers to high-level visual perception, and whether this is accompanied by neuroplastic changes. The current event-related potential (ERP) study showed that training-induced increased sensitivity to a low-level feature, namely low spatial frequency (LSF), alters neural processing of this feature in high level visual stimuli. Specifically, neural activity related to face processing (N170), was decreased for low (trained) but not high (untrained) SF content in faces following LSF training. These novel results suggest that: (1) SF discrimination learning transfers from simple stimuli to complex objects; and that (2) training the use of specific SF information affects neural processing of facial information. These findings may open up a new avenue to improve face recognition skills in individuals with atypical SF processing, such as in cataract or Autism Spectrum Disorder (ASD).

Keywords: ERP, face processing, spatial frequency, learning, neuroplasticity, ASD

INTRODUCTION

Perception of visual stimuli improves with training, but is in general highly specific for the trained stimulus set or feature. For example, learning to distinguish individuals in one set of face identities does not transfer to other face identities (e.g., Hancock et al., 2000), or across emotional expressions (Calder et al., 2000). This is generally also true for low-level features: training improves performance on a wide range of perceptual tasks (see Fine and Jacobs, 2002; Watanabe and Sasaki, 2015 for review) including discrimination of orientation (e.g., Schoups et al., 2001), texture (Karni and Sagi, 1991), coherent motion (Watanabe et al., 2001) and spatial frequency (SF; Fiorentini and Berardi, 1980), but does not transfer to other stimulus dimensions (Yu et al., 2004), stimuli (Fahle, 2004) or visual field locations (e.g., Karni and Sagi, 1991; Shiu and Pashler, 1992).

However, it remains unknown to what extent training-induced improved sensitivity of low-level visual features (such as spatial frequency (SF), the number of black-to-white transitions in an image) transfers to complex stimuli. Here, we study whether improved sensitivity to Low SF (LSF) content, achieved by learning to discriminate black-white stripes (gratings), affects neural LSF processing in faces. LSF information in faces contains the pivotal global information necessary for proficient holistic face processing (Goffaux et al., 2005; Peters et al., 2013). In adult face perception, information carried by different SF bands is combined following a coarse-to-fine sequence (Goffaux et al., 2011; see Ruiz-Soler and Beltran, 2006 for review). LSF conveys highly important coarse information (e.g., emotional expressions) that is first extracted, before more fine-grained High SF (HSF) information is examined for further facial cues (related to for example facial age; see LSF- and HSF-filtered faces in right panel of **Figure 1B**).

If training LSF sensitivity indeed enhances an optimized use of information in LSF content during face processing, such an approach may lead to new skill training development to improve (emotional) face recognition abilities. Such training could aid individuals with Autism Spectrum Disorder (ASD), who have a detrimental bias towards processing information conveyed by HSF over LSF ranges, resulting in hampered recognition of faces and emotional expressions (Deruelle et al., 2004, 2008; Vlamings et al., 2010). Although there are training programs available to improve face processing skills in children with ASD (Silver and Oakes, 2001; Tanaka et al., 2003), learning a particular set of faces does not transfer easily to other face identities, expressions or general context. Moreover, face learning is a slow process (Faja et al., 2008), compared to learning of low-level visual features such as SF (e.g., Fiorentini and Berardi, 1980; Huang et al., 2008). Finally, low-level feature learning effects are long-lasting, causing a neural reorganization in the visual system (Karni and Sagi, 1993; Schoups et al., 2001), essential to training programs aiming for long-term improvements in face perception skills.

The present study investigates whether such a learning transfer is feasible. To this end, we examined four unresolved questions related to SF training:

1. Do learning effects, established by training to discriminate simple stimuli, transfer to complex objects such as faces? Therefore, we trained subjects to discriminate small LSF differences between black-white stripes (gratings) and examined whether this improved LSF sensitivity for gratings affected face processing. The extent to which learning low-level features of simple stimuli transfers to high-level object processing is (to our knowledge) yet unknown. Nevertheless, we speculate that improvements in discrimination of LSF gratings will transfer to real-world objects such as faces.
2. Does increased SF sensitivity solely transfer to processing image information in the trained SF ranges, or also to other ranges? More specifically, will LSF training transfer to low-pass (LSF) but not high-pass (HSF) filtered faces? We investigated this question by comparing neural processing of LSF and HSF faces before and after SF training. Learning-induced improvements in SF discrimination between gratings are specific for the trained SF range (Fiorentini and Berardi, 1980; Huang et al., 2008). In the same vein, we expect that training-induced LSF sensitivity will only affect processing of face images containing the trained SF band. Thus, we assume exclusive training effects for LSF- but not for HSF-faces in the present study.
3. How is such training-induced modification of LSF processing in faces reflected at the neural level? To assess neural markers of LSF learning in face perception, we recorded event-related potentials (ERP) while subjects performed the same face perception tasks before and after 3 days of LSF discrimination training (**Figure 1A**). The most prominent ERP component indexing face processing is the N170, a negative peak occurring at occipito-temporal sites around 170 ms post stimulus onset (Eimer, 2000). The N170 is earlier and stronger for faces containing LSF compared to HSF content (Goffaux et al., 2005; Vlamings et al., 2009; Peters et al., 2013). The neural correlates of SF discrimination training are not investigated yet, which hinders a straightforward prediction of training-related N170 modulations. Nevertheless, we hypothesize that improvements in neural LSF processing will be guided by the same neural mechanisms that attain more efficient orientation processing: orientation learning paradigms show that improved orientation discrimination results from a narrowing of the tuning-curves of orientation-selective visual neurons (Yang and Maunsell, 2004). Such a steeper slope of the tuning curve increases the neuron's selectivity, resulting in a reduced number of responding neurons. Since ERPs reflect activity at the neural population level, narrowing of the tuning curves would hence lead to a lower ERP activity. Although exact mechanisms remain elusive, we assume that LSF discrimination learning induces a narrowing of tuning curves in SF-selective neurons, akin to the neural tuning observed in orientation learning. Therefore, we expect that neural tuning induced by LSF discrimination training will be reflected by reduced N170 responses during LSF processing in face images.
4. Is the effect of SF learning on face processing hemifield specific? Like other low-visual feature learning effects, SF improvements are specific for the trained visual field location (Fiorentini and Berardi, 1980; Huang et al., 2008). That is, even after prolonged training, SF discrimination accuracy is at pre-training level for gratings presented at untrained retinotopic locations, suggesting that learning takes places in early, retinotopically organized brain areas such as V1 (Karni and Sagi, 1993). To examine whether similar retinotopic specificities occur for training-induced alterations in face processing, LSF discrimination training was always performed in the left hemifield, whereas faces were presented in the left (trained) as well as right (untrained) hemifield. We assume that face processing is only modified for faces presented in the trained hemifield. Although we expect that the N170 is modified accordingly (i.e., only reduced N170 responses for LSF faces in the left hemifield), we would like to note that the N170 does not reflect hemifield location. That is, the N170 is generated in left and right face-selective higher-

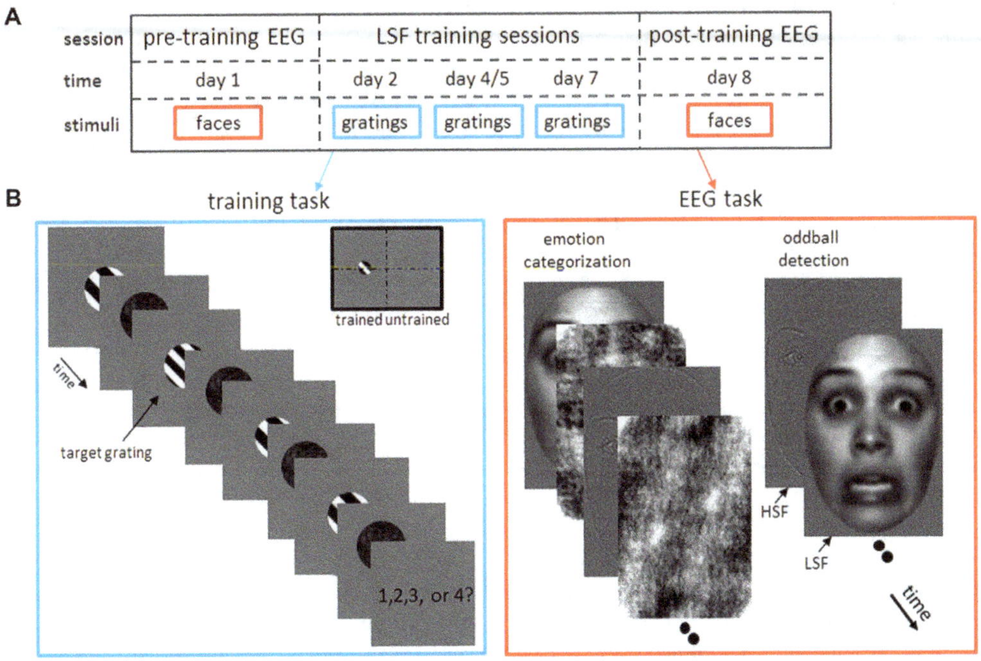

FIGURE 1 | Experimental design. (A) Timeline of the experimental protocol. After a pre-training ("baseline") electroencephalogram (EEG) measurement on day 1, subjects participated in behavioral sessions on day 2, 4 or 5 and 7 in which they trained low spatial frequency (LSF) discrimination on grating stimuli. Finally, a post-training EEG was acquired on day 8, while subject performed an emotion categorization and oddball detection task identical to the pre-training EEG measurements. **(B)** Tasks in the LSF training (left) and EEG (right) sessions. Left: LSF discrimination skills were trained by detecting the odd one out target grating which SF was increasingly similar to the reference gratings as performance improved (i.e., staircase tracking 84% accuracy). In this example trial, the grating with a different SF than the fixed SF (2 cpa) of the reference gratings, is the second grating in the row. Therefore, the correct answer is "2". In catch trials, where two target gratings were shown, participants pressed the spacebar (instead of the number corresponding to the position of the deviant grating). Gratings were always presented in the left hemifield, to allow comparisons between trained (left hemifield) and untrained (right hemifield) visual field locations. Right: in the EEG measurements, subjects performed an emotion categorization (left image series) and oddball detection (right) task on low-pass (LSF) and high-pass filtered (HSF) faces. Note that faces were presented at the same position as the gratings in the training task (trained hemifield) or at the mirror location in the opposite hemifield (untrained hemifield).

visual areas (Ghuman et al., 2014), regardless whether the faces is presented in the left or right hemifield. Therefore, the N170 might be influenced by neuroplastic changes in lower visual areas in both hemispheres, and moreover, both left- and right-hemispheric N170 activity might be affected by LSF training. The right hemispheric lateralization of face perception (Ojemann et al., 1992) might however make the training effects more pronounced for N170 responses in the right hemisphere.

In sum, we expect that LSF training will improve LSF sensitivity, leading to skilled processing of LSF (but not HSF) content in faces. At the neural level, this is reflected by a reduced N170 after training for LSF faces presented in the trained hemifield. Such a training-induced reduction is not expected for HSF faces, or LSF faces presented in the untrained hemifield. Overall, our findings confirm our expectations, suggesting the following answers to the questions raised above: (1) Improved LSF sensitivity acquired by learning to discriminate SF variations in simple stimuli (gratings) does transfer to complex objects such as faces. (2) This increased LSF sensitivity exclusively modifies processing of LSF and not HSF information in faces. (3) At the neural level, such training-induced modifications of LSF processing in faces are mirrored in reduced post-training N170 responses. (4) The observed N170 effect is specific for the trained retinotopic location (i.e., the N170 reduction only occurs for LSF faces presented in the trained hemifield).

MATERIALS AND METHODS

Participants

Twenty healthy adults (10 males; age 18–30) with normal or corrected-to-normal visual acuity participated in two ERP measurements and three (n = 13) or 4 (n = 7) psychophysical training sessions for financial compensation or as part of their Psychology curriculum. One participant did not complete the last session and the corresponding electroencephalogram (EEG) data were therefore excluded from further analyses. This study was carried out in accordance with the recommendations of the local ethics committee of the Faculty of Psychology and Neuroscience, Maastricht University with written informed consent from all subjects. All subjects gave written informed consent in accordance with the Declaration of Helsinki.

Experimental Procedure

Figure 1A illustrates the timeline of the experiment: on day 1, a baseline ERP measurement ("pre-training EEG") was performed, in which the subject performed an emotion categorization task and oddball detection task on HSF and LSF faces presented in the left or right hemifield (see **Figure 1B** and below). Subsequently, subjects participated in 25-min sessions on day 2, 4 and 7 in which they trained LSF discrimination on grating stimuli presented in the left visual field (**Figure 1B**). Eight participants received the second training on day 5 instead of day 4. The SF difference between the target and reference gratings was adapted to the participant's performance (staircase tracking 84% accuracy), resulting in improved LSF sensitivity as subjects learned to discriminate very fine varieties in LSF content. Finally, a second EEG measurement ("post-training EEG") was carried out on day 8, in which subject performed the same tasks as in the pre-training EEG session. Task order in the EEG sessions was counterbalanced across participants.

All subjects were individually tested. They were comfortably seated in a dimly lit room shielded by a Faraday cage and monitored by cameras. Subjects were reminded throughout the sessions to maintain fixation at the middle of the screen (and limit unnecessary movements and eyeblinks during EEG recordings). Stimuli were presented at a 21″ CRT screen, (1280 × 1024 × 32 screen resolution; refresh rate 75 Hz) using the Presentation software package (v. 12.1; Neurobehavioral Systems, San Francisco, CA, USA). Subjects viewed the stimuli at a distance of 106 cm, and viewing position was stabilized using a chin-rest.

Stimuli and Tasks

LSF Discrimination Training

Participants trained SF discrimination in a four Alternative Forced Choice task, in which they had to indicate which of the four sequentially presented gratings had a different SF (Fine and Jacobs, 2000; see left panel of **Figure 1B**). Each trial began with a 500 ms presentation of a fixation cross at the middle of a blank screen. Then, a sequence of four black-white, square-wave gratings (4.6° * 4.6° visual angle; 100% contrast) was presented at 4° eccentricity on the left horizontal meridian. Each grating had a random phase and was immediately followed by a randomly scrambled phase noise mask of the same size. Both stimuli were presented for 67 ms, followed by a 200 ms interval in which only the fixation-cross was present.

Importantly, three reference gratings had a SF of 2 cycles/degree of visual angle (cpa; reference SF), whereas the SF of the fourth grating (target grating) had a higher or lower SF (target SF), with higher or lower SF being randomly selected for each trial. This difference in SF varied across trials controlled by an adaptive staircase procedure targeting a discrimination accuracy of 84% (staircase step size 0.05% cpa; Wetherill and Levitt, 1965). The SF difference was 30% for the first trial of the first session. The starting levels for the subsequent sessions were determined based on the just noticeable difference (JND) achieved on the previous session (except for the first seven subjects who were tracked at 79, 84, 87 and 89% correct performance in session 1–4 respectively; this was corrected in the analyses by scaling obtained differences according to tracked performance). The presentation order of target and reference gratings was randomly selected for each trial. After presentation of the fourth grating and mask, a fixation cross was shown until participants responded (maximally for 1.5 s). Subjects were instructed to respond as fast and accurately as possible by pressing the keyboard keys "1" "2" "3" or "4" to indicate the target as the 1st, 2nd, 3rd or 4th grating, respectively. Participants received feedback on their response by brief (200 ms) coloring of the fixation cross (green for correct, red for incorrect or miss).

To improve task performance, we included 7% catch trials, in which two target and two reference gratings were presented. In this case, participants were required to press the spacebar. Catch trials were excluded from analyses and did not influence staircase accuracy. Note that at the beginning and throughout the session, subjects were instructed to maintain fixation at the fixation cross throughout the experiment. Training sessions lasted 25 min (400 trials) excluding self-paced breaks every 2 min.

EEG: Oddball Detection Task

We investigated the influence of SF training on neural processing of facial expressions using an oddball task. This orthogonal (i.e., unrelated to face perception) task ensured a continuous attention to the stimuli, yet enabled us to study face processing that occurs without any imposed task constraint that could bias facial perception. Sixty grayscale front-view photographs of Caucasian faces (50% male) with neutral (n = 30) or fearful (n = 30) expression, and four houses (odd-ball targets) served as stimuli. Face stimuli were selected from the NimStim Face Set (Tottenham et al., 2009) and subsequently trimmed to remove neck and hairline. Furthermore, all stimuli (5.4° * 3.8°) were equal in mean luminance and root mean square contrast and were presented on a homogeneous gray background of the same luminance. The SF content of each stimulus was unfiltered (broad-pass SF or BSF), or filtered with a high-pass (HSF; 6 cpa) or low-pass (LSF; 2 cpa) cut-off (see Peters et al., 2013 for details). Faces were presented at the same position as the gratings in the training task (trained hemifield) or at the mirror location in the opposite hemifield (untrained hemifield). Finally, 50 neutral faces (LSF or HSF filtered) with inverted (180° rotation) orientation were presented in each hemifield, in order to test effect of training on perception of inverted faces. All stimuli (50 trials per conditions) were in random order presented for 200 ms (Inter Stimulus Interval = 700–1100 ms) at the horizontal meridian at 4° eccentricity left or right of center. During the task, subjects were instructed to maintain fixation at the cross in the middle of the screen and press the spacebar as soon as a house was shown on the screen. Presentation of oddball trials (n = 32) was dispersed across the task (spacing between 11–19 stimuli). The inverted and fearful faces were presented (together with the neutral upright faces) in two separate, consecutive runs for three subjects, whereas all conditions were randomly presented in one run for all other subjects. The total task lasted about 20 min.

EEG: Emotion Categorization Task

The emotion categorization task employed the same stimuli as the oddball detection task, excluding inverted faces and houses. In this task, however, a scrambled version of one of the (randomly selected) face stimuli was presented immediately after the stimulus mask in order to keep stimulus processing time identical between conditions. For mask creation, phase of the face images was scrambled in the Fourier domain via random permutation, which preserves orientation content (Dakin et al., 2002). The face and mask were presented for 150 ms each, after which a fixation cross was shown 800 ms. Subjects were instructed to indicate as fast and accurately as possible whether the face had fearful or neutral emotional expression by pressing the "F" or "J", respectively. Half of the subjects applied the reversed button order. Subsequently, participants received feedback on their response by brief (200 ms) coloring of the fixation cross (green for correct, red for incorrect, and the word "faster" for a missing response), followed by a 300 ms fixation cross. Each face was presented twice in each condition (60 trials per condition), resulting in 720 trials per session in total (360 trials per hemifield). Stimulus onset markers were not recorded in the post-training session of one subject, which missing values in the ANOVA were therefore replaced with the condition mean. The total task lasted about 20 min, including five short, self-paced breaks.

EEG Recording

The EEG was recorded (sampling rate 500 Hz; band-pass filter of 0.01–200 Hz) from 35 AgCl scalp electrodes (extended International 10/20 system; Easycap, BrainProducts) with reference electrodes placed at the mastoids. Signals were collected using the left mastoid as reference and re-referenced off-line to the average activity of all electrodes. Horizontal and vertical electrooculograms (EOG) were recorded with bipolar electrodes placed at the external canthi and above and below the left eye. Electrode impedance was kept below 5 kOhm for all electrodes.

Data Analysis

Behavioral Data

Individual performance thresholds on SF discrimination were estimated for each training day. JNDs were computed as the geometric average of the last 14 reversal points in the staircase (Wetherill and Levitt, 1965). The first session JND of one subject with insufficient reversal points was replaced by group mean JND. Improvement of LSF sensitivity was assessed by contrasting normalized JNDs of the first and third session of all subjects with a paired *t*-tested.

Reaction times of the emotion categorization task were filtered (i.e., responses below 350 ms after stimulus onset and outliers 3 standard deviations below or above condition mean were excluded) before entering the data into a repeated-measures ANOVA with SF (LSF, HSF), emotion (fear, neutral), hemifield presentation (trained, untrained stimulus position) and time (pre-training, post-training) as within-subject factors. Finally, to assess task performance, we computed d-primes indexing changes in the sensitivity of fearful facial expression detection. D-primes (d') were subjected to repeated-measures ANOVA with SF (LSF, HSF), hemifield presentation (trained, untrained stimulus position) and time (pre-training, post-training) as within-subject factors. *Post hoc* paired *t*-tests were Bonferroni corrected.

EEG Analyses

EEG data were epoched (−200 to 900 ms, relative to stimulus onset), band-pass filtered (0.01–30 Hz; and 50 Hz Notch filter) and baseline corrected (200 ms pre-stimulus interval) using Vision Analyser (Brain Products GmbH., Munich, Germany). Artifacts from horizontal eye movements and blinks were reduced with the algorithm of Gratton et al. (1983). Trials with artifacts (i.e., samples exceeding ±75 μV, a change in voltage of 50 μV per ms, or a difference of 200 μV per 200 ms) were excluded from subsequent analyses.

For each subject-specific averaged EEG epoch of a condition, N170 peak latency and amplitude at maximal negative amplitude between 140 and 230 ms after stimulus onset were extracted for electrode PO7 (right) and PO8 (left hemisphere). In addition, mean N170 amplitudes were extracted to analyze the mean amplitude (178–182 ms) in the emotion categorization task and upward N170 slope (140–170 ms) in the oddball detection task. We opted to analyze mean amplitudes rather than subject- and condition-specific peak amplitudes to avoid averaging distortions by the trial-to-trial latency jitter in the emotion category task (e.g., Luck, 2014). Furthermore, the analysis of the upward slope was not planned *a priori*, but based on potential differences in the grand averages. Amplitudes and latencies were submitted to separate repeated-measures ANOVAs with SF (LSF, HSF), hemifield presentation (trained, untrained stimulus position) and time (pre-training, post-training) as within-subject factors. Note that we averaged across emotion (fear, neutral) for peak analyses to reduce the number of factors, since a first set of analyses did not show any interactions between emotion, SF and time. All ANOVA results were Greenhouse–Geisser corrected (but uncorrected degrees of freedom are reported) and were performed in SPSS 24 (SPSS INC, Chicago, IL, USA). Main effects and interactions that are not reported did not reach significance.

RESULTS

LSF Discrimination Training

Participants improved LSF sensitivity across training sessions, as indicated by a lower JND in the third compared to first training session ($t_{(18)} = 4.08$; $p = 0.0007$). **Figure 2** shows this gradual decrease in required SF difference across concatenated sessions.

On average, participants could detect more than twice as small differences between the SF of the target and reference gratings in the third (mean JND SF difference = 25.4%) compared to first

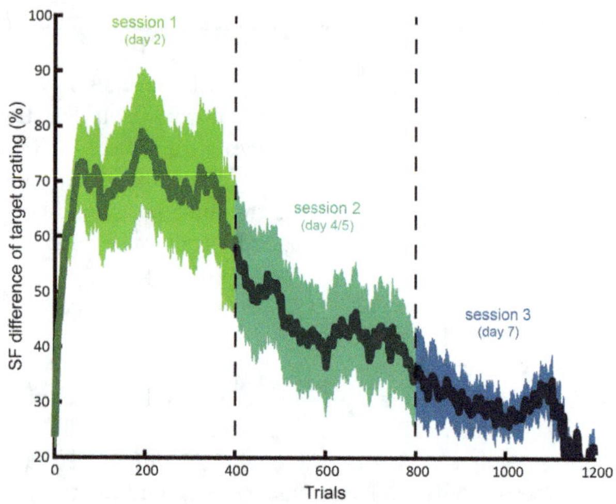

FIGURE 2 | Average learning curve for the LSF training. The difference between the SF of the target and reference (as percentage of the SF reference grating with 2 cpa SF) as a function of concatenated trials of session 1, 2 and 3. The shaded area indicates standard error of the mean.

(mean difference = 67.8%) session. The fourth session (n = 7) did not seem to result in further learning, as suggested by no further decrease of JND in the fourth compared to third session ($t_{(6)}$ = 0.88; $p > 0.4$).

Likewise, reaction times decreased from 674 (SE = 32) in the first to 576 (SE = 40) ms in the third session ($t_{(18)}$ = 2.31; p = 0.03). Furthermore, RTs in the third and fourth session did not differ ($t_{(6)}$ = 0.95; $p > 0.3$), suggesting that learning plateaued in the fourth session.

EEG: Oddball Detection Task

Task performance on the oddball task was excellent, with a mean accuracy of 96.8% (SE = 0.9). Accuracy did not differ between pre- and post-training ($t_{(18)}$ = 0.43; p = 0.8). One subject had only 80% accuracy in the post-training session and was therefore excluded from subsequent analyses for this task.

N170 peak latencies were faster in pre- compared to post-training ($F_{(1,17)}$ = 12.5, p = 0.003) for electrode PO7, whereas no main effects or interactions were present for peak latencies at PO8 (**Figure 3A**).

Analyses of N170 peak activity revealed an interaction between time and SF, which was significant for electrode PO7 ($F_{(1,17)}$ = 5.3, p = 0.03) and a tendency at PO8 ($F_{(1,17)}$ = 3.4, p = 0.08). *Post hoc* comparisons for PO7 did not survive Bonferroni correction. However, planned comparisons revealed the expected time*SF interaction per hemifield at electrode PO8: the N170 tended to be higher for LSF than HSF faces in the trained (left) hemifield before ($t_{(17)}$ = 2.1, p = 0.05) but not after ($p > 0.5$) training. Such an effect was not present for stimuli presented in the untrained (right) hemifield (p's > 0.1). Notably, this differential learning effect between LSF and HSF faces presented in the trained hemifield is already present in the upward slope of the N170 at PO8: mean activity was higher for LSF than HSF faces in the trained hemifield before ($t_{(17)}$ = 2.3, p = 0.03) but not after ($p > 0.3$) training. Such an effect was not present for stimuli presented in the untrained hemifield (p's > 0.2).

EEG: Emotion Categorization Task

Participants performed the task fast (632.9 ms; SE = 19.7 ms) and accurately (mean accuracy of 74.7%; SE = 2.6%; mean d' = 1.6; SE = 0.14). Reaction times revealed an interaction between emotional expression and SF ($F_{(1,18)}$ = 13.0, p = 0.02). The only *post hoc* comparison that survived Bonferroni correction revealed that LSF neutral faces were on average 16 ms faster recognized than HSF neutral faces ($t_{(18)}$ = 3.0; p = 0.08).

No main effects or interactions were observed for d': although the training-induced increase in sensitivity was twice as high for LSF compared to HSF faces (d' post- minus pre-training difference for LSF = 0.19 for HSF = 0.09), variance was too high to obtain significant differences.

As illustrated by **Figure 3B**, N170 peak latency at PO8 was shorter for LSF faces compared to HSF faces ($F_{(1,18)}$ = 4.6, p = 0.046). Furthermore, stimuli presented in the trained hemifield were faster processed than stimuli in the untrained hemifield ($F_{(1,18)}$ = 64.3, $p < 0.001$). However, SF, time and hemifield showed no interactions. In contrast, peak latencies at PO7 were faster for left (trained) compared to right hemifield ($F_{(1,18)}$ = 84.4, $p < 0.001$), but this effect did not interact with time, nor were any other effects observed.

For electrode PO8, mean activity in the N170 window was affected by hemifield ($F_{(1,18)}$ = 25.0, p = 0.0001), SF ($F_{(1,18)}$ = 17.1, p = 0.001) and interactions between hemifield and SF ($F_{(1,18)}$ = 5.6, p = 0.03), time, hemifield and SF ($F_{(1,18)}$ = 7.3, p = 0.015) and a tendency for an interaction between time and SF ($F_{(1,18)}$ = 4.1, p = 0.06). To interpret the two- and three-way interactions, we performed additional ANOVAs per hemifield with SF and time as factors. Results showed that ERPs elicited by stimuli presented in the untrained hemifield were affected by SF content of the face image ($F_{(1,18)}$ = 17.7, p = 0.01), but no effects of time. In contrast, stimulus presentation in the trained hemifield was influenced by an interaction between SF and time ($F_{(1,18)}$ = 10.8, p = 0.04): compared to pre-training, mean activity in the post-training was reduced for LSF faces ($t_{(18)}$ = 2.2; p = 0.045) but not for HSF faces ($t_{(18)}$ = 0.5; $p > 0.5$). In sum, results showed that LSF training reduced neural activity in the N170 window, but only for stimuli with *LSF content* presented in the *trained hemifield.* This selective influence of training is reflected in **Figure 3C** showing mean differential activity as a function of hemifield presentation and SF content.

For mean N170 activity at electrode PO7, we observed an interaction between hemifield and SF ($F_{(1,18)}$ = 9.7, p = 0.06). *Post hoc* tests revealed that activity in the untrained hemifield was smaller for LSF than HSF faces ($t_{(18)}$ = 3.7; p = 0.002), whereas activity did not differ in the trained hemifield ($t_{(18)}$ = 0.7; $p > 0.1$).

In sum, the N170 in the right hemisphere was reduced in the post-training compared to pre-training session. Notably, this

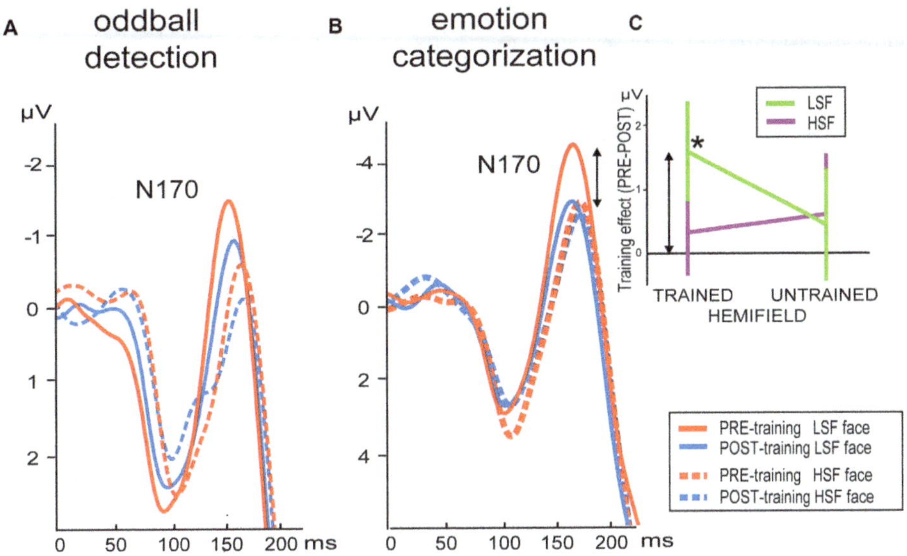

FIGURE 3 | Grand average waveforms of LSF and HSF faces presented in the trained hemifield in the pre- and post-training session elicited at electrode PO8 in the (A) oddball detection and **(B)** emotion categorization task. **(C)** Differential mean N170 activation between the pre- minus post-training per hemifield stimulation (*x*-axis) and SF content in the emotion categorization task (arrows indicate the correspondence between activity shown in **B,C**). Note that the training-induced difference (*) is only present for LSF faces presented in the trained hemifield. Error bars indicate standard error of the mean.

decreased processing was only observed for faces containing LSF information. Moreover, this learning effect was not only specific for trained SF, but also for trained location: the learning-related decrease in LSF processing was only present when faces were presented at the same location as the gratings in the LSF discrimination training sessions. In contrast, no differences between pre- and post-training ERP were observed for LSF faces presented in the untrained hemifield.

DISCUSSION

For fast and proficient face processing, facial cues conveyed by information in the LSF range are essential (Goffaux et al., 2005, 2011). Improving LSF processing might therefore increase face processing abilities. Our results showed that training-induced improvement in LSF discrimination of low-level stimuli indeed transfers to LSF processing in faces, which is accompanied by enduring changes at the neural level.

Participants learned to discriminate increasingly small SF variations in LSF gratings in a discrimination task. After only three training sessions (25 min., 400 trials), the JND between target and reference SF dropped from ~68% to ~25%, indicating a fast and strong increase in LSF sensitivity. Interestingly, this improvement in LSF perception was neurally reflected by a decrease in N170 amplitude. This reduction was exclusively observed for *LSF* faces in the *trained* hemifield in the post-training emotion categorization task. This is in line with psychophysical observations that SF learning is restricted to trained SF range and retinotoptic location (Fiorentini and Berardi, 1981). Similar learning-specific effects were also present in an oddball task, yet less pronounced. This discrepancy could result from several differences between the categorization and oddball detection task. Fast and accurate categorization of emotional expressions required more intensive processing than the passive perception in the oddball task, which could underlie the more pronounced expression of LSF training effects. That is, whereas LSF content is important for proficient, configural processing in general, it is known to play an even more pivotal role in assessing emotional expressions (Vlamings et al., 2009). Moreover, the categorization task put a high demand on attentional resources, since emotional expressions had to be correctly identified within 150 ms. This higher demand on attention resources might have contributed to lateralization towards the right hemisphere in the categorization task (Heilman and Van Den Abell, 1980), compared to the more distributed effects in the easy oddball task. Increased attentional processing might have also boosted neural face (LSF-) processing in the categorization task. The higher amplitude of the N170 in the categorization compared to the detection task (**Figure 3**), despite being elicited by identical face stimuli, corroborates the idea that attention differences might play a role in the observed task differences.

To our knowledge, there are only a few studies that investigated perceptual learning with EEG and none of them studied the transfer of learning effects to other stimulus categories. The majority of studies reported a decreased occipital N1 across sessions of training in line discrimination (Song et al., 2002; Qu et al., 2010). More complex results were observed in a visual texture segmentation task, showing that learning-related Visual Evoked Potential decreased for stimulus configurations where global and local orientations conflicted, but not for conflict-free configurations (Casco et al., 2004). Our reduced early neurophysiological activity is in agreement with previous findings using electrophysiology (Yang and Maunsell, 2004) and fMRI (Zhang et al., 2010) suggesting that learning narrows the tuning-curves of feature-selective visual neurons. A steeper slope of the tuning curve changes the neuron's discrimination threshold, resulting in a sparser response (i.e., reduced number of responding neurons) at the neural population level, culminating in reduced ERPs. Such a tuning mechanism is a likely candidate to explain the reduced LSF processing in face images, resulting from the improved LSF sensitivity induced by LSF discrimination training.

Peak latencies and amplitudes were differently affected. In line with previous results (Goffaux et al., 2005; Flevaris et al., 2008; Peters et al., 2013), we observed earlier N170 peaks for LSF compared to HSF faces. This effect cannot be driven by other low-level stimulus differences, as contrast and luminance were equalized between LSF and HSF faces. Rather, this effect indicates that facial information in LSF ranges is processed faster than those in HSF ranges. Neuroimaging studies in adults suggest that LSF content in faces is not only processed faster, but also processed via different neural pathways than HSF content (Vuilleumier et al., 2003; Rotshtein et al., 2007). That is, LSF information travels via the middle occipital gyrus to an area in the fusiform gyrus specialized in face processing (the so-called fusiform face area; Kanwisher et al., 1997), where it converges with HSF information coming from inferior occipital and temporal areas (Rotshtein et al., 2007). This differential processing might be a continuation from the distinct magno- and parvocellular pathways running from retina to early visual areas which are specialized for processing coarse and fine details respectively (e.g., De Valois et al., 1982; Hess, 2004). Peak latency was not influenced by LSF training, corroborating previous findings suggesting that learning-related adaptations are reflected in reduced visual activity rather than faster processing in visual cortex (Song et al., 2002; Casco et al., 2004).

In sum, our results show—to our knowledge for the first time—that training effects based on an orthogonal task using low-level stimuli, transfer to a higher-level object processing task. That is, the training employed a fundamentally different stimulus type (gratings) and task (LSF discrimination) than the experiment in which we observed the transfer effects (face images in an oddball detection and emotion categorization task). The present study only investigated face perception, but LSF training effects might transfer to other stimuli as well. Although adequate LSF processing is particularly important for holistic face perception, it might aid configural object processing in general. Similar to our face perception expertise, acquired expertise on other object classes appears to be guided by holistic processing (e.g., Richler et al., 2011) and proficient use of LSF information (Viggiano et al., 2006). Further research could investigate whether the current LSF learning paradigm may transfer to other object classes for which configural processing is important.

Interestingly, SF learning affected neural face processing after training was finished, suggesting that training effects caused a long-lasting neural reorganization. These findings can have important implications for treatment of atypical vision. Various conditions, such as ASD (Deruelle et al., 2004, 2008; Vlamings et al., 2010), pervasive developmental disorder (Boeschoten et al., 2007) and cataract (Ellemberg et al., 1999) are associated with deteriorated HSF and/or LSF processing. Our results suggest that the neural LSF and HSF processing pathways in such individuals can be optimized by SF discrimination training, resulting in improved processing of the SF ranges that convey the most important information (e.g., LSF content in faces). SF (and orientation) decomposition is a fundamental step in vision, affecting all further visual processing stages. Improving such a cardinal aspect of vision could constitute a highly generic training approach that might complement existing specific face training programs in promoting face processing skills in atypical development.

AUTHOR CONTRIBUTIONS

JP and CK conceived and designed the experiments. JP and CB: data acquisition and analyses. JP, CB and CK wrote the manuscript.

ACKNOWLEDGMENTS

We thank Joel Reithler for comments on the manuscript. This research was supported by an NWO-VICI (453-07-004) grant to CK.

REFERENCES

Boeschoten, M. A., Kenemans, J. L., van Engeland, H., and Kemner, C. (2007). Face processing in pervasive developmental disorder (PDD): the roles of expertise and spatial frequency. *J. Neural Transm. (Vienna)* 114, 1619–1629. doi: 10.1007/s00702-007-0780-y

Calder, A. J., Young, A. W., Keane, J., and Dean, M. (2000). Configural information in facial expression perception. *J. Exp. Psychol. Hum. Percept. Perform.* 26, 527–551. doi: 10.1037/0096-1523.26.2.527

Casco, C., Campana, G., Grieco, A., and Fuggetta, G. (2004). Perceptual learning modulates electrophysiological and psychophysical response to visual texture segmentation in humans. *Neurosci. Lett.* 371, 18–23. doi: 10.1016/j.neulet.2004.08.005

Dakin, S. C., Hess, R. F., Ledgeway, T., and Achtman, R. L. (2002). What causes nonmonotonic tuning of fMRI response to noisy images? *Curr. Biol.* 12, R476–R477; author reply R478. doi: 10.1016/s0960-9822(02)00960-0

Deruelle, C., Rondan, C., Gepner, B., and Tardif, C. (2004). Spatial frequency and face processing in children with Autism and asperger syndrome. *J. Autism Dev. Disord.* 34, 199–210. doi: 10.1023/b:jadd.0000022610.09668.4c

Deruelle, C., Rondan, C., Salle-Collemiche, X., Bastard-Rosset, D., and Da Fonséca, D. (2008). Attention to low-and high-spatial frequencies in categorizing facial identities, emotions and gender in children with autism. *Brain Cogn.* 66, 115–123. doi: 10.1016/j.bandc.2007.06.001

Eimer, M. (2000). The face-specific N170 component reflects late stages in the structural encoding of faces. *Neuroreport* 11, 2319–2324. doi: 10.1097/00001756-200007140-00050

Ellemberg, D., Lewis, T. L., Maurer, D., Lui, C. H., and Brent, H. P. (1999). Spatial and temporal vision in patients treated for bilateral congenital cataracts. *Vision Res.* 39, 3480–3489. doi: 10.1016/s0042-6989(99)00078-4

Fahle, M. (2004). Perceptual learning: a case for early selection. *J. Vis.* 4, 879–890. doi: 10.1167/4.10.4

Faja, S., Aylward, E., Bernier, R., and Dawson, G. (2008). Becoming a face expert: a computerized face-training program for high-functioning individuals with autism spectrum disorders. *Dev. Neuropsychol.* 33, 1–24. doi: 10.1080/87565640701729573

Fine, I., and Jacobs, R. A. (2000). Perceptual learning for a pattern discrimination task. *Vision Res.* 40, 3209–3230. doi: 10.1016/s0042-6989(00)00163-2

Fine, I., and Jacobs, R. A. (2002). Comparing perceptual learning across tasks: a review. *J. Vis.* 2, 190–203. doi: 10.1167/2.2.5

Fiorentini, A., and Berardi, N. (1980). Perceptual learning specific for orientation and spatial frequency. *Nature* 287, 43–44. doi: 10.1038/287043a0

Fiorentini, A., and Berardi, N. (1981). Learning in grating waveform discrimination: specificity for orientation and spatial frequency. *Vision Res.* 21, 1149–1158. doi: 10.1016/0042-6989(81)90017-1

Flevaris, A. V., Robertson, L. C., and Bentin, S. (2008). Using spatial frequency scales for processing face features and face configuration: an ERP analysis. *Brain Res.* 1194, 100–109. doi: 10.1016/j.brainres.2007.11.071

Ghuman, A. S., Brunet, N. M., Li, Y., Konecky, R. O., Pyles, J. A., Walls, S. A., et al. (2014). Dynamic encoding of face information in the human fusiform gyrus. *Nat. Commun.* 5:5672. doi: 10.1038/ncomms6672

Goffaux, V., Hault, B., Michel, C., Vuong, Q. C., and Rossion, B. (2005). The respective role of low and high spatial frequencies in supporting configural and featural processing of faces. *Perception* 34, 77–86. doi: 10.1068/p5370

Goffaux, V., Peters, J., Haubrechts, J., Schiltz, C., Jansma, B., and Goebel, R. (2011). From coarse to fine? Spatial and temporal dynamics of cortical face processing. *Cereb. Cortex* 21, 467–476. doi: 10.1093/cercor/bhQ92

Gratton, G., Coles, M. G. H., and Donchin, E. (1983). A new method for off-line removal of ocular artifact. *Electroencephalogr. Clin. Neurophysiol.* 55, 468–484. doi: 10.1016/0013-4694(83)90135-9

Hancock, P. J., Bruce, V. V., and Burton, A. M. (2000). Recognition of unfamiliar faces. *Trends Cogn. Sci.* 4, 330–337. doi: 10.1016/S1364-6613(00)01519-9

Heilman, K. M., and Van Den Abell, T. (1980). Right hemisphere dominance for attention: the mechanism underlying hemispheric asymmetries of inattention (neglect). *Neurology* 30, 327–330. doi: 10.1212/wnl.30.3.327

Hess, R. F. (2004). "Spatial scale in visual processing," in *The Visual Neurosciences*, eds L. M. Chalupa and J. S. Werner (Cambridge, MA: MIT Press), 1043–1059.

Huang, C. B., Zhou, Y., and Lu, Z. L. (2008). Broad bandwidth of perceptual learning in the visual system of adults with anisometropic amblyopia. *Proc. Natl. Acad. Sci. U S A* 105, 4068–4073. doi: 10.1073/pnas.0800824105

Kanwisher, N., McDermott, J., and Chun, M. M. (1997). The fusiform face area: a module in human extrastriate cortex specialized for face perception. *J. Neurosci.* 17, 4302–4311.

Karni, A., and Sagi, D. (1991). Where practice makes perfect in texture discrimination: evidence for primary visual cortex plasticity. *Proc. Natl. Acad. Sci. U S A* 88, 4966–4970. doi: 10.1073/pnas.88.11.4966

Karni, A., and Sagi, D. (1993). The time course of learning a visual skill. *Nature* 365, 250–252. doi: 10.1038/365250a0

Luck, S. J. (2014). *An Introduction to the Event-Related Potential Technique.* 2nd Edn. Cambridge, MA: The MIT Press.

Ojemann, J. G., Ojemann, G. A., and Lettich, E. (1992). Neuronal activity related to faces and matching in human right nondominant temporal cortex. *Brain* 115, 1–13. doi: 10.1093/brain/115.1.1

Peters, J. C., Vlamings, P., and Kemner, C. (2013). Neural processing of high and low spatial frequency information in faces changes across development: qualitative changes in face processing during adolescence. *Eur. J. Neurosci.* 37, 1448–1457. doi: 10.1111/ejn.12172

Qu, Z., Song, Y., and Ding, Y. (2010). ERP evidence for distinct mechanisms of fast and slow visual perceptual learning. *Neuropsychologia* 48, 1869–1874. doi: 10.1016/j.neuropsychologia.2010.01.008

Richler, J. J., Cheung, O. S., and Gauthier, I. (2011). Holistic processing predicts face recognition. *Psychol. Sci.* 22, 464–471. doi: 10.1177/0956797611401753

Rotshtein, P., Vuilleumier, P., Winston, J., Driver, J., and Dolan, R. (2007). Distinct and convergent visual processing of high and low spatial frequency information in faces. *Cereb. Cortex* 17, 2713–2724. doi: 10.1093/cercor/bhl180

Ruiz-Soler, M., and Beltran, F. S. (2006). Face perception: an integrative review of the role of spatial frequencies. *Psychol. Res.* 70, 273–292. doi: 10.1007/s00426-005-0215-z

Schoups, A., Vogels, R., Qian, N., and Orban, G. (2001). Practising orientation identification improves orientation coding in V1 neurons. *Nature* 412, 549–553. doi: 10.1038/35087601

Shiu, L. P., and Pashler, H. (1992). Improvement in line orientation discrimination is retinally local but dependent on cognitive set. *Percept. Psychophys.* 52, 582–588. doi: 10.3758/bf03206720

Silver, M., and Oakes, P. (2001). Evaluation of a new computer intervention to teach people with autism or Asperger syndrome to recognize and predict emotions in others. *Autism* 5, 299–316. doi: 10.1177/1362361301005003007

Song, Y., Ding, Y., Fan, S., and Chen, L. (2002). An event-related potential study on visual perceptual learning under short-term and long-term training conditions. *Neuroreport* 13, 2053–2057. doi: 10.1097/00001756-200211150-00013

Tanaka, J., Lincoln, S., and Hegg, L. (2003). "A framework for the study and treatment of face processing deficits in autism," in *The Development of Face Processing*, eds H. Leder and G. Swartzer (Berlin: Hogrefe Publishers), 101–119.

Tottenham, N., Tanaka, J., Leon, A. C., McCarry, T., Nurse, M., Hare, T. A., et al. (2009). The NimStim set of facial expressions: judgments from untrained research participants. *Psychiatry Res.* 168, 242–249. doi: 10.1016/j.psychres.2008.05.006

De Valois, R. L., Albrecht, D. G., and Thorell, L. G. (1982). Spatial frequency selectivity of cells in macaque visual cortex. *Vision Res.* 22, 545–559. doi: 10.1016/0042-6989(82)90113-4

Viggiano, M. P., Righi, S., and Galli, G. (2006). Category-specific visual recognition as affected by aging and expertise. *Arch. Gerontol. Geriatr.* 42, 329–338. doi: 10.1016/j.archger.2005.08.003

Vlamings, P.H.J.M., Goffaux, V., and Kemner, C. (2009). Is the early modulation of brain activity by fearful facial expressions primarily mediated by coarse low spatial frequency information? *J. Vis.* 9:12. doi: 10.1167/9.5.12

Vlamings, P. H. J. M., Jonkman, L. M., van Daalen, E., van der Gaag, R. J., and Kemner, C. (2010). Basic abnormalities in visual processing affect face processing at an early age in autism spectrum disorder. *Biol. Psychiatry* 68, 1107–1113. doi: 10.1016/j.biopsych.2010.06.024

Vuilleumier, P., Armony, J. L., Driver, J., and Dolan, R. J. (2003). Distinct spatial frequency sensitivities for processing faces and emotional expressions. *Nat. Neurosci.* 6, 624–631. doi: 10.1038/nn1057

Watanabe, T., Náñez, J. E., and Sasaki, Y. (2001). Perceptual learning without perception. *Nature* 413, 844–848. doi: 10.1038/35101601

Watanabe, T., and Sasaki, Y. (2015). Perceptual learning: toward a comprehensive theory. *Annu. Rev. Psychol.* 66, 197–221. doi: 10.1146/annurev-psych-010814-015214

Wetherill, G. B., and Levitt, H. (1965). Sequential estimation of points on a psychometric function. *Br. J. Math. Stat. Psychol.* 18, 1–10. doi: 10.1111/j.2044-8317.1965.tb00689.x

Yang, T., and Maunsell, J. H. (2004). The effect of perceptual learning on neuronal responses in monkey visual area V4. *J. Neurosci.* 24, 1617–1626. doi: 10.1523/JNEUROSCI.4442-03.2004

Yu, C., Klein, S. A., and Levi, D. M. (2004). Perceptual learning in contrast discrimination and the (minimal) role of context. *J. Vis.* 4, 169–182. doi: 10.1167/4.3.4

Zhang, J., Meeson, A., Welchman, A. E., and Kourtzi, Z. (2010). Learning alters the tuning of functional magnetic resonance imaging patterns for visual forms. *J. Neurosci.* 30, 14127–14133. doi: 10.1523/JNEUROSCI.2204-10.2010

10

Cognitive Training Sustainably Improves Executive Functioning in Middle-Aged Industry Workers Assessed by Task Switching: A Randomized Controlled ERP Study

Patrick D. Gajewski[1], Gabriele Freude[2] and Michael Falkenstein[1,3]*

[1] *Ageing Research Group, Leibniz Research Centre for Working Environment and Human Factors (IfADo), Technical University of Dortmund, Dortmund, Germany,* [2] *Federal Institute for Occupational Safety and Health, Berlin, Germany,* [3] *Institute for Working, Learning and Aging, Bochum, Germany*

Edited by:
Soledad Ballesteros, National University of Distance Education, Spain

Reviewed by:
Philip D. Zelazo, University of Minnesota, USA
Marco Calabria, Pompeu Fabra University, Spain

***Correspondence:**
Patrick D. Gajewski
gajewski@ifado.de

Recently, we reported results of a cross-sectional study investigating executive functions in dependence of aging and type of work. That study showed deficits in performance and electrophysiological activity in middle-aged workers with long-term repetitive and unchallenging work. Based on these findings, we conducted a longitudinal study that aimed at ameliorating these cognitive deficits by means of a trainer-guided cognitive training (CT) in 57 further middle-aged workers with repetitive type of work from the same factory. This study was designed as a randomized controlled trail with pre- (t1), post- (t2), and a 3-month follow-up (t3) measure. The waiting control group was trained between t2 and t3. The training lasted 3 months (20 sessions) and was evaluated with the same task switching paradigm used in the previous cross-sectional study. The CT improved performance in accuracy at the behavioral level and affected the electrophysiological correlates of retrieval of stimulus-response sets (P2), response selection (N2), and error detection (Ne), thus unveiling the neuronal background of the behavioral effects. The same training effects were observed in the waiting control group after CT at t3. Moreover, at t3, most of the behavioral and electrophysiological training-induced changes were found stable. Hence, CT appears to be an important intervention for compensating cognitive deficits in executive functions in middle-aged employees with cognitively unchallenging work.

Keywords: aging, work, cognitive training, task switching, ERPs, N2, Ne, ERN

INTRODUCTION

The continuous aging of the society leads to an increasing average age of the workforce and an increase in the pensionable age at least in the majority of western countries (Ilmarinen, 2006). In addition, the working demands have changed in recent years: while physical work and physical demands have diminished successively, mental work and psychological work demands have increased (see Hagger et al., 2010, for an overview). Also, there has been an increasing trend for highly specialized work which in turn implies a larger amount of repetitive work which is done under increasing time pressure and worry about job loss due to globalization and cost pressure

(Sparks et al., 2001; De Cuyper et al., 2008). This raises the problem whether and to which extent such modern working environments have a negative (or positive) impact on cognitive skills, and particularly so in older employees. Even more important is the issue of potential interventions that may ameliorate cognitive changes due to age and work and hence increase the workability of older employees.

It is well-known that extended cognitive engagement has a positive effect on cognition (Hultsch et al., 1999; Schooler et al., 1999; Wilson et al., 1999; Schooler and Mulatu, 2001; Singh-Manoux et al., 2003; Stern, 2009). Cognitively demanding work is an important cognitive stimulation supporting cognitive functions (Alvarado et al., 2002; Bosma et al., 2002; Wild-Wall et al., 2009; Marquié et al., 2010) which also lowers the risk of dementia in older age (Stern et al., 1994; Andel et al., 2005; Lee et al., 2010; Swaab and Bao, 2011).

In a longitudinal study, Schooler et al. (1999) investigated the effects of complex and cognitive demanding work on cognitive performance across 20 years. The authors showed that demanding jobs improved cognitive performance, particularly in older employees. Potter et al. (2008) observed a similar beneficial effect of demanding work in a sample of about 1000 older workers across a time range of 7 years, whereas tedious physical job demands tended to impair cognition in the workers regardless of age, intelligence, and education. Furthermore, in a recent longitudinal study, Marquié et al. (2010) analyzed performance in cognitive tasks as a function of cognitive work demands in about 3000 workers. The authors could show that the more cognitively stimulating the work the higher the scores in tests of episodic memory, attention and speed of processing. More importantly, cognitively stimulating work leads even to an increase in cognitive performance in the tested employees over 10 years despite their increasing age.

In the previous cross-sectional study (Gajewski et al., 2010b), we assessed cognitive functions of young and middle-aged blue-collar workers who have been working for a long time either under repetitive or under flexible working conditions. Both groups of middle-aged employees were matched regarding age- and education. In particular, we aimed at investigating the status of cognitive control functions involved in a memory-based task-switching task, namely task preparation, working memory, and error processing. These functions were investigated by analyzing a specific ERP-component which reflects the cortical activity underlying different aspects of processing during task switching. We observed no age- and work-related impairments when the relevant task was indicated by a cue which reduced the working memory load. Age differences were apparent when memory demands were higher, i.e., when the task sequence had to be maintained across a large number of trials (memory-based task switching). Importantly, the older workers with long-term repetitive work showed the strongest deficits in performance. These behavioral impairments were accompanied by specific findings in the ERP, namely attenuation of preparation, reduction of working memory capacity, and diminished error detection. In contrast, the older workers with long-term flexible work showed small or no performance and ERP detriments when compared to young workers but differed considerably from their contemporary, repetitive working colleagues. These results are in line with the literature reporting negative impact of long-term unchallenging work on cognition.

Nonetheless, since our previous study was a cross-sectional one, the impairment of cognition in the workers with long-term repetitive work could also be due to early selection mechanisms, i.e., workers with relatively low cognitive skills prefer work in such repetitive jobs. While this is unlikely, given that the deficit was only seen in the demanding memory-based switching condition, it cannot be excluded. Therefore, a longitudinal study would be necessary to control for possible confounding variables and to analyze the time-course of cognitive functions across decades in workers with different working conditions. More useful, however, would be a longitudinal study which examines methods to improve cognitive functions (Stern, 2009; Gajewski and Falkenstein, 2015b). More specifically, it should be analyzed whether the cognitive deficits and their electrophysiological correlates found in our previous study could be ameliorated by cognitive training (CT).

Indeed, in the literature the most often reported type of formal CT is training of a specific function that focuses on one domain only, for example memory (Jaeggi et al., 2008), attention (Green and Bavelier, 2008), visual search (Becic et al., 2008), dual task (Bherer et al., 2005), or task switching (Karbach and Kray, 2009). In most studies the training effects were restricted to the trained function and did not transfer to other functions (e.g., Willis and Schaie, 1986; Willis et al., 2006), while some reports showed also transfer effects on non-trained activities (e.g., Gopher et al., 1994; Ball et al., 2007; Caserta et al., 2007; Cassavaugh and Kramer, 2009; Edwards et al., 2009; Karbach and Kray, 2009). Yet, the trained function could be influenced by an implicit involvement of non-explicitly trained functions.

As a consequence from the training literature it appears beneficial to conduct training that involves several fluid functions relevant for work and daily life (Kramer and Morrow, 2008). In most CT studies, test-like tasks or games which target different cognitive functions were trained via PC (computerized cognitive training; CCT) for an extended time. Recent meta-analyses suggest that CCT leads to improvements in various cognitive functions and also transfers to untrained cognitive tasks or even everyday situations (far transfer) in healthy older adults (Karbach and Verhaeghen, 2014; Kelly et al., 2014; Lampit et al., 2014; Ballesteros et al., 2015; Gajewski and Falkenstein, 2015b).

ERPs in the Task Switching Paradigm

Studies evaluating training-related effects using electrophysiological measures are scarce despite the advantage of this method to investigate distinct processing steps from stimulus analysis across memory activation, decision making to response-related processes. In the present study, we focus primarily on cognitive processes associated with particular ERP components: retrieval of stimulus-response sets (P2), response selection (N2), allocation of cognitive resources to the task (P3b) and response-related processes like response monitoring (Nc) and error detection (Ne). The P2 is a frontocentral positive wave with latency of about 170–200 ms that has been associated with evaluation of task relevant stimuli and retrieval of S-R mappings (Kieffaber and Hetrick, 2005; Gajewski et al., 2008; Adrover-Roig and Barceló, 2010). Larger P2 amplitudes may reflect enhanced target processing under difficult conditions such as task switch trials where larger P2 amplitudes were related to slower responses (Finke et al., 2011). Moreover, P2 latency was positively correlated with reaction times (RTs), supporting the interpretation of P2 as an index of S-R retrieval (Kieffaber and Hetrick, 2005).

Following the P2 the frontocentral negativity, the N2, with a latency of about 280–320 ms occurs. The N2 was mainly associated with mismatch (Folstein and Van Petten, 2008, for review), cognitive control of response (Hämmerer et al., 2014), conflict processing (Van Veen and Carter, 2002; Yeung and Cohen, 2006), decision making (Ritter et al., 1979), and response selection (Gajewski et al., 2008). In task switch trials interference processing between conflicting task-sets (i.e., S-R sets) was often associated with larger N2 amplitude and longer latency than in non-switch trials (Gajewski et al., 2010a, 2011; Karayanidis et al., 2011). This process seems to be sensitive to training as the N2 increased substantially after 4 months of CT in seniors (Gajewski and Falkenstein, 2012).

The P3b is a large positive wave with parietal maximum peaking at about 300 to 600 ms after stimulus onset that is associated with context updating (Donchin and Coles, 1988), allocation of cognitive resources (Kok, 2001), working memory (Polich, 2007), and outcome of a decision process (Nieuwenhuis et al., 2005; Verleger et al., 2006). The P3b was frequently reported in task switching studies with larger amplitudes in non-switch than task switch trials (e.g., Barceló et al., 2000; Lorist et al., 2000; Rushworth et al., 2002; Jost et al., 2008; Gajewski and Falkenstein, 2011). Training effects on the P3b are inconsistent. However, generally larger P3b amplitude was associated with better performance (Polich and Lardon, 1997; Hillman et al., 2006).

During response execution an error may occur. Such response errors are usually followed by a negative wave with a frontocentral maximum, the error negativity (Ne; Falkenstein et al., 1991), or error-related negativity (ERN; Gehring et al., 1993) which is thought to reflect the detection of errors or incorrect response tendencies. The Ne is seen as the result of a comparison process between the expected and the actual outcome, leading to behavioral readjustment and reflects a precondition for successful learning (Falkenstein et al., 2000; Holroyd and Coles, 2002). It has also been shown that the Ne is smaller for older than younger participants, suggesting a weakening of action monitoring processes in older adults (Band and Kok, 2000; Falkenstein et al., 2001). After correct responses, a smaller negativity is seen, called Nc or CRN (Yordanova et al., 2004) which is thought to reflect response monitoring (Allain et al., 2004).

The Present Study

The aim of the longitudinal part of the cross-sectional study reported by Gajewski et al. (2010b) was to ameliorate cognitive decline found in middle-aged assembly line workers, as outlined above. In the present study, CT as a crucial method for improving fluid cognition as reported in the literature (Strobach and Karbach, 2016) was applied. We used a formal paper- and computer-based CT which was found to be effective in improving cognitive functions in healthy older subjects as measured with behavior as well as electrical brain activity in the previous training study (Gajewski and Falkenstein, 2012; Wild-Wall et al., 2012). The training was not focused on a particular cognitive function but aimed at affecting a broad spectrum of cognitive abilities with different training tasks. The CT contained both several paper and pencil tasks (Mental Activation Training, MAT; Lehrl et al., 1994) and a number of computer-based tasks from commercial packages. The tasks were selected to target different cognitive functions such as attention, working memory, inhibition, and dual-task performance. The training format was two sessions per week (lasting 1.5 h each) for 3 months in groups guided by a skilled teacher. Fifty-seven middle-aged workers with highly repetitive work finished this study. The participants were randomly assigned to the training group and a Waiting Control Group. The latter received a combined cognitive, relaxation, and stress management training after the Cognitive Training Group finished the training, i.e., after both groups were post-measured. The offer of the combined training was aimed to keep the motivation of the waiting group high and to reduce dropouts and also to assess effects of the stress management training (which will be reported elsewhere). Moreover, this design allows additional validation of CT effects in a second sample. Apart from behavioral data we aimed at analyzing a number of ERPs which may be affected by CT.

Following hypotheses were formulated: Existing evidence indicates that CT is a useful tool for enhancing cognitive functions (Strobach and Karbach, 2016). Thus, CT should be particularly helpful in restoring cognitive deficits in individuals with long-term repetitive and unchallenging type of work. To measure the effects of CT, the same difficult memory-based task switching paradigm was used as in the previous study that revealed cognitive impairments in assembly line workers (Gajewski et al., 2010b). This task should be suitable to detect even marginal training-induced changes in executive functioning in middle-aged healthy workers. According to the findings of our previous training study with healthy seniors (Gajewski and Falkenstein, 2012), we expected improvement of accuracy in this task, whereas no changes in speed were expected. Moreover, performance effects should be accompanied by specific enhancements in ERP activity. Specifically, we expect an enlargement of N2 and P3b amplitudes after the training, indicating more efficient response selection, and working memory processes, as well as increased Ne/ERN, suggesting improved error detection that would corroborate our previous results. In respect to the P2, we also expect larger amplitudes after CT as enhanced performance was associated with larger P2 amplitudes (Wild-Wall et al., 2012). We do not have any specific expectations regarding the long-term effect of training assessed by the follow-up measure. Finally, we do not expect any beneficial effects of a combined relaxation and CT over a pure CT on executive functions, as relaxation alone was not associated with cognitive effects (Gajewski and Falkenstein, 2012).

MATERIALS AND METHODS

Participants

From the 60 participants 57 healthy male volunteers aged from 40 to 57 (M = 46.5, SD = 4.5) finished the study and completed all measures. None of the individuals participated in the cross-sectional study conducted previously (Gajewski et al., 2010b). Eleven participants were left- or both handed. They had normal or corrected-to-normal vision. Five participants finished Primary school (4th grade), 34 secondary general school (10th grade), 13 intermediate secondary school (10th grade), and 5 grammar school (gymnasium, 12th grade). Twenty-eight participants worked in double shifts (early and late shift), 20 participants worked in a night shifts only. Early and night shift employees were trained together in the afternoon after the early shift was finished. Late shift employees were trained before the late shift began. All participants received a payment for their participation. This study was carried out in accordance with the recommendations of the local ethics committee of the Leibniz association with written informed consent from all subjects. All subjects gave written informed consent in accordance with the Declaration of Helsinki. The protocol was approved by the local ethics committee of the Leibniz association.

Study Design

The schedule of trainings and measurements is presented in **Figure 1**. The study was designed as a randomized controlled trial with pre-, post-measure, and a follow-up measures. After the pre-measure (t1), participants were randomly assigned to the cognitive training (COG) and a Waiting Control Group. After the 20 sessions of the CT were finished (t2) both groups were tested again. Thereafter the Control Group received a stress management and relaxation training (REL) in the first eight sessions and in the remaining 12 sessions qualitatively the same (though shorter) cognitive training (REL + COG). After the combined training was finished both groups were measured again (t3), providing a follow-up measure for the COG group and an assessment of the training changes in the combined training group (REL + COG). Note, though the main focus was on the effects of the COG-group relative to the control between t1 and t2 and the long-term effect of training assessed at t3, we also report the effects of the combined intervention to investigate whether the training effects were similar to that for the COG group. Before, after the training and 3 months after the end of the training several paper and pencil and computer-based psychometric tests were applied. Here, we report only the results of the PC-based task switching paradigm.

Cognitive Training

The CT lasted 3 months with two sessions per week and 1.5 h per session (20 sessions in total). The training aimed at enhancing general cognitive abilities and was not designed to improve a particular cognitive function. Thus, the training consisted of a paper and pencil and a number of commercial and non-commercial PC-based exercises. A number of training packages listed below were already used and described in a previous study (cf. appendix in Gajewski and Falkenstein, 2012).

During the first month the so-called MAT (Lehrl et al., 1994) was applied. MAT is a paper-based CT to increase basic cognitive functions such as short-term memory and speed of information processing. In the subsequent weeks, the participants were trained with selected tasks taken from commercial and non-commercial internet-based software packages[1,2,3,4,5]. The difficulty level of the training tasks was continuously adapted to the participants' individual abilities either by the program or by the trainer.

Each session comprised different exercises that aimed to train crucial cognitive functions like perceptual speed, attention, and memory. For example, the training package FreshMinder2 includes games that require fast responding to specific stimuli like colored balloons, fast selecting digits in ascending order, memorizing and delayed recalling of faces, repeating of sound sequences, matching of letters, memorizing shopping lists, counting bricks in 3-D figures, memorizing and recalling of schematic paths, etc.

The package Ahano peds consists of units with different difficulty levels. The freely available program includes an eye-hand coordination task, money counting task, detection of word repetitions in a text, block tapping task, memorizing abstract figures etc. The package Mentaga consists of exercises enhancing vigilance, perceptual speed, spatial cognition, and eye–hand coordination. Finally, the package Mental-Aktiv offers a number of memory tasks using digits, letters, colors and figures and exercises to train speed of processing. The specific tasks from those packages were chosen on the basis of their validity for the targeted functions as well as the fun they induced during exercising.

Additional sessions took place at the end of the program for those participants who missed the regular sessions.

Task Switch Task

The same task was used as in a number of previous reports (Gajewski et al., 2010b; Gajewski and Falkenstein, 2012, 2015a; Schapkin et al., 2014). Briefly, the stimuli in the task switching paradigm consisted of the digits 1–9, excluding the number 5. The digits were presented in white on a black computer screen 3 mm above the white fixation point (10 mm diameter). Each digit was presented in small (7 mm × 10 mm) and in large (12 mm × 18 mm) size. A cue (16 mm × 32 mm) indicating the relevant task was presented 3 mm below the fixation point. The cue "NUM" (German "Numerisch," numeric) indicated a numerical task (greater or less than 5), "GER" (German "Geradzahligkeit," parity) the parity task (odd vs. even), "SCH" (German "Schrift," font) the font-size task (small vs. large). The cue was presented in the single tasks only. In the memory-based mixed block (see below) three letters X were presented

[1]www.brain-trainer.de

[2]www.happyneuron.de

[3]www.ahano.de

[4]www.freshminder.de

[5]www.mentaga.de

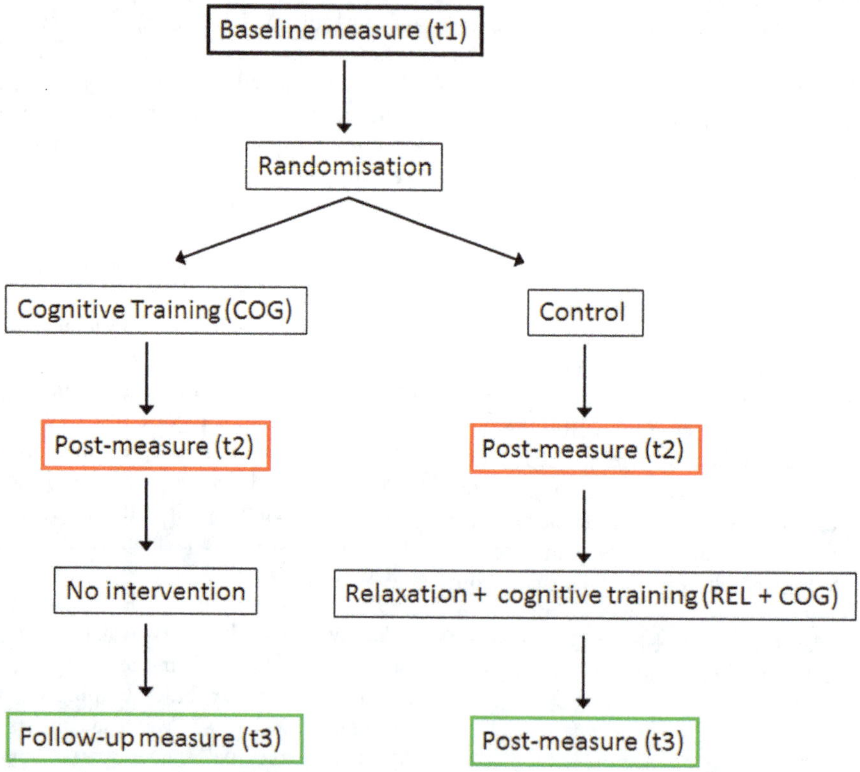

FIGURE 1 | A scheme of the study design.

instead of the informative cue. Responses consisted of pressing one of two buttons which were mounted in a response box. The buttons should be pressed with the index fingers. The stimulus–response mapping of the three tasks was overlapping, that is, responses according to 'smaller than five,' 'even,' and 'small size' were assigned to the left key and 'larger than five,' 'odd,' and 'large size' to the right key. This assignment was counterbalanced across participants.

Procedure

A schematic example of a trial is shown in **Figure 2**.

The same procedure was used as in the previous studies that used this task (Gajewski et al., 2010b; Gajewski and Falkenstein, 2012, 2015a; Schapkin et al., 2014). Shortly, a trial started with a presentation of the fixation point for 300 ms. In the single task blocks, a cue stimulus was presented for 1300 ms which remained visible when the digit was presented. A response had to be given within 2500 ms after target-onset. Five hundred milliseconds after the response a feedback was displayed for 500 ms. In case of a correct response a plus sign, after a false response a minus sign was displayed. After that the next cue was shown. The response-cue interval (RCI) was set to 1000 ms and included the response-feedback delay and the feedback.

At the beginning of the session participants performed three single task blocks with a fixed task NUM, GER, and SCH consisting of 34 trials each. The single task blocks were used to become familiar with the different task rules before the mixed block was run and to assess baseline performance in a task without a concurrent task.

In the memory-based mixed block, the three tasks were presented in mixed order and the participants were instructed to switch the task after every three trials in the following order "NUM–NUM–NUM–GER–GER–GER–SCH–SCH–SCH" etc. while a dummy cue "XXX" instead of a cue was presented, i.e., participants had to keep the trial sequence in mind. When three consecutive errors were made or no response within the 2500 ms interval was given, cues were presented for the next three trials, helping the participants to find the track. The mixed block consisted of 126 trails.

The frequency of task switch in the memory-based block amounted to 33.3% of trials. The participants were given written instructions explaining the task. The instructions encouraged quick and accurate responses.

EEG Recording

The same recording parameters were used as in our previous studies (Gajewski et al., 2010b; Gajewski and Falkenstein, 2012, 2015a). Briefly, EEG was recorded from 32 scalp electrodes according to the extended 10–20 system and mounted on an elastic cap. The montage included 8 midline sites and 12 sites on each hemisphere and two mastoid electrodes (M1 and M2). The EEG was re-referenced offline to linked mastoids. The horizontal and vertical EOG was recorded bipolarly from electrodes at both eyes. Eye movement artifacts were corrected

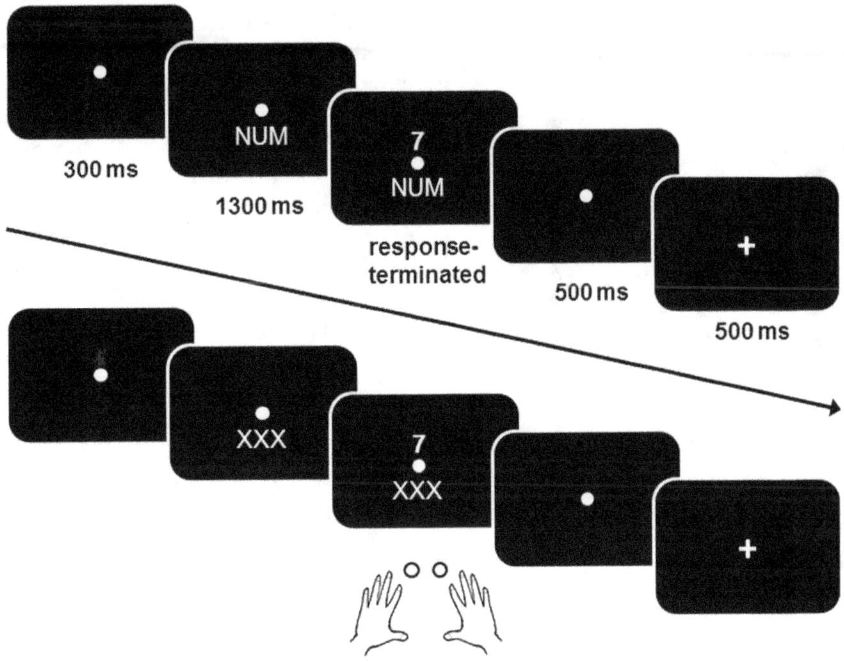

FIGURE 2 | Schematic illustration of a trial in the single (practice) block and a mixed task block (bottom). In contrast to the single block, no explicit cue was presented in the mixed block.

using the correction algorithm of Gratton et al. (1983). Electrode impedance was kept below 10 kΩ. The amplifier bandpass was 0.01–140 Hz. EEG and EOG were sampled continuously with a rate of 2048 Hz. Offline, the EEG was downscaled to a sampling rate of 1000 Hz and cut in stimulus-locked by using the software Vision Analyzer (Brain Products, Munich). Epochs in which the amplitude exceeded ±150 μV were rejected. The ERPs were filtered digitally offline with a 17 Hz low and 0.05 Hz high pass.

Data Analysis

Excluded from the RT analysis were: the first trial of each test block, trials with responses faster than 100 ms or slower than 2500 ms and error trials. RTs and error rates (ERs) were subjected to an ANOVA design including within-subject factors Task-Set Transition (non-switch vs. switch), Session (pre-test (t1) vs. post-test (t2)) and the between-subject factor Group (training vs. control).

As the design was not fully balanced (CT between t1 and t2 and combined training between t2 and t3, see **Figure 1**) the follow-up effect in the COG was assessed by planned comparisons t2 vs. t3 and t1 vs. t3 within this group. ANOVAs were conducted with the two within-subject factors Task-Set Transition and Session without the between subject factor Group. A significant effect of Session between t1 and t3 and lack of difference between t2 and t3 would suggest a training-induced change that persists until the follow-up measure.

The training effect in the combined training group (REL + COG) was assessed by planned comparisons between t2 and t3 and t1 vs. t2. Similar to the planned comparisons used in the COG group, ANOVAs with the two within-subject factors Task-Set Transition and Session within this group were conducted. A substantial training effect would be found when a change occurs between t2 and t3 whereas no difference will be found between t1 and t2 (effect of repeated measures).

Behavioral and ERP data were analyzed from the memory-based mixing block. The length of the epoch in the target-locked ERP was 1100 ms, and 600 ms in the response-locked ERP. The ERP analysis was restricted to the post-target and post-response ERPs at the midline electrodes (Cz and Pz) as the targeted components P2, N2, P3b, and Nc/Ne are usually maximum at the midline. Moreover, *a priori* selection of these electrodes considerably reduced the complexity of the reported effects. In contrast to our previous studies, we analyzed the P2 at Cz and not at Fz as the P2 amplitude was clearly maximum at Cz. The P2 was measured as the most positive peak between 150 and 300 ms. N2, P3b, and Ne were analyzed at the same electrodes as in the previous reports (Gajewski et al., 2010b; Gajewski and Falkenstein, 2012, 2015a). The N2 was measured as the most negative peak at Cz in the time range 150–400 ms after target-onset. The P3b was measured at Pz in the time range 300–600 ms after target-onset. P2, N2, and P3b were measured in correct trials relative to 100 ms baseline prior to target - onset. Nc and Ne were measured in as the most negative peak in the time range 0–150 ms after the response relative to the 100 ms pre-response baseline. Nc and Ne were collapsed across non-switch and switch trials to get at least six error trials per subject (Steele et al., 2016). The ERPs were analyzed in the same way as the behavioral data.

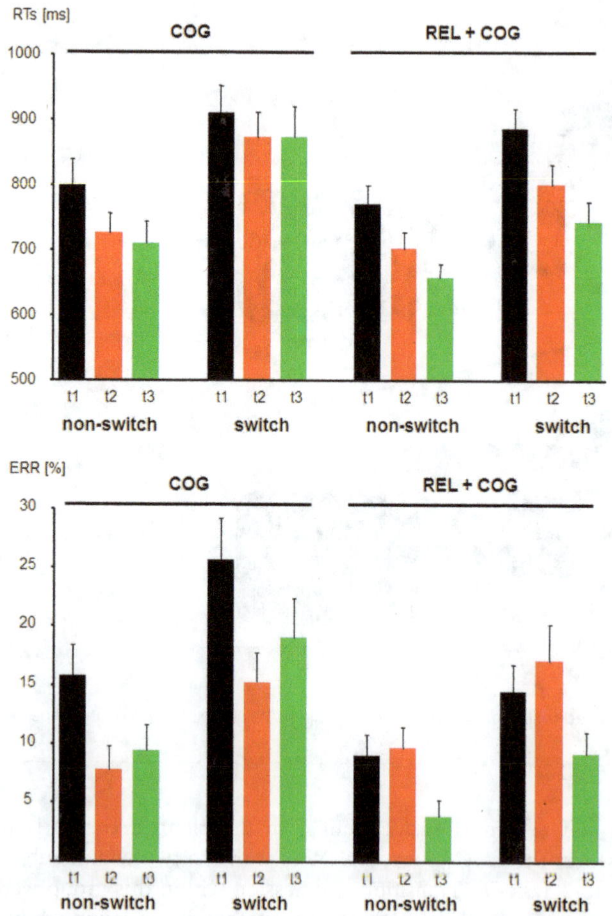

FIGURE 3 | Behavioral data. Reaction times **(Top)** and error rates **(Bottom)** as a function of Task-Set Transition (non-switch and switch) in the Cognitive Training Group (between t1 and t2; COG) and Waiting Control Group (REL + COG). T3 in the COG group reflects the follow-up measure, whereas t3 in the REL + COG reflects effect of the combined relaxation and cognitive training.

RESULTS

Behavioral Data

Mean RTs and ERs for the non-switch and switch trials for the training and the Control Group are presented in **Figure 3**.

For the analysis of response times, error trials (8.5 and 6.0%) and outliers (0.9 and 0.4%) for the training and Control Group, respectively, were discarded.

Reaction Times

For the group comparison between t1 and t2 the mean RTs in non-switch trials were shorter than in switch trials (750 vs. 868 ms), reflecting substantial switch costs [$F(1,56) = 66.8$, $p < 0.0001$, $\eta^2 = 0.544$]. The factor Session was significant due to faster RTs in the post- than pre-measure [776 vs. 846 ms; $F(1,56) = 8.8$, $P < 0.005$, $\eta^2 = 0.137$]. None of these factors were modulated by the factor Group.

The follow-up effect in the COG group assessed by the comparison between the Sessions t2 and t3 confirmed again an effect of Task-Set transition [$F(1,25) = 39.1$, $p < 0.0001$, $\eta^2 = 0.610$] but no effect of Session nor interaction between Task-Set Transition and time were significant (both F's < 1). The comparison between t3 and t1 showed, apart from the effect of Task-Set Transition [$F(1,25) = 24.2$, $p < 0.0001$, $\eta^2 = 0.493$], only trends for the effect of Session [$F(1,25) = 2.7$, $p = 0.114$, $\eta^2 = 0.097$] and the interaction of both factors [$F(1,25) = 2.5$, $p = 0.123$, $\eta^2 = 0.092$], suggesting no stable change of RTs due to training.

In order to assess a possible training effect in the REL + COG group, t2 was compared with t3. ANOVA yielded an effect of Task-Set Transition [$F(1,30) = 40.8$, $p < 0.0001$, $\eta^2 = 0.557$], which was not modulated by time-point ($F < 1$). However, there was a trend of Session, suggesting faster RTs at t3 than at t2 in this group [701 vs. 740 ms, $F(1,30) = 3.4$, $p = 0.076$, $\eta^2 = 0.101$]. For the comparison t2 vs. t1 the effect of Task-Set Transition was again significant [$F(1,30) = 62.3$, $p < 0.0001$, $\eta^2 = 0.675$] as well as the effect of Session [$F(1,30) = 11.0$, $p < 0.005$, $\eta^2 = 0.269$]. The interaction did not reach significance [$F(1,30) = 1.4$, $p = 0.245$, $\eta^2 = 0.045$]. Basically, no changes in speed due to training were observed. RT reductions were merely due to repeated measures.

Error Rates

The main effect of Task-Set Transition was significant [$F(1,56) = 76.5$, $p < 0.0001$, $\eta^2 = 0.577$], suggesting switch costs in accuracy (10.5 vs. 18.1%, for non-switch and switch trials, respectively). The ER was lower at t2 than t1 resulting in the effect of Session [12.4 vs. 16.2%; $F(1,56) = 5.9$, $p < 0.05$, $\eta^2 = 0.096$]. Importantly, the factor Session was modulated by Group [$F(1,56) = 12.2$, $p < 0.001$, $\eta^2 = 0.179$] due to a reduction of ERs from t1 to t2 in the COG group from (20.7 to 11.5%) and a slight increase in the Control Group (11.7 vs. 13.4%).

The follow-up analysis in the COG group revealed an effect of Task-Set Transition [$F(1,25) = 49.8$, $p < 0.0001$, $\eta^2 = 0.666$] and no effect of Session or interaction of both factors (both F's < 1). Comparison between t3 and t1 yielded an effect of Task-Set Transition [$F(1,25) = 36.7$, $p < 0.0001$, $\eta^2 = 0.595$] and an effect of Session [$F(1,25) = 4.7$, $p < 0.05$, $\eta^2 = 0.159$], whereas no interaction between Task-Set Transition and Session was found ($F < 1$).

After the training between t2 and t3 the REL + COG group showed apart from the expected effect of Task-Set Transition [$F(1,30) = 36.5$, $p < 0.0001$, $\eta^2 = 0.549$] a main effect of Session [$F(1,30) = 10.7$, $p < 0.005$, $\eta^2 = 0.264$], whereas the interaction Session × Task-Set Transition did not reach significance [$F(1,30) = 1.4$, $p = 0.236$, $\eta^2 = 0.049$]. The comparison t1 vs. t2 did not reveal effect of Session or interaction Session × Task-Set Transition and showed merely the effect of Task-Set Transition [$F(1,30) = 33.2$, $p < 0.0001$, $\eta^2 = 0.518$].

In order to analyze which participants benefitted from the CT we split the COG group in low and high performers (i.e., lower vs. higher ERs at t1 in task switch condition than the median). The analysis revealed an interaction Session × Performance [$F(1,24) = 10.1$, $p < 0.005$, $\eta^2 = 0.297$], and a second order interaction Session × Task-Set Transition × Performance [$F(1,24) = 13.8, p < 0.001, \eta^2 = 0.365$], suggesting that the low performers improved the accuracy after training particularly in task switch trials between t1 and t2 (41.2 vs. 20.1%), whereas high performers did not (10.0 vs. 10.4%) improve. The benefit was less pronounced in non-switch trials (23.6 vs. 12.9% in the low performers and 8 vs. 3.3% in the high performers). Moreover, age was differentially associated with training gains. Younger trainees (40–47 years) benefitted strongly from the training (14% accuracy improvement) than their older colleagues (47–57 years, 2% improvement), resulting in an interaction Age Group × Session [$F(1,24) = 5.5, p < 0.05, \eta^2 = 0.187$].

In sum, the ERs were reduced in the COG group after training. This reduction remained unchanged during the follow-up measure. In the Waiting Control Group, no changes were found between t1 and t2 but again a clear reduction of ERs was observed after the combined training at t3. No specific changes of local switch effects in accuracy due to training were seen. Initial low performers benefitted more from the training than high performers, particularly in task switching trials. Younger trainees improved their accuracy after training more than the older ones.

ERP Data

Grand averages for target-locked ERP-waveforms at Cz and Pz for the two groups are shown in **Figures 4** and **5**.

In order to focus on training-related changes of executive functions, only effects or interactions including Task-Set Transition, Session, and Group were reported in the following.

ERPs

P2

The ANOVA analyzing effect of the COG training relative to the Waiting Control Group revealed a trend for an interaction Session × Group for P2 latency [$F(1,56) = 4.2, p < 0.05, \eta^2 = 0.069$]. This interaction was due to reduced P2 latency at t2 relative to t1 in the COG group (158 vs. 167 ms), whereas no such effect was observed in the Control Group (161 vs. 158 ms). Also, there was a trend for the interaction Session × Group × Task-Set Transition [$F(1,56) = 3.2, p = 0.078, \eta^2 = 0.055$], suggesting that the latency reduction was mainly due to task switch (14 ms) and hardly in non-switch trials (5 ms). P2 amplitude showed an effect of Session [$F(1,56) = 10.7, p < 0.005, \eta^2 = 0.161$], indicating a general reduction of P2 at t2 compared to t1 (5.3 vs. 4.7 μV) that was additionally modulated by the factor Group [$F(1,56) = 9.6, p < 0.005, \eta^2 = 0.147$]. This interaction was based on the amplitude reduction between t1 and t2 in the COG group (5.4 vs. 4.2 μV) while no changes in the Waiting Control Group were observed (5.1 vs. 5.1 μV). The assessment of the follow-up effect for P2 latency and amplitude (t2 vs. t3) yielded no effect of Session nor interaction Session × Task-Set Transition (all F's < 1). However, the comparison between t1 and t3 revealed a substantial effect of Session for P2 amplitude (5.4 vs. 3.9 μV; $F(1,23) = 19.0, p < 0.0001, \eta^2 = 0.354$) but not for P2 latency ($F < 1$).

Comparison between the Sessions t2 and t3 for the Waiting Control Group (REL + COG) showed for the P2 latency a main effect of Task-Set Transition due to delayed P2 in non-switch than switch trials [168 vs. 159 ms; $F(1,30) = 6.0, p < 0.05, \eta^2 = 0.167$] and an interaction Task-Set Transition and Session [$F(1,30) = 4.7, p < 0.05, \eta^2 = 0.127$] due to later P2 latency at t3 than t2 for non-switch (178 vs. 159 ms) and a shorter latency at t3 than t2 for task switch trials (155 vs. 162 ms). The P2 amplitude showed a large reduction after the combined REL + COG training (5.2 vs. 3.6 μV ms), resulting in a main effect of Session [$F(1,30) = 54.5, p < 0.0001, \eta^2 = 0.645$]. No effect of Task-Set Transition or interaction Task-Set Transition × Session was found (Both F's < 1). Finally, in order to assess possible effects of repeated measures comparison between t1 and t2 was conducted. ANOVA showed no significant effects or interactions either for P2 latency or amplitude.

In sum, the P2 amplitude was substantially reduced and the latency partly shortened both after the pure cognitive training (COG) and the combined relaxation and cognitive training (REL + COG). The P2 amplitude reduction remained stable during the follow-up measure.

N2

ANOVA analysing effects of the CT on the N2 latency showed an effect of Task-Set Transition [$F(1,56) = 5.9, p < 0.05, \eta^2 = 0.096$], reflecting prolonged N2 latency in switch vs. non-switch trials (283 vs. 272 ms). There was a strong trend of Session [$F(1,56) = 3.8, p = 0.054, \eta^2 = 0.065$] due to shorter latency at t2 than at t1 (172 vs. 184 ms). The interaction Session × Group did not reach significance [$F(1,56) = 2.3, p = 0.13, \eta^2 = 0.040$].

In respect to N2 amplitude a main effect of Session indicated a larger (more negative) N2 at t2 than at t1 [−1.0 vs. −0.5 μV; $F(1,56) = 6.2, p < 0.05, \eta^2 = 0.100$]. Most importantly, Session was modulated by Group [$F(1,56) = 5.7, p < 0.05, \eta^2 = 0.092$], suggesting a N2 increase after COG training at t2 relative to t1 (−1.9 vs. −1.0 μV) while no difference in the Waiting Control Group was observed (−0.1 vs. −0.1 μV). The follow-up measure in the COG group showed no significant effects or interactions on N2 latency, whereas N2 amplitude was significantly reduced at t3 relative to t2 (−0.6 vs. −1.9 μV), resulting in an effect of Session [$F(1,23) = 12.1, p < 0.005, \eta^2 = 0.345$]. Comparison between t1 and t3 did not yield any significant effects or interactions on N2 amplitude.

Assessment of the training effects in the REL + COG group showed an effect of Session on N2 latency [$F(1,56) = 6.5, p < 0.05, \eta^2 = 0.183$], indicating a shorter N2 latency at t3 than at t2 (248 vs. 267 ms). No further effect or interaction reached significance. Comparison between t1 and t2 reflecting effects of repeated measure showed merely an effect of Task-Set Transition due to larger N2 in task switch than non-switch trials [−0.3 vs. 0.1 μV; $F(1,56) = 5.8, p < 0.05, \eta^2 = 0.157$]. No effects of Session or interaction Session × Task-Set Transition was found.

In sum, N2 amplitude was increased after CT whereas no difference was found in the Waiting Control Group. However, the effect on N2 amplitude diminished in the follow-up measure. No significant training effect on N2 latency in the COG group was found. However, the N2 latency was shorter in the REL + COG group after training.

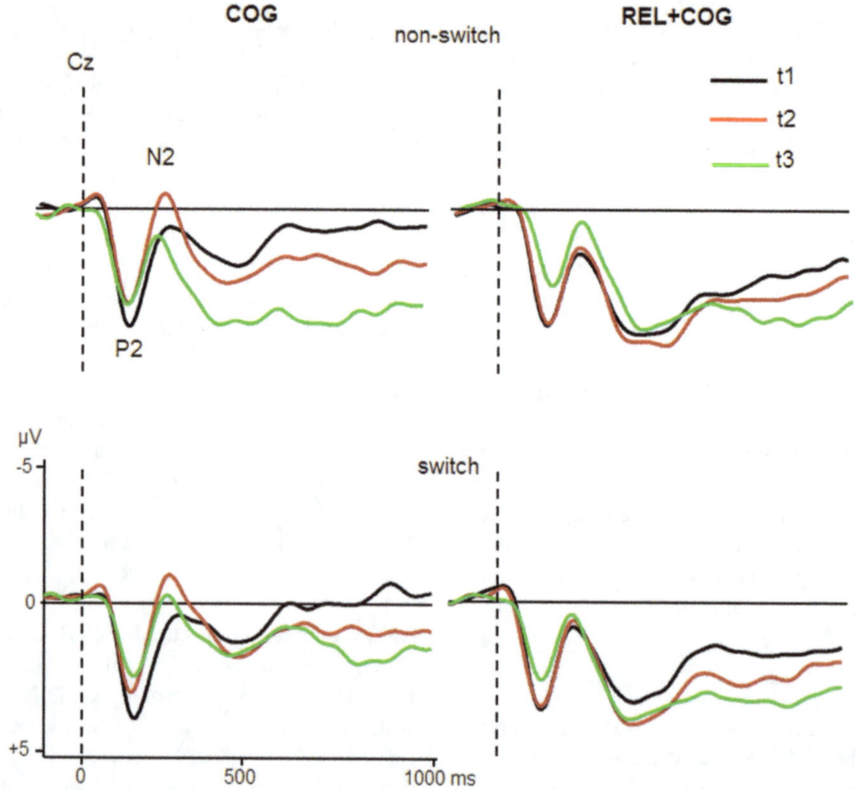

FIGURE 4 | ERPs at Cz of the COG and the Waiting Control Group (REL + COG) as a function of Task-Set transition for the Sessions t1 (black), t2 (red), and t3 (green). See caption of **Figure 3** and the study design for more information.

P3b

ANOVA did not show any effects or interactions on P3b latency. Analysis of P3b amplitude revealed an effect of Task-Set Transition, indicating smaller P3b in switch than non-switch trials [5.1 vs. 5.9 µV; $F(1,56) = 12.8$, $p < 0.001$, $\eta^2 = 0.187$] and a trend of Session, showing a slight increase in P3b amplitude at t2 compared to t1 [6.2 vs. 6.8 µV; $F(1,56) = 3.5$, $p = 0.06$, $\eta^2 = 0.059$]. There was no interaction with Group (*F*'s < 1). However, the main effect of Group showed a larger P3b in the control than in the training group [6.5 vs. 4.5 µV; $F(1,56) = 6.5$, $p < 0.05$, $\eta^2 = 0.105$]. The follow-up measure showed no substantial changes of the P3b between t2 and t3.

The ANOVA analysing the effects of the combined training (REL + COG) yielded an effect of Session, indicating P3b reduction from t2 to t3 [6.9 vs. 5.8 µV; $F(1,30) = 7.5$, $p < 0.01$, $\eta^2 = 0.201$]. No effects on P3b latency were found. Finally, the comparison t1 vs. t2 in this group showed apart from the standard effect of Task-Set Transition [6.9 vs. 6.0 µV; $F(1,31) = 8.8$, $p < 0.01$, $\eta^2 = 0.222$] a trend of Session, suggesting P3b increase from t1 to t2 [6.2 vs. 6.8 µV; $F(1,31) = 3.7$, $p = 0.06$, $\eta^2 = 0.108$].

Taken together, the P3b amplitude and latency did not vary consistently as a function of training. Its amplitude increased at t2 and decreased at t3. The Waiting Control Group showed generally larger P3b amplitude than the COG group.

Nc and Ne

The correct response negativity (Nc) and error negativity (Ne) at Cz (**Figure 6**) were pooled across switch and non-switch trials. There were 24 participants in each group that made a sufficient number of erroneous responses. There were no effects or interactions on Nc or Ne latency.

The ANOVA including the factors Response Correctness (Nc, Ne), Session and Group showed an effect of Correctness [$F(1,46) = 26.8$, $p < 0.0001$, $\eta^2 = 0.368$] with larger amplitudes in error than correct trials (−3.1 vs. −1.0 µV), an interaction Correctness and Session [$F(1,46) = 6.6$, $p < 0.05$, $\eta^2 = 0.125$] due to larger increase in the Ne (−2.6 vs. −3.6 µV) than Nc (−1.3 vs. −0.7 µV) between t1 and t2. Most importantly, the interaction of all three factors was also significant [$F(1,46) = 4.6$, $p < 0.05$, $\eta^2 = 0.091$], indicating a larger increase in the Ne after the CT whereas no difference was found for the Control Group. Comparison between t1 and t2 for Ne in the COG group confirmed this result [−1.8 vs. −3.6 µV; $F(1,23) = 4.3$, $p < 0.05$, $\eta^2 = 0.158$], whereas no difference between t1 and t2 was found in the Waiting Control Group (−3.4 vs. −3.6 µV; $F < 1$). The Ne amplitude in the COG group remained at the same level in the follow-up measure (−3.7 µV; $F < 1$). An additional comparison between t1 and t3 revealed a trend [−1.8 vs. −3.6 µV; $F(1,20) = 3.5$, $p = 0.07$, $\eta^2 = 0.150$].

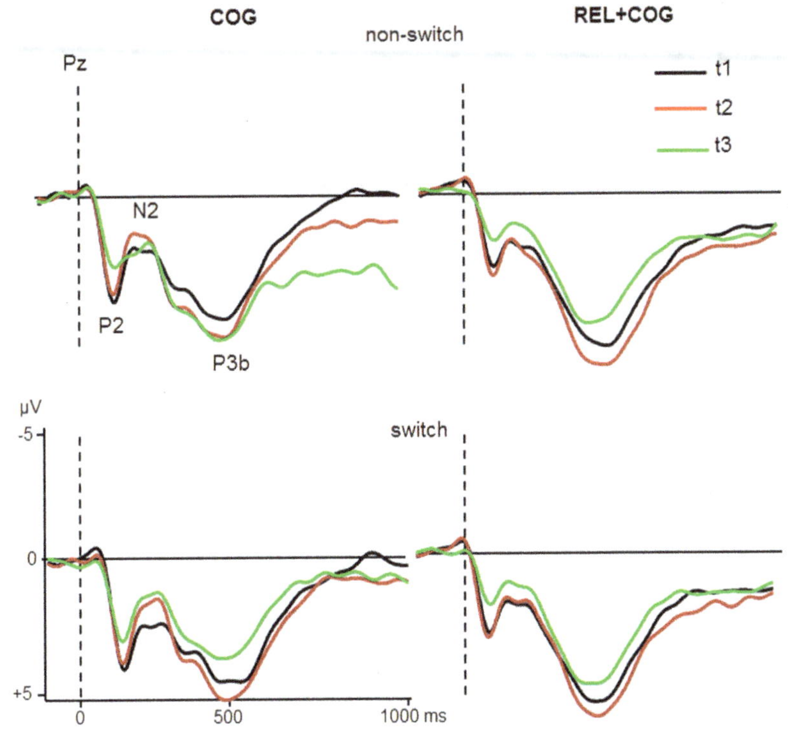

FIGURE 5 | ERPs at Pz of the COG and the Waiting Control Group (REL + COG) as a function of Task-Set transition for the Sessions t1 (black), t2 (red), and t3 (green). See caption of **Figure 3** and the study design for more information.

For the combined REL + COG group, the ANOVA showed again an effect of Correctness due to larger amplitude in error than correct trials [−5.6 vs. −1.2 μV; $F(1,18) = 19.5$, $p < 0.0001$, $\eta^2 = 0.520$], an effect of Session, suggesting an amplitude increase between t2 and t3 [−2.6 vs. −4.2 μV; $F(1,18) = 4.8$, $p < 0.05$, $\eta^2 = 0.210$] and an interaction Correctness × Session [$F(1,18) = 7.1$, $p < 0.05$, $\eta^2 = 0.284$], showing a strong increase in the Ne between t2 and t3 [−3.8 vs. −7.3 μV; $F(1,18) = 6.3$, $p < 0.05$, $\eta^2 = 0.259$], while the Nc showed similar amplitudes at t2 and t3 (−1.4 vs. −1.0). The comparison between t1 and t3 corroborated the training-related increase in the Ne [$F(1,18) = 15.4$, $p < 0.001$, $\eta^2 = 0.448$], which cannot be attributed to repeated measures as indicated by the non-significant comparison between t1 and t2 ($F < 1$).

In sum, the Ne after erroneous responses was, as expected, larger than the Nc after correct responses. The Ne (but not the Nc) was larger after the CT and remained stable during the follow-up measure while no changes were found in the Waiting Control Group. However, after the combined training (REL + COG) this group also showed a strong enhancement of the Ne.

DISCUSSION

The aim of the present study was the enhancement of executive control processes in middle-aged industry employees with unchallenging, repetitive type of work by a 3 months, trainer-guided CT or a combined relaxation/stress management and cognitive intervention. Pre- and post measure in the Cognitive Training and the Waiting Control Group allowed assessing the effects of the CT. A follow-up measure was included to assess the residual effects of training 3 months after the training was finished. The Waiting Control Group received a combined relaxation and CT (REL + COG) lasting also 3 months after the post-measure was completed. The effects of the combined training were evaluated after the training was finished.

Training effects were assessed using a complex memory based task switching paradigm which was shown to be sensitive to a number of cognitive or physical interventions (Gajewski and Falkenstein, 2012, 2015a). In accordance with the previous study with seniors (Gajewski and Falkenstein, 2012) CT substantially improved the accuracy in this task, whereas RTs were not affected. The new finding of the present study is that this improvement remained stable 3 months after the training ended. An additional support for this finding provided the Waiting Control Group showing a similar improvement in accuracy after the REL + COG training. However, one point may be problematic for the interpretation of training effects in the present study. At first glance the different ERs at t1 between the groups may question the real training effect as the chance to reduce ERs was rather higher in the COG group due to poorer initial performance than in the REL + COG group (despite randomization procedure). However, the statistical analysis showed unequivocally significant

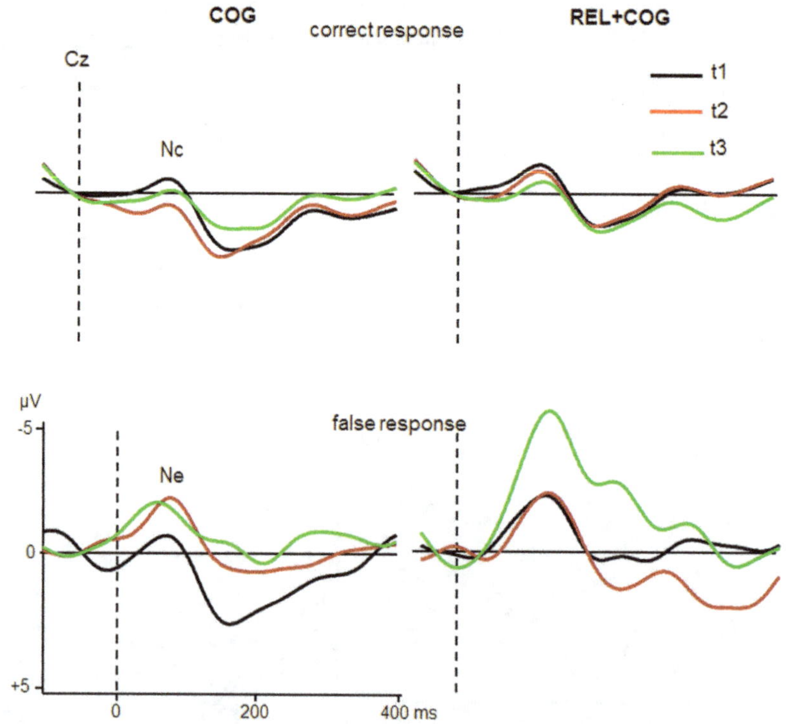

FIGURE 6 | Nc and Ne at Cz of the COG and the Waiting Control Group (REL + COG) for correct (Top) and false response **(Bottom)** as a function Sessions t1 (black), t2 (red), and t3 (green). See caption of **Figure 3** and the study design for more information.

improvement in accuracy both in the COG group as well as in the REL +COG group. In other words, the REL + COG group did not reduce ERs between t1 and t2 but reduced it significantly after training, indicating no effects of repeated measures and a real effect of training even if the initial accuracy was high.

Electrophysiological data allowed further insights in the specific processing steps and cognitive subcomponents influenced by training. The target-locked ERPs provide a number of interesting findings concerning effects of the CT. First, the amplitude of the P2 was consistently reduced and its latency shortened both after CT alone and after combined training. This attenuation remained stable during the follow-up measure and was not caused by repeated measures. Its reduced amplitude and latency after training may reflect less effort during task-set retrieval that leads to a faster activation of task relevant stimulus-response sets (c.f. Finke et al., 2011; Schapkin et al., 2014).

The next process which was influenced by training in the present study was the frontocentral N2. Our previous study with seniors already showed the sensitivity of the N2 to CT (Gajewski and Falkenstein, 2012). Apart from the usually observed effects of a larger N2 in task switch than non-switch trials, the N2 amplitude was increased both after the pure CT and the combined cognitive and relaxation training. The enhanced N2 suggests a more intense response selection and may be the origin of the improved accuracy. No training effects on N2 latency were found. A surprising finding in this study was the reduction in the amplitude enhancement after a 3-month training free period. This may suggest either an adaptation effect of neuronal structures underlying response selection or alternatively an index of gradual decay of the training induced effect. Both possibilities should be considered in future studies.

The P3b showed a lower amplitude in switch vs. non-switch trials, which was consistently reported previously (Barceló et al., 2000; Rushworth et al., 2002; Jost et al., 2008; Gajewski and Falkenstein, 2011, 2012, 2015a; Karayanidis et al., 2011). However, the P3b did not vary as a function of training. Its amplitude was generally increased during pre-measure and reduced during follow-up measure but this effect was probably not related to the training but rather due to the repeated application of the same task and corresponding adaptation effects. As the P3b is a conglomerate of diverse neuronal mechanisms (e.g., Polich, 2007) a simpler paradigm like Oddball paradigm may be more appropriate to analyze P3b changes in the course of CT.

Finally, the most consistent results associated with training was provided by the analysis of error negativity Ne. The Ne was expectedly more pronounced than the corresponding negativity during correct responses. Most importantly, the Ne (but not the Nc) was substantially increased after CT in both groups (COG, COG + REL) and remained stable during the follow-up measure for the COG group while no changes were found in the Waiting Control Group. These results corroborate findings obtained in our previous study with seniors (Gajewski and Falkenstein, 2012). The improvement of accuracy was previously interpreted as a consequence of the enhancement of the response selection process reflected by the N2. This may lead to higher awareness about the correct response which in turn produces a strong signal if the expectation to respond correctly was violated.

The present study extended previous results obtained with middle-aged employees of the same big car factory that showed cognitive impairments in assembly line workers compared to flexibly working employees responsible for service, maintenance and repair of machines (Gajewski et al., 2010b). The assembly line employees showed increased ERs and RTs in the same task as in the present study and reduced P3b and Ne relative to their flexible working colleagues. In the present study, the initial cognitive status of the participants was comparable to the performance of those of the previous study as the participants were derived from the same population of middle-aged assembly line workers. The training effects obtained in the present study indicate that 3 months of cognitive or combined relaxation training is able to reduce cognitive decline and to elevate cognitive performance to the level of flexibly working employees.

Unfortunately, these findings do not allow drawing conclusions regarding the employability of the elderly workers as no far transfer tasks related to the work were used. However, it is plausible to assume that the observed gains of cognitive functions may improve the ability to learn new contents and work processes, enhance self-confidence and help to strengthen individual potential at work. Therefore, future studies in occupational environments should also evaluate far transfer by measurements of work efficiency, individual performance at work, risk of workplace injuries and work-related illness.

In summary, CT appears a most promising tool for improving mental fitness and employability in older workers. Future CT studies in occupational environments should evaluate far transfer by measurements of work efficiency, individual performance at work, risk of workplace injuries and work-related illness.

Limitations

The present study has a number of limitations which have to be acknowledged. Firstly, much effort has been invested to acquire the sample, as a large number of industry workers of this car factory were not willing to participate in the relatively time-consuming study before or after their work. Therefore, we assume that the study population was not fully representative of the factory population. Secondly, the age of the participants was rather homogeneous (mid forty). It would be interesting to analyze training effects in older employees, beyond sixties as older workers may show larger cognitive deficits which may be restored to improve or maintain their quality of life and employability until their retirement. Thirdly, the experimental design was not fully balanced and the training effects in the COG and REL + COG Group not directly comparable. Fourthly, the effects of CT were not specific to the switch ability as no differential effects in non-switch and switch trials were found. Reduction of local switch costs would be indicative for improvements in the switch ability, whereas performance enhancement in non-switch trials would be indicative for improvements in mixing costs. Indeed, mixing costs are a more sensitive parameter in respect to physical or CT (Gajewski and Falkenstein, 2012, 2015a). In other words, it is quite possible that other functions were improved by the training as a wide range of cognitive abilities was trained. Our assumption is that CT does not affect the switch ability *per se* but rather enhance updating of relevant task information and working memory capacity that improve the ability to maintain a long task sequence as in the current paradigm and to activate the relevant task-set at the right time point. This was supported by the observation that the errors in this paradigm are mainly due to lapses in the representation of the task sequence and activating the wrong task-set. Finally, and related to the previous point, the CT was qualitatively heterogeneous and trained a large number of cognitive functions. Therefore, it is not possible to determine which specific training regime was effective to affect the data of our study and which trainings were fully ineffective. Nevertheless, as this study was conducted in an applied context, controlling of a large number of confounding factors was not possible. Future studies with more controlled training regimes should be conducted to establish the most efficient training conditions in respect to duration, intensity, and content.

CONCLUSION

The present study was designed to compensate cognitive deficits in middle-aged workers with unchallenging work. Training-related gains in cognitive performance were observed in an improved accuracy, suggesting enhanced maintenance of a complex task sequence in working memory. This performance benefit was accompanied by a number of electrophysiological effects, like amplitude decrease and latency reduction of a frontocentral P2 related to retrieval of task-sets and latency decrease and amplitude increase of the frontocentral N2 associated with selection of a correct response. The P2 effect persisted 3 months after the training was finished, whereas the N2 amplitude effect disappeared.

Furthermore, an increase in error negativity (Ne) associated with error detection and monitoring was found which also persisted after a 3 months training-free period. In contrast, no performance and ERP effects in the Control Group were observed. Though, after the Waiting Control Group received the combined cognitive and relaxation training, the same performance and ERP changes were observed as in the Cognitive Training Group, suggesting that these effects are unequivocally due to training and not to the effect of repeated measures. These findings suggest that formal CT may indeed ameliorate cognitive decline that is also reflected in a sustained improvement of brain activity.

AUTHOR CONTRIBUTIONS

PG: Conception and design, data analysis, interpretation of the data, writing, and final approval. GF and MF: Conception and design, interpretation of the data, writing, and final approval.

and Social Affairs, BMAS. The publication of this article was supported by the Open Access Fund of the Leibniz Association and by the Open Access Fund of the Technical University of Dortmund.

ACKNOWLEDGMENTS

We thank Dr. Thomas Koiky and Dieter Welwei for assistance in organizing the study, Claudia Wipking, Ines Mombrei, Christiane Westedt and Rita Willemssen for conducting the testing, Rita Pfeiffer for conducting the training and Ludger Blanke for developing the software and technical support.

REFERENCES

Adrover-Roig, D., and Barceló, F. (2010). Individual differences in aging and cognitive control modulate the neural indexes of context updating and maintenance during task switching. *Cortex* 46, 434–450. doi: 10.1016/j.cortex.2009.09.012

Allain, S., Carbonnell, L., Falkenstein, M., Burle, B., and Vidal, F. (2004). The modulation of the Ne-like wave on correct responses foreshadows errors. *Neurosci. Lett.* 372, 161–166. doi: 10.1016/j.neulet.2004.09.036

Alvarado, B. E., Zunzunegui, M. V., del Ser, T., and Beland, F. (2002). Cognitive decline is related to education and occupation in a Spanish elderly cohort. *Aging Clin. Exp. Res.* 14, 132–142. doi: 10.1007/BF03324426

Andel, R., Crowe, M., Pedersen, N. L., Mortimer, J., Crimmins, E., Johansson, B., et al. (2005). Complexity of work and risk of Alzheimer's disease: a population-based study of Swedish twins. *J. Gerontol. B Psychol. Sci. Soc. Sci.* 60, 251–258. doi: 10.1093/geronb/60.5.P251

Ball, K., Edwards, J. D., and Ross, L. A. (2007). The impact of speed of processing training on cognitive and everyday functions. *J. Gerontol. B Psychol. Sci. Soc. Sci.* 62, 19–31. doi: 10.1093/geronb/62.special_issue_1.19

Ballesteros, S., Kraft, E., Santana, S., and Tziraki, C. (2015). Maintaining older brain functionality: a targeted review. *Neurosci. Biobehav. Rev.* 55, 453–477. doi: 10.1016/j.neubiorev.2015.06.008

Band, G. P., and Kok, A. (2000). Age effects on response monitoring in a mentalrotation task. *Biol. Psychol.* 51, 201–221. doi: 10.1016/S0301-0511(99)00038-1

Barceló, F., Muñoz-Céspedes, J. M., Pozo, M. A., and Rubia, F. J. (2000). Attentional set shifting modulates the target P3b response in the Wisconsin card sorting test. *Neuropsychologia* 38, 1342–1355. doi: 10.1016/S0028-3932(00)00046-4

Becic, E., Boot, W. R., and Kramer, A. F. (2008). Training older adults to search more effectively: scanning strategy and visual search in dynamic displays. *Psychol. Aging* 23, 461–466. doi: 10.1037/0882-7974.23.2.461

Bherer, L., Kramer, A. F., Peterson, J. S., Colcombe, S., Erickson, K., and Becic, E. (2005). Training effects on dual-task performance: are there age-related differences in plasticity of attentional control? *Psychol. Aging* 20, 95–709. doi: 10.1037/0882-7974.20.4.695

Bosma, H., van Boxtel, M. P., Ponds, R. W., Houx, P. J., Burdorf, A., and Jolles, J. (2002). Mental work demands protect against cognitive impairment: MAAS prospective cohort study. *Exp. Aging Res.* 29, 33–45. doi: 10.1080/03610730303710

Caserta, R. J., Young, J., and Janelle, C. M. (2007). Old dogs, new tricks: training the perceptual skills of senior tennis players. *J. Sport Exerc. Psychol.* 29, 479–497. doi: 10.1123/jsep.29.4.479

Cassavaugh, N., and Kramer, A. F. (2009). Transfer of computer-based cognitive training to simulated driving in older adults. *Appl. Ergon.* 40, 943–952. doi: 10.1016/j.apergo.2009.02.001

De Cuyper, N., Bernhard-Oettel, C., Berntson, E., Witte, H. D., and Alarco, B. (2008). Employability and employees' well-being: mediation by job insecurity. *Appl. Psychol.* 57, 488–509. doi: 10.1111/j.1464-0597.2008.00332.x

Donchin, E., and Coles, M. G. H. (1988). Is the P300 component a manifestation of context updating? *Behav. Brain Sci.* 11, 357–374. doi: 10.1017/S0140525X00058027

Edwards, J. D., Myers, C., Ross, L. A., Roenker, D. L., Cissell, G. M., McLaughlin, A. M., et al. (2009). The longitudinal impact of cognitive speed of processing training on driving mobility. *Gerontologist* 49, 485–494. doi: 10.1093/geront/gnp042

Falkenstein, M., Hohnsbein, J., and Hoormann, J. (1991). Effects of crossmodal divided attention on late ERP components. II. Error processing in choice reaction tasks. *Electroencephalogr. Clin. Neurophysiol.* 78, 447–455. doi: 10.1016/0013-4694(91)90062-9

Falkenstein, M., Hoormann, J., Christ, S., and Hohnsbein, J. (2000). ERP components on reaction errors and their functional significance: a tutorial. *Biol. Psychol.* 51, 87–107. doi: 10.1016/S0301-0511(99)00031-9

Falkenstein, M., Hoormann, J., and Hohnsbein, J. (2001). Changes of error-related ERPs with age. *Exp. Brain Res.* 138, 258–262. doi: 10.1007/s002210100712

Finke, M., Barceló, F., Garolera, M., Cortinas, M., Garrido, G., Pajares, M., et al. (2011). Impaired preparatory re-mapping of stimulus-response associations and rule-implementation in schizophrenic patients—the role for differences in early processing. *Biol. Psychol.* 87, 358–365. doi: 10.1016/j.biopsycho.2011.04.006

Folstein, J. R., and Van Petten, C. (2008). Influence of cognitive control and mismatch on the N2 component of the ERP: a review. *Psychophysiology* 45, 152–170.

Gajewski, P. D., and Falkenstein, M. (2011). Diversity of the P3 in the task-switching paradigm. *Brain Res.* 1411, 87–97. doi: 10.1016/j.brainres.2011.07.010

Gajewski, P. D., and Falkenstein, M. (2012). Training-induced improvement of response selection and error detection in aging assessed by task switching: effects of cognitive, physical and relaxation training. *Front. Hum. Neurosci.* 6:130. doi: 10.3389/fnhum.2012.00130

Gajewski, P. D., and Falkenstein, M. (2015a). Lifelong physical activity and executive functions in older age assessed by memory based task switching. *Neuropsychologia* 73, 195–207. doi: 10.1016/j.neuropsychologia.2015.04.031

Gajewski, P. D., and Falkenstein, M. (2015b). "Lifestyle and interventions for improving cognitive performance in older adults," in *Performance Psychology: Perception, Action, Cognition, and Emotion*, eds M. Raab, B. Lobinger, S. Hoffmann, A. Pizzera, and S. Laborde (Oxford: Elsevier), 189–203.

Gajewski, P. D., Hengstler, J., Golka, K., Falkenstein, M., and Beste, C. (2011). The Met-allele of the BDNF Val66Met polymorphism enhances task switching in elderly. *Neurobiol. Aging* 32, 2327.e7-19. doi: 10.1016/j.neurobiolaging.2011.06.010

Gajewski, P. D., Kleinsorge, T., and Falkenstein, M. (2010a). Electrophysiological correlates of residual switch costs. *Cortex* 46, 1138–1148. doi: 10.1016/j.cortex.2009.07.014

Gajewski, P. D., Stoerig, P., and Falkenstein, M. (2008). ERP—correlates of response selection in a response conflict paradigm. *Brain Res.* 1189, 127–134. doi: 10.1016/j.brainres.2007.10.076

Gajewski, P. D., Wild-Wall, N., Schapkin, S. A., Erdmann, U., Freude, U., and Falkenstein, M. (2010b). Effects of aging and job demands on cognitive flexibility assessed by task switching. *Biol. Psychol.* 85, 187–199. doi: 10.1016/j.biopsycho.2010.06.009

Gehring, W. J., Goss, B., Coles, M. G. H., and Meyer, D. E. (1993). A neural system for error detection and compensation. *Psychol. Sci.* 4, 385–390. doi: 10.1118/1.4868459

Gopher, D., Weil, M., and Bareket, T. (1994). Transfer of skill from a computer game trainer to flight. *Hum. Factors* 36, 387–405.

Gratton, G., Coles, M. G. H., and Donchin, E. (1983). A new method for off-line removal of ocular artifact. *Electroencephalogr. Clin. Neurophysiol.* 55, 468–484. doi: 10.1016/0013-4694(83)90135-9

Green, C. S., and Bavelier, D. (2008). Exercising your brain: a review of human brain plasticity and training-induced learning. *Psychol. Aging* 23, 692–701. doi: 10.1037/a0014345

Hagger, M. S., Wood, C., Stiff, C., and Chatzisarantis, N. L. D. (2010). Ego depletion and the strength model of self-control: a meta-analysis. *Psychol. Bull.* 136, 495–525. doi: 10.1037/a0019486

Hämmerer, D., Müller, V., and Li, S. C. (2014). Performance monitoring across the lifespan: still maturing post-conflict regulation in children and declining task-set monitoring in older adults. *Neurosci. Biobehav. Rev.* 46, 105–123. doi: 10.1016/j.neubiorev.2014.06.008

Hillman, C. H., Kramer, A. F., Belopolsky, A. V., and Smith, D. P. (2006). A cross-sectional examination of age and physical activity on performance and event-related brain potentials in a task switching paradigm. *Int. J. Psychophysiol.* 59, 30–39. doi: 10.1016/j.ijpsycho.2005.04.009

Holroyd, C. B., and Coles, M. G. H. (2002). The neural basis of human error processing: reinforcement learning, dopamine, and the error-related negativity. *Psychol. Rev.* 109, 679–709. doi: 10.1037/0033-295X.109.4.679

Hultsch, D. F., Hertzog, C., Small, B. J., and Dixon, R. A. (1999). Use it or lose it: engaged lifestyle as a buffer of cognitive decline in aging? *Psychol. Aging* 14, 245–263. doi: 10.1037/0882-7974.14.2.245

Ilmarinen, J. (2006). The ageing workforce—challenges for occupational health. *Occup. Med.* 56, 362–364. doi: 10.1093/occmed/kql046

Jaeggi, S. M., Buschkuehl, M., Jonides, J., and Perrig, W. J. (2008). Improving fluid intelligence with training on working memory. *Proc. Natl. Acad. Sci. U.S.A.* 105, 6829–6833. doi: 10.1073/pnas.0801268105

Jost, K., Mayr, U., and Rösler, F. (2008). Is task switching nothing but cue priming? Evidence from ERPs. *Cogn. Affect. Behav. Neurosci.* 8, 74–84. doi: 10.3758/CABN.8.1.74

Karayanidis, F., Whitson, L. R., Heathcote, A., and Michie, P. T. (2011). Variability in proactive and reactive cognitive control processes across the adult lifespan. *Front. Psychol.* 2:318. doi: 10.3389/fpsyg.2011.00318

Karbach, J., and Kray, J. (2009). How useful is executive control training? Age differences in near and far transfer of task-switching training. *Dev. Sci.* 12, 978–990. doi: 10.1111/j.1467-7687.2009.00846.x

Karbach, J., and Verhaeghen, P. (2014). Making working memory work: a meta-analysis of executivecontrol and working memory training in older adults. *Psychol. Sci.* 25, 2027–2037. doi: 10.1177/0956797614548725

Kelly, M. E., Loughrey, D., Lawlor, B. A., Robertson, I. H., Walsh, C., and Brennan, S. (2014). The impact of exercise on the cognitive functioning of healthy older adults: asystematic review and meta-analysis. *Ageing Res. Rev.* 16, 12–31. doi: 10.1016/j.arr.2014.05.002

Kieffaber, P. D., and Hetrick, W. P. (2005). Event-related potential correlates of task switching and switch costs. *Psychophysiology* 42, 56–71. doi: 10.1111/j.1469-8986.2005.00262.x

Kok, A. (2001). On the utility of P3 amplitude as a measure of processing capacity. *Psychophysiology* 38, 557–577. doi: 10.1017/S0048577201990559

Kramer, A. F., and Morrow, D. (2008). "Cognitive training and expertise," in *Cognitive Aging: A Primer*, 2nd Edn, eds D. Park and N. Schwarz (New York, NY: Psychology Press).

Lampit, A., Hallock, H., and Valenzuela, M. J. (2014). Computerized cognitive training in cognitively healthy older adults: a systematic review and meta-analysis of effect modifiers. *PLoS Med.* 11:e1001756. doi: 10.1371/journal.pmed.1001756

Lee, Y., Back, J. H., Kim, J., and Byeon, H. (2010). Multiple socioeconomic risks and cognitive impairment in older adults. *Dement. Geriatr. Cogn. Disord.* 29, 523–529. doi: 10.1159/000315507

Lehrl, S., Lehrl, M., and Weickmann, E. (1994). *MAT Gehirnjogging, Einführung in das Mentale AktivierungsTraining.* Ebersberg: Vless Verlag.

Lorist, M. M., Klein, M., Nieuwenhuis, S., De Jong, R., Mulder, G., and Meijman, T. F. (2000). Mental fatigue and task control: planning and preparation. *Psychophysiology* 37, 614–625. doi: 10.1111/1469-8986.3750614

Marquié, J. C., Duarte, L. R., Bessieres, P., Dalm, C., Gentil, C., and Ruidavets, B. (2010). Higher mental stimulation at work is associated with improved cognitive functioning in both young and older workers. *Ergonomics* 53, 1287–1301. doi: 10.1080/00140139.2010.519125

Nieuwenhuis, S., Aston-Jones, G., and Cohen, J. D. (2005). Decision making, the P3, and the locus coeruleus-norepinephrine system. *Psychol. Bull.* 131, 510–532. doi: 10.1037/0033-2909.131.4.510

Polich, J. (2007). Updating P300: an integrative theory of P3a and P3b. *Clin. Neurophysiol.* 118, 2128–2148. doi: 10.1016/j.clinph.2007.04.019

Polich, J., and Lardon, M. T. (1997). P300 and long-term physical exercise. *Electroencephalogr. Clin. Neurophysiol.* 103, 493–498. doi: 10.1016/S0013-4694(97)96033-8

Potter, G. G., Helms, M. J., and Plassman, B. L. (2008). Associations of job demands and intelligence with cognitive performance among men in late life. *Neurology* 70, 1803–1808. doi: 10.1212/01.wnl.0000295506.58497.7e

Ritter, W., Simson, R., Vaughan, H. G. Jr., and Friedman, D. (1979). A brain event related to the making of a sensory discrimination. *Science* 203, 1358–1361. doi: 10.1126/science.424760

Rushworth, M. F., Passingham, R. E., and Nobre, A. C. (2002). Components of switching intentional set. *J. Cogn. Neurosci.* 14, 1139–1150. doi: 10.1162/089892902760807159

Schapkin, S. A., Gajewski, P. D., and Freude, G. (2014). Age differences in memory-based task switching with and without cues: an ERP study. *J. Psychophysiol.* 28, 187–201. doi: 10.1027/0269-8803/a000125

Schooler, C., and Mulatu, M. S. (2001). The reciprocal effects of leisure time activities and intellectual functioning in older people: a longitudinal analysis. *Psychol. Aging* 16, 466–482. doi: 10.1037/0882-7974.16.3.466

Schooler, C., Mulatu, M. S., and Oates, G. (1999). The continuing effects of substantively complex work on the intellectual functioning of older workers. *Psychol. Aging* 14, 483–506. doi: 10.1037/0882-7974.14.3.483

Singh-Manoux, A., Richards, M., and Marmot, M. (2003). Leisure activities and cognitive function in middle age: evidence from the Whitehall II study. *J. Epidemiol. Comm. Health* 57, 907–913. doi: 10.1136/jech.57.11.907

Sparks, K., Faragher, B., and Cooper, C. L. (2001). Well-being and occupational health in the 21st century workplace. *J. Occup. Organiz. Psychol.* 74, 489–509. doi: 10.1348/096317901167497

Steele, V. R., Anderson, N. E., Claus, E. D., Bernat, E. M., Rao, V., Assaf, M., et al. (2016). Neuroimaging measures of error-processing: extracting reliable signals from event-related potentials and functional magnetic resonance imaging. *Neuroimage* 132, 247–260. doi: 10.1016/j.neuroimage.2016.02.046

Stern, Y. (2009). Cognitive reserve. *Neuropsychologia* 47, 2015–2028. doi: 10.1016/j.neuropsychologia.2009.03.004

Stern, Y., Gurland, B., Tatemichi, T. K., Tang, M. X., Wilder, D., and Mayeux, R. (1994). Influence of education and occupation on the incidence of Alzheimer's disease. *JAMA* 271, 1004–1010. doi: 10.1001/jama.1994.03510370056032

Strobach, T., and Karbach, J. (2016). *Cognitive Training: An Overview of Features and Applications.* Berlin: Springer-Verlag. doi: 10.1007/978-3-319-42662-4

Swaab, D. F., and Bao, A. M. (2011). (Re-) activation of neurons in aging and dementia: lessons from the hypothalamus. *Exp. Gerontol.* 46, 178–184. doi: 10.1016/j.exger.2010.08.028

Van Veen, V., and Carter, C. S. (2002). The timing of action-monitoring processes in the anterior cingulate cortex. *J. Cogn. Neurosci.* 14, 593–602. doi: 10.1162/08989290260045837

Verleger, R., Jaskowski, P., and Wascher, E. (2006). Evidence for an integrative role of P3b in linking reaction to perception. *Int. J. Psychophysiol.* 19, 165–181. doi: 10.1027/0269-8803.19.3.165

Wild-Wall, N., Falkenstein, M., and Gajewski, P. D. (2012). Neural correlates of changes in a visual search task due to cognitive training. *Neural Plast.* 2012:529057. doi: 10.1155/2012/529057

Wild-Wall, N., Gajewski, P. D., and Falkenstein, M. (2009). Kognitive leistungsfähigkeit älterer arbeitnehmer. *Z. Gerontol. Geriatr.* 42, 299–304. doi: 10.1007/s00391-009-0045-5

Willis, S. L., and Schaie, K. W. (1986). Training the elderly on the ability factors of spatial orientation and inductive reasoning. *Psychol. Aging* 1, 239–247. doi: 10.1037/0882-7974.1.3.239

Willis, S. L., Tennstedt, S. L., Marsiske, M., Ball, K., Elias, J., Koepke, K. M., et al. (2006). ACTIVE study group. long-term effects of cognitive training on everyday functional outcomes in older adults. *JAMA* 296, 2805–2814. doi: 10.1001/jama.296.23.2805

Wilson, R. S., Beckett, L. A., Bennett, D. A., Albert, M. S., and Evans, D. A. (1999). Change in cognitive function in older persons from a community population: relation to age and Alzheimer disease. *Arch. Neurol.* 56, 1274–1279. doi: 10.1001/archneur.56.10.1274

Yeung, N., and Cohen, J. D. (2006). Impact of cognitive deficits on conflict monitoring. Predictable dissociations between the error related negativity and N2. *Psychol. Sci.* 17, 164–171. doi: 10.1111/j.1467-9280.2006.01680.x

Yordanova, J., Falkenstein, M., Hohnsbein, J., and Kolev, V. (2004). Parallel systems of error processing in the brain. *Neuroimage* 22, 590–602. doi: 10.1016/j.neuroimage.2004.01.040

11

Music Games: Potential Application and Considerations for Rhythmic Training

Valentin Bégel[1,2], Ines Di Loreto[3], Antoine Scilles[2] and Simone Dalla Bella[1,4,5,6]**

[1]Euromov Laboratory, University of Montpellier, Montpellier, France, [2]NaturalPad, Montpellier, France, [3]Homme, Environnement et Technologies de l'Information, Université de Technologie de Troyes, Troyes, France, [4]Institut Universitaire de France, Paris, France, [5]International Laboratory for Brain, Music and Sound Research (BRAMS), Montreal, QC, Canada, [6]Department of Cognitive Psychology, Wyższa Szkoła Finansów i Zarzadzanią w Warszawie (WSFiZ), Warsaw, Poland

Edited by:
Louis Bherer,
Université de Montréal, Canada

Reviewed by:
Katja Kornysheva,
University College London,
United Kingdom
Michael Thaut,
Colorado State University,
United States

***Correspondence:**
Valentin Bégel
valentin.begel@umontpellier.fr
Simone Dalla Bella
simone.dalla-bella@umontpellier.fr

Rhythmic skills are natural and widespread in the general population. The majority can track the beat of music and move along with it. These abilities are meaningful from a cognitive standpoint given their tight links with prominent motor and cognitive functions such as language and memory. When rhythmic skills are challenged by brain damage or neurodevelopmental disorders, remediation strategies based on rhythm can be considered. For example, rhythmic training can be used to improve motor performance (e.g., gait) as well as cognitive and language skills. Here, we review the games readily available in the market and assess whether they are well-suited for rhythmic training. Games that train rhythm skills may serve as useful tools for retraining motor and cognitive functions in patients with motor or neurodevelopmental disorders (e.g., Parkinson's disease, dyslexia, or ADHD). Our criteria were the peripheral used to capture and record the response, the type of response and the output measure. None of the existing games provides sufficient temporal precision in stimulus presentation and/or data acquisition. In addition, games do not train selectively rhythmic skills. Hence, the available music games, in their present form, are not satisfying for training rhythmic skills. Yet, some features such as the device used, the interface or the game scenario provide good indications for devising efficient training protocols. Guidelines are provided for devising serious music games targeting rhythmic training in the future.

Keywords: rhythm, serious game, rehabilitation, movement, training

INTRODUCTION

Musical Rhythm as a Training Tool

Humans display a natural tendency to move, spontaneously or deliberately, to the beat of rhythmic auditory stimuli, such as music (Repp, 2005; Repp and Su, 2013). This activity is widespread and is typically participatory. It manifests, for example, in dance, synchronized sport, and in group activities (e.g., waving together at a rock concert). Synchronization to a musical beat is sustained by a complex neuronal network, including perceptual regions (the superior temporal gyrus; Thaut, 2003; Chen et al., 2008a; Schwartze and Kotz, 2013), motor regions (e.g., the basal ganglia and the cerebellum; Grahn and Brett, 2007; Chen et al., 2008b; Grahn and Rowe, 2009), as well as sensorimotor integration areas (e.g., premotor cortex; Chen et al., 2006; Zatorre et al., 2007; Kornysheva and Schubotz, 2011). Disruption of these neuronal networks due to brain damage or neurodevelopmental disorder affects auditory-motor synchronization to a musical beat (Corriveau and Goswami, 2009; Bégel et al., 2017), as well as other functions such as speech. For example, difficulties encountered by individuals who stutter in speech production extend to non-verbal sensorimotor skills (Watkins et al., 2008; Falk et al., 2015). In speech production tasks, individual who stutter display reduced activity in brain regions that are also responsible for beat tracking and synchronization to a musical beat such as the basal ganglia (Civier et al., 2013), and the cerebellum (Brown et al., 2005).

Notably, tracking the beat does not require mandatorily an explicit motor response. In perceptual tasks, when detecting a deviation from the beat in an isochronous sequence (anisochrony detection; Ehrlé and Samson, 2005; Dalla Bella et al., 2017b), or detecting if a metronome is aligned or not to the beat (Beat Alignement Task, Iversen and Patel, 2008), the beat is extracted from the auditory signal to perform the judgment. Interestingly, beat extraction in the absence of an explicit motor response recruits motor regions of the brain, such as the basal ganglia (Grahn and Brett, 2007; Grahn and Rowe, 2009), or premotor cortex (Chen et al., 2008a,b). It is worth noting that processing sequences with an underlying beat engages partly separate mechanisms (beat-based timing), as compared to treating single durations (duration-based timing; Coull et al., 2011). The former rely on basal-ganglia-cortical mechanisms, while the latter are more associated to cerebellar-cortical pathways (Grube et al., 2010; Teki et al., 2011). For the purposes of this short review we focus in particular on the training of rhythmic skills engaging beat-based mechanisms.

Because mere listening to an auditory rhythm, for example conveyed via music, activates movement-related areas of the brain, training with rhythmic stimuli may be beneficial to (re)activate the motor system in the damaged and in the healthy brain. There are a few examples of the beneficial effects of rhythm on motor behavior. Rhythmic auditory stimulation can be used as a tool to retrain gait in Parkinson disease (e.g., for increasing speed and stride length; Thaut et al., 1996; Thaut and Abiru, 2010; Benoit et al., 2014; Dalla Bella et al., 2015, 2017a), to improve arm function in stroke (Thaut et al., 1997, 2002, 2007), or to enhance physical performance in sport (e.g., by reducing oxygen consumption in cycling; Hoffmann et al., 2012; Bardy et al., 2015). Positive effects of rhythmic training are not confined to motor behavior, but can extend to perception (Benoit et al., 2014; Dalla Bella et al., 2015). Stimulation using auditory rhythms shows promise also for training speech perception in children with Developmental Language Disorders (e.g., for syntax processing, Przybylski et al., 2013; Schön and Tillmann, 2015). In sum, previous studies point to beneficial effects of a rhythmic training protocol on movement and cognition. In addition, as rhythmic skills are linked to other cognitive abilities such as working memory and reading skills (Tierney and Kraus, 2013; Woodruff Carr et al., 2014), rhythmic training may foster improvements of more general cognitive abilities, which play a critical role in language learning and literacy (Schwartze and Kotz, 2013; Gordon et al., 2015; Kotz and Gunter, 2015). Ultimately, these beneficial effects of rhythmic training are likely to have positive consequences for health and well-being, such as promoting an active lifestyle, by reducing motor and cognitive decline in patient populations or reducing the need for healthcare services.

Serious Games

A great deal of work over the last two decades has been devoted to devise and promote games for training patients and for rehabilitation. This stream of research has been encouraged by low-cost and widespread new technologies offering unprecedented opportunities to implement training protocols. An increasing number of technologies are designed to improve health and well-being, from smartphone applications to control dietetics (Withings *Wi-Fi Scales*) to movement-based rehabilitation tools using motion capture (Zhou and Hu, 2008; Weiss et al., 2009; Chang et al., 2011). Among them, video games provide a way to entertain people while targeting serious goals, such as the rehabilitation of impaired movement skills (e.g., *Hammer and Planks,* Di Loreto et al., 2013; *Nintendo Wii* games, Saposnik et al., 2010) or cognitive re-entrainment (e.g., *RehaCom,* Fernández et al., 2012) in neurological diseases (for a review and classification of serious games in health, see Rego et al., 2010). In particular, movement-based rehabilitation games exploiting motion capture devices such as the *Wii* or the *Kinect* are a promising way to use technology in the context of re-education (for a review see Webster and Celik, 2014). This method is referred to as "Exergaming". Note that video games for entertainment may also be used in a serious manner. For example, off-the-shelf video games are often used by physicians for therapeutic purposes, such as *Nintendo Wii* or *Kinect* games (Lange et al., 2009; Barry et al., 2014; Karahan et al., 2015). Exergaming has been proven as efficient in stroke (Webster and Celik, 2014), Parkinson's disease (Harris et al., 2015), as well as in healthy elderly adults (Sun and Lee, 2013).

During the last 5 years, studies have focused on the cognitive and neuronal underpinnings of the benefits linked to health-targeted serious games (Connolly et al., 2012). On top of the physical and physiological benefits associated with serious games (e.g., via dedicated physiotherapeutic exercises), the effects of this type of training extend to cognition. Cognitive functions such as language and memory can also be enhanced by serious games, an effect which is likely to be accompanied by plastic changes of the brain. For example, structural brain changes associated with learning have been observed due to the use of videogames (Anguera et al., 2013). These promising results indicate that implementing training protocols via serious games may be particularly valuable for enhancing brain functions as well as for therapy and rehabilitation.

In summary, serious games and rhythmic stimulation are promising tools that can be exploited to improve or retrain movement and cognition. We propose that a training of rhythm skills implemented in a serious game would be a means to set up training protocols which may serve rehabilitation of different patient populations. The aim of this review article is to provide an overview of the existing rhythm games and to assess whether they could be well-suited for training purposes. We conducted a survey in which we used criteria such as the precision of the recorded response or the modality of the stimuli provided to evaluate the benefits and limitations of each game.

LIMITS AND ADVANTAGES OF THE EXISTING RHYTHM GAMES

To the best of our knowledge, only one music-based training program that uses a game setting has been successfully devised for arm rehabilitation in stroke patients (Friedman et al., 2011, 2014). However, this protocol is not training rhythmic skills *per se* but is rather a music-based adaptation of a standard rehabilitation protocol (i.e., conventional tabletop exercises therapy; Dickstein et al., 1986). To examine whether existing games involving rhythm conveyed by auditory stimuli could be potentially used as training tools, we selected games based on the following inclusion criteria. First, the game has to focus on rhythmic skills. The player must be instructed to synchronize movement (or voice) with stimuli (auditory or visual) which can be predicted on the basis of their temporal structure (i.e., the underlying beat). To our knowledge, no rhythm games currently on the market use purely perceptual tasks, in which the player's task is to judge the rhythmic features of music. All the games presented below involve movement synchronized to auditory or visual cues. Second, the game device must record the temporal precision of the player's responses. The scores, levels, difficulty and feedback given to the player must depend on her/his temporal precision in performing the movement. Once the games were selected, they were categorized by: (a) the peripheral used to capture and record the response; (b) the type of response that is recorded; and (c) the output. The peripheral is important to judge if the game is readily usable for training (e.g., in a clinical context). In addition, note that most of the studies in cognitive psychology of rhythm use finger tapping, since this is a simple and objective way to study rhythmic skills (Repp, 2005; Repp and Su, 2013), but other reponses are possible (e.g., full-body motion). Finally, the output is relevant as it indicates whether the games provide a feedback (an outcome measure or score) on the precision of the performance reflecting a participant's rhythmic skills. These categories are helpful for evaluating the therapeutic potential of each game. For example, a game requiring finger tapping is likely to have a different effect on behavior than a game requiring full body motion, such as dance.

Twenty-seven games on a variety of devices (Wii, PlayStation, PC, Tablet/Smartphone, Xbox, Gameboy) fulfilling the aforementioned criteria were considered for the analysis (see **Table 1**). These games were classified in four categories as indicated below.

Games that Involve Full Body Movements Recorded via an External Interface (e.g., Kinect, Wii)

Here we refer mostly to dance games (e.g., *Just Dance*). These games have interesting applications in physiotherapy for patients with spinal cord injury, traumatic brain injury and stroke (Lange et al., 2009). They focus more on physical exercise and activity than on rhythm *per se*. Indeed, the ability of these games to record and score the rhythmic precision of the player is rather poor. Because these games focus on discrete movements/actions instead of repeated movements (i.e., rhythmic) they cannot be used for delivering specific training of rhythmic skills. For example, *Just Dance* consists in reproducing movements that are illustrated through images displayed on the screen. The player's score depends on the precision of the movements as compared to a model action sequence. The player has to execute the movements in a given temporal window. Yet, the task is not purely rhythmic and synchronization to the musical beat is not recorded. In spite of the fact that these games do not measure rhythmic skills *per se*, they provide a motivating setting to perform dance while monitoring the player's movements. Adding a rhythm component to some of these games, as in the case of dance, may be a valuable strategy to translate them into a training program.

Games that Involve Rhythmic Finger Tapping on a Tablet

An example of these games is *Beat Sneak Bandit*. Here, the player has to tap precisely to the beat in order to make the character progress, avoid the enemies and so forth. This kind of feature is used in serious games dedicated to learning, such as *Rhythm Cat*, designed to learn music rhythm notation. For the purposes of training rhythmic skills, one major drawback of these games is that the timing precision of the software is very poor. The time window in which a response is considered as good is very wide (i.e., up to several hundreds of milliseconds) and the temporal variability of the recording is high. In addition, no feedback on the rhythmic performance of the player is provided.

Computer or Console Games that Involve Finger Tapping on Keys

These games can be played on a keyboard, using a joystick, or on special devices. One of the most famous is *Guitar Hero*. In this game the player plays on a guitar replica with five keys, and has to push the keys in correspondence of images presented on a screen. Rhythm precision of the responses is recorded and used to compute a performance score. The response must appear in a specific temporal window to be considered as good. The same concept is used in many PC games, but keyboards key (e.g., arrows) are used instead of guitar replica. As in the case of tablet games, the main weakness of these games is their low temporal precision in recording rhythmic performance (around 100 ms in *Guitar Hero*). Nevertheless, these games are interesting as they represent a good starting point to develop serious-game applications aimed at training rhythmic skills.

Console Games Involving Singing

In these games, the player is asked to sing in synchrony with the music. This is not a rhythmic task *per se*, but the performance involves a rhythmic component. As in classical karaoke, lyrics are presented on the screen. In this case, a feedback (score) is provided to the player while she/he sings and a final global score is given at the end of the performance, including temporal precision (the response must appear in a given temporal window to be considered as good) but also pitch precision. Here, the potential benefit for health rests upon the fact that singing is

TABLE 1 | List of the reviewed rhythm-based games.

Game	Peripheral	Type of response recorded	Output
Dance revolution/dancing stage	Dance pad (PS2, PC)	Impacts of feet (PS2)/fingers (PC)	Incrementing score
Donkey konga	Bongos	Impacts of hands	Incrementing score
Dancing with the star	Wiimote, Nunchuk (Wii), keyboard (PC)	Hands movement (Wiimote), Key tapping (PC)	Incrementing score
DJ hero	Turntable replica (Wii, PS 2 and 3, Xbox 360)	Hands and fingers movement on the Turntable	Incrementing score
Everyone sing	Microphone (Wii, PS 3, Xbox 360)	Voice	Incrementing score
Guitar hero	Guitar replica, joystick (Wii, PS 3, Xbox 360), keyboard (PC), screen (tablet, Androïd)	Left-hand key tapping, right-hand key moving up and down (Wii, PS3, Xbox 360), screen tapping (tablet), joystick button pressing (Wiimote, pS3, Xbox 360)	Incrementing score
Just dance	Wiimote (Wii), PS camera, PS move (PS4, PS3), Kinect (Xbox 360, Xbox one)	Hand movement (Wiimote), all-body movement (PS move, PS camera, Kinect)	Incrementing score
Rhythm paradise (USA: Rhythm Heaven Fever)	Nintendo DS, Wiimote	Finger tapping on the screen, hand movement (stylus; DS), key tapping (Wii)	Incrementing score
Rock band	Guitar, Drums replica, Microphone (Wii, Xbox 360, PS3), Tactile screen (Iphone, Ipod Touch), Nintendo DS, PSP	Left-hand key tapping, right-hand key moving up and down (mediator-like), feet impact (bass drum), drumsticks impact (Wii, PS3, Xbox 360, Nintendo DS, PSP), screen tapping (Iphone, Ipod), joystick button pressing (Wiimote, pS3, Xbox 360), voice (microphone)	Incrementing score
140	Keyboard (PC)	Key pressing	Progression in a level
Osu	Mouse (PC)	Key pressing	Incrementing score
Beatmania	Turntable replica (Arcade, PS1, PS2), Nintendo gameboy	Hands and fingers movement on the Turntable (Arcade, PS1, PS2), key pressing (Gameboy color)	Incrementing score
Patapon	PSP	Key tapping	Progression in a level
Rhythm cat	Tablet, Smartphone	Screen tapping, holding, swiping	Incrementing score
Groove coaster zero	Tablet, Smartphone	Screen tapping, holding, swiping	Incrementing score
Igobeat	Tablet, Smartphone	Screen tapping, holding, swiping	Incrementing score
Beat brite	Tablet, Smartphone	Screen tapping, holding, swiping	Incrementing score
Online PC games	Keyboard	Screen tapping	Progression in a level/Incrementing score

The last row concerns online PC games (available at www.musicgames.co/games-by-category/rhythm-games/) having similar characteristics.

a good way to restore speech abilities (e.g., fluency) in aphasia following stroke (for example, see Norton et al., 2009).

Even though some of the aforementioned games present good ground for training rhythmic skills, their main drawback is that their temporal precision when recording movement relative to the beat is rather poor. Thus, the output measures provided by these games are insufficient to isolate rhythmic features of the performance (e.g., variability of the motor performance, precision of the synchronization with the beat, etc.). Moreover, in none of these games the rhythmic complexity of musical stimuli has been manipulated. Difficulty is manipulated only through the amount of responses required during the game (e.g., number of visual tags which the player has to react to) which is not a rhythmical feature. For example, using music with various degrees of beat saliency would allow introducing rhythm-based difficulty levels in the game. This has the advantage that rhythms with increased complexity could be presented progressively throughout the game, thus potentially leading to improved beat-tracking skills.

CONCLUSION

We reviewed 27 rhythm-based games already in the market that could be used in a rhythmic training protocol. Unfortunately, based on our criteria, none of the aforementioned games is satisfying for this purpose. First, in most of the games, the task consists in reacting to visual stimulations while music is presented. Thus rhythmic skills are not selectively trained. Second, the number of stimuli, instead of the rhythmic characteristics of the music, is varied to change the difficulty of the game. Third, in spite of the fact that the regularity of rhythmic patterns can influence the performance in the game, the response provided by the player is not targeted at the rhythmic aspects of the stimuli. For example, the player touches the screen at the right moment to catch objects or makes full-body movements to imitate model-actions in dance games. In addition, note that the reviewed games do not offer opportunities for controlled functional movement training. For example, none of them provide a guidance to achieve desired movement trajectories. This problem may be overcome in the future by providing relevant feedback when the player approaches optimal movement trajectories (e.g., via sonification, Effenberg et al., 2016). The tasks implemented in these games are vaguely reminiscent of implicit timing tasks (Lee, 1976; Zelaznik et al., 2002; Coull and Nobre, 2008). Explicit and implicit timing have been treated as relatively independent processes in cognitive neuroscience (Zelaznik et al., 2002; Coull and Nobre, 2008; Coull et al., 2011). The former is associated with tasks requiring voluntary motor production (e.g., synchronized tapping tasks; Repp, 2005; Repp and Su, 2013) or overt estimation of stimulus duration (e.g., duration discrimination; Grondin, 1993). In contrast, implicit timing is tested with tasks unrelated to timing (e.g., avoiding a vehicle when crossing the road), but in which temporal prediction affects the performance (judging the time before the vehicle reaches us; Lee, 1976; for more details, see Nobre et al., 2007; Coull and Nobre, 2008; Coull, 2009). In particular, temporal prediction fostered by a regular temporal pattern (e.g., a metronome) of sensory stimuli improves performance in non-temporal tasks (e.g., working memory, Cutanda et al., 2015; pitch judgment, Jones et al., 2002; language judgments, Przybylski et al., 2013).

Despite the available music games are not explicitely targeted at rhythmic training, they may still foster training timing implicitly, in combination with other more explicit processes (e.g., focusing on spatial and pitch accuracy). There is evidence that the implicit dimension of timing may be more robust than explicit timing, for example in beat deafness (Bégel et al., 2017). It is possible that participants with timing disorders (e.g., Parkinson's disease or developmental stuttering; Grahn and Brett, 2009; Falk et al., 2015) may still be able to capitalize on partly spared implicit timing functions to re-learn rhythmic skills via a training program. Note, however, that so far beneficial effects of rhythm-based training protocols typically made use of explicit timing tasks (e.g., walking with an auditory rhythm; e.g., Lim et al., 2005; Spaulding et al., 2013; Benoit et al., 2014). This may suggest that tasks which recruit explicit timing mechanisms may be a particularly good candidate to build a successful protocol for rhythmic training. In only one of the reviewed games (*Beat Sneak Bandit*), the goal was to tap to the beat of music, which is an explicit timing task. In sum, almost all of the reviewed games do not require participants to perform explicitly rhythmic tasks. Yet, they are likely to engage implicit timing mechanisms. Whether training rhythm implicitely in the context of a music game can lead to positive effects comparable to those found with explicit rhythmic tasks deserves further enquiry.

In summary, the games currently on the market, albeit they are not optimal for rhythmic training, provide at least interesting ideas that might pave the ground to devise successful training programs. Games on portable devices (e.g., tablets or smartphones) using tapping to the beat provide the simplest solution to implement a rhythm training protocol. They are low-cost while offering a motivating and user-friendly environment to train rhythmic skills with a playful interface. Although this solution has some potential, there are two problems. The precision of movement recording relative to the beat, and the ensuing measures of rhythm precision, need significant improvement. To deal with these issues, methods used to analyze synchronization to the beat in the neurosciences of rhythm (Kirschner and Tomasello, 2009; Pecenka and Keller, 2009; Woodruff Carr et al., 2014; Dalla Bella et al., 2017b) should be applied to games designed for rhythm training. In addition, estimations of timekeeper and motor implementation variance (e.g., based on tapping performance) might allow to refine the feedback on the performance (e.g., Schulze and Vorberg, 2002; for a review see, Wing, 2002). This will ensure that a precise feedback on the rhythmic performance can be provided and that the stimuli and game progression can be tailored to individual learning curves. Moreover, to ensure that the training program specifically targets rhythmic skills, stimulus (or response) will have to be varied in terms of rhythmic difficulty. This can be achieved, for example, by selecting musical excerpts based on their rhythmic complexity. Using stimuli with increasing difficulty in beat tracking (e.g., with a less salient beat) throughout the game might allow to progressively fine tune the player's rhythmic skills. These guidelines should be taken into account in the future to devise efficient protocols for training rhythmic skills via serious music games.

AUTHOR CONTRIBUTIONS

VB and SDB conceived the study; VB conducted the survey; VB, IDL and AS contributed to data analysis; all authors contributed to the writing of the manuscript.

ACKNOWLEDGMENTS

We wish to thank two reviewers for their insightful comments on a first draft of the manuscript.

REFERENCES

Anguera, J. A., Boccanfuso, J., Rintoul, J. L., Al-Hashimi, O., Faraji, F., Janowich, J., et al. (2013). Video game training enhances cognitive control in older adults. *Nature* 501, 97–101. doi: 10.1038/nature12486

Bardy, B. G., Hoffmann, C. P., Moens, B., Leman, M., and Dalla Bella, S. (2015). Sound-induced stabilization of breathing and moving. *Ann. N Y Acad. Sci.* 1337, 94–100. doi: 10.1111/nyas.12650

Barry, G., Galna, B., and Rochester, L. (2014). The role of exergaming in Parkinson's disease rehabilitation: a systematic review of the evidence. *J. Neuroeng. Rehabil.* 11:33. doi: 10.1186/1743-0003-11-33

Bégel, V., Benoit, C.-E., Correa, A., Cutanda, D., Kotz, S. A., and Dalla Bella, S. (2017). "Lost in time" but still moving to the beat. *Neuropsychologia* 94, 129–138. doi: 10.1016/j.neuropsychologia.2016.11.022

Benoit, C.-E., Dalla Bella, S., Farrugia, N., Obrig, H., Mainka, S., and Kotz, S. A. (2014). Musically cued gait-graining improves both perceptual and motor timing in Parkinson's disease. *Front. Hum. Neurosci.* 8:494. doi: 10.3389/fnhum.2014.00494

Brown, S., Ingham, R. J., Ingham, J. C., Laird, A. R., and Fox, P. T. (2005). Stuttered and fluent speech production: an ALE meta-analysis of functional neuroimaging studies. *Hum. Brain Mapp.* 25, 105–117. doi: 10.1002/hbm.20140

Chang, Y. J., Chen, S. F., and Huang, J. D. (2011). A kinect-based system for physical rehabilitation: a pilot study for young adults with motor disabilities. *Res. Dev. Disabil.* 32, 2566–2570. doi: 10.1016/j.ridd.2011.07.002

Chen, J. L., Zatorre, R. J., and Penhune, V. B. (2006). Interactions between auditory and dorsal premotor cortex during synchronization to musical rhythms. *Neuroimage* 32, 1771–1781. doi: 10.1016/j.neuroimage.2006.04.207

Chen, J. L., Penhune, V. B., and Zatorre, R. J. (2008a). Moving on time: brain network for auditory-motor synchronization is modulated by rhythm complexity and musical training. *J. Cogn. Neurosci.* 20, 226–239. doi: 10.1162/jocn.2008.20018

Chen, J. L., Penhune, V. B., and Zatorre, R. J. (2008b). Listening to musical rhythms recruits motor regions of the brain. *Cereb. Cortex* 18, 2844–2854. doi: 10.1093/cercor/bhn042

Civier, O., Bullock, D., Max, L., and Guenther, F. H. (2013). Computational modeling of stuttering caused by impairments in a basal ganglia thalamo-cortical circuit involved in syllable selection and initiation. *Brain Lang.* 126, 263–278. doi: 10.1016/j.bandl.2013.05.016

Connolly, T. M., Boyle, E. A., MacArthur, E., Hainey, T., and Boyle, J. M. (2012). A systematic literature review of empirical evidence on computer games and serious games. *Comput. Educ.* 59, 661–686. doi: 10.1016/j.compedu.2012.03.004

Corriveau, K. H., and Goswami, U. (2009). Rhythmic motor entrainment in children with speech and language impairments: tapping to the beat. *Cortex* 45, 119–130. doi: 10.1016/j.cortex.2007.09.008.

Coull, J. T. (2009). Neural substrates of mounting temporal expectation. *PLoS Biol.* 7:e1000166. doi: 10.1371/journal.pbio.1000166

Coull, J. T., Cheng, R. K., and Meck, W. H. (2011). Neuroanatomical and neurochemical substrates of timing. *Neuropsychopharmacology* 36, 3–25. doi: 10.1038/npp.2010.113

Coull, J. T., and Nobre, A. C. (2008). Dissociating explicit timing from temporal expectation with fMRI. *Curr. Opin. Neurobiol.* 18, 137–144. doi: 10.1016/j.conb.2008.07.011

Cutanda, D., Correa, Á., and Sanabria, D. (2015). Auditory temporal preparation induced by rhythmic cues during concurrent auditory working memory tasks. *J. Exp. Psychol. Hum. Percept. Perform.* 41, 790–797. doi: 10.1037/a0039167

Dalla Bella, S., Benoit, C.-E., Farrugia, N., Schwartze, M., and Kotz, S. A. (2015). Effects of musically cued gait training in Parkinson's disease: beyond a motor benefit. *Ann. N Y Acad. Sci.* 1337, 77–85. doi: 10.1111/nyas.12651

Dalla Bella, S., Benoit, C.-E., Farrugia, N., Keller, P. E., Obrig, H., Mainka, S., et al. (2017a). Gait improvement via rhythmic stimulation in Parkinson's disease is linked to rhythmic skills. *Sci. Rep.* 7:42005. doi: 10.1038/srep42005

Dalla Bella, S., Farrugia, N., Benoit, C. -E., Begel, V., Verga, L., Harding, E., et al. (2017b). BAASTA: battery for the assessment of auditory sensorimotor and timing abilities. *Behav. Res. Methods* 49, 1128–1145. doi: 10.3758/s13428-016-0773-6

Di Loreto, I., Lange, B., Seilles, A., Andary, S., and Dyce, W. (2013). "Game design for all: the example of hammer and planks a game for rehabilitation purposes or a game for all?" in *4th International Conference on Serious Games Development and Applications (SGDA), LNCS 323 8101*, (Norway), 70–75.

Dickstein, R., Hocherman, S., Pillar, T., and Shaham, R. (1986). Stroke rehabilitation. three exercise therapy approaches. *Phys. Ther.* 66, 1233–1238.

Effenberg, A. O., Fehse, U., Schmitz, G., Krueger, B., and Mechling, H. (2016). Movement sonification: effects on motor learning beyond rhythmic adjustments. *Front. Neurosci.* 10:219. doi: 10.3389/fnins.2016.00219

Ehrlé, N., and Samson, S. (2005). Auditory discrimination of anisochrony: influence of the tempo and musical backgrounds of listeners. *Brain Cogn.* 58, 133–147. doi: 10.1016/j.bandc.2004.09.014

Falk, S., Müller, T., and Dalla Bella, S. (2015). Non-verbal sensorimotor timing deficits in children and adolescents who stutter. *Front. Psychol.* 6:847. doi: 10.3389/fpsyg.2015.00847

Fernández, E., Bringas, M. L., Salazar, S., Rodríguez, D., García, M. E., and Torres, M. (2012). Clinical impact of RehaCom software for cognitive rehabilitation of patients with acquired brain injury. *MEDICC Rev.* 14, 32–35. doi: 10.1590/s1555-79602012000400007

Friedman, N., Chan, V., Reinkensmeyer, A. N., Beroukhim, A., Zambrano, G. J., Bachman, M., et al. (2014). Retraining and assessing hand movement after stroke using the musicglove: comparison with conventional hand therapy and isometric grip training. *J. Neuroeng. Rehabil.* 11:76. doi: 10.1186/1743-0003-11-76

Friedman, N., Reinkensmeyer, D., and Bachman, M. (2011). A real-time interactive MIDI glove for domicile stroke rehabilitation. *Lect. Notes Comp. Sci.* 6764, 151–158. doi: 10.1007/978-3-642-21619-0_20

Gordon, R. L., Shivers, C. M., Wieland, E. A., Kotz, S. A., Yoder, P. J., and McAuley, J. D. (2015). Musical rhythm discrimination explains individual differences in grammar skills in children. *Dev. Sci.* 18, 635–644. doi: 10.1111/desc.12230

Grahn, J. A., and Brett, M. (2007). Rhythm and beat perception in motor areas of the brain. *J. Cogn. Neurosci.* 19, 893–906. doi: 10.1162/jocn.2007.19.5.893

Grahn, J. A., and Brett, M. (2009). Impairment of beat-based rhythm discrimination in Parkinson's disease. *Cortex* 45, 54–61. doi: 10.1016/j.cortex.2008.01.005

Grahn, J. A., and Rowe, J. B. (2009). Feeling the beat: premotor and striatal interactions in musicians and nonmusicians during beat perception. *J. Neurosci.* 29, 7540–7548. doi: 10.1523/JNEUROSCI.2018-08.2009

Grondin, S. (1993). Duration discrimination of empty and filled intervals marked by auditory and visual signals. *Percept. Psychophys.* 54, 383–394. doi: 10.3758/bf03205274

Grube, M., Cooper, F. E., Chinnery, P. F., and Griffiths, T. D. (2010). Dissociation of duration-based and beat-based auditory timing in cerebellar degeneration. *Proc. Natl. Acad. Sci. U S A* 107, 11597–11601. doi: 10.1073/pnas.0910473107

Harris, D. M., Rantalainen, T., Muthalib, M., Johnson, L., and Teo, W.-P. (2015). Exergaming as a viable therapeutic tool to improve static and dynamic balance among older adults and people with idiopathic Parkinson's disease: a systematic review and meta-analysis. *Front. Aging Neurosci.* 7:167. doi: 10.3389/fnagi.2015.00167

Hoffmann, C. P., Torregrosa, G., and Bardy, B. G. (2012). Sound stabilizes locomotor-respiratory coupling and reduces energy cost. *PLoS One* 7:e45206. doi: 10.1371/journal.pone.0045206

Iversen, J. R., and Patel, A. D. (2008). "The beat alignment test (BAT): surveying beat processing abilities in the general population," in *Proceedings of the 10th International Conference on Music Perception & Cognition (ICMPC10), August 2008, Sapporo, Japan*, ed. K. Miyazaki (Adelaide: Causal Productions), 465–468.

Jones, M. R., Moynihan, H., MacKenzie, N., and Puente, J. (2002). Temporal aspects of stimulus-driven attending in dynamic arrays. *Psychol. Sci.* 13, 313–319. doi: 10.1111/1467-9280.00458

Karahan, A. Y., Tok, F., Taşkin, H., Küçüksaraç, S., Basaran, A., and Yildirim, P. (2015). Effects of exergames on balance, functional mobility and quality of life of geriatrics versus home exercise programme: randomized controlled study. *Cent. Eur. J. Public Health* 23, S14–S18. doi: 10.21101/cejph.a4081

Kirschner, S., and Tomasello, M. (2009). Joint drumming: social context facilitates synchronization in preschool children. *J. Exp. Child Psychol.* 102, 299–314. doi: 10.1016/j.jecp.2008.07.005

Kornysheva, K., and Schubotz, R. I. (2011). Impairment of auditory-motor timing and compensatory reorganization after ventral premotor cortex stimulation. *PLoS One* 6:e21421. doi: 10.1371/journal.pone.0021421

Kotz, S. A., and Gunter, T. C. (2015). Can rhythmic auditory cuing remediate language-related deficits in Parkinson's disease? *Ann. N Y Acad. Sci.* 1337, 62–68. doi: 10.1111/nyas.12657

Lange, B., Flynn, S., and Rizzo, A. (2009). Initial usability assessment of off-the-shelf video game consoles for clinical game-based motor rehabilitation. *Phys. Ther. Rev.* 14, 355–363. doi: 10.1179/108331909x12488667117258

Lee, D. N. (1976). A theory of visual control of braking based on information about time-to-collision. *Perception* 5, 437–459. doi: 10.1068/p050437

Lim, I., Van Wegen, E., de Goede, C., Deutekom, M., Nieuwboer, A., Willems, A., et al. (2005). Effects of external rhythmical cueing on gait in patients with Parkinson's disease: a systematic review. *Clin. Rehabil.* 19, 695–713. doi: 10.1191/0269215505cr906oa

Nobre, A. C., Correa, A., and Coull, J. T. (2007). The hazards of time. *Curr. Opin. Neurobiol.* 17, 465–470. doi: 10.1016/j.conb.2007.07.006

Norton, A., Zipse, L., Marchina, S., and Schlaug, G. (2009). Melodic intonation therapy: shared insights on how it is done and why it might help. *Ann. N Y Acad. Sci.* 1169, 431–436. doi: 10.1111/j.1749-6632.2009.04859.x

Pecenka, N., and Keller, P. E. (2009). Auditory pitch imagery and its relationship to musical synchronization. *Ann. N Y Acad. Sci.* 1169, 282–286. doi: 10.1111/j.1749-6632.2009.04785.x

Przybylski, L., Bedoin, N., Krifi-Papoz, S., Herbillon, V., Roch, D., Léculier, L., et al. (2013). Rhythmic auditory stimulation influences syntactic processing in children with developmental language disorders. *Neuropsychology* 27, 121–131. doi: 10.1037/a0031277

Rego, P., Moreira, P., and Reis, L. (2010). "Serious games for rehabilitiation: a survey and classification towards a taxonomy," in *5th Iberian Conference on Information Systems and Technologies (CISTI)*, (Santiago de Compos tela), 1–6.

Repp, B. H. (2005). Sensorimotor synchronization: a review of the tapping literature. *Psychon. Bull. Rev.* 12, 969–992. doi: 10.3758/bf03206433

Repp, B. H., and Su, Y.-H. (2013). Sensorimotor synchronization: a review of recent research (2006–2012). *Psychon. Bull. Rev.* 20, 403–452. doi: 10.3758/s13423-012-0371-2

Saposnik, G., Teasell, R., Mamdani, M., Hall, J., McIlroy, W., Cheung, D., et al. (2010). Effectiveness of virtual reality using Wii gaming technology in stroke rehabilitation: a pilot randomized clinical trial and proof of principle. *Stroke* 41, 1477–1484. doi: 10.1161/STROKEAHA.110.584979

Schön, D., and Tillmann, B. (2015). Short- and long-term rhythmic interventions: perspectives for language rehabilitation. *Ann. N Y Acad. Sci.* 1337, 32–39. doi: 10.1111/nyas.12635

Schulze, H. H., and Vorberg, D. (2002). Linear phase correction models for synchronization: parameter identification and estimation of parameters. *Brain Cogn.* 48, 80–97. doi: 10.1006/brcg.2001.1305

Schwartze, M., and Kotz, S. A. (2013). A dual-pathway neural architecture for specific temporal prediction. *Neurosci. Biobehav. Rev.* 37, 2587–2596. doi: 10.1016/j.neubiorev.2013.08.005

Spaulding, S. J., Barber, B., Colby, M., Cormack, B., Mick, T., and Jenkins, M. E. (2013). Cueing and gait improvement among people with Parkinson's disease: a meta-analysis. *Arch. Phys. Med. Rehabil.* 94, 562–570. doi: 10.1016/j.apmr.2012.10.026

Sun, T. L., and Lee, C. H. (2013). An impact study of the design of exergaming parameters on body intensity from objective and gameplay-based player experience perspectives, based on balance training exergame. *PLoS One* 8:e69471. doi: 10.1371/journal.pone.0069471

Teki, S., Grube, M., Kumar, S., and Griffiths, T. D. (2011). Distinct neural substrates of duration-based and beat-based auditory timing. *J. Neurosci.* 31, 3805–3812. doi: 10.1523/JNEUROSCI.5561-10.2011

Thaut, M. H. (2003). Neural basis of rhythmic timing networks in the human brain. *Ann. N Y Acad. Sci.* 999, 364–373. doi: 10.1196/annals.1284.044

Thaut, M. H., and Abiru, M. (2010). Rhythmic auditory stimulation in rehabilitation of movement disorders: a review of current research. *Music Percept.* 27, 263–269. doi: 10.1525/mp.2010.27.4.263

Thaut, M. H., Kenyon, G. P., Hurt, C. P., McIntosh, G. C., and Hoemberg, V. (2002). Kinematic optimization of spatiotemporal patterns in paretic arm training with stroke patients. *Neuropsychologia* 40, 1073–1081. doi: 10.1016/s0028-3932(01)00141-5

Thaut, M. H., Leins, A. K., Rice, R. R., Argstatter, H., Kenyon, G. P., McIntosh, G. C., et al. (2007). Rhythmic auditor y stimulation improves gait more than NDT/Bobath training in near-ambulatory patients early poststroke: a single-blind, randomized trial. *Neurorehabil. Neural Repair* 21, 455–459. doi: 10.1177/1545968307300523

Thaut, M. H., McIntosh, G. C., Rice, R. R., Miller, R. A., Rathbun, J., and Brault, J. M. (1996). Rhythmic auditory stimulation in gait training for Parkinson's disease patients. *Mov. Disord.* 11, 193–200. doi: 10.1002/mds.870110213

Thaut, M. H., McIntosh, G. C., and Rice, R. R. (1997). Rhythmic facilitation of gait training in hemiparetic stroke rehabilitation. *J. Neurol. Sci.* 151, 207–212. doi: 10.1016/s0022-510x(97)00146-9

Tierney, A. T., and Kraus, N. (2013). The ability to tap to a beat relates to cognitive, linguistic and perceptual skills. *Brain Lang.* 124, 225–231. doi: 10.1016/j.bandl.2012.12.014

Watkins, K. E., Smith, S. M., Davis, S., and Howell, P. (2008). Structural and functional abnormalities of the motor system in developmental stuttering. *Brain* 131, 50–59. doi: 10.1093/brain/awm241

Webster, D., and Celik, O. (2014). Systematic review of kinect applications in elderly care and stroke rehabilitation. *J. Neuroeng. Rehabil.* 11:108. doi: 10.1186/1743-0003-11-108

Weiss, P. L., Sveistrup, H., Rand, D., and Kizony, R. (2009). Video capture virtual reality: a decade of rehabilitation assessment and intervention. *Phys. Ther. Rev.* 14, 307–321. doi: 10.1179/108331909x12488667117339

Wing, A. M. (2002). Voluntary timing and brain function: an information processing approach. *Brain Cogn.* 48, 7–30. doi: 10.1006/brcg.2001.1301

Woodruff Carr, K., White-Schwoch, T., Tierney, A. T., Strait, D. L., and Kraus, N. (2014). Beat synchronization predicts neural speech encoding and reading readiness in preschoolers. *Proc. Natl. Acad. Sci. U S A* 111, 14559–14564. doi: 10.1073/pnas.1406219111

Zatorre, R. J., Chen, J. L., and Penhune, V. B. (2007). When the brain plays music: auditory-motor interactions in music perception and production. *Nat. Rev. Neurosci.* 8, 547–558. doi: 10.1038/nrn2152

Zelaznik, H. N., Spencer, R., and Ivry, R. B. (2002). Dissociation of explicit and implicit timing in repetitive tapping and drawing movements. *J. Exp. Psychol. Hum. Percept. Perform.* 28, 575–588. doi: 10.1037/0096-1523.28.3.575

Zhou, H., and Hu, H. (2008). Human motion tracking for rehabilitation—A survey. *Biomed. Signal Process. Control* 3, 1–18. doi: 10.1016/j.bspc.2007.09.001

12

Cognitive and Brain Plasticity Induced by Physical Exercise, Cognitive Training, Video Games, and Combined Interventions

Soledad Ballesteros[1,2*], *Claudia Voelcker-Rehage*[3] and *Louis Bherer*[4,5,6]

[1] *Studies on Aging and Neurodegenerative Diseases Research Group, Universidad Nacional de Educación a Distancia (UNED), Madrid, Spain,* [2] *Department of Basic Psychology II, Universidad Nacional de Educación a Distancia (UNED), Madrid, Spain,* [3] *Institute of Human Movement Science and Health, Technische Universität Chemnitz, Chemnitz, Germany,* [4] *Department of Medicine, Université de Montréal, Montreal, QC, Canada,* [5] *Montreal Heart Institute, Montreal, QC, Canada,* [6] *Institut Universitaire de Gériatrie de Montréal, Montreal, QC, Canada*

Edited by:
Shuhei Yamaguchi,
Shimane University, Japan

Reviewed by:
Hasan Ayaz,
Drexel University, United States

Correspondence:
Soledad Ballesteros
mballesteros@psi.uned.es

Keywords: cognitive training, lifespan, multi-domain intervention, neuroplasticity, physical training, randomized controlled trial, video games, working memory

Editorial on the Research Topic

Cognitive and Brain Plasticity Induced by Physical Exercise, Cognitive Training, Video Games, and Combined Interventions

This Research Topic (RT) focused on recent research conducted in the field of cognitive and brain plasticity induced by physical activity, different types of cognitive training, including computerized interventions, learning therapy, video games, and combined intervention approaches as well as other forms of brain stimulation that target brain activity, including electroencephalography and neurofeedback. It contains 49 contributions to the topic, including original research articles (37), clinical trials (2), reviews (5), mini-reviews (2), hypothesis and theory (1), and corrections (2).

The premise of neuroplasticity on enhancing cognitive functioning among healthy as well as cognitively impaired individuals across the lifespan, and the potential of harnessing these processes to prevent cognitive decline attract substantial scientific and public interest. Indeed, the systematic evidence base for cognitive training, video games, physical exercise, and other forms of brain stimulation such as entrain brain activity is growing rapidly, thus paving the way for research geared at better understanding the underlying mechanisms and translation to clinical practice (Raz and Lindenberger, 2013). Studies in this field might contribute to improve our knowledge on cognitive and brain plasticity and be of great help for designing effective cognitive-enhancement interventions (see Karbach and Schubert, 2013). It is well-known that brain plasticity and its role in brain adaptation across the lifespan are influenced by other changes occurring as a result of environmental factors, personality variables and genetic and epigenetic factors (see Ballesteros et al., 2015). To date, most cognitive training studies have focused on measuring gains immediately after training, typically demonstrating effects on the trained tasks or closely-related transfer measures (i.e., near transfer). Yet the potency of cognitive training depends on evidence of: (1) far transfer from training to untrained functions; (2) the durability of training effects, including what booster regimens are needed to maintain cognitive benefits in young and older adults; and (3) the extent to which cognitive training can affect clinically meaningful outcomes.

Researchers are increasingly using cognitive training platforms and video games to investigate its impact on cognition and brain plasticity. Video game play is a very popular leisure activity. An interesting preliminary question is why consumers choose to download smartphones applications (apps) offering brain training. Torous et al. noticed that there is much interest in brain training apps among US younger people. Results from an online via internet survey with more than 3,000 participants suggest a high level of interest in these sort of programs. However, the data pointed out to the importance of expectations as both naïve participants as well as application-exposed participants showed a positive perception of brain training. These results suggest that people expect to improve with the use of brain-training apps. Importantly, brain training should focus on scientific research efficacy and generalizable benefits not in expectations of improvement (see Torous et al. correction).

Training with video games has shown to enhance moderately perceptual and cognitive functions in young and older individuals (for meta-analyses, see Lampit et al., 2014; Toril et al., 2014). Video games are inexpensive, gratifying and fun. Regular and occasional video game players reported significantly higher levels of well-being, but gaming could potentially lead to addiction, sedentary lifestyle and social isolation. Maximizing the benefits of video games will require studies dealing with questions such as: (1) what benefits should be expected from specific types of games; (2) how to account for individual differences; and (3) how to address expectancy bias and placebo effects in study designs. Physical activity has been repeatedly shown to improve cognitive functioning in all age groups, particularly in older adults. This Frontiers RT includes articles that investigate (1) the dose-response relationships of different types of exercise as well as the long-term effects of exercise on various cognitive domains, (2) the analysis of functional and structural as well as behavioral data, (3) the association between acute and chronic exercise effects, and (4) the potential of combining physical and cognitive exercise for enhancing cognitive performance and brain health.

In sum, the major aim of this RT is, therefore, to provide the interested reader with an objective picture of the state of the art on the influence of different types of interventions on cognition and brain state across the lifespan. Special emphasis is placed mainly in randomized controlled trials and longitudinal intervention studies conducted to assess possible transfer effects to cognitive and brain health in older adults.

COGNITIVE TRAINING IN YOUNG AND OLDER ADULTS WITH TRADITIONAL METHODS, COMPUTER-BASED ACTIVITIES, AND VIDEO GAMES

Several articles included in this Frontiers RT are longitudinal studies that have used different types of cognitive training programs to improve different aspects of cognition, including working memory, executive control and other cognitive functions in young and older adults. Other series of articles in this issue dealt with neurophysiological (ERPs) and neurofeedback (NFB) methods as a form of brain stimulation.

In their hypothesis and theory paper, Moreau et al. critically discuss pervasive statistical flaws in intervention designs for training-induced cognitive enhancement. That is (i) lack of power; (ii) sampling error; (iii) continuous variable splits; (iv) erroneous interpretations of correlated gain scores; (v) single transfer assessments; (vi) multiple comparisons; and (vii) publication bias. Similarly Cremen and Carson asked, "Have standard tests of cognitive function been misappropriated in the study of cognitive enhancement?" They argue that the latent constructs to which tests of cognitive functions relate are not usually subject to a sufficient level of analytic scrutiny. In addition they consider their neurophysiological correlates. Using linear mixed models, they found the efficacy of training and some maintenance effects. The individual characteristics considered contributed in some cases to explain the effects of training.

Lawton compared three intervention conditions in dyslexic second grade school children. Two of them target temporal dynamics of either the auditory or visual pathways, and the third condition consisted of a reading control group. The results pointed to the lack of synchronization of the activity of the magnocellular with the parvocellular visual pathway as the main cause of dyslexia, not the phonological deficits. Lawton proposed that visual movement direction-discrimination could be used as a tool for the successful treatment of this deficit Nouchi et al.

Nouchi et al. conducted a RCT to investigate whether the "Learning Therapy" (LT) improved a wide range of cognitive functions in older adults. They found benefits of LT on inhibition of executive functions. The article of Borella et al. explored in older adults whether age, education, vocabulary and baseline performance in a working memory task predict the short- and long-term gains and transfer effects of a verbal WM training. The authors selected four studies of the research group that adopted the verbal WM training procedure. Using linear mixed models, they found the efficacy of training and some maintenance effects. The individual characteristics considered contributed in some cases to explain the effects of training. Maraver et al. provided computerized training to groups of young adults to investigate the effects of training on WM or inhibitory control (IC) as compared to two-control groups, one passive and the other active, which performed non-executive control tasks. The trained groups improved in the trained task. More important were the pattern of near transfer effects as a function of the type of training. Only the IC group showed far transfer to reasoning (Raven test). Interestingly, these findings were obtained with just six training sessions. Schmicker et al. asked whether training young adults either attentional filtering or memory storage would influence decision-making assessed with the Iowa Gambling Task. All participants improved their performance in the trained task but decision-making was more influenced by training to filter out irrelevant information than by training to store items in WM. It seems that selective attention is more important for enhancing efficiency in decision-making.

Video games are perhaps the most popular computerized intervention approach to train different aspects of cognition. So far, the results of intervention studies are mixed with some studies reporting improvements after training in several aspects of cognition (e.g., Basak et al., 2008; Anguera et al., 2013; Ballesteros et al., 2014) while others have not found positive effects (e.g., Ackerman et al., 2010; Owen et al., 2010; Boot et al., 2013). Palaus et al. reviewed the relationship between the use of video games and their neural correlates. The final selection included 100 articles that provided functional data and 22 that measured structural brain changes. The authors established some links between the neural and cognitive aspects, including attention, cognitive control, visuospatial abilities, cognitive workload, and reward processing.

Toril et al. conducted an intervention study with experimental and control groups to investigate whether cognitively healthy older adults trained with non-action video games improve visuospatial working memory and episodic memory and whether these possible enhancements would persist 3 months after the end of training. The group trained with games showed post-training improvements in visuospatial working memory, and in short-term memory and episodic memory. Some results were maintained during a 3-month follow-up period. The authors concluded that older adults still retain some degree of plasticity and that video games seem to be an effective tool to improve some memory functions in aging. In contrast, the RCT conducted by Buitenweg et al. with healthy older adults assigned to a frequent or to an infrequent switching experimental condition, or to the active control group showed significant time effects on multiple transfer tasks in all three groups, probably as a result of expectancy and motivation. The authors concluded that the therapeutic value of using available training games to train the aging brain is modest. Possibly the use of different methods such as stimulating social interaction and training in groups by individual-adjusted variable exercises would produce better results.

Another type of training that becomes more popular involves the use of music or rhythm within a cognitive or video game setup. For example, rhythmic training has been successfully used to improve motor performance (e.g., gait) as well as cognitive and language skills. Begel et al. reviewed the games readily available in the market in order to see if it can be used for cognitive training in populations with motor or neurodevelopmental disorders (e.g., Parkinson's disease, ADHD). They concluded that none of the existing games provides sufficient temporal precision in stimulus presentation and/or data acquisition and that the available music games are not satisfying for implementing a rhythmic training protocol. The authors also provide guidelines for serious music games targeting rhythmic training in the future. The rational for rhythmic training is supported by some studies. An example is the study of Pollok et al. that used transcranial direct current stimulation to study potential superior synchronization in professional drummers compared to non-musician controls. Their data support the hypothesis that the posterior parietal cortex is involved in auditory-motor synchronization and extend previous findings by showing that its functional significance varies with musical expertise.

Effects of working memory training and training-related alterations in neural activity on dual-tasking in older adults were investigated by Heinzel et al. The training group participated in 12 sessions of an adaptive n-back training. At pre and post-measurement, a multimodal dual-task was performed in all participants to assess transfer effects. While no transfer to single-task performance was found, dual-task costs decreased at post measurement in the training, but not in the control group. Neural activity that changed in left dorsolateral prefrontal cortex (DLPFC) during one-back predicted post-training auditory dual-task costs, while neural activity changes in right DLPFC during three-back predicted visual dual-task costs. Results might indicate an improvement in central executive processing that could facilitate both working memory and dual-task coordination.

Teasdale et al. investigated whether individuals with MCI can benefit from a training program and improve their overall driving performance in a driving simulator. Therefore, older drivers with MCI participated in five training sessions in a simulator. They revealed gradual and significant decrease in the number of errors, indicating learning and safer driving and therewith the possibility to maintain driving skills and safe driving in MCI individuals. Another clinical population with which cognitive training is often used is patients that suffered from stroke, which often results in cognitive impairments in working memory, attention, and executive function. Van de Ven et al. conducted a systematic review of the evidence for computer-based cognitive training of executive dysfunctions after stroke. They reported that cognitive training could lead to improvement in tasks similar to the training (near transfer) and in tasks dissimilar to the training (far transfer). Studies evaluated neural effects and found changes in both functional and structural connectivity. The authors concluded that for most studies reporting positive findings, including neural changes, future research should address existing methodological limitations.

COMBINED MULTI-DOMAIN INTERVENTIONS

Some studies looked at the effect of combining multi-domain intervention, such as different cognitive domains or cognitive intervention combined to fitness training regimes. For instance, Fraser et al. examined the dual-task benefits of combined physical and cognitive training in a sample of sedentary older adults, but failed to demonstrate a more beneficial effect of a combined physical and cognitive training as compared to physical and computer training combined with a respective control group (stretch and cognitive/computer training). Küper et al. used electrophysiology (ERP) to examine the effects of multi-domain cognitive training on performance in an untrained cue-based task switch paradigm featuring Stroop color words. Older adults were assigned to either a 4-month multi-domain cognitive training, a passive no-contact control group or an active (social) control group. Only the cognitive training group showed an increase in response accuracy at posttest, irrespective of task and trial type. Cognitive training was also associated with an overall increase in N2 amplitude and a decrease of P2 latency on single trials suggesting enhanced response selection and improved access to relevant stimulus-response mappings.

Recently, movement based video games (exergames) have been introduced to have the capability to improve cognitive function in older adults. During exergaming, participants are required to perform physical activities while being simultaneously surrounded by a cognitively challenging environment. Ordnung et al. investigated the effects of an exergame training over 6 weeks on cognitive, motor, and sensory functions in healthy old participants. However, gains in the trained exergames did not result in specific performance improvements.

NEUROFEEDBACK (NFB) AND ELECTROPHYSIOLOGICAL STUDIES

Neurofeedback (NFB) is becoming a popular method aimed at improving cognitive and behavioral performance and it is used as a treatment intervention. The goal of this type of intervention is to induce changes in the power of certain electroencephalography (EEG) bands to produce beneficial changes in cognition and motor activity. Rogala et al. reviewed the evidence that support the validity of several NFB protocols. The article highlights that the methodology used in most of the reviewed experiments did not enable proper targeting of the brain regions that control the desired cognitive changes and made a series of recommendations for improving the NFB training efficacy. Paluch et al. conducted an experiment using EEG-NFB with young adults and conclude that the activity from the EEG electrodes might be overwhelmed by the easier to control electro-miographyc signals. The authors advice the NFB community to develop, validate and implement efficient automatic artifact detection algorithms. Cowley et al. presented the results of a RCT intervention that used NFB therapy for adults with Attention Deficit/Hyperactivity Disorder (ADHD/ADD). Preliminary results suggest that NFB improved self-reported ADHD symptoms, but did not show transfer of leaning in a computerized attention test (T.O.V.A.). Hudak et al. reported an effect of NFB in reducing impulsive behavior via the strengthening of frontal lobe functioning. The randomized, controlled functional near-infrared spectroscopy (fNIRS) NFB intervention study tested its efficacy in an ADHD adult subgroup with high impulsivity. The reduction in the commission of errors on a no-go task, and an increase in prefrontal oxygenated hemoglobin concentration in the experimental group only, together with other findings suggest the potential of NFB in reducing impulsive behaviors by improving frontal lobe functioning. In addition, the authors argued that the use of virtual reality with NFB might improve the ecological validity of the training situation. This could affect positively transfer of the just acquired skills to real life.

Peters et al. investigated in an event–related potential (ERP) study conducted with young adults whether spatial frequency training modulates neural face perception. Interestingly, the authors showed that training effects based on a task using low-level stimuli, transfer to performance on a higher-level object-processing task. Interestingly, training the use of specific spatial frequency information was found to affect neural processing of facial information. These findings may have practical application to improve face recognition in people with atypical spatial frequency processing, including people suffering from cataracts or Autism Spectrum Disorder.

Gajewski et al. conducted a RCT to investigate the deficits in performance and EEG activity in workers with repetitive and unchallenging work. The results showed that the 3-month training protocol improved accuracy performance and affected the electrophysiological correlates of retrieval of stimulus-response sets (P2), response selection (N2), and error detection (Ne). Importantly, at the 3-month follow-up assessment most of the induced changes at the behavioral and EEG levels were maintained. It appears that cognitive training is useful for improving executive functions in workers with unchallenging work.

Wei et al. investigated whether structural differences in the hippocampus could explain sex difference in a 3D mental rotation task. Males had a larger anterior hippocampus and gray matter volume of the right anterior hippocampus was significantly correlated with performance in a 3D mental rotation task and could explain sex differences in mental rotation. Results suggest that the structural difference between males' and females' right anterior hippocampus was a neurobiological substrate for the sex difference in 3D mental rotation.

Hallock et al. presented the results of a meta-analysis that included 14 published studies that investigated the effects of cognitive training on measures of cognition and function measures in patients that have suffered traumatic brain injury (TBI). They showed a small but significant effect of cognitive training with no evidence of publication bias and a moderate effect size for overall functional outcomes and possible publication bias. In addition, the authors found significant effects only for executive function and verbal memory. The findings indicated that training is moderately effective in improving cognition and function in TBI patients.

FITNESS EFFECTS ON COGNITION AND BRAIN ANATOMY

It is well-accepted that an active cognitive and physical lifestyle can reduce the risk of cognitive decline and dementia with aging (Valenzuela and Sachdev, 2006; Ngandu et al., 2015). Physical training promotes cognitive and functional brain plasticity in older adults (Nagamatsu et al., 2012; Kattenstroth et al., 2013). An important question is whether cognitive and physical training may increase white matter integrity (WMI), which is deteriorated in cognitive impaired patients. Fissler et al. did not find evidence that short-term cognitive or physical training were related to changes in WMI (hippocampus and prefrontal white matter tracks) in older adults at risk of dementia despite activity-related cognitive changes. However, the authors found positive associations between the two targeted training outcomes and WMI. This result opens the path for a potential of long-term activities to affect WMI. The article of Fletcher et al. tested the hypothesis that if cardiorespiratory fitness counteracts the negative effects of aging; the regions that show the greatest age-related volumetric loss should show the largest beneficial effects of physical exercise. The structural magnetic resonance imaging (MRI) data from 54 healthy elders showed that lower fitness and older age are associated with atrophy in different brain areas, but the profiles of age and fitness effects were not totally overlapping. While brain areas such as the precentral gyrus, the superior temporal sulcus, and some parts of the medial temporal lobe were affected by both fitness and aging, other areas (regions of the frontal, parietal, and temporal cortex) were only affected by aging while other brain regions in the basal ganglia were only affected by fitness. These results support the idea that aging and fitness have differential effects on the brain and leads to the conclusion that fitness couldn't revert all the negative effects of aging.

Wengaard et al. investigated the association of physical fitness, measured as maximal oxygen uptake (VO2max), muscle mass, weekly training, and cognitive function in the executive domains of selective attention and inhibitory control, in healthy male high-school students. Only maximal oxygen uptake was positively associated with cognitive function. Kleemeyer et al. addressed the theme of neural specificity (understood as the degree to which neural representations of different types of stimuli can be distinguished). Neural specificity declines with aging and its reduction is associated with lower cognitive performance (Park et al., 2010). The authors concluded that physical activity might protect against age-related declines in neural specificity. The study tested the hypothesis that exercise-induced improvements in fitness would be related to greater neural specificity in a group of 52 older adults randomly assigned to a high-intensity training group or to a low-intensity training group. The hypothesis was confirmed by the results of an fMRI experiment in which the participants were presented with pictures of faces and buildings. Participants whose physical fitness improved more also showed more changes in neural specificity. Hsu et al. conducted a 6-month RCT to investigate the impact of aerobic exercise (AE) training in older adults on fronto-parietal network connectivity. The results suggested that AT improve mobility in older adults with mild subcortical ischemic cognitive impairments (see Hsu et al. correction).

Rehfeld et al. compared the effects of an 18-month dancing intervention and traditional health fitness training on volumes of hippocampal subfields and balance abilities. Both, members of the dance-intervention and members of the fitness intervention revealed hippocampal volume increases mainly in the left hippocampus. The dancers showed additional increases in the left dentate gyrus and the right subiculum. Moreover, only the dancers achieved a significant increase in the balance composite score. Hence, dancing constitutes a promising candidate in counteracting the age-related decline in physical and mental abilities. Kandola et al. performed a review on how aerobic exercise is associated with cognitive enhancements and stimulates a cascade of neuroplastic mechanisms that support improvements in hippocampal functioning. Therefore, they summarized the animal and human literature. Using the examples of schizophrenia and major depressive disorder, they proposed the utility and implementation of an aerobic intervention to the clinical domain.

Panda et al. investigated how meditation alters the default mode network (DMN) using simultaneous EEG and functional MRI to compare the spatial extents and temporal dynamics of the DMN during rest and meditation. They found alterations in the duration of the DMN microstate in meditators highlighting the role of meditation practice in producing durable changes in temporal dynamics of the DMN. Su et al. also studied the effect of mindfulness training and its modulation on pain perception. They compare participants' brain-behavior response before and after a 6-week mindfulness-based stress reduction (MBSR) training course on mindfulness in relation to pain modulation using pain questionnaires and resting-state fMRI. They observed that the pain-afflicted group experienced significantly less pain after the mindfulness treatment than before, in conjunction with increased brain connectivity. These results suggest that mindfulness training can modulate the brain network dynamics underlying the subjective experience of pain. Cakmak et al. investigated the potential structural cortical plasticity in Sufi Whirling Dervishes, a form of physically active meditation. Results demonstrated significantly thinner cortical areas for Sufi Whirling Dervishes subjects compared with the control group in the DMN as well as in motion perception and discrimination areas of the brain.

Dordevic et al. conducted a feasibility study to assess the effect of 1-month of slackline-training on different components of balancing ability and its transfer effects on non-visual-dependent spatial orientation abilities. The training group performed significantly better on the closed-eyes conditions of the clinical balance test and in the vestibular condition of the orientation test, probably caused by a positive influence of slackline-training on the vestibular system function. Beck et al. investigated whether and how academic achievements in children can benefit from specific types of motor activities (e.g., fine and gross) integrated in to learning activities, here math lessons. They conducted a 6-week within school cluster-randomized intervention study. The study demonstrates that motor enriched learning activities can improve mathematical performance, particularly in normal math performers (but less in low math performers).

Godde and Volcker-Rehage conducted an intervention study to investigate whether a walking intervention and a motor control intervention reduce the cognitive brain resources that people recruited while performing motor tasks. Brain activation was assessed pre and post-intervention while the participants were imagining forward and backward walking. The results showed a positive association between initial motor status and activation decrease in the dorsolateral prefrontal cortex from pre-to-post assessment in both trained groups, suggesting that training effects might improve situations where people have to perform motor and cognitive tasks at the same time.

Condello et al. performed a cross-sectional study and investigated whether physical activity (PA) habits may positively impact performance of the orienting and executive control networks in community-dwelling older adults and diabetics, who are at risk of cognitive dysfunction. Results suggest that high PA levels exert beneficial, but differentiated effects on processing speed and attentional networks performance in aging individuals that partially counteract the detrimental effects of advancing age and diabetic status. Nadeau et al. assessed the impact of a 3-month aerobic exercise training using a stationary bicycle on a set of gait parameters and executive functions in sedentary Parkinson's disease (PD) patients and healthy controls. Aerobic capacity, as well as performance of motor learning and on cognitive inhibition, increased significantly in both groups after the training regimen, but only PD patients improved their walking speed and cadence. In PD patients, training-related improvements in aerobic capacity correlated positively with improvements in walking speed. Gait improvements seem to be specific to the type of motor activity practiced during exercise (i.e., pedaling), where improvements in cognitive inhibition were rather unspecific to the type of training (i.e., improvement of cardiovascular capacity).

Tan et al. investigated the cortical structural and functional differences in athletes and novices by comparing gray matter volumes and resting-state functional connectivity in 21 basketball players and 21 novices with MRI techniques. They found larger gray matter volume in basketball players than in novices in many regions (anterior insula, inferior frontal gyrus, inferior parietal lobule, and right anterior cingulate cortex). They also reported higher functional connectivity in the DMN, salience network and executive control network in basketball players compared to novices. Yu et al. investigated the effects of modified constraint induced movement therapy (CIMT) in acute subcortical cerebral infarction. The results showed positive effects immediatelly after treatment but long-term effects were not found.

In a very interesting review, Stillman et al. used a macroscopic lens to identify potential brain and behavioral/socioemotional mediators of the association between physical activity and cognitive function. They first summarized what is known regarding cellular and molecular mechanisms, and then discussed evidence for brain systems and behavioral/socioemotional pathways by which physical activity could impact cognition. The review proposes a number of potential moderator and mediators of the relationship between physical activity and cognitive performances. This review offers a theoretical context that could be useful to organize the current scientific knowledge regarding physical activity and brain structure and functions. It could also lead to a more complete characterization of the processes by which physical activity influences neurocognitive function, as well as a greater variety of targets for modifying neurocognitive function in clinical contexts.

Finally, some studies adopted the approach of studying acute exercise effects. For instance, Spring et al. investigation revealed that cardiovascular exercise could reduce movement related cortical potentials assessed with EEG while performing a knee extension task, which was related to muscle alterations and resulted in the inability to produce a maximal voluntary contraction.

Lundbye-Jensen et al. investigated whether acute exercise protocols following motor skill practice in a school setting can improve long-term retention of motor memory in preadolescent children and were able to show that acute intense intermittent exercise performed immediately after motor skill acquisition facilitates long-term motor memory in pre-adolescent children, presumably by promoting memory consolidation.

To summarize, the series of review and research articles that compose this Frontiers RT provide comprehensive information on the importance of different types of interventions as a way of enhancing some cognitive functions across the lifespan. We hope that this RT will prompt a critical "thinking" in the context of the scientific community on the possibilities of improving cognition and well-being, providing clues for conducting further research intervention studies in the next years. We also hope that the information included in this RT will move the scientific community to generate new research projects directed to overcome some shortcomings appearing in the field of neuroplasticity, promoting cognitive enhancement and improving a the quality of life of young and older adults.

AUTHOR CONTRIBUTIONS

All authors listed have made a substantial, direct and intellectual contribution to the work, and approved it for publication.

ACKNOWLEDGMENTS

Grants from Ministerio de Economía y Competitividad (PSI2013- 41409-R; PSI2016-80337-R) supported SB.

REFERENCES

Ackerman, P. L., Kanfer, R., and Caldrwood, C. (2010). Use or lose it? Wii Brain exercise practice and reading for domain knowledge. *Psychol. Aging* 25, 753–766. doi: 10.1037/a0019277

Anguera, J. A., Boccanfuso, J., Rintoul, J. L., Alhashimi, O., Faraji, F., Janowich, J., et al. (2013). Video game training enhances cognitive control in older adults. *Nature* 501, 97–101. doi: 10.1038/nature.12486

Ballesteros, S., Kraft, E., Santana, S., and Tziraki, C. (2015). Maintaining older brain functionality: a targeted review. *Neurosci. Biobehav. Rev.* 55, 453–477. doi: 10.1016/j.neubiorev.2015.06.008

Ballesteros, S., Prieto, A., Mayas, J., Toril, P., Pita, C., Ponce de León, L., et al. (2014). Training dults with non-action video games enhances cognitive functions that decline with aging: a randomized controlled trial. *Front. Aging Neurosc.* 6:277. doi: 10.3389/fnagi.2014.00277

Basak, C., Boot, W. R., Voss, M. W., and Kramer, A. F. (2008). Can training in a real time strategy game attenuate cognitive decline in older adults? *Psychol. Aging* 12, 765–777. doi: 10.1037/a0013494

Boot, W. R., Champion, M., Blakely, D. P., Wright, T., Souders, D. J., and Charness, N. (2013). Video-games as a mean to reduce age-related cognitive decline: attitudes, compliance and effectiveness. *Front. Psychol.* 4:31. doi: 10.3389/fpsyg.2013.00031

Karbach, J., and Schubert, T. (2013). Training induced cognitive and neural plasticity. *Front. Human. Neurosci.* 7:48. doi: 10.3389/fnhum.2013.00048

Kattenstroth, J. C., Kalisch, T., Holt, S., Tegenthoff, M., and Dinse, H. R. (2013). Six monthsof dance intervention enhances postural, sensorimotor, and cognitiveperformance in elderly without affecting cardio-respiratory functions. *Front. Aging Neurosci.* 5:5. doi: 10.3389/fnagi.2013.00005

Lampit, A., Halloxk, H., and Valenzuela, M. (2014). Computarized cognitive training in cognitively healthy older adults: a systematic review and meta-analysis of effects modifiers. *PLoS Med.* 11:e1001756. doi: 10.1371/journal.pmed.1001756

Nagamatsu, L. S., Handy, T. C., Hsu, C. L., Voss, M., and Liu-Ambrose, T. (2012). Resistance training promotes cognitive and functional brain plasticity in seniors with probable cognitive mild impairment. *Arch. Inter. Med.* 172, 666–668. doi: 10.1001/archinternmed.2012.379

Ngandu, T., Lehtisalo, J., Solomon, A., Levalähti, E., Ahtilouto, O., Antikainen, R., et al. (2015). A 2 year multidomain intervention of diet, exercise, cognitive training, and vascular risk monitoring versus control to prevent cognitive decline in at-risk elderly people (FINGER). A randomized controlled trial. *Lancet* 385, 2255–2263. doi: 10.1016/S0140-6736(15)60461-5

Owen, A. M., Hampshire, A., Stenton, R., Dajani, S., Burns, A. S., et al. (2010). Putting brain training to test. *Nature* 465, 775–778. doi: 10.1038/nature09042

Park, J., Carp, J., Hebrank, A., Park, D. C., and Polk, T. A. (2010). Neural specificity predicts fluid processing ability in older adults. *J. Neurosci.* 30, 9253–9259. doi: 10.1523/JNEUROSC.0853-10.2010

Raz, N., and Lindenberger, U. (2013). Life-span plasticity of the brain and cognition: from questions to evidence and back. *Neurosci. Biobehav. Rev.* 37, 2195–2200. doi: 10.1016/jneubeorev.2013.10.003

Toril, P., Reales, J. M., Mayas, J., and Ballesteros, S. (2014). Brain training with video games enhances cognition of older adults: a meta-analytic study. *Psychol. Aging* 29, 706–716. doi: 10.1037/a0037507

Valenzuela, M. J., and Sachdev, P. (2006). Brain reserve and cognitive decline: a non-parametric systematic review. *Psychol. Med.* 36, 1065–1073. doi: 10.1017/S0033291706007747

13

Sex Differences in Gray Matter Volume of the Right Anterior Hippocampus Explain Sex Differences in Three-Dimensional Mental Rotation

Wei Wei[1,2,3], *Chuansheng Chen*[4], *Qi Dong*[3] *and Xinlin Zhou*[3]*

[1] Advanced Technology Innovation Center for Future Education, Beijing Normal University, Beijing, China, [2] Department of Psychology and Behavioral Sciences, Zhejiang University, Hangzhou, China, [3] State Key Laboratory of Cognitive Neuroscience and Learning, Beijing Normal University, Beijing, China, [4] Department of Psychology and Social Behavior, University of California, Irvine, CA, USA

Edited by:
Claudia Voelcker-Rehage, Chemnitz University of Technology, Germany

Reviewed by:
Rachael D. Seidler, University of Michigan, USA
Chris Lange-Küttner, London Metropolitan University, UK

***Correspondence:**
Xinlin Zhou
zhou_xinlin@bnu.edu.cn

Behavioral studies have reported that males perform better than females in 3-dimensional (3D) mental rotation. Given the important role of the hippocampus in spatial processing, the present study investigated whether structural differences in the hippocampus could explain the sex difference in 3D mental rotation. Results showed that after controlling for brain size, males had a larger anterior hippocampus, whereas females had a larger posterior hippocampus. Gray matter volume (GMV) of the right anterior hippocampus was significantly correlated with 3D mental rotation score. After controlling GMV of the right anterior hippocampus, sex difference in 3D mental rotation was no longer significant. These results suggest that the structural difference between males' and females' right anterior hippocampus was a neurobiological substrate for the sex difference in 3D mental rotation.

Keywords: sex difference, mental rotation, anterior hippocampus, brain structure

INTRODUCTION

The hippocampus plays an important role in spatial processing. The "place cells" in the hippocampus are the core part in the "GPS" of the brain that processes spatial information (O'Keefe, 1976; Fyhn et al., 2004; Sargolini et al., 2006). Both animal and human studies have shown that the hippocampal volume is related to spatial ability. For example, homing pigeons have larger hippocampi than non-homing pigeons (Rehkämper et al., 1988). The birds that need to store their food have larger hippocampi than the ones who do not (Krebs et al., 1989; Sherry et al., 1989). In terms of the mammals, the rats that store their food in a distributed manner have larger hippocampi than the ones that store their food in one central location (Jacobs and Spencer, 1994).

Human studies also showed that the hippocampus plays an important role in spatial processing (for a recent summary see Lee et al., 2012). First, patients who suffered from developmental topographical disorders (DTD) have damages to the hippocampus (in addition to the retrosplenial cortex, fusiform gyrus, and lingual gyrus) and show impaired performance on navigation tasks (Aguirre and D'Esposito, 1999; Iaria and Barton, 2010). Damages to the hippocampus also result in a deficit in spatial working memory (Abrahams et al., 1997; Bohbot et al., 1998; Holdstock et al., 2000). Second, neuroimaging studies found that the hippocampus is activated by navigation tasks (Maguire et al., 1998; Mellet et al., 2000; Hartley et al., 2003; Iaria et al., 2003, 2008) and spatial memory tasks (Maguire, 1997; Burgess et al., 2002). Moreover, when performing the spatial memory task, only spatial strategies (but not non-spatial strategies) elicited activation in the hippocampus (Iaria et al., 2003; Bohbot et al., 2004). Third, the size of the hippocampus may change dynamically due to a long-term or sustained demand of spatial processing. Experienced taxi drivers have larger posterior hippocampi than the control subjects (Maguire et al., 2000). Spatial navigation training has been found to increase the gray matter of the hippocampus (Lövdén et al., 2010, 2012; Kühn and Gallinat, 2014; Kühn et al., 2014).

Neuroimaging studies have further shown differentiated functions of the anterior and posterior hippocampus (Chua et al., 2007; Ghetti et al., 2010; DeMaster and Ghetti, 2013). Based on the results of 54 previous studies, Lepage et al. (1998) proposed the Hippocampus Encoding/Retrieval (HIPER) Model that specifies the anterior hippocampus's role in acquiring or encoding new visuospatial information and the posterior hippocampus's role in retrieval. Subsequent studies have further supported this model (Strange and Dolan, 2001; Hartley et al., 2003; Kumaran and Maguire, 2005; Maguire et al., 2006a; Iaria et al., 2007). Most of the previous studies had focused on spatial memory and have thus implicated the posterior hippocampus for such a function. For example, the "place cells" were found only in the posterior hippocampus in monkeys (Colombo et al., 1998). Taxi drivers' constant retrieval of city maps can lead to increased gray matter volume (GMV) of the posterior hippocampus (Woollett and Maguire, 2011).

If the hippocampus plays a crucial role in visuospatial processing (in particular, the anterior hippocampus's role in spatial information encoding), would its structural variations explain one of the most well-documented sex differences—that in visuospatial processing? Decades of behavioral research have shown that sex differences in visuospatial ability are stable across different age groups (Voyer et al., 1995) and that males' advantage is particularly obvious in mental rotation (Linn and Petersen, 1985; Maeda and Yoon, 2013; Reilly and Neumann, 2013; Lütke and Lange-Küttner, 2015). Moreover, compared to 2-dimensional (2D) mental rotation, 3-dimensional (3D) mental rotation (which requires more spatial processing) has a larger and more consistent sex effect across age groups (Peters et al., 1995; Roberts and Bell, 2003; for a meta-analysis, see Linn and Petersen, 1985). Overall, sex differences are robust based on large-scale studies (e.g., 109,612 men and 88,509 women in Maylor et al., 2007, study; 90,000 women and 111,000 men in Lippa et al., 2010 study) and meta-analysis studies (Geiser et al., 2008; Maeda and Yoon, 2013; Reilly and Neumann, 2013). These sex differences are so robust that only special experimental designs (e.g., positive instructions to women, different delivery modes) or training would reduce or sometimes eliminate them (Goldstein et al., 1990; Peters et al., 1995; Roberts and Bell, 2003; Peters, 2005; Feng et al., 2007; Monahan et al., 2008; Moè, 2009; Glück and Fabrizii, 2010; Tzuriel and Egozi, 2010; Maeda and Yoon, 2013).

In support of a possible neural basis of sex differences in mental rotation, especially, 3D mental rotation, neuroimaging studies have found structural and functional differences between male and female hippocampi. Structurally, the total volume of the hippocampus was larger for females than for males (Giedd et al., 1997; Goldstein et al., 2001). Males showed a significant correlation between the size of the hippocampus and age (from 18 years to 42 years), which was not significant for females (Pruessner et al., 2001; Suzuki et al., 2005), suggesting that the growth of the hippocampus occurred earlier in females (Giedd et al., 1997). Functionally, when performing a navigation task, males have been found to depend more on the hippocampus, whereas females depend more on the parietal and frontal lobes (Grön et al., 2000). Thus far, however, no study has examined whether structural differences in the hippocampus would account for sex differences in 3D mental rotation.

In the current study, we examined the relationship between GMV of the hippocampus (especially its anterior part) and sex differences in 3D mental rotation. The anterior part is particularly relevant because mental rotation tasks mainly involve the encoding of spatial information, rather than the retrieval of previously stored spatial information. We hypothesized that males would have larger volumes in the anterior hippocampus than would females, and such a difference would explain a large part of sex differences in 3D mental rotation.

MATERIALS AND METHODS

Participants

Participants were 431 college students (192 males and 239 females, mean age = 19.9 years, ranging from 18 to 24 years) from Beijing Normal University. No participants had a history of neurological or psychiatric disorders or head injury. This study was approved by the Institutional Review Board of the Imaging Center for Brain Research in the Institute of Cognitive Neuroscience and Learning at Beijing Normal University.

MRI Acquisition

Whole brain structural MRI scans were performed on a Siemens 3T Trio scanner (Munich, Germany) by using a T1-weighted three-dimensional gradient echo sequence (TR = 2350 ms, TE = 3.39 ms; flip angle = 7°; field of view = 100 mm; matrix = 256 × 256; voxel size = 1 mm × 1 mm × 1 mm).

Behavioral Tasks

The three-dimensional mental rotation task was based on Shepard's mental rotation task (Shepard and Metzler, 1971; Peters et al., 1995). Participants were presented one 3D picture as the target and four as answer choices, and they were asked to select the answer that matched the target after rotation. This task had 24 items, which were divided into two 3-min blocks. The total score was analyzed.

Motor-Free Visual Perception Test, Third Edition (MVPT-3) was used to test the general visual perception ability (Colarusso and Hammill, 1972). Five categories of visual perception were measured: spatial relationship, visual closure, visual discrimination, visual memory and figure ground. Total score was analyzed. This task was used to control the general visual perception ability.

Raven's Advanced Progressive Matrices (RAPM; Raven and Court, 1998) was used to assess general intelligence. Subjects were given 30 min to complete as many items as possible. For each test item, subjects were asked to select from several alternatives of the missing segment that would complete a larger pattern. The number of correct trials was analyzed.

Data Analysis

Structural Whole Brain Analysis

Data were analyzed by using voxel-based morphometry (VBM) implemented in Statistical Parametric Mapping (SPM5, Wellcome Department of Cognitive Neurology) and executed in MATLAB (R2012b, Mathworks, Sherborn, MA, USA). Following the procedures described by Ashburner and Friston (2000) and Good et al. (2001), we conducted the following steps of data pre-processing: extraction of the brain, spatial normalization into the stereotactic space by using the standard SPM gray template, segmentation into gray and white matter and CSF compartments, and correction for volume changes induced by spatial normalization (modulation). The spatially normalized images were written in voxels of 1 mm × 1 mm × 1 mm. The smoothing with a 12 mm full width at half maximum (FWHM) isotropic Gaussian kernel was applied. In the current study, the GMV was analyzed. Two-sample t-test was used to investigate sex differences in GMV of the hippocampus.

Structural ROI Analysis

The current study focused only on the hippocampus arch, which can be divided into three parts: anterior, middle and posterior hippocampus. This segmentation method has been commonly used to study the different parts of hippocampus arch (Huang et al., 2013; Travis et al., 2014; for a review see Malykhin and Coupland, 2015). The segmentation process was executed in MATLAB (Mathworks, Sherborn, MA, USA). A sagittal view of the hippocampus from Anatomical Automatic Labeling (AAL) was projected onto a plane and the maximum values in the right-left direction and the top-down direction were calculated. After marking the hippocampus into four quarters, it was divided into the anterior, middle, and posterior parts, with the ratios of 1:2:1 (Duvernoy, 2005), which were then used as the mask for structural ROI analysis. To control for sex differences in overall brain size, the whole brain GMV was used as a covariate. A separate analysis was conducted without controlling for the whole brain GMV (see Supplementary Material).

Statistical analysis of the behavioral data was conducted in SPSS (SPSS Inc., Chicago, IL, USA).

RESULTS

Behavioral Results

The behavioral tasks showed that males performed better than females on the 3D mental rotation task ($F_{(1,429)} = 5.95, p = 0.015, d = 0.234$). This sex difference became even slightly greater ($F_{(1,427)} = 7.65$, $p = 0.006$, $d = 0.254$), after controlling for general visual perception and intelligence (RAPM) even though these two correlates did not show significant sex differences (for visual perception, $F_{(1,429)} = 2.77$, $p = 0.097$; and for RAPM, $F_{(1,429)} = 2.43, p = 0.120$; see **Table 1**).

Structural ROI Analysis

The structural ROI analysis involved six brain areas (bilateral anterior, middle and posterior hippocampus), so we used Bonferroni correction to adjust for the significance thresholds: $p = 0.05/6 = 0.008$. Controlling for the whole brain GMV, the GMV of the anterior hippocampus was significantly larger for males than for females ($F_{(1,428)} = 14.92$, $p < 0.008$, for the left hemisphere, and $F_{(1,428)} = 13.44$, $p < 0.008$, for the right hemisphere), whereas the posterior hippocampus was significantly larger for females than males ($F_{(1,428)} = 24.32$, $p < 0.008$, for the left hemisphere, and $F_{(1,428)} = 9.59, p < 0.008$, for the right hemisphere; see **Table 2** and Supplementary Table 1S). There was no significant sex difference in GMV of the middle hippocampus ($F_{(1,428)} = 0.001$, *n.s.*, for the left hemisphere; $F_{(1,428)} = 0.01$, *n.s.*, for the right hemisphere). After controlling for the whole brain GMV, there also were no significant sex differences in GMV of the whole left hippocampus ($F_{(1,428)} = 0.07$, *n.s.*) and the whole right hippocampus ($F_{(1,428)} = 0.19$, *n.s.*).

Table 3 shows the correlations between GMVs of the different parts of the hippocampus and the scores of 3D mental rotation and the other two cognitive tasks after controlling for the whole brain GMV (see Supplementary Table 2S). The results showed that GMVs of the left and right anterior hippocampus were significantly correlated with performance on the 3D mental rotation task (left, $r = 0.14, p < 0.008$; right, $r = 0.19, p < 0.008$; see **Figure 1** and Supplementary Figure 1S). After controlling for visual perception, the correlations between 3D mental rotation and the GMVs of the left and right anterior hippocampus

TABLE 1 | Mean scores (and standard deviations) and sex differences for the three behavioral tasks.

Task	Measure	Mean (SD)		F
		Male	Female	Sex
3-D mental rotation	Number of correct items in 6 min	20.34 (8.92)	18.42 (7.43)	5.95*
MVTP	Total score	42.79 (4.37)	43.49 (4.24)	2.77
Raven's advanced progressive matrices	Number of correct items in 30 min	36.65 (4.67)	37.28 (3.71)	2.43

Note: *$p < 0.05$.

TABLE 2 | Mean scores (and standard error) and sex differences in gray matter volumes (mm³) of the left and right anterior, middle and posterior hippocampus (with the gray matter volume of the whole brain as a covariate).

	Sex		*F*	*p*
	Male	Female		
Left				
Anterior	1202.93 (4.21)	1180.06 (3.77)	14.92	**0.0001**
Middle	2458.53 (10.52)	2458.69 (9.43)	0.0001	0.99
Posterior	585.90 (4.07)	612.86 (3.64)	24.32	**0.000001**
Right				
Anterior	1211.27 (5.22)	1185.55 (4.68)	13.44	**0.0003**
Middle	2346.08 (9.92)	2347.33 (8.89)	0.01	0.93
Posterior	564.98 (3.77)	580.66 (3.37)	9.59	**0.002**

Note: The critical p value after Bonferroni correction was 0.008 (0.05/6 ROIs). Significant p values are in bold.

remained significant (left, $r = 0.14$, $p < 0.008$; right, $r = 0.19$, $p < 0.008$). After controlling for intelligence, the correlation between 3D mental rotation and the GMVs of the right anterior hippocampus remained significant (right, $r = 0.17$, $p < 0.008$). After controlling for both visual perception and intelligence, the correlation between 3D mental rotation and the GMV of the right anterior hippocampus also remained significant (right, $r = 0.18$, $p < 0.008$). The correlations between mental rotation and the GMV of the left anterior hippocampus ($r = 0.12$, controlling for either intelligence alone or both intelligence and visual perception) were no longer significant after Bonferroni correction.

ANCOVA was conducted to test whether the sex difference in 3D mental rotation could be explained by sex differences in GMVs of the hippocampus. After controlling for GMVs of the right anterior hippocampus and the whole brain, the sex difference in 3D mental rotation was no longer significant ($F_{(1,427)} = 3.04$, $p = 0.070$). The change in sex difference was statistically significant ($t = 3.47$, $p < 0.01$).

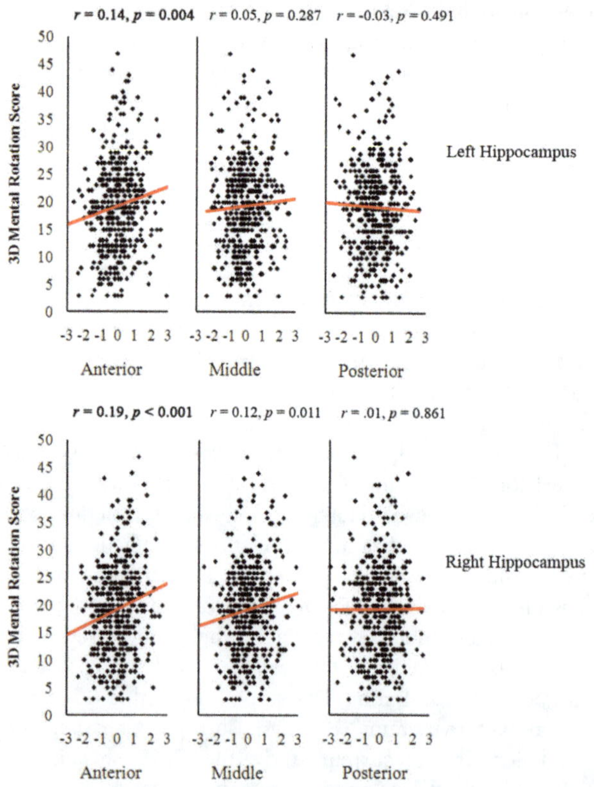

FIGURE 1 | Scatter plots between gray matter volumes (GMV) of anterior, middle and posterior hippocampus and 3-dimensional (3D) mental rotation performance (with the GMV of the whole brain as a covariate). The critical *p* value after Bonferroni correction was 0.008 (0.05/6 ROIs). Significant *p* values are in bold.

Whole-Brain Analysis

To supplement the structural ROI analysis, we conducted a whole-brain analysis in SPM. Sex differences in the whole brain GMV are shown in **Table 4**. Correlation analysis confirmed that the structure of left and right anterior hippocampus was correlated with 3D mental rotation ($p < 0.05$, FWE-corrected for multiple comparison, peak, left: $x = -34$, $y = -9$, $z = -19$, $t = 3.80$; right: $x = 35$, $y = -9$, $z = -17$, $t = 4.69$; see **Figure 2**). In addition, GMV in the calcarine was significantly and positively associated with 3D mental rotation ($p < 0.05$,

TABLE 3 | Correlation coefficients between gray matter volumes of the left and right hippocampus and behavioral performance (with the gray matter volume of the whole brain as a covariate).

	Left			Right		
	Anterior	Middle	Posterior	Anterior	Middle	Posterior
3-D mental rotation						
r	**0.14**	0.05	−0.03	**0.19**	0.12	0.01
p	**0.004**	0.287	0.491	**0.000**	0.011	0.861
MVTP						
r	0.08	0.10	0.01	0.07	0.07	0.04
p	0.119	0.045	0.881	0.156	0.135	0.43
Raven's advanced progressive matrices						
r	0.12	−0.00	0.02	0.11	0.00	0.08
p	0.015	0.989	0.629	0.028	0.943	0.087

Note: The critical p value after Bonferroni correction was 0.008 (0.05/6 ROIs). Significant p values are in bold.

TABLE 4 | Loci showing significant sex differences in gray matter volume based on the whole brain analysis ($p < 0.001$, FWE-corrected for multiple comparisons, cluster size >200).

Brain region	Brodmann area	Cluster size	Coordinates			*t* value	$P_{corrected}$
Brain areas showing greater gray matter volumes in males than in females							
Right lingual	BA 17	21,486	12	−92	−13	13.06	<0.000001
	BA 17		53	−66	−22	12.43	<0.000001
	BA 17		43	−76	−17	11.49	<0.000001
	BA 30		9	−54	8	5.91	0.0004
Right hippocampus	BA 36	3467	12	−7	−34	9.09	<0.000001
	BA 36		19	−3	−31	8.88	<0.000001
Left precuneus	BA 30	2132	−4	−49	16	7.73	<0.000001
Left cerebellum		2041	−29	−73	−19	8.09	<0.000001
		1107	−30	−39	−56	10.3	<0.000001
		1013	−20	−59	−33	7.75	<0.000001
Left fusiform	BA 20	495	−30	−3	−44	6.69	0.000005
Right rectus	BA 47	453	20	13	−15	8.05	<0.000001
Right putamen		430	24	0	5	7.07	<0.000001
Right paracentral lobule	BA 5	416	4	−40	75	9.22	<0.000001
	BA 5		0	−27	76	7.96	<0.000001
	BA 5		−3	−44	72	6.68	0.000006
Right precuneus	BA 30		5	−47	14	7.69	<0.000001
Left amygdala		316	−23	−3	−25	6.37	0.00003
Left lingual	BA 18	209	−9	−84	−3	6.28	0.00005
	BA 18		−6	−74	0	5.98	0.0002
Brain areas showing greater gray matter volumes in females than males							
Right thalamus		2381	3	−15	0	8.84	<0.000001
Left caudate		1709	−8	8	11	8.37	<0.000001
Right caudate		1284	8	6	9	7.72	0.00003
Right cerebellum		464	50	−75	36	8.17	0.000002
Left cerebellum		381	−51	−72	−35	8.37	<0.000001

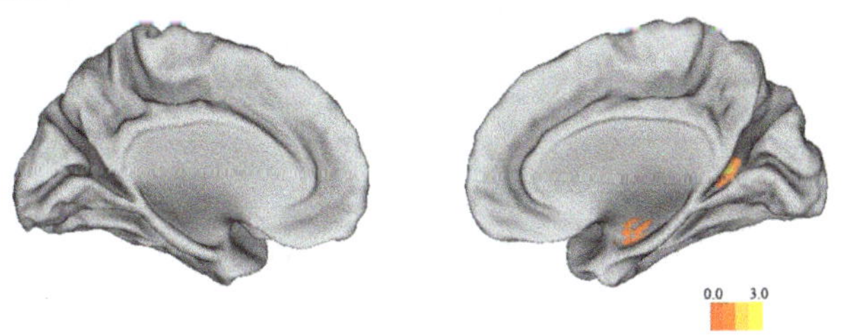

FIGURE 2 | The correlation map between 3D mental rotation performance and GMV of the whole brain ($p < 0.05$, FWE-corrected for multiple comparisons, cluster size >50).

FWE-corrected for multiple comparison, cluster size >50; **Table 5**).

DISCUSSION

In the present study, we found that, compared to females, males performed better in 3D mental rotation and had greater GMV in the anterior hippocampus. The GMV of the right anterior hippocampus was significantly correlated with 3D mental rotation performance, even after controlling for visual perception and general intelligence. The sex difference in 3D mental rotation disappeared after controlling for GMV of the right anterior hippocampus.

Sex Differences in Spatial Abilities

Our behavioral results were consistent with many previous studies that showed a stable male advantage in spatial ability, especially in 3D mental rotation. This male advantage may have had an evolutionary origin because of males' role in hunting, for which a good sense of direction and a superior ability in spatial relations (throwing spears at the games) had been critical (Geary, 1995; Ecuyer-Dab and Robert, 2004). In modern-day life, males may no longer need to hunt, but they still prefer activities involving spatial processing such video games and sports (Okagaki and Frensch, 1994; Ozel et al., 2004; Robert and Héroux, 2004; Cherney and London, 2006), which may have continued to help males gain an advantage in spatial ability. Males and females have also been found to use different strategies when performing a navigation task, with males using spatial strategies and females using both verbal and spatial strategies (Merrill et al., 2016).

It is worth mentioning that, although Raven's Progressive Matrices test also involves spatial processing and mental rotation, it did not show sex differences in our study. This result is consistent with previous studies (e.g., Raven, 1938; Eysenck and Kamin, 1981; Wei et al., 2012; Lütke and Lange-Küttner, 2015). There are at least two possible reasons. First, Raven's Progressive Matrices aims to test general intelligence, so it includes measures of both visuospatial ability and reasoning. Using structural equation modeling, Schweizer et al. (2007) showed that the component of reasoning explained 46% of the

TABLE 5 | Loci showing positive correlations between 3-dimensional (3D) mental rotation and gray matter volumes based on the whole brain analysis ($p < 0.05$, FWE-corrected for multiple comparisons, cluster size >50).

Brain region	Brodmann area	Cluster size	Coordinates			*t* value	$P_{corrected}$
Right calcarine	BA 30	397	23	−55	8	5.01	0.03
Right anterior hippocampus		393	35	−9	−17	4.69	0.03
	BA 28	66	24	4	−23	4.51	0.03

variance of the total score, whereas mental rotation explained only 7% (Schweizer et al., 2007). Second, Raven's mental rotation task involves only 2D rotation, which has smaller sex differences than 3D rotation (Peters et al., 1995; Roberts and Bell, 2003; Lütke and Lange-Küttner, 2015).

Neural Basis of Sex Differences in Spatial Abilities

Sex difference in spatial processing has been associated with the volume and activation of the hippocampus. In nonhuman animals, the sex that is responsible for searching for food and nesting has a larger hippocampus (Clayton et al., 1997, and for a review see Lee et al., 1998). Our results showed that compared to females, males had a larger anterior hippocampus, which accounted for their advantage in 3D mental rotation. Consistently, previous research has linked a larger anterior hippocampus to better performance in encoding new spatial information (Maguire et al., 2006b). Our results on the role of the anterior hippocampus in mental rotation are consistent with the HIPER model (Lepage et al., 1998). According to this model, the anterior hippocampus is responsible for acquiring or encoding new visuospatial information, more specifically, coding information for head directions and angular features (Maguire et al., 1998), and registering new and abstract spatial environment (Save et al., 1992; Hartley et al., 2003; Sperling et al., 2003; Jackson and Schacter, 2004; Maguire et al., 2006b; Chua et al., 2007; Iaria et al., 2007; Doeller et al., 2008). Functional MRI studies also found that imagination tasks activated anterior hippocampus more than did memory tasks (Addis et al., 2007, 2009). The 3D mental rotation task seems to meet the requirements of this particular type of spatial information processing because it involves head directions and angular features and the 3D figures were likely to be new and abstract to the participants. Therefore, it seems likely that the anterior hippocampus subserves 3D mental rotation as tested in our project. Furthermore, it was the right anterior hippocampus that had a high correlation with 3D mental rotation after controlling for covariates. Consistent with such hemispheric specialization, previous fMRI studies have found that navigation tasks activate the right anterior hippocampus (Maguire et al., 1998; Mellet et al., 2000; Iaria et al., 2003, 2009; Doeller et al., 2008) and lesion studies have found that damages to the right anterior hippocampus impair spatial memory while damages to the left anterior hippocampus impair verbal memory (Abrahams et al., 1997; Bohbot et al., 1998). In sum, structural differences between males and females in the right anterior hippocampus seem to explain sex differences in 3D mental rotation.

Interestingly, the sex difference in the posterior hippocampus was opposite of that in the anterior hippocampus. Consequently, the whole hippocampus did not show sex difference in GMV. Some of the previous studies, however, have shown sex difference in the total GMV of the hippocampus (Giedd et al., 1997; Goldstein et al., 2001). One possible reason is age differences between studies. Goldstein et al. (2001) found that females in their 30 s (mean = 36.3 years of age) showed a larger hippocampus than their male counterparts and Pruessner et al. (2001) found that males in their 30 s began to show a decrease in their hippocampus. Our participants were all college students. Indeed previous studies found sex differences in developmental trajectories of the size of the hippocampus (Giedd et al., 1997; Pruessner et al., 2001; Suzuki et al., 2005).

It should be mentioned that, although our study focused on the hippocampus's role in 3D mental rotation, our whole-brain analysis also found that the right calcarine was associated with 3D mental rotation. The calcarine sulcus is an important part of the primary visual cortex (V1; Sereno et al., 1995), which is important for all types of visual processing, but its specific role in 3D mental rotation needs further research. In addition to these two regions, previous studies found that mental rotation also elicited activation in other brain regions, but with mixed results on sex differences. One study found that males activated the frontal gyrus, cingulate cortex and occipital gyrus more than did females (Semrud-Clikeman et al., 2012), whereas another study found that females activated the middle temporal gyrus, frontal gyrus and primary motor cortex more than did males (Kucian et al., 2005). These cross-study differences in other brain regions may have been due to different levels of difficulty of the tasks (Roberts and Bell, 2003) or the particular paradigms used in different studies. Previous studies also found that the parietal lobe, rather than the hippocampus, had the highest correlation with spatial ability (Corbetta et al., 2000; Koscik et al., 2009; Hänggi et al., 2010). There are three possible explanations. First, the hippocampus is involved during the early brief stage of the spatial tasks (Iaria et al., 2003; Etchamendy et al., 2012), and thus its activation may be overshadowed by later stages of processing. Event-related potentials (ERP) studies also showed a late posterior negativity related to mental rotation tasks (Peronnet and Farah, 1989; Heil, 2002). Second, there are sex differences in neural bases of spatial processing, which might have complicated previous findings: males depend more on the hippocampus for spatial processing, whereas females depend more on the parietal and frontal lobes (Grön et al., 2000). Third, as mentioned earlier, task differences (using spatial or verbal strategies) affect the involvement of the hippocampus (Iaria et al., 2003; Bohbot et al., 2004).

Finally, although this study found significant sex differences in 3D mental rotation which could be accounted for by structural differences in the right anterior hippocampus, we should recognize that the brain is plastic and the structure of the hippocampus could be changed through training (Lövdén et al., 2010; Kühn and Gallinat, 2014; Kühn et al., 2014), even in the case of the aging brain (Kempermann et al., 1998; Maguire et al., 2000, 2006a; Lövdén et al., 2012). Training has been found to improve spatial ability (Sanchez, 2012; Sorby et al., 2013) and reduce or eliminate its sex difference (Terlecki and Newcombe, 2005; Feng et al., 2007; Spence et al., 2009; Tzuriel and Egozi, 2010). In addition, some researchers have also found that the GMV of females' posterior hippocampus changes with menstrual cycle, showing increases from the early follicular phase to the late follicular phase (Lisofsky et al., 2015). Such an influence should be considered in future research of sex differences in the hippocampus, especially the posterior hippocampus.

AUTHOR CONTRIBUTIONS

CC, QD and XZ designed the study. WW analyzed the data. WW, CC and XZ wrote the manuscript.

ACKNOWLEDGEMENTS

This research was supported by the National Key Basic Research Program of China (no. 2014CB846100), two grants from the Natural Science Foundation of China (nos. 31521063 and 31271187), a grant from Advanced Technology Innovation Center for Future Education, Beijing Normal University, and the 111 Project (B07008). We thank Chunhui Chen, Qinghua He, Jin Li, Mingxia Zhang, Bi Zhu, Xuemei Lei, and many others for helping collect the data.

REFERENCES

Abrahams, S., Pickering, A., Polkey, C. G., and Morris, R. E. (1997). Spatial memory deficits in patients with unilateral damage to the right hippocampal formation. *Neuropsychologia* 35, 11–24. doi: 10.1016/s0028-3932(96)00051-6

Addis, D. R., Pan, L., Vu, M. A., Laiser, N., and Schacter, D. L. (2009). Constructive episodic simulation of the future and the past: distinct subsystems of a core brain network mediate imagining and remembering. *Neuropsychologia* 47, 2222–2238. doi: 10.1016/j.neuropsychologia.2008.10.026

Addis, D. R., Wong, A. T., and Schacter, D. L. (2007). Remembering the past and imagining the future: common and distinct neural substrates during event construction and elaboration. *Neuropsychologia* 45, 1363–1377. doi: 10.1016/j.neuropsychologia.2006.10.016

Aguirre, G. K., and D'Esposito, M. (1999). Topographical disorientation: a synthesis and taxonomy. *Brain* 122, 1613–1628. doi: 10.1093/brain/122.9.1613

Ashburner, J., and Friston, K. J. (2000). Voxel-based morphometry—the methods. *Neuroimage* 11, 805–821. doi: 10.1006/nimg.2000.0582

Bohbot, V. D., Iaria, G., and Petrides, M. (2004). Hippocampal function and spatial memory: evidence from functional neuroimaging in healthy participants and performance of patients with medial temporal lobe resections. *Neuropsychology* 18, 418–425. doi: 10.1037/0894-4105.18.3.418

Bohbot, V. D., Kalina, M., Stepankova, K., Spackova, N., Petrides, M., and Nadel, L. (1998). Spatial memory deficits in patients with lesions to the right hippocampus and to the right parahippocampal cortex. *Neuropsychologia* 36, 1217–1238. doi: 10.1016/s0028-3932(97)00161-9

Burgess, N., Maguire, E. A., and O'Keefe, J. (2002). The human hippocampus and spatial and episodic memory. *Neuron* 35, 625–641. doi: 10.1016/s0896-6273(02)00830-9

Cherney, I. D., and London, K. (2006). Gender-linked differences in the toys, television shows, computer games and outdoor activities of 5-to 13-year-old children. *Sex Roles* 54, 717–726. doi: 10.1007/s11199-006-9037-8

Chua, E. F., Schacter, D. L., Rand-Giovannetti, E., and Sperling, R. A. (2007). Evidence for a specific role of the anterior hippocampal region in successful associative encoding. *Hippocampus* 17, 1071–1080. doi: 10.1002/hipo.20340

Clayton, N. S., Reboreda, J. C., and Kacelnik, A. (1997). Seasonal changes of hippocampus volume in parasitic cowbirds. *Behav. Processes* 41, 237–243. doi: 10.1016/s0376-6357(97)00050-8

Colarusso, R. P., and Hammill, D. D. (1972). *Motor-Free Visual Perception Test.* Novato, CA: Academic Therapy Publications.

Colombo, M., Fernandez, T., Nakamura, K., and Gross, C. G. (1998). Functional differentiation along the anterior-posterior axis of the hippocampus in monkeys. *J. Neurophysiol.* 80, 1002–1005.

Corbetta, M., Kincade, J. M., Ollinger, J. M., McAvoy, M. P., and Shulman, G. L. (2000). Voluntary orienting is dissociated from target detection in human posterior parietal cortex. *Nat. Neurosci.* 3, 292–297. doi: 10.1038/73009

DeMaster, D. M., and Ghetti, S. (2013). Developmental differences in hippocampal and cortical contributions to episodic retrieval. *Cortex* 49, 1482–1493. doi: 10.1016/j.cortex.2012.08.004

Doeller, C. F., King, J. A., and Burgess, N. (2008). Parallel striatal and hippocampal systems for landmarks and boundaries in spatial memory. *Proc. Natl. Acad. Sci. U S A* 105, 5915–5920. doi: 10.1073/pnas.0801489105

Duvernoy, H. M. (2005). *The Human Hippocampus: Functional Anatomy, Vascularization and Serial Sections With MRI.* Berlin: Springer Science & Business Media.

Ecuyer-Dab, I., and Robert, M. (2004). Have sex differences in spatial ability evolved from male competition for mating and female concern for survival? *Cognition* 91, 221–257. doi: 10.1016/j.cognition.2003.09.007

Etchamendy, N., Konishi, K., Pike, G. B., Marighetto, A., and Bohbot, V. D. (2012). Evidence for a virtual human analog of a rodent relational memory task: a study of aging and fMRI in young adults. *Hippocampus* 22, 869–880. doi: 10.1002/hipo.20948

Eysenck, H. J., and Kamin, L. (1981). *Intelligence: The Battle for the Mind.* Berlin: Springer.

Feng, J., Spence, I., and Pratt, J. (2007). Playing an action video game reduces gender differences in spatial cognition. *Psychol. Sci.* 18, 850–855. doi: 10.1111/j.1467-9280.2007.01990.x

Fyhn, M., Molden, S., Witter, M. P., Moser, E. I., and Moser, M.-B. (2004). Spatial representation in the entorhinal cortex. *Science* 305, 1258–1264. doi: 10.1126/science.1099901

Geary, D. C. (1995). Sexual selection and sex differences in spatial cognition. *Learn. Individ. Differ.* 7, 289–301. doi: 10.1016/1041-6080(95)90003-9

Geiser, C., Lehmann, W., and Eid, M. (2008). A note on sex differences in mental rotation in different age groups. *Intelligence* 36, 556–563. doi: 10.1016/j.intell.2007.12.003

Ghetti, S., DeMaster, D. M., Yonelinas, A. P., and Bunge, S. A. (2010). Developmental differences in medial temporal lobe function during memory encoding. *J. Neurosci.* 30, 9548–9556. doi: 10.1523/JNEUROSCI.3500-09.2010

Giedd, J. N., Castellanos, F. X., Rajapakse, J. C., Vaituzis, A. C., and Rapoport, J. L. (1997). Sexual dimorphism of the developing human brain. *Prog.*

Neuropsychopharmacol. Biol. Psychiatry 21, 1185–1201. doi: 10.1016/s0278-5846(97)00158-9

Glück, J., and Fabrizii, C. (2010). Gender differences in the Mental Rotations Test are partly explained by response format. *J. Individ. Differ.* 31, 106–109. doi: 10.1027/1614-0001/a000019

Goldstein, D., Haldane, D., and Mitchell, C. (1990). Sex differences in visual-spatial ability: the role of performance factors. *Mem. Cognit.* 18, 546–550. doi: 10.3758/bf03198487

Goldstein, J. M., Seidman, L. J., Horton, N. J., Makris, N., Kennedy, D. N., Caviness, V. S., et al. (2001). Normal sexual dimorphism of the adult human brain assessed by *in vivo* magnetic resonance imaging. *Cereb. Cortex* 11, 490–497. doi: 10.1093/cercor/11.6.490

Good, C. D., Johnsrude, I., Ashburner, J., Henson, R. N., Friston, K. J., and Frackowiak, R. S. (2001). Cerebral asymmetry and the effects of sex and handedness on brain structure: a voxel-based morphometric analysis of 465 normal adult human brains. *Neuroimage* 14, 685–700. doi: 10.1006/nimg.2001.0857

Grön, G., Wunderlich, A. P., Spitzer, M., Tomczak, R., and Riepe, M. W. (2000). Brain activation during human navigation: gender-different neural networks as substrate of performance. *Nat. Neurosci.* 3, 404–408. doi: 10.1038/73980

Hänggi, J., Buchmann, A., Mondadori, C. R., Henke, K., Jäncke, L., and Hock, C. (2010). Sexual dimorphism in the parietal substrate associated with visuospatial cognition independent of general intelligence. *J. Cogn. Neurosci.* 22, 139–155. doi: 10.1162/jocn.2008.21175

Hartley, T., Maguire, E. A., Spiers, H. J., and Burgess, N. (2003). The well-worn route and the path less traveled: distinct neural bases of route following and wayfinding in humans. *Neuron* 37, 877–888. doi: 10.1016/s0896-6273(03)00095-3

Heil, M. (2002). The functional significance of ERP effects during mental rotation. *Psychophysiology* 39, 535–545. doi: 10.1111/1469-8986.3950535

Holdstock, J., Mayes, A., Cezayirli, E., Isaac, C., Aggleton, J., and Roberts, N. (2000). A comparison of egocentric and allocentric spatial memory in a patient with selective hippocampal damage. *Neuropsychologia* 38, 410–425. doi: 10.1016/s0028-3932(99)00099-8

Huang, Y., Coupland, N. J., Lebel, R. M., Carter, R., Seres, P., Wilman, A. H., et al. (2013). Structural changes in hippocampal subfields in major depressive disorder: a high-field magnetic resonance imaging study. *Biol. Psychiatry* 74, 62–68. doi: 10.1016/j.biopsych.2013.01.005

Iaria, G., and Barton, J. J. (2010). Developmental topographical disorientation: a newly discovered cognitive disorder. *Exp. Brain Res.* 206, 189–196. doi: 10.1007/s00221-010-2256-9

Iaria, G., Bogod, N., Fox, C. J., and Barton, J. J. (2009). Developmental topographical disorientation: case one. *Neuropsychologia* 47, 30–40. doi: 10.1016/j.neuropsychologia.2008.08.021

Iaria, G., Chen, J. K., Guariglia, C., Ptito, A., and Petrides, M. (2007). Retrosplenial and hippocampal brain regions in human navigation: complementary functional contributions to the formation and use of cognitive maps. *Eur. J. Neurosci.* 25, 890–899. doi: 10.1111/j.1460-9568.2007.05371.x

Iaria, G., Lanyon, L. J., Fox, C. J., Giaschi, D., and Barton, J. J. (2008). Navigational skills correlate with hippocampal fractional anisotropy in humans. *Hippocampus* 18, 335–339. doi: 10.1002/hipo.20400

Iaria, G., Petrides, M., Dagher, A., Pike, B., and Bohbot, V. D. (2003). Cognitive strategies dependent on the hippocampus and caudate nucleus in human navigation: variability and change with practice. *J. Neurosci.* 23, 5945–5952.

Jackson, O. III, and Schacter, D. L. (2004). Encoding activity in anterior medial temporal lobe supports subsequent associative recognition. *Neuroimage* 21, 456–462. doi: 10.1016/j.neuroimage.2003.09.050

Jacobs, L. F., and Spencer, W. D. (1994). Natural space-use patterns and hippocampal size in kangaroo rats. *Brain Behav. Evol.* 44, 125–132. doi: 10.1159/000113584

Kempermann, G., Kuhn, H. G., and Gage, F. H. (1998). Experience-induced neurogenesis in the senescent dentate gyrus. *J. Neurosci.* 18, 3206–3212.

Koscik, T., O'Leary, D., Moser, D. J., Andreasen, N. C., and Nopoulos, P. (2009). Sex differences in parietal lobe morphology: relationship to mental rotation performance. *Brain Cogn.* 69, 451–459. doi: 10.1016/j.bandc.2008.09.004

Krebs, J. R., Sherry, D. F., Healy, S. D., Perry, V. H., and Vaccarino, A. L. (1989). Hippocampal specialization of food-storing birds. *Proc. Natl. Acad. Sci. U S A* 86, 1388–1392. doi: 10.1073/pnas.86.4.1388

Kucian, K., Loenneker, T., Dietrich, T., Martin, E., and Von Aster, M. (2005). Gender differences in brain activation patterns during mental rotation and number related cognitive tasks. *Psychol. Sci.* 47, 112–131.

Kühn, S., and Gallinat, J. (2014). Amount of lifetime video gaming is positively associated with entorhinal, hippocampal and occipital volume. *Mol. Psychiatry* 19, 842–847. doi: 10.1038/mp.2013.100

Kühn, S., Gleich, T., Lorenz, R. C., Lindenberger, U., and Gallinat, J. (2014). Playing Super Mario induces structural brain plasticity: gray matter changes resulting from training with a commercial video game. *Mol. Psychiatry* 19, 265–271. doi: 10.1038/mp.2013.120

Kumaran, D., and Maguire, E. A. (2005). The human hippocampus: cognitive maps or relational memory? *J. Neurosci.* 25, 7254–7259. doi: 10.1523/JNEUROSCI.1103-05.2005

Lee, D. W., Miyasato, L. E., and Clayton, N. S. (1998). Neurobiological bases of spatial learning in the natural environment: neurogenesis and growth in the avian and mammalian hippocampus. *Neuroreport* 9, R15–R27. doi: 10.1097/00001756-199805110-00076

Lee, A. C., Yeung, L.-K., and Barense, M. D. (2012). The hippocampus and visual perception. *Front. Hum. Neurosci.* 6:91. doi: 10.3389/fnhum.2012.00091

Lepage, M., Habib, R., and Tulving, E. (1998). Hippocampal PET activations of memory encoding and retrieval: the HIPER model. *Hippocampus* 8, 313–322. doi: 10.1002/(SICI)1098-1063(1998)8:4<313::AID-HIPO1>3.0.CO;2-I

Linn, M. C., and Petersen, A. C. (1985). Emergence and characterization of sex differences in spatial ability: a meta-analysis. *Child Dev.* 56, 1479–1498. doi: 10.2307/1130467

Lippa, R. A., Collaer, M. L., and Peters, M. (2010). Sex differences in mental rotation and line angle judgments are positively associated with gender equality and economic development across 53 nations. *Arch. Sex. Behav.* 39, 990–997. doi: 10.1007/s10508-008-9460-8

Lisofsky, N., Mårtensson, J., Eckert, A., Lindenberger, U., Gallinat, J., and Kühn, S. (2015). Hippocampal volume and functional connectivity changes during the female menstrual cycle. *Neuroimage* 118, 154–162. doi: 10.1016/j.neuroimage.2015.06.012

Lövdén, M., Schaefer, S., Noack, H., Kanowski, M., Kaufmann, J., Tempelmann, C., et al. (2010). Performance-related increases in hippocampal N-acetylaspartate (NAA) induced by spatial navigation training are restricted to BDNF Val homozygotes. *Cereb. Cortex* 21, 1435–1442. doi: 10.1093/cercor/bhq230

Lövdén, M., Schaefer, S., Noack, H., Bodammer, N. C., Kühn, S., Heinze, H. J., et al. (2012). Spatial navigation training protects the hippocampus against age-related changes during early and late adulthood. *Neurobiol. Aging* 33, 620.e9–620.e22. doi: 10.1016/j.neurobiolaging.2011.02.013

Lütke, N., and Lange-Küttner, C. (2015). Keeping it in three dimensions: measuring the development of mental rotation in children with the rotated colour cube test (RCCT). *Int. J. Dev. Sci.* 9, 95–114. doi: 10.3233/dev-14154

Maeda, Y., and Yoon, S. Y. (2013). A meta-analysis on gender differences in mental rotation ability measured by the Purdue spatial visualization tests: visualization of rotations (PSVT: R). *Educ. Psychol. Rev.* 25, 69–94. doi: 10.1007/s10648-012-9215-x

Maguire, E. A. (1997). Hippocampal involvement in human topographical memory: evidence from functional imaging. *Philos. Trans. R. Soc. Lond. B Biol. Sci.* 352, 1475–1480. doi: 10.1098/rstb.1997.0134

Maguire, E. A., Burgess, N., Donnett, J. G., Frackowiak, R. S., Frith, C. D., and O'Keefe, J. (1998). Knowing where and getting there: a human navigation network. *Science* 280, 921–924. doi: 10.1126/science.280.5365.921

Maguire, E. A., Gadian, D. G., Johnsrude, I. S., Good, C. D., Ashburner, J., Frackowiak, R. S., et al. (2000). Navigation-related structural change in the hippocampi of taxi drivers. *Proc. Natl. Acad. Sci. U S A* 97, 4398–4403. doi: 10.1073/pnas.070039597

Maguire, E. A., Nannery, R., and Spiers, H. J. (2006a). Navigation around London by a taxi driver with bilateral hippocampal lesions. *Brain* 129, 2894–2907. doi: 10.1093/brain/awl286

Maguire, E. A., Woollett, K., and Spiers, H. J. (2006b). London taxi drivers and bus drivers: a structural MRI and neuropsychological analysis. *Hippocampus* 16, 1091–1101. doi: 10.1002/hipo.20233

Malykhin, N. V., and Coupland, N. J. (2015). Hippocampal neuroplasticity in major depressive disorder. *Neuroscience* 309, 200–213. doi: 10.1016/j.neuroscience.2015.04.047

Maylor, E. A., Reimers, S., Choi, J., Collaer, M. L., Peters, M., and Silverman, I. (2007). Gender and sexual orientation differences in cognition across adulthood: age is kinder to women than to men regardless of sexual orientation. *Arch. Sex. Behav.* 36, 235–249. doi: 10.1007/s10508-006-9155-y

Mellet, E., Bricogne, S., Tzourio-Mazoyer, N., Ghaëm, O., Petit, L., Zago, L., et al. (2000). Neural correlates of topographic mental exploration: the impact of route versus survey perspective learning. *Neuroimage* 12, 588–600. doi: 10.1006/nimg.2000.0648

Merrill, E. C., Yang, Y., Roskos, B., and Steele, S. (2016). Sex differences in using spatial and verbal abilities influence route learning performance in a virtual environment: a comparison of 6- to 12-year old boys and girls. *Front. Psychol.* 7:258. doi: 10.3389/fpsyg.2016.00258

Moè, A. (2009). Are males always better than females in mental rotation? Exploring a gender belief explanation. *Learn. Individ. Differ.* 19, 21–27. doi: 10.1016/j.lindif.2008.02.002

Monahan, J. S., Harke, M. A., and Shelley, J. R. (2008). Computerizing the mental rotations test: are gender differences maintained? *Behav. Res. Methods* 40, 422–427. doi: 10.3758/BRM.40.2.422

Okagaki, L., and Frensch, P. A. (1994). Effects of video game playing on measures of spatial performance: gender effects in late adolescence. *J. Appl. Dev. Psychol.* 15, 33–58. doi: 10.1016/0193-3973(94)90005-1

O'Keefe, J. (1976). Place units in the hippocampus of the freely moving rat. *Exp. Neurol.* 51, 78–109. doi: 10.1016/0014-4886(76)90055-8

Ozel, S., Larue, J., and Molinaro, C. (2004). Relation between sport and spatial imagery: comparison of three groups of participants. *J. Psychol.* 138, 49–64. doi: 10.3200/jrlp.138.1.49-64

Peronnet, F., and Farah, M. J. (1989). Mental rotation: an event-related potential study with a validated mental rotation task. *Brain Cogn.* 9, 279–288. doi: 10.1016/0278-2626(89)90037-7

Peters, M. (2005). Sex differences and the factor of time in solving Vandenberg and Kuse mental rotation problems. *Brain Cogn.* 57, 176–184. doi: 10.1016/j.bandc.2004.08.052

Peters, M., Laeng, B., Latham, K., Jackson, M., Zaiyouna, R., and Richardson, C. (1995). A redrawn Vandenberg and Kuse mental rotations test-different versions and factors that affect performance. *Brain Cogn.* 28, 39–58. doi: 10.1006/brcg.1995.1032

Pruessner, J., Collins, D., Pruessner, M., and Evans, A. (2001). Age and gender predict volume decline in the anterior and posterior hippocampus in early adulthood. *J. Neurosci.* 21, 194–200.

Raven, J. C. (1938). *Progressive Matrices: A Perceptual Test of Intelligence.* London: HK Lewis.

Raven, J. C., and Court, J. H. (1998). *Raven's Progressive Matrices and Vocabulary Scales.* Oxford, UK : Oxford Psychologists Press.

Rehkämper, G., Haase, E., and Frahm, H. D. (1988). Allometric comparison of brain weight and brain structure volumes in different breeds of the domestic pigeon, Columba livia fd (fantails, homing pigeons, strassers). *Brain Behav. Evol.* 31, 141–149. doi: 10.1159/000116581

Reilly, D., and Neumann, D. L. (2013). Gender-role differences in spatial ability: a meta-analytic review. *Sex Roles* 68, 521–535. doi: 10.1007/s11199-013-0269-0

Robert, M., and Héroux, G. (2004). Visuo-spatial play experience: forerunner of visuo-spatial achievement in preadolescent and adolescent boys and girls? *Infant Child Dev.* 13, 49–78. doi: 10.1002/icd.336

Roberts, J. E., and Bell, M. A. (2003). Two-and three-dimensional mental rotation tasks lead to different parietal laterality for men and women. *Int. J. Psychophysiol.* 50, 235–246. doi: 10.1016/s0167-8760(03)00195-8

Sanchez, C. A. (2012). Enhancing visuospatial performance through video game training to increase learning in visuospatial science domains. *Psychon. Bull. Rev.* 19, 58–65. doi: 10.3758/s13423-011-0177-7

Sargolini, F., Fyhn, M., Hafting, T., McNaughton, B. L., Witter, M. P., Moser, M.-B., et al. (2006). Conjunctive representation of position, direction and velocity in entorhinal cortex. *Science* 312, 758–762. doi: 10.1126/science.1125572

Save, E., Poucet, B., Foreman, N., and Buhot, M.-C. (1992). Object exploration and reactions to spatial and nonspatial changes in hooded rats following damage to parietal cortex or hippocampal formation. *Behav. Neurosci.* 106, 447–456. doi: 10.1037/0735-7044.106.3.447

Schweizer, K., Goldhammer, F., Rauch, W., and Moosbrugger, H. (2007). On the validity of Raven's matrices test: does spatial ability contribute to performance? *Pers. Individ. Dif.* 43, 1998–2010. doi: 10.1016/j.paid.2007.06.008

Semrud-Clikeman, M., Fine, J. G., Bledsoe, J., and Zhu, D. C. (2012). Gender differences in brain activation on a mental rotation task. *Int. J. Neurosci.* 122, 590–597. doi: 10.3109/00207454.2012.693999

Sereno, M. I., Dale, A., Reppas, J., Kwong, K., Belliveau, J., Brady, T., et al. (1995). Borders of multiple visual areas in humans revealed by functional magnetic resonance imaging. *Science* 268, 889–893. doi: 10.1126/science.7754376

Shepard, R. N., and Metzler, J. (1971). Mental rotation of three-dimensional objects. *Science* 171, 701–703. doi: 10.1126/science.171.3972.701

Sherry, D. F., Vaccarino, A. L., Buckenham, K., and Herz, R. S. (1989). The hippocampal complex of food-storing birds. *Brain Behav. Evol.* 34, 308–317. doi: 10.1159/000116516

Sorby, S., Casey, B., Veurink, N., and Dulaney, A. (2013). The role of spatial training in improving spatial and calculus performance in engineering students. *Learn. Individ. Differ.* 26, 20–29. doi: 10.1016/j.lindif.2013.03.010

Spence, I., Yu, J. J., Feng, J., and Marshman, J. (2009). Women match men when learning a spatial skill. *J. Exp. Psychol. Learn. Mem. Cogn.* 35, 1097–1103. doi: 10.1037/a0015641

Sperling, R., Chua, E., Cocchiarella, A., Rand-Giovannetti, E., Poldrack, R., Schacter, D. L., et al. (2003). Putting names to faces: successful encoding of associative memories activates the anterior hippocampal formation. *Neuroimage* 20, 1400–1410. doi: 10.1016/S1053-8119(03)00391-4

Strange, B. A., and Dolan, R. J. (2001). Adaptive anterior hippocampal responses to oddball stimuli. *Hippocampus* 11, 690–698. doi: 10.1002/hipo.1084

Suzuki, M., Hagino, H., Nohara, S., Zhou, S.-Y., Kawasaki, Y., Takahashi, T., et al. (2005). Male-specific volume expansion of the human hippocampus during adolescence. *Cereb. Cortex* 15, 187–193. doi: 10.1093/cercor/bhh121

Terlecki, M. S., and Newcombe, N. S. (2005). How important is the digital divide? The relation of computer and videogame usage to gender differences in mental rotation ability. *Sex Roles* 53, 433–441. doi: 10.1007/s11199-005-6765-0

Travis, S. G., Huang, Y., Fujiwara, E., Radomski, A., Carter, R., Seres, P., et al. (2014). High field structural MRI reveals specific episodic memory correlates in the subfields of the hippocampus. *Neuropsychologia* 53, 233–245. doi: 10.1016/j.neuropsychologia.2013.11.016

Tzuriel, D., and Egozi, G. (2010). Gender differences in spatial ability of young children: the effects of training and processing strategies. *Child Dev.* 81, 1417–1430. doi: 10.1111/j.1467-8624.2010.01482.x

Voyer, D., Voyer, S., and Bryden, M. P. (1995). Magnitude of sex differences in spatial abilities: a meta-analysis and consideration of critical variables. *Psychol. Bull.* 117, 250–270. doi: 10.1037/0033-2909.117.2.250

Wei, W., Lu, H., Zhao, H., Chen, C., Dong, Q., and Zhou, X. (2012). Gender differences in children's arithmetic performance are accounted for by gender differences in language abilities. *Psychol. Sci.* 23, 320–330. doi: 10.1177/0956797611427168

Woollett, K., and Maguire, E. A. (2011). Acquiring "the Knowledge" of London's layout drives structural brain changes. *Curr. Biol.* 21, 2109–2114. doi: 10.1016/j.cub.2011.11.018

14

Attentional Filter Training but Not Memory Training Improves Decision-Making

Marlen Schmicker[1,2], Patrick Müller[1,2], Melanie Schwefel[1,2] and Notger G. Müller[1,2,3]*

[1]Neuroprotection Laboratory, German Center for Neurodegenerative Diseases (DZNE), Magdeburg, Germany, [2]Otto von Guericke University, Magdeburg, Germany, [3]Center for Behavioral Brain Sciences, Magdeburg, Germany

Edited by:
Soledad Ballesteros, Universidad Nacional de Educación a Distancia (UNED), Spain

Reviewed by:
Tracy L. Luks, University of California, San Francisco, USA
Ben Godde, Jacobs University Bremen, Germany

***Correspondence:**
Marlen Schmicker
marlen.schmicker@dzne.de

Decision-making has a high practical relevance for daily performance. Its relation to other cognitive abilities such as executive control and memory is not fully understood. Here we asked whether training of either attentional filtering or memory storage would influence decision-making as indexed by repetitive assessments of the Iowa Gambling Task (IGT). The IGT was developed to assess and simulate real-life decision-making (Bechara et al., 2005). In this task, participants gain or lose money by developing advantageous or disadvantageous decision strategies. On five consecutive days we trained 29 healthy young adults (20–30 years) either in working memory (WM) storage or attentional filtering and measured their IGT scores after each training session. During memory training (MT) subjects performed a computerized delayed match-to-sample task where two displays of bars were presented in succession. During filter training (FT) participants had to indicate whether two simultaneously presented displays of bars matched or not. Whereas in MT the relevant target stimuli stood alone, in FT the targets were embedded within irrelevant distractors (bars in a different color). All subjects within each group improved their performance in the trained cognitive task. For the IGT, we observed an increase over time in the amount of money gained in the FT group only. Decision-making seems to be influenced more by training to filter out irrelevant distractors than by training to store items in WM. Selective attention could be responsible for the previously noted relationship between IGT performance and WM and is therefore more important for enhancing efficiency in decision-making.

Keywords: decision-making, distractor inhibition, filter training, Iowa Gambling Task, working memory

INTRODUCTION

In everyday life we have to make decisions all the time. Successful decision-making requires the ability to make decisions that are unpleasant at the moment, but are advantageous in the long run. The Iowa Gambling Task (IGT) can be considered as a proxy to this real-life function. Performing advantageously on this task depends on, as in real-life, dealing with uncertainty in a context of punishment and reward (Brevers et al., 2013). The IGT was originally designed for patients with lesions of the ventromedial prefrontal cortex (Bechara et al., 1994, 1997). Subjects have to pick cards from four different decks to maximize their monetary gain (Bechara et al., 1994). Of these four decks, two decks offer the opportunity to obtain large gains but are also associated with greater losses (disadvantageous: A and B), whereas the other two decks result in small wins but also smaller losses (advantageous: C and D). The decks further differ in their payoff scheme.

Decks A and C involve frequent losses; decks B and D infrequent losses. Normal subjects develop a tendency towards advantageous decisions and improve their performance after picking up ~100 cards (Overman and Pierce, 2013). The behavior of choosing the cards depends on cognitive processes and emotional states (Bechara and Damasio, 2005). The somatic marker hypothesis assumes that decision processes are influenced by emotion-based signals arising from the body to guide human behavior (Damasio et al., 1991). Other studies have suggested a stronger association with cognition and have reported correlations with executive functions (working memory (WM), inhibition, set-shifting) and intelligence (Webb et al., 2014), but others do no support these findings (Toplak et al., 2010).

The extent to which subjects are able to develop advantageous decision strategies in the sequential learning task seems to be related to WM. In a dual task, participants were not able to develop implicit learning strategies under concurrent high WM load. Their IGT performance was lower than with no/low WM load (Cui et al., 2015). In the past few years, researchers have tried to investigate individual differences in WM performance and their relation to decision-making. Subjects with high WM capacity develop a more advantageous strategy than those with low WM capacity (Bagneux et al., 2013). However, the results of studies concerning decision-making and its relation to WM are very inconsistent. To resolve this discrepancy one could ask whether cognitive load and the ability to inhibit irrelevant information influence IGT performance. A recent study investigated the cognitive load effects of divided and full attention on deck selection in the IGT (Hawthorne and Pierce, 2015). They found that a disadvantageous strategy in the divided attention group and limited cognitive resources were responsible for bad decisions. However, the role of attention in decision-making has yet to be properly researched, especially regarding individual differences in distractor inhibition abilities. Gansler et al. (2011) modulated a structural equation model to predict IGT performance. The authors showed that successful IGT performance demands different cognitive functions, and the prediction from attention was twice as strong as the prediction from other executive functions.

The inconsistent results regarding the relationship between WM and decision-making led us to the question whether a third cognitive component could moderate the relation between WM and the IGT. Based on the correlation between WM updating tasks and decision-making (Achtziger et al., 2014), we assumed that an attentional selection component inherent in these updating tasks may be the reason for the close relation. Another empirical evidence for this theory was the finding that subjects with high WM capacity are better able to filter out irrelevant items in a visual WM paradigm (Vogel et al., 2005). The role of selective attention in WM was also emphasized by other authors (Conway and Engle, 1996; Cowan, 1999) and was confirmed by the finding of overlapping neuronal correlates (Awh and Jonides, 2001; Awh et al., 2006). These observations led us to ask whether selective attention is the reason for the inconsistent results on the relation between WM and decision making. In order to investigate the relation between selective attention and decision making further, we employed a cognitive training paradigm aimed at inducing transfer effects from selective attention to decision making (Moreau et al., 2016). We asked whether this selective attentional training would influence IGT performance more than WM storage training. So far, only emotion regulation strategies have been shown to facilitate decision-making (Martin and Delgado, 2011). Here, we designed a task that—like in memory updating—required selective attention. We developed two variants of a difference detection paradigm that stressed either memory storage or selective attention demands. One group performed the selective attention (filter) training, the other performed the memory storage training. In a prior study (Schmicker et al., 2016), we had compared transfer effects of both training regimes on WM performance and observed stronger transfer effects of the selective attention training program. We now asked how the different trainings influenced IGT performance. We assumed that training of the core function of selective attention would enhance the tendency to make advantageous decisions as indexed by higher IGT gains more than memory storage training.

MATERIALS AND METHODS

Sample

Twenty-nine young, healthy subjects (24.31 years ± 2.9, 15 female) took part in the study. All participants were right-handed and had correct or corrected to normal vision. The study protocol was approved by the ethics committee of the University of Magdeburg (Germany). All subjects gave their written informed consent in accordance with the Declaration of Helsinki to participate in the study and were paid 100 € for complete participation. In addition, they were paid an amount of money that was calculated as the mean of the gain from five IGT sessions (mean: 20.94 €; range: 14.20 €–29.90 €). The participants were divided into two training groups: 15 subjects (8 female) received the filter training (FT), and 14 subjects (7 female) received the memory training (MT). The groups were matched according to their age and performance in attention and WM.

Design

During the training (training days 1–5; Monday to Friday), half of the subjects received 60 min of memory storage training (MT), while the other half trained selective attention by having to filter out irrelevant stimuli for 60 min (FT). In the middle of each training session, a break was used to present the IGT (**Figure 1**).

Experimental Tasks

Training

In MT (**Figure 2A**) participants had to compare two arrays presented consecutively with a delay of 900–1400 ms at the center of the screen. The arrays consisted of 4–6 horizontal and vertical bars (1.43° × 0.29°) of one color (either red or green). They were shown after a black square-shaped cue had been presented. The task was to decide whether there was a

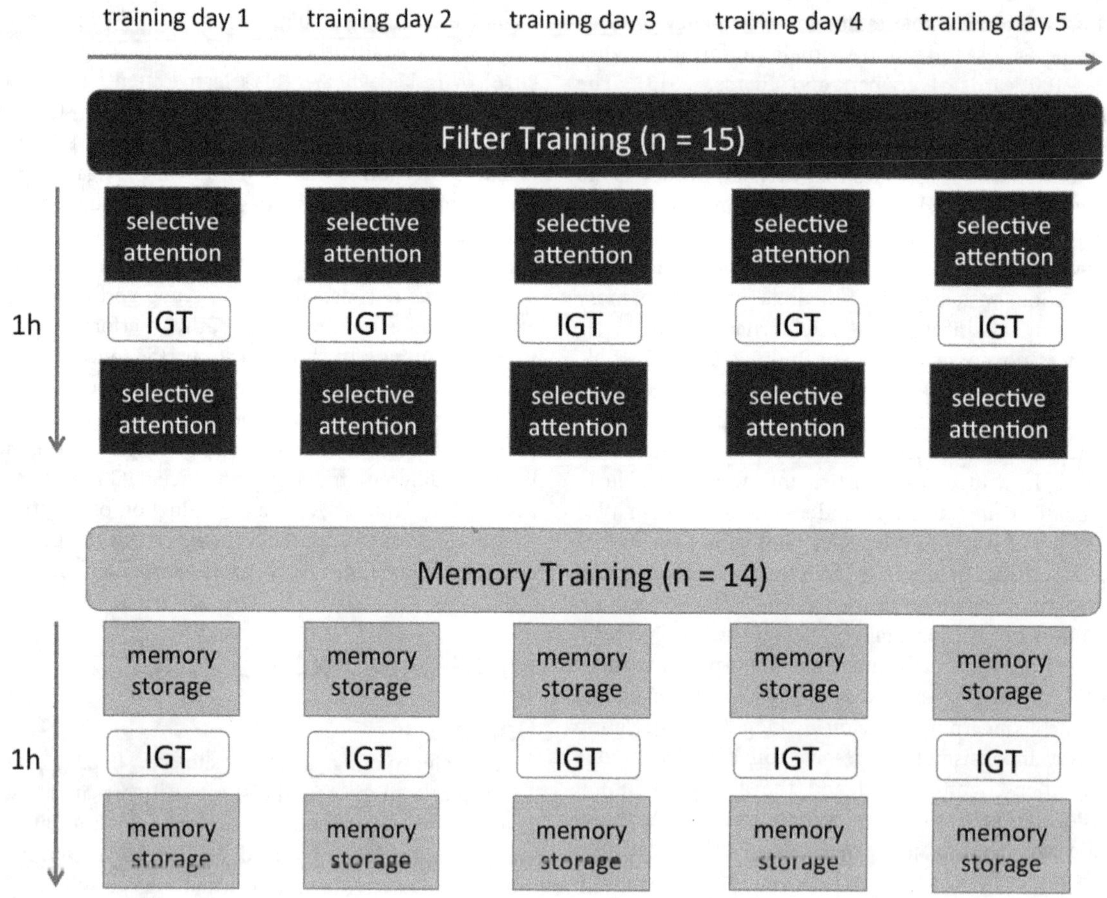

FIGURE 1 | Study design. Memory Training (MT) consists of trials with memory storage demand. Filter Training (FT) trials were designed to train selective attention. The Iowa Gambling Task (IGT) was performed during a break between the first and the second 100 trials.

bar direction change in one of the presented stimuli. Hence, the MT training lacked the necessity to filter out irrelevant distractors.

In FT participants had to compare two simultaneously presented arrays of colored bars (**Figure 2B**). In these trials, a red or green cue instructed them to compare either only the red or green bars of the double array while ignoring bars of the other color. The arrays consisted of 4–6 relevant bars and the same amount of irrelevant distractors. All bar arrays were presented within a 4° × 9.3° rectangle against a gray background and were placed 1.79° to the right and left of the central fixation cross. The participants were instructed to decide whether the simultaneously presented arrays matched in terms of the orientation of the bars in the relevant color. This condition did not demand memory storage.

MT and FT subjects pressed one of two buttons to respond. In half of the trials, the orientation of one target changed, and in the other half of the trials, no orientation change occurred. Seventy two trials of each were presented in each of the three conditions. The different trials were randomized within four blocks (runs) and presented in a counterbalanced order across participants.

528 training trials were created for the training sessions. Every daily session consisted of 200 training trials in a randomized order. The trainings sessions became more difficult over the week by successively increasing the number of presented bars within one array (for more details, see Schmicker et al., 2016).

Iowa Gambling Task

Each of the training days included a short break after 100 training trials in FT or MT. During this break all subjects performed the IGT. Apart from our interest in the impact of our different training protocols on decision-making, the IGT implementation was also intended to keep our subjects motivated by providing them with additional reward. The repeated application of the IGT entails the possibility of practice effects within the IGT so that improvements in IGT scores cannot be solely attributed to transfer effects induced by FT or MT, respectively. Note, however, that these practice effects cannot account for group differences as the IGT assessment did not differ across groups. Group differences, which were the main focus of this study, must, therefore, be related to the different cognitive training protocols. We used the computerized version of the original IGT, which is identical to the reward structure and instructions of

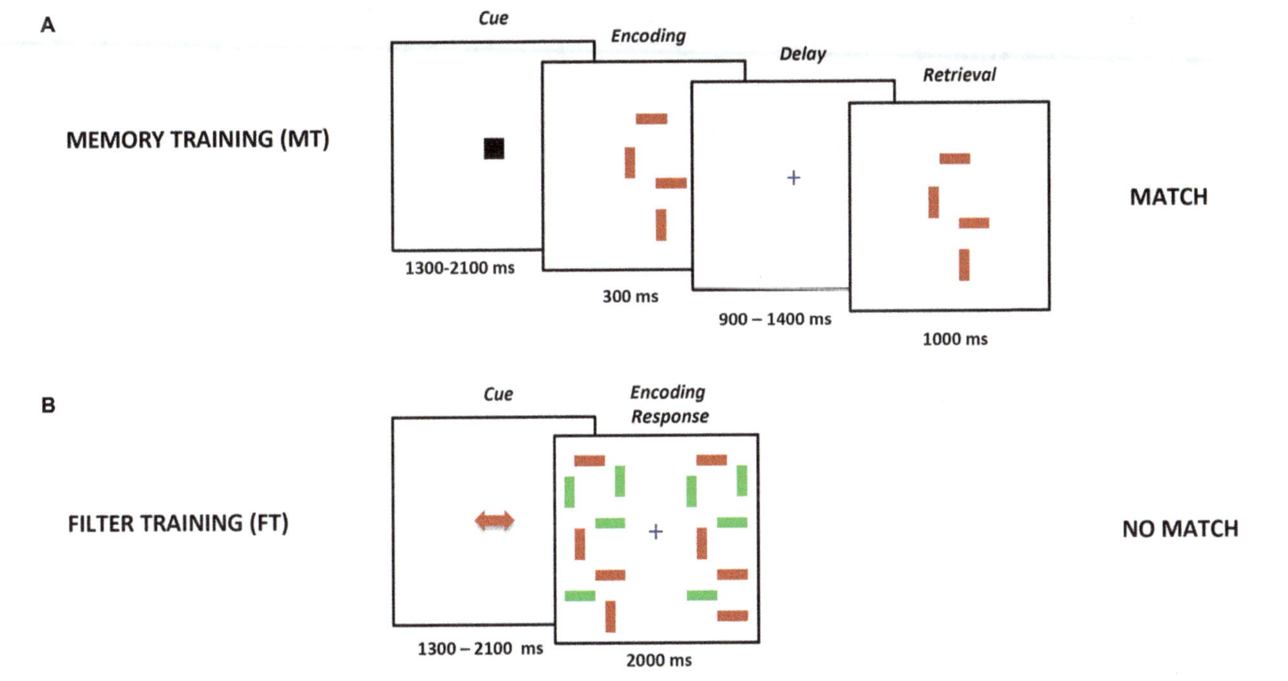

FIGURE 2 | Schematic design of the bar paradigm. (A) Subjects had to remember (MT) or **(B)** compare (FT) the direction of the bars in either the cued color (with distractors) or independent from the color (without distractors).

the IGT established by Bechara et al. (1994) presented with the Software Inquisit 4.0.8.0[1]. Before the task every subject was given a fictitious amount of money (20 Euro). Four card decks were presented on the screen, and participants were instructed to select a card by clicking with the mouse cursor on one of the decks to increase their gain of money. Additional information occurred at the bottom of the screen. The reward was reported in green letters, the penalty in red letters, and the total score in a black font. The obtained gain of money was paid out at the end of the study.

Data Analysis

We analyzed correct answers and reaction times as outcomes for the two training conditions in the bar paradigm. For IGT data, we recorded the total gain of one session for each subject. First, we examined the correlations of the IGT score (training day 1) with correct answers in MT and FT. Second, we investigated the training effects for both training groups and analyzed correct answers and reaction times for the five training days using one-way repeated measures ANOVA and t-tests for both groups. Third, we compared the change in the IGT score of both training groups together and separately in each group in one-way repeated measures ANOVAs (with five levels), with group as the between-subject factor. In addition, we performed paired t-tests for each group comparing training day 1 and training day 5 with a hypothesis defined *a priori*. Afterwards, the training success in MT and FT was correlated to test if training success correlated with IGT changes (day 5–day 1) for all subjects together and both groups separately.

[1]http://www.millisecond.com

RESULTS

Cognitive Training Effects

To address the question whether FT and MT affected the performance within the trained task, we analyzed performance changes within the five training days. FT trials were more difficult than MT trials (FT: 61.97% ± 2.19%, MT: 78.59% ±1.71%; $t_{(1,28)} = 10.15$, $p < 0.001$). Performance in the trained conditions increased for both groups (MT, FT) during the five sessions (**Figure 3**). For both groups, we found a main effect of training sessions in correct answers (MT: $F_{(4,9)} = 5.43$, $p = 0.017$; $\eta_p^2 = 0.707$; FT: $F_{(4,8)} = 4.65$, $p = 0.031$; $\eta_p^2 = 0.699$) and reaction times (MT: $F_{(4,9)} = 5.40$, $p = 0.017$; $\eta_p^2 = 0.706$; FT: $F_{(4,8)} = 4.63$, $p = 0.031$; $\eta_p^2 = 0.698$). One-sample t-tests for day 1 and day 5 performances showed significant t-values ($p < 0.05$) for both. Correct responses increased for all subjects (4.5% for MT, 7.8% for FT), while reactions time decreased (61 ms for MT, 134 ms for FT) during training.

IGT Changes during Cognitive Training

The main focus of this article is on how the two different training protocols impacted decision-making performance. IGT scores were repeatedly measured during the 5-session-training period for both groups (see **Figure 4** and **Table 1**). In a between-subject ANOVA with five levels, no main or interaction effect was observed for the factor group. Because of our *a priori*

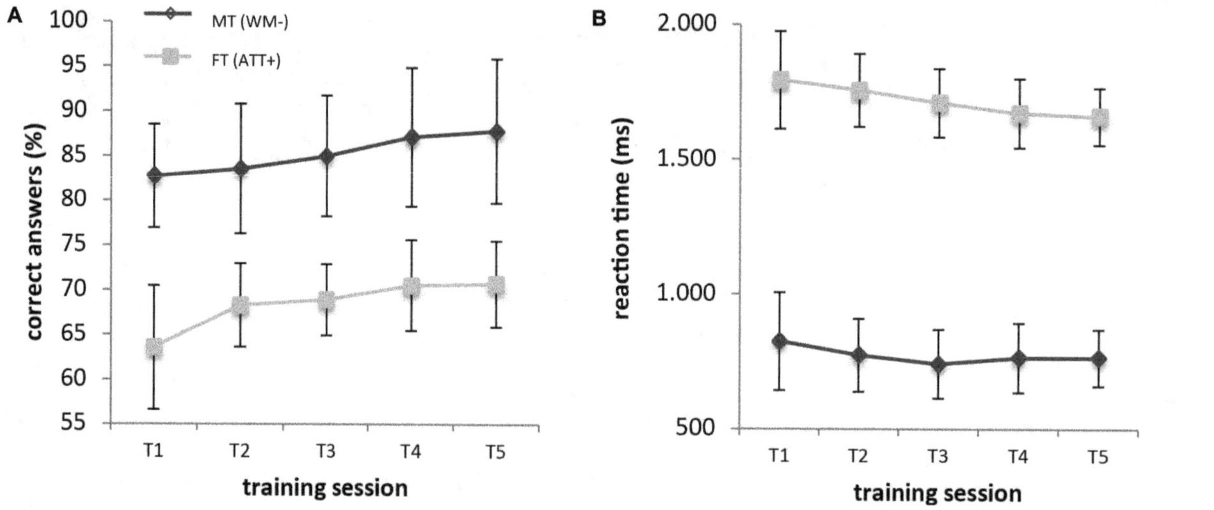

FIGURE 3 | Increase in working memory (WM; MT) and filtering (FT) training. Mean values and standard errors of correct responses **(A)** and reaction times **(B)** are visualized.

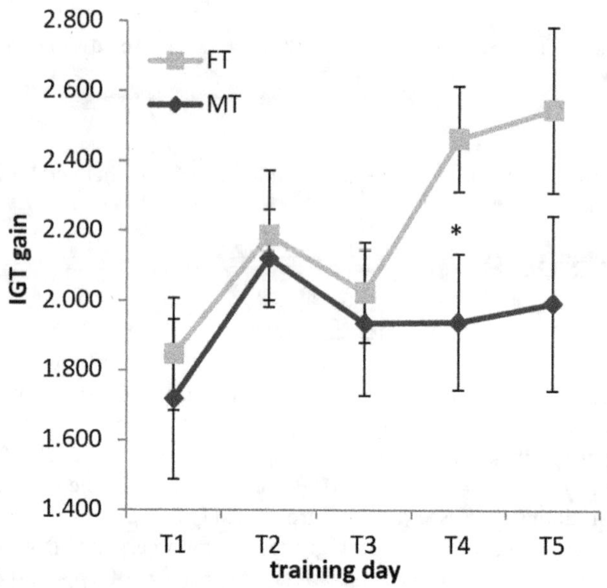

FIGURE 4 | Increase in IGT gain during the training week. Mean values and standard errors for all days (1–5) and both training groups (FT, MT) are visualized. *$p < 0.05$.

defined hypotheses, we calculated ANOVAs for each group. For the factor "days", no main effect was observed for the MT group, but there was a main effect for the FT group (MT: $F_{(4,9)} = 0.20$, $p = 0.661$; $\eta_p^2 = 0.015$; FT: $F_{(4,8)} = 6.90$, $p = 0.020$; $\eta_p^2 = 0.330$). Subjects who had been trained on filtering out distractors won 7.00 € (SD: 11.21 €) more in the last gambling session (training day 5). MT subjects increased their winnings by 2.75 € (SD: 14.93). A one-sample *t*-test showed significant mean differences for the FT group ($t_{(1,14)} = -2.42$, $p < 0.030$) but no significant increase for the MT group ($t_{(1,13)} = -0.69$, $p = 0.50$). Additionally, Cohen's *d* was calculated. We found a large effect size for the FT group and a small *d* for MT (see **Table 1**).

Performed *t*-tests for independent samples revealed significant mean differences between the FT and MT group on day 4 ($t_{(1,27)} = -2.14$, $p < 0.041$). The FT group had a 5.24 € higher gain than the MT group. For training day 5, a two-sample *t*-test did not reach significance due to a higher variance in the values, but Cohen's *d* showed a moderate effect for both days. All means, standard deviations and effect sizes are presented in **Table 1**.

We did not find any correlations of the training success in FT and MT with IGT changes.

DISCUSSION

The current study investigated the relationship between WM storage, selective attention and decision-making by testing whether training of either memory storage or attentional filtering influences performance in the IGT. During training, performance increased in the two trained tasks. Regarding IGT performance, for the first three training days, there was no difference between both training groups. Starting with training day 4, moderate effect sizes reflect that subjects who received FT made more advantageous decisions in the IGT than those in the MT group. FT participants also won a significant higher amount of money between day 1 and day 5 than MT participants, which is emphasized by a strong effect size.

These findings suggest different impacts of the trained tasks on decision-making in the IGT. During FT subjects learn to ignore irrelevant items during the encoding process (Schmicker et al., 2016). How does this capability induce effects on learning in decision-making? Knowing that additional cognitive load increases disadvantageous deck selection in the IGT (Hawthorne and Pierce, 2015), the increased ability to filter out irrelevant information after FT may have freed attentional resources for

TABLE 1 | Mean gain in Iowa Gambling Task (IGT) over five training days.

	MT		FT					
IGT training day	**Mean**	**SD**	**Mean**	**SD**	**FT-MT**	***t***	***p***	***d***
Day 1	1717	855	1846	623	128	−0.47	0.65	0.17
Day 2	2121	523	2186	718	65	−0.28	0.78	0.10
Day 3	1935	778	2023	941	87	−0.27	0.79	0.10
Day 4	1939	729	2463	585	524	−2.14	0.04*	**0.79**
Day 5	1992	937	2546	916	553	−1.61	0.12	**0.59**
Day 5–day 1	275		–		–	−0.69	0.50	0.31
Day 5–day 1	–		700		–	−2.42	0.03*	**0.89**

Statistical results for t-values (t) and significance (p) for group mean differences between (FT-MT) and within (day 5–day 1) groups are reported. Means and standard deviations are stated in €-cent. Significant differences are marked with a star. Cohen's d was calculated with the standard formula using the pooled standard deviations. Strong effect sizes are highlighted in bold type. Fourteen subjects received the memory training (MT), 15 participants were trained with the filter training (FT).

goal-driven decisions in the IGT. Alternatively or in addition, FT may have enhanced not only the top-down control of distracting information but also that of emotions and effective emotional control has been shown to favor advantageous decisions in the IGT (Martin and Delgado, 2011). The sensory marker hypothesis (Bechara and Damasio, 2005) claims that prior emotional processes induced by gains or losses influence implicit and explicit knowledge for advantageous decisions. Assuming an attentional control mechanism for these sensory markers, learning to filter out irrelevant information could extend to the suppression of strong emotions (Brevers et al., 2013) produced by salient bottom-up stimuli (high losses, high gains). In turn, attention could be guided towards less (emotionally) salient stimuli allowing for an advantageous strategy during decision-making. Considering that successful attentional filtering is associated with activity in posterior middle frontal gyrus (McNab and Klingberg, 2008) and training of attentional filtering enhances activity in this area (Schmicker et al., 2016), one can assume that emotion-related neural signals from the amygdala or thalamus (John et al., 2016) are better controlled by this frontal region after FT. Therefore, learning to inhibit emotions might favor more rational decisions. However, a direct neural evidence for this assumed role of attentional filtering in decision-making still needs to be provided and future research should address whether learning to inhibit distracting information extends to the successful suppression of emotional salient stimuli resulting in advantageous decision-making. Alternatively, the frontal activity observed in the cited earlier studies and ascribed there to attentional control might be related to motor imagery during the preparation of finger movements for responding, especially as the activity increases emerged in rather posterior, premotor areas (Hanakawa et al., 2008).

Why did the MT group fail to show an increase in IGT performance? First, our previous training study (Schmicker et al., 2016) indicates that MT subjects do not effectively differentiate between relevant and irrelevant information and, therefore, store unnecessary content. Relating this inefficient strategy to decision-making, subjects may have stored information or emotional markers that were irrelevant for a gainful gambling behavior. In other words, simply improving information storage does not make decisions better.

Second, mood can modulate decision processes and, therefore, IGT performance (Bagneux et al., 2013). Fatigue or boredom induced by the less demanding MT tasks may have made participants more susceptible to emotionally attributed stimuli and to avoid them. Harm avoidance is a personality trait that has been shown to cause an inability to filter out irrelevant distractors (especially for emotion-attributed stimuli) and could lead to disadvantageous behavior (Most et al., 2005). Alternatively, the more effortful FT tasks might have simply increased the arousal levels with which subjects addressed the IGT. In contrast the easier MT task with its behavioral ceiling effects may have not been challenging enough to induce transfer effects. Future research should therefore make use of a more challenging memory storage training, for example one that includes constant updating processes. Finally, the lack of a passive control group and the small sample size limits the possibility to draw conclusions regarding possible unspecific effects of the active interventions on IGT behavior. Therefore, based on the present results we cannot specify further which processes underlay the FT induced effects on the IGT.

In sum our results indicate that training of attentional control entails better decisions in the IGT. Whether this finding relates to decision-making in real-life has not yet to be shown. Also, the link between the ability to inhibit emotional reactions and to inhibit distracting information during decision-making needs more elaboration. It would be interesting to investigate neural correlates of FT in decision-making and whether the effects can be transferred to IGT performance in independent measurements and to decision-making in everyday life.

AUTHOR CONTRIBUTIONS

MaS designed the experiment, collected and analyzed the data and drafted the article. MeS supported the development of the paradigm and the data collection. PM and NGM contributed to the discussion of content-related issues and to the critical revision of the article.

ACKNOWLEDGMENTS

This work was funded by Deutsche Forschungsgemeinschaft (DFG) grant Mu1364/4.

REFERENCES

Achtziger, A., Alós-Ferrer, C., Hügelschäfer, S., and Steinhauser, M. (2014). The neural basis of belief updating and rational descion making. *Soc. Cogn. Affect. Neurosci.* 9, 55–62. doi: 10.1093/scan/nss099

Awh, E., and Jonides, J. (2001). Overlapping mechanisms of attention and spatial working memory. *Trends Cogn. Sci.* 5, 119–126. doi: 10.1016/s1364-6613(00)01593-x

Awh, E., Vogel, E. K., and Oh, S. H. (2006). Interactions between attention and working memory. *Neuroscience* 139, 201–208. doi: 10.1016/j.neuroscience.2005.08.023

Bagneux, V., Thomassin, N., Gonthier, C., and Roulin, J.-L. (2013). Working memory in the processing of the iowa gambling task: an individual differences approach. *PLoS One* 8:e81498. doi: 10.1371/journal.pone.0081498

Bechara, A., and Damasio, A. R. (2005). The somatic marker hypothesis: a neural theory of economic decision. *Games Econ. Behav.* 52, 336–372. doi: 10.1016/j.geb.2004.06.010

Bechara, A., Damasio, A. R., Damasio, H., and Anderson, S. W. (1994). Insensitivity to future consequences following damage to human prefrontal cortex. *Cognition* 50, 7–15. doi: 10.1016/0010-0277(94)90018-3

Bechara, A., Damasio, H., Tranel, D., and Damasio, A. R. (1997). Deciding advantageously before knowing the advantageous strategy. *Science* 275, 1293–1295. doi: 10.1126/science.275.5304.1293

Bechara, A., Damasio, H., Tranel, D., and Damasio, A. R. (2005). The Iowa Gambling Task and the somatic marker hypothesis: some questions and answers. *Trends Cogn. Sci.* 9, 159–162. doi: 10.1016/j.tics.2005.02.002

Brevers, D., Bechara, A., Cleeremans, A., and Noël, X. (2013). Iowa Gambling Task (IGT): twenty years after- gambling disorder and IGT. *Front. Psychol.* 4:665. doi: 10.3389/fpsyg.2013.00665

Conway, A. R., and Engle, R. W. (1996). Individual differences in working memory capacity: more evidence for a general capacity theory. *Memory* 4, 577–590. doi: 10.1080/741940997

Cowan, N. (1999). "An embedded-processes model of working memory," in *Models of Working Memory: Mechanisms of Active Maintenance and Executive Control*, eds A. Miyake and P. Shah (Cambridge, MA: Cambridge University Press), 62–101.

Cui, J.-F., Wang, Y., Shi, H.-S., Liu, L.-L., Chen, X.-J., and Chen, Y.H. (2015). Effects of working memory load on uncertain decision-making: evidence from the Iowa Gambling Task. *Front. Psychol.* 6:162. doi: 10.3389/fpsyg.2015.00162

Damasio, A. R., Tranel, D., and Damasio, H. (1991). "Somatic markers and the guidance of behaviour: theory and preliminary testing," in *Frontal Lobe Function and Dysfunction*, eds H. S. Levin, H. M. Eisenberg and A. L. Benton (New York, NY: Oxford University Press), 217–229.

Gansler, D. A., Jerram, M. W., Vannorsdall, T. D., and Schretlen, D. J. (2011). Does the Iowa Gambling Task measure executive function? *Arch. Clin. Neuropsychol.* 26, 706–717. doi: 10.1093/arclin/acr082

Hanakawa, T., Dimyan, M. A., and Hallett, M. (2008). Motor planning, imagery and execution in the distributed motor network: a time-course study with functional MRI. *Cereb. Cortex* 18, 2775–2788. doi: 10.1093/cercor/bhn036

Hawthorne, M. J., and Pierce, B. H. (2015). Disadvantageous deck selection in the iowa gambling task: the effect of cognitive load. *Eur. J. Psychol.* 11, 335–348. doi: 10.5964/ejop.v11i2.931

John, Y. J., Zikopoulos, B., Bullock, D., and Barbas, H. (2016). The emotional gatekeeper: a computational model of attentional selection and suppression through the pathway from the amygdala to the inhibitory thalamic reticular nucleus. *PLoS Comput. Biol.* 12:e1004722. doi: 10.1371/journal.pcbi.1004722

Martin, L. N., and Delgado, M. R. (2011). The influence of emotion regulation on decision-making under risk. *J. Cogn. Neurosci.* 23, 2569–2581. doi: 10.1162/jocn.2011.21618

McNab, F., and Klingberg, T. (2008). Prefrontal cortex and basal ganglia control access to working memory. *Nat. Neurosci.* 11, 103–107. doi: 10.1038/nn2024

Moreau, D., Kirk, I. J., and Waldie, K. E. (2016). Seven pervasive statistical flaws in cognitive training interventions. *Front. Hum. Neurosci.* 10:153. doi: 10.3389/fnhum.2016.00153

Most, A. B., Chun, M. M., Widders, D. M., and Zald, D. (2005). Attentional rubbernecking: cognitive control and personality in emotion-induced blindness. *Psychon. Bull. Rev.* 12, 654–661. doi: 10.3758/bf03196754

Overman, W. H., and Pierce, A. (2013). Iowa Gambling Task with non-clinical participants: effects of using real + virtual cards and additional trials. *Front. Psychol.* 4:935. doi: 10.3389/fpsyg.2013.00935

Schmicker, M., Schwefel, M., Vellage, A. K., and Müller, N. G. (2016). Training of attentional filtering, but not of memory storage, enhances working memory efficiency by strengthening the neuronal gatekeeper network. *J. Cogn. Neurosci.* 28, 636–642. doi: 10.1162/jocn_a_00922

Toplak, M. E., Sorge, G. B., Benoit, A., West, R. F., and Stanovich, K. E. (2010). Decision-making and cognitive abilities: a review of associations between Iowa Gambling Task performance, executive functions and intelligence. *Clin. Psychol. Rev.* 30, 562–581. doi: 10.1016/j.cpr.2010.04.002

Vogel, E. K., McCollough, A. W., and Machizawa, M. G. (2005). Neural measures reveal individual differences in controlling access to working memory. *Nature* 438, 500–503. doi: 10.1038/nature04171

Webb, C. A., DelDonno, S., and Killgore, W. D. (2014). The role of cognitive versus emotional intelligence in Iowa Gambling Task performance: what's emotion got to do with it? *Intelligence* 44, 112–119. doi: 10.1016/j.intell.2014.03.008

15

Video Game Training Enhances Visuospatial Working Memory and Episodic Memory in Older Adults

Pilar Toril [1,2], José M. Reales [1,3], Julia Mayas [1,2] and Soledad Ballesteros [1,2]*

[1] *Studies of Aging and Neurodegenerative Diseases Research Group, Universidad Nacional de Educación a Distancia (UNED), Madrid, Spain,* [2] *Department of Basic Psychology II, Universidad Nacional de Educación a Distancia (UNED), Madrid, Spain,* [3] *Department of Methodology of the Behavioral Sciences, Universidad Nacional de Educación a Distancia (UNED), Madrid, Spain*

Edited by:
Rachael D. Seidler, University of Michigan, USA

Reviewed by:
Marian Berryhill, University of Nevada, Reno, USA
Corey Bohil, University of Central Florida, USA

***Correspondence:**
Pilar Toril
pilartoril@psi.uned.es

In this longitudinal intervention study with experimental and control groups, we investigated the effects of video game training on the visuospatial working memory (WM) and episodic memory of healthy older adults. Participants were 19 volunteer older adults, who received 15 1-h video game training sessions with a series of video games selected from a commercial package (*Lumosity*), and a control group of 20 healthy older adults. The results showed that the performance of the trainees improved significantly in all the practiced video games. Most importantly, we found significant enhancements after training in the trained group and no change in the control group in two computerized tasks designed to assess visuospatial WM, namely the Corsi blocks task and the Jigsaw puzzle task. The episodic memory and short-term memory of the trainees also improved. Gains in some WM and episodic memory tasks were maintained during a 3-month follow-up period. These results suggest that the aging brain still retains some degree of plasticity, and that video game training might be an effective intervention tool to improve WM and other cognitive functions in older adults.

Keywords: brain plasticity, cognitive aging, episodic memory, training, video games, visuospatial working memory

INTRODUCTION

Age-related brain changes occurring mainly in the prefrontal cortex and the medial temporal lobe system (including the hippocampus and the cerebellum) are associated with cognitive declines (Raz et al., 2005) in several functions, including processing speed (Salthouse, 1996), peripheral vision (Muiños and Ballesteros, 2014), dynamic visual acuity (Muiños and Ballesteros, 2015), working memory (WM), executive control functioning, and episodic memory (e.g., Baltes and Lindenberger, 1997; Hoyer and Verhaeghen, 2006; Nilsson, 2003; Park and Gutchess, 2002; Rönnlund et al., 2005). However, other cognitive functions, including implicit memory, verbal abilities and world knowledge, are mostly spared with age (e.g., Park et al., 2002; Mitchell and Bruss, 2003; Craik and Bialystok, 2006; Osorio et al., 2010; Ballesteros et al., 2013; Ballesteros and Mayas, 2015). Experience-related changes induced by the modification of the social environment, physical activity, and cognitive training affect brain structure and function (for a recent review see, Ballesteros et al., 2015a). Research on brain plasticity in older adults and its relationship to experiential changes is currently attracting substantial public interest (Raz and Lindenberger, 2013). However, several studies have found brain plasticity not only in healthy older adults, but also in patients suffering chronic traumatic brain injury (Sacco et al., 2011), schizophrenia (Fisher et al., 2010), and intellectual disability (Söderqvist et al., 2012). Recently, research on training-induced changes in brain and behavior has attracted a great interest in cognitive neuroscience across lifespan, especially in the older age. Studies on this field might contribute to improve our knowledge on brain plasticity and result of a great help for designing effective interventions (see Karbach and Schubert, 2013).

Training intervention studies suggest that the older human brain maintains a certain level of neural plasticity (Bialystok and Craik, 2006; Li et al., 2006, 2008). Based on this idea, an active line of research concerns ways of maintaining and/or improving cognitive skills (Green and Bavelier, 2003), delaying cognitive and brain declines as much as possible (Hertzog et al., 2008; Park and Reuter-Lorenz, 2009; Park and Bischof, 2013; Reuter-Lorenz and Park, 2014). The observed increase in neural volume in response to cognitive training is an indicator of brain plasticity (see, Boyke et al., 2009; Park and Bischof, 2013). Based on the assumption that the older brain retains at least some degree of plasticity and still has the capacity to modify its structural and functional patterns to meet new environmental demands, researchers are intensively exploring different types of intervention for older adults.

One of the most popular computerized intervention approaches is training older adults with video games. Some intervention studies have reported improvements in the trained group but not in the control group in several cognitive functions, including processing speed (e.g., Clark et al., 1987; Dustman et al., 1992; Ballesteros et al., 2014), visuo-motor coordination (Drew and Waters, 1986), attention (e.g., Goldstein et al., 1997; Belchior, 2008; Mayas et al., 2014), memory (e.g., Craik et al., 2007; Smith et al., 2009; Hampstead et al., 2012), WM (e.g., Edwards et al., 2005; Erickson et al., 2007; Anguera et al., 2013), and global cognitive function (Torres, 2008). By contrast, other studies have failed to find any positive effects of training with video games on cognition (e.g., Ackerman et al., 2010; Owen et al., 2010; Boot et al., 2013a).

Video games are designed with two aims: enjoyment and sustained player engagement (Anguera and Gazzaley, 2015). They can be classified as simple (non-action games) and complex (action games). Complex video games are fast, intense, unpredictable, and require more perceptual and cognitive skills than non-action games (e.g., Green and Bavelier, 2003; Feng et al., 2007). Some researchers have used complex video games to train older adults (e.g., Basak et al., 2008; Stern et al., 2011), while others have used non-action games, which seem more appropriate for older adults (e.g., Torres, 2008; van Muijden et al., 2012; Ballesteros et al., 2014).

An important question in this context is whether training with video games transfers to other untrained cognitive functions. This is a critical issue for its practical significance, but remains debatable. A systematic review conducted to examine the effectiveness of computer-based interventions in cognitively healthy older adults found that video game training improved processing speed and global cognition but was less efficient for improving executive functions (Kueider et al., 2012). More recently, we conducted a meta-analysis to examine the hypothesis that training older adults with video games enhances their cognitive functioning (Toril et al., 2014). The studies included in this meta-analysis were 20 experimental video game training interventions with pre- and post-training measures, published between 1986 and 2013. The mean effect size was moderate [0.37 (SE 0.05) with a 95% CI of between 0.26 and 0.48]. The results indicated that training older adults with video games produces moderate positive effects on several cognitive functions (e.g., reaction time (RT), attention, memory and global cognition), but does not improve executive functions. This meta-analytic study (see also Lampit et al., 2014) also found that these positive results were moderated by variables such as the age of the trainees and the frequency or length of the training program (the amount of time needed to induce cognitive improvement).

WM is a capacity-limited system that stores and processes information needed for ongoing cognition. This capacity-limited workspace is necessary to keep things in mind while performing complex tasks such as comprehension and reasoning (Baddeley and Hitch, 1974). This key component of cognition, central to many cognitive functions, including concentration, problem solving, and impulse control, declines significantly with age (e.g., Park et al., 2002; Bopp and Verhaeghen, 2005; Park and Reuter-Lorenz, 2009). Many recent reviews and longitudinal computerized cognitive training studies have investigated the effectiveness of computerized training approaches aimed at improving WM (e.g., Dahlin et al., 2008; Perrig et al., 2009; Klingberg, 2010; Shipstead et al., 2010, 2012; Takeuchi et al., 2010; Boot et al., 2011; Morrison and Chein, 2011). Unfortunately, the results of these studies are at best mixed, with some articles reporting the effectiveness of WM training (e.g., Borella et al., 2010; Klingberg, 2010; Morrison and Chein, 2011), while others concluded that it is ineffective (e.g., Shipstead et al., 2010; Redick et al., 2013; Ballesteros et al., 2014).

Several recent meta-analytic studies (Karbach and Verhaeghen, 2014; Lampit et al., 2014; Toril et al., 2014) have noticed the great variability in the interventions in terms for example of the intensity and duration of the training regimes, whether they are carried out at home or in the presence of the trainer, and the age of the participants. Our meta-analytic study (Toril et al., 2014) showed that a small number of training sessions is more effective than a large number, possibly because older adults get tired and lose motivation after many training sessions. We also found that the benefits of training increased with the age of participants. The lower baseline scores of the older participants can explain this result. Lampit et al. (2014) also found that computerized cognitive training can improve the cognitive performance of healthy older adults, but that its effectiveness varies across domains. They suggested that training more than three times per week is ineffective. Karbach and Verhaeghen (2014) examined the effects of executive-function and WM training in older adults, suggesting that the inconsistencies of the results were due to differences in the type, intensity, and duration of the intervention, and to the methods used to compare different studies. Their results suggest that WM and executive-function training produces significant and large improvements in the performance of the trained tasks and reliable small to medium-sized transfer effects in the process trained, at least in healthy older adults.

A recent randomized controlled trial study conducted to investigate the effects of training older adults with non-action video games on a series of cognitive functions that decline with age and on subjective wellbeing (Ballesteros et al., 2014) found significant improvements in the experimental group after training in processing speed, attention, immediate and delayed visual recognition memory, as well as a tendency to improve in some dimensions (affection and assertiveness) of the wellbeing scale. However, visuospatial WM and executive control did not improve after training. Overall, these pre-/post-training results support the view that training older adults with non-action video games improves some cognitive abilities but not others. Moreover, the assessment conducted after a 3-month no-contact interval showed that the benefits in processing speed, attention and long-term memory vanished and that only the effects on wellbeing were maintained 3 months later (see Ballesteros et al., 2015b). However, participants in the trained group showed no transfer to either executive control or spatial WM from pre-test to 3-month follow-up. These results suggest that cognitive plasticity can be induced in healthy older adults, but that periodic boosting sessions are needed to maintain the training benefits.

In view of the importance of WM for the daily life activities of older adults, we designed this longitudinal intervention study taking into account the results of our previous study (Ballesteros et al., 2014, 2015b) and the findings of several recently published meta-analyses (Karbach and Verhaeghen, 2014; Lampit et al., 2014; Toril et al., 2014). The program was composed of 15 1-h sessions. An important variable is the number of video games included in the training schedule (see Toril et al., 2014), and we therefore selected just six non-action video games to train mainly WM. Importantly, all the participants in the experimental group were trained in group sessions at the municipal senior center and in the presence of an experimenter (as recommended by Kelly et al., 2014 and Lampit et al., 2014).

The goal of the present study was to investigate whether cognitively healthy older adults could benefit from training with non-action video games. We addressed two main questions. First, would training older adults with non-action video games improve their visuospatial WM as well as short- and long-term memory? Secondly, would any improvements persist after a 3-month no-contact period? Based on the results of previous studies, we hypothesized that: (1) video game training would improve the visuospatial WM of older adults; (2) the effects of training would transfer to episodic memory; and (3) memory improvements would persist 3 months after finishing the training program.

MATERIALS AND METHODS

Participants

Forty cognitively healthy volunteer older adults were recruited from a municipal senior center in the Madrid suburbs to participate in this training study. They all had normal or corrected-to-normal vision and hearing and informed that they did not have previous experience with video games. After signing a consent form, participants were randomly assigned either to the trained (experimental) group or to the control group. Participants in both groups regularly attended cultural activities at the senior center (e.g., painting classes, lectures, cultural visits). The control group continued their routine lifestyle activities at the senior center. The study was approved by the Ethics Committee of the Universidad Nacional de Educación a Distancia. The inclusion criteria were to obtain a score of 26 or above on the Mini-Mental State Examination (MMSE; Folstein et al., 1975) and a normal score on the Information subscale of the Wechsler Adult Intelligence Scale (WAIS III; Wechsler, 1999). The two groups did not differ in age, years of education, or in the Information subscale and MMSE scores (all $ps > 0.05$). In the experimental group, one participant declined to participate after screening for medical reasons. Thus, 19 participants in the training group and 20 in the control group completed the study. Demographic data for each group are displayed in **Table 1**.

Study Design

The study was a 2 (group: experimental, control) × 3 (session: pre-training, post-training, 3-month follow-up) mixed factorial design. Group was the between-subjects factor and session was the within-subjects factor. To investigate the effectiveness of the intervention to improve and/or maintain both visuospatial WM and short- and long-term memory, participants performed a series of tests and experimental tasks designed to assess these types of memory: digit span forward and backward, Corsi blocks, Jigsaw puzzle task, and immediate and delayed visual episodic memory tasks (Faces I and II, and Family Pictures I and II from Wechsler Memory Scale, WMS III). The Corsi blocks and the Jigsaw puzzle tasks were programmed using E-Prime 2.0 (Psychology Software Tools Inc., Pittsburg, PA, USA). Long-term memory was assessed with tests from the WMS-III (Wechsler, 1997), and the Digit Span tasks were extracted from WAIS III (Wechsler, 1999).

Training Schedule and Overview of the Training Program

Participants assigned to the experimental group completed 15 1-h training sessions at the community senior center in the presence of the experimenter over a period of 7–8 weeks. In each training session, participants played six video games twice

TABLE 1 | Demographic information about participants in each group.

Characteristics	Experimental mean (SD)	Control mean (SD)	*p*	*F*
Age (Years)	69.95 (6.73)	73.20 (6.48)	0.13	2.36
Education (Years)	13.37 (3.27)	12.85 (3.36)	0.62	0.23
MMSE	28.31 (1.00)	27.75 (1.48)	0.17	1.92
Information	18.42 (2.61)	16.95 (3.06)	0.11	2.58

Note: Means and Standard deviations (SD) by group; MMSE, Mini-Mental State Examination.

each. The games were selected from *Lumosity*[1], a web-based cognitive training platform[2]; they were *Speed Match, Memory matrix, Rotation matrix, Face memory, Money comb* and *Lost in migration.* The session score for each participant on each game was calculated as the mean score of the first and second time they played the game. The session RT for each participant on each game was calculated as the mean performance of the first and second time they played the game. The control group did not receive training but met the experimenter periodically (once a month) in the senior center to talk about their activities and other general topics related to aging. The video games used in this study are described below.

Speed Match

In this game, a symbol is displayed on the computer screen, followed immediately by another. The trainee has to decide whether the two symbols are the same, indicating their choice by pressing one of two keys (same, different) as fast as possible.

Memory Matrix

A matrix varying in size is displayed in the center of the screen with a pattern of colored squares followed by a blank matrix. The player has to reproduce the pattern by clicking on the squares that were colored.

Rotation Matrix

This game is similar to the previous one, except that the matrix is rotated between the coding phase and the response phase. The player has to mentally rotate the encoded matrix, and click on the correct positions of the colored squares.

Face Memory

Different faces appear on the screen continuously, one after another, and the player has to decide whether the face on the screen matches the one shown one (1-back), two (2-back), or three (3-back) faces before.

Moneycomb

In this game, a honeycomb appears in the center of screen and a sequence of tokens of different values is presented briefly inside it. The task consists of clicking on the correct tiles of the honeycomb to reveal the tokens in the correct order (from lowest to highest value).

Lost in Migration

In this game, a static flock of birds appears in the center of the screen. The goal is to identify the direction in which the bird in the middle of the flock is flying (right, left, upward, downward) by pressing one of the four arrow keys on the keyboard as fast as possible.

Participants received points based on their performance on each video game. Some of the games also recorded response times. None of the participants in the study reported that they had any previous experience of playing video games.

Assessment Tasks and Procedures

Assessment tasks fell into one of the following three domains: visuospatial WM, short-term memory and episodic memory.

Visuospatial Working Memory Tasks

Visuospatial WM (Baddeley and Hitch, 1974) was assessed with the Corsi blocks and the Jigsaw-puzzle task.

Corsi Blocks Task

The original Corsi Blocks task (Milner, 1971) consisted of a set of nine identical blocks (3 cm × 3 cm × 3 cm) unevenly positioned on a wooden board (23 cm × 28 cm). The participant had to point to the blocks in their order of presentation. The length of the sequence increased until recall was no longer correct in terms of order or position (Berch et al., 1998). In this study, we used the same computerized version of the Corsi task as in our previous study (Ballesteros et al., 2014) with four levels of increasing difficulty (2, 3, 4 and 5 cube positions) and 10 trials per level. The stimuli were black squares on a 3 × 3 matrix that appeared one after the other, for 1 s each. The positions in each sequence were selected randomly, with the restriction that stimuli could not appear in the same position in two consecutive sequences. In each trial, the participant reproduced the previously presented sequence of cubes (the black squares in the 3 × 3 matrix) by writing down their order of presentation on a separate response sheet. To familiarize participants with the task, they performed a practice block of trials. The final score was the proportion of correct sequences obtained at each difficulty level.

Jigsaw-Puzzle Task

The original pencil-and-paper Jigsaw-Puzzle task was developed to assess active visuospatial abilities (Richardson and Vecchi, 2002). We designed a computerized version of this task with puzzles consisting of 4, 6 or 9 pieces. Each piece was numbered and the participant had to write down on a response sheet the number corresponding to the pieces in the correct spatial positions. The stimuli were 15 pictures with similar visual complexity (mean = 2.4, SD = 0.32) and familiarity (mean = 4.3, SD = 0.26) selected from the Snodgrass and Vanderwart (1980) picture set. Each picture was fragmented into 4, 6 and 9 pieces to produce 45 different puzzles. The pictures were enlarged to fit a 12 cm × 12 cm area and were cut into four 6 cm × 6 cm pieces, six 6 cm × 4 cm pieces, or nine 3 cm × 3 cm pieces using Adobe Photoshop CC (Adobe Systems Software, Ireland Ltd.). We generated three different counterbalanced orders. Different pictures were used at pre-test, post-test and follow-up assessments. Participants were presented with 15 puzzles representing all possible combinations and number of pieces. The response sheets contained grids of the same size as the original pictures with the appropriate number of squares (4, 6, 9 squares). We used two puzzles as practice items and their results were not included in the analysis. For each trial, a fragmented picture appeared on the computer screen and the participant

[1]http://www.lumosity.com

[2]The authors confirm that they did not have any contact with the *Lumosity* cognitive training platform at any time during the study, which was conducted independently.

wrote down on the response sheet the appropriate numbers to form a spatially correct picture. The jigsaw was presented on the computer screen for 90 s. Participants were allowed to correct errors within that time. Performance was assessed in terms of the proportion of correct puzzles per level (4, 6 and 9 pieces).

Short-Term Memory

Short-term memory was assessed with the Digit Span Test of the WAIS III scale (Wechsler, 1999).

Digit Span Test

This test has two parts: Digit span forward and Digit span backward. For each part, the test administrator says a series of numbers aloud at the rate of one per second. The participant then repeats the numbers in the same order (digit span forward) or in reverse order (digit span backward). Both tests begin with a series of two numbers. For digits forward, the test continues up to a maximum of eight numbers. For digits backward, the test continues up to a maximum of seven numbers. Participants are given two trials at each length and the test continues until the participant fails both trials at one length. In both the forward and the backward task, the score was the maximum number of correctly remembered digits.

Immediate and Delayed Episodic Memory Tests

The **Faces and Family Pictures** subtests of the WMS-III were used to assess visual episodic memory. For immediate recognition and inmediate recall, we used Faces I and Family Pictures I, respectively. Delayed recognition and recall was assessed 25 min later using Faces II for delayed recognition and Family Pictures II for delayed recall.

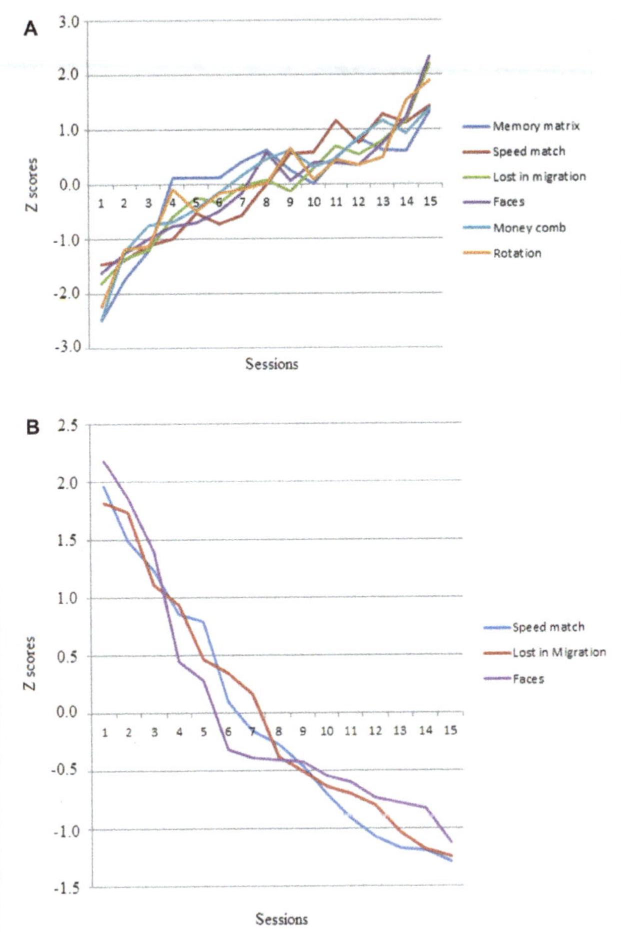

FIGURE 1 | (A) Average performance scores obtained in the six non-action video games across the 15 sessions in Z scores (mean 0; standard deviation 1). **(B)** Average response times of four video games across the training sessions in Z scores.

RESULTS

Video Game Practice Effects

Although the main dependent variables of this intervention study were the scores obtained on the memory tests, we also analyzed performance on the video games to evaluate whether the trained participants improved as a consequence of playing the video games. Video game performance showed significant improvements (accuracy and response times) across the 15 training sessions (see **Figures 1A,B**). **Figure 1A** shows the positive linear trend of the mean number of correct responses as a function of session. **Figure 1B** presents the mean response times for the video games that recorded response times. The mean scores of each game at the beginning and end of the training period were compared using regression analysis, with Training Session as the predictor variable and RT and Game Score as the criterion variables. Performance on all games improved after training. R^2 coefficients were high and accounted for more than 80% of the variance of the model in the six games. The ANOVAS for the previous analyses showed that all R^2 coefficients were statistically significant. This means that Training Session was a reliable predictor of Score and RT in the six games. **Table 2** summarizes the results.

Effects of Video Game Training on Visuospatial Working Memory Tasks and Other Memory Tests

We investigated whether training with video games improved memory abilities that decline with age, especially visuospatial WM and episodic memory. We addressed two questions. The first was whether training older adults with video games would transfer to performance on a series of memory tasks (transfer effects). The second was whether these possible enhancements would remain after a 3-month no-contact period (maintenance). To answer these questions, we investigated whether group (trained vs. control) interacted with session (pre-test, post-test, follow-up) with regard to performance on the different memory tests. Statistical analyses were conducted using Bonferroni correction for main effects and interactions in all tasks.

Jigsaw-Puzzle Task

A Group (2) × Session (3) × Level of fragmentation (3) mixed ANOVA with Group as the between-subjects factor and Session

TABLE 2 | Determination coefficients (R^2), *F* and *p* values for the six video games.

Videogame	DV	R^2	R^2 (corr)	F	p
Memory matrix	Score	0.699	0.675	30.14	0.00
Speed match	Score	0.952	0.949	260.64	0.00
	RT	0.951	0.948	254.91	0.00
Lost in migration	Score	0.921	0.914	150.65	0.00
	RT	0.954	0.951	271.49	0.00
Faces	Score	0.896	0.888	112.42	0.00
	RT	0.813	0.798	56.44	0.00
Money comb	Score	0.866	0.856	84.34	0.00
Rotation matrix	Score	0.840	0.828	68.45	0.00

Note. DV, Dependent variable; R^2, Regression coefficient; R^2corr, corrected regression coefficient; F, F values of ANOVAs; p, p values.

and Level of fragmentation as the within-subjects factor was performed on the proportion of correct puzzles completed at each level of fragmentation. The results showed that the main effect of Group was statistically significant ($F_{(1,37)}$ = 12.10, *MSe* = 3.03, p = 0.001, η_p^2 = 0.84). The trained group performed better (mean = 0.52, SD = 0.17) than the control group (mean = 0.33, SD = 0.17). Session was also statistically significant ($F_{(2,74)}$ = 8.71, *MSe* = 0.32, p = 0.001, η_p^2 = 0.19). Participants performed better at post-test (mean = 0.41, SD = 0.12) than at pre-test (mean = 0.36, SD = 0.18), but there was no difference between post-test and 3-month follow-up (p = 0.29). Level of fragmentation was also significant ($F_{(2,74)}$ = 207.56, *MSe* = 12.70, p = 0.001, η_p^2 = 0.84), showing that performance deteriorated with higher levels of fragmentation (level 4, mean = 0.75, SD = 0.18; level 6, mean = 0.43, SD = 0.24; level 9, mean = 0.09, SD = 0.12). The two-way Session by Group interaction was statistically significant ($F_{(2,74)}$ = 13.30, *MSe* = 0.49, p = 0.001, η_p^2 = 0.26), showing that the trained group performed better at post-test (mean = 0.61, SD = 0.13) than the control group (mean = 0.32, SD = 0.13). The trained group performed better (mean = 0.55, SD = 0.13) at the 3-month follow-up assessment (p = 0.001) than the control group (mean = 0.32, SD = 0.13), while the performance of the control group did not differ between sessions. No other interaction was significant (all $p > 0.05$); see **Figure 2** (bottom right).

Corsi Blocks Task

A Group (2) × Session (3) × Corsi level (2, 3, 4 and 5 blocks) mixed ANOVA with Group as the between-subjects factor and Session and Corsi level as within-subjects factors were conducted on the proportion of correct sequences per level. The results showed that the main effect of Group was statistically significant ($F_{(1,37)}$ = 10.04, *MSe* = 3.55, p = 0.001, η_p^2 = 0.21), showing that the trained group (mean = 0.62, SD = 0.17) outperformed the control group (mean = 0.45, SD = 0.17). The main effect of Session was also statistically significant ($F_{(2,74)}$ = 5.43, *MSe* = 0.24, p = 0.001, η_p^2 = 0.12), with better performance at post-test (mean = 0.58, SD = 0.12) than at pre-test (mean = 0.50, SD = 0.18). There were significant differences between pre-test and post-test assessments (p = 0.01). Moreover, there were marginally significant differences (p = 0.054) between post-test (mean = 0.58, SD = 0.12) and 3-month follow-up (mean = 0.53, SD = 0.12), while performance at pre-test and 3-month follow-up (p = 0.57) did not differ. The main factor of Corsi level was also significant ($F_{(3,37)}$ = 285.84, *MSe* = 12.84, p = 0.001, η_p^2 = 0.88), showing that performance deteriorated as the number of blocks increased (Corsi 2, mean = 0.89, SD = 0.06; Corsi 3, mean = 0.67, SD = 0.18; Corsi 4, mean = 0.46, SD = 0.24; Corsi 5, mean = 0.12, SD = 0.12). The two-way Session by Group interaction was also statistically significant ($F_{(2,74)}$ = 5.25, *MSe* = 0.23, p = 0.001, η_p^2 = 0.12). The analysis of this interaction showed that there were significant differences (p = 0.001) between pre- and post-test in the trained group (mean pre-test = 0.55, SD = 0.21; mean post-test = 0.70, SD = 0.17), but a reverse trend was observed in the control group (p = 1.00). There were also significant differences (p = 0.01) in the trained group between post-test and 3-month follow-up (mean post-test = 0.70, SD = 0.17; mean follow-up = 0.62, SD = 0.17), with lower performance at the 3-month follow-up. Differences between pre- and post-test were not significant (p = 1.00) in the control group (mean pre-test = 0.45, SD = 0.22; mean post-test = 0.46, SD = 0.17). The two-way Group by Level interaction was also significant ($F_{(3,111)}$ = 5.67, *MSe* = 0.24, p = 0.001, η_p^2 = 0.13). The analysis of this interaction showed that there were significant differences ($ps < 0.05$) between groups at all Corsi levels. In the trained group, the means for each level were: level 2 = 0.94, SD = 0.08; level 3 = 0.78, SD = 0.17; level 4 = 0.60, SD = 0.26; level 5 = 0.17, SD = 0.13. In the control group the means were: level 2 = 0.84, SD = 0.08; level 3 = 0.54, SD = 0.17; level 4 = 0.32, SD = 0.26; level 5 = 0.07, SD = 0.13). Although the trained group performed better than the control group in this task, performance deteriorated in both groups as the number of blocks increased; see **Figure 2** (bottom left).

Digit Forward Test

The ANOVA conducted with Group (2) and Session (3) on the numbers of correct digits reportedly showed that Session was significant ($F_{(2,74)}$ = 3.97, *MSe* = 1.23, p = 0.02, η_p^2 = 0.09), with better performance at post-test (mean = 5.38, SD = 0.87) than at pre-test (mean = 5.05, SD = 0.74), but there were no significant differences between post-test and 3-month follow-up (p = 1.00). The trained group performed better at post-test than at pre-test (p = 0.02), but there was no difference between post-test and 3-month follow-up (p = 1.00). Group as a main factor was not significant (p = 0.37), as the performance of the trained group (mean = 5.35, SD = 0.69) was similar to that of the control group (mean = 5.15, SD = 0.71). No other factors or interactions were significant (all $ps > 0.05$); see **Figure 2** (top left).

Digit Backward Test

An ANOVA with Group (2) and Session (3) was conducted on the numbers of correct digits reported. The main factor of Group was significant ($F_{(1,37)}$ = 5.09, *MSe* = 8.78, p = 0.03, η_p^2 = 0.12), showing that the trained group performed better (mean = 4.29, SD = 0.73) than the control group (mean = 3.75,

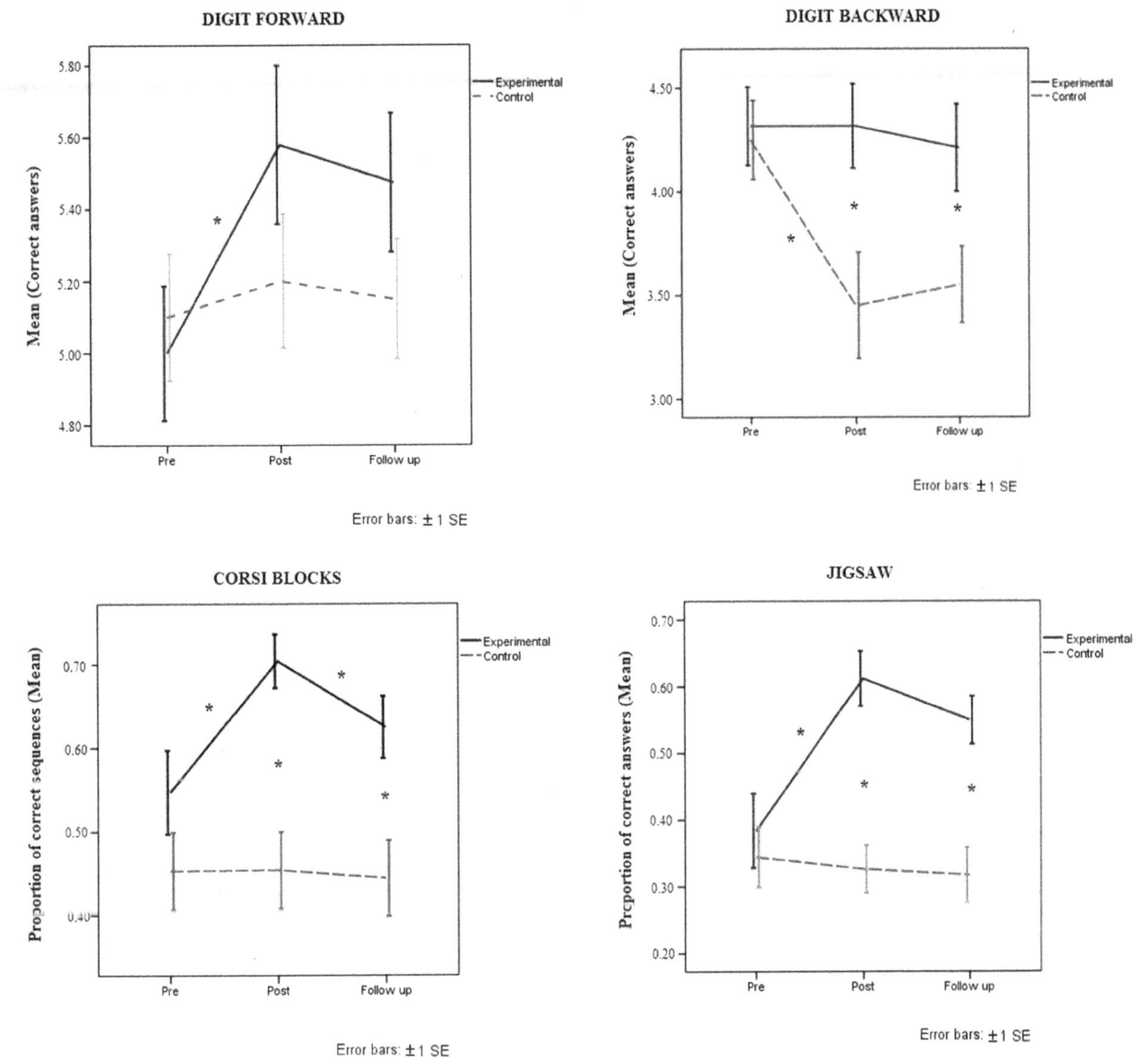

FIGURE 2 | Top: Mean performance of trained and control groups at pre-test, post-test and follow-up assessments in Digits forward (left) and Digits backward (right). **Bottom:** Mean performance of trained and control groups at pre-test, post-test and follow-up assessments in the working memory (WM) tasks (left: Corsi blocks; right: Jigsaw puzzle tasks). Error bars represent ± SE. *$p < 0.05$.

SD = 0.67). The main effect of Session ($F_{(2,74)} = 5.24$, $MSe = 1.96$, $p = 0.001$, $\eta_p^2 = 0.12$) was significant. Performance at pre-test was better than at post-test (mean pre-test = 4.28, SD = 0.81; mean post-test = 3.88, SD = 0.93). The control group performed worse at post-test than at pre-test. The two-way Group by Session interaction was also significant ($F_{(2,74)} = 4.69$, $MSe = 1.75$, $p = 0.01$, $\eta_p^2 = 0.11$). Simple effects analysis showed no significant differences in the trained group between pre-test, post-test and 3-month follow-up evaluations ($p = 1.00$). Participants performed similarly in the three assessment sessions (mean = 4.31, SD = 0.82; mean = 4.31, SD = 0.80; mean = 4.26, SD = 0.87, for pre-test, post-test and 3-month follow-up, respectively). By contrast, there were significant differences in the control group between pre- and post-test ($p = 0.001$) due to poorer performance at post-test (mean post-test = 3.45; SD = 1.14) than at pre-test (mean = 4.25, SD = 1.14), but there were no differences ($p = 1.00$) between post-test and 3-month follow-up; see **Figure 2** (top right).

Episodic Memory Test (Faces)

The results of the episodic memory tests are shown in **Figure 3** and **Table 3**.

Faces I

An ANOVA with Group (2) and Session (3) was performed on the recognition scores (Faces I). The analysis showed that Group was not significant although there was a trend in that direction ($p = 0.07$). Session was significant ($F_{(2,74)} = 4.37$,

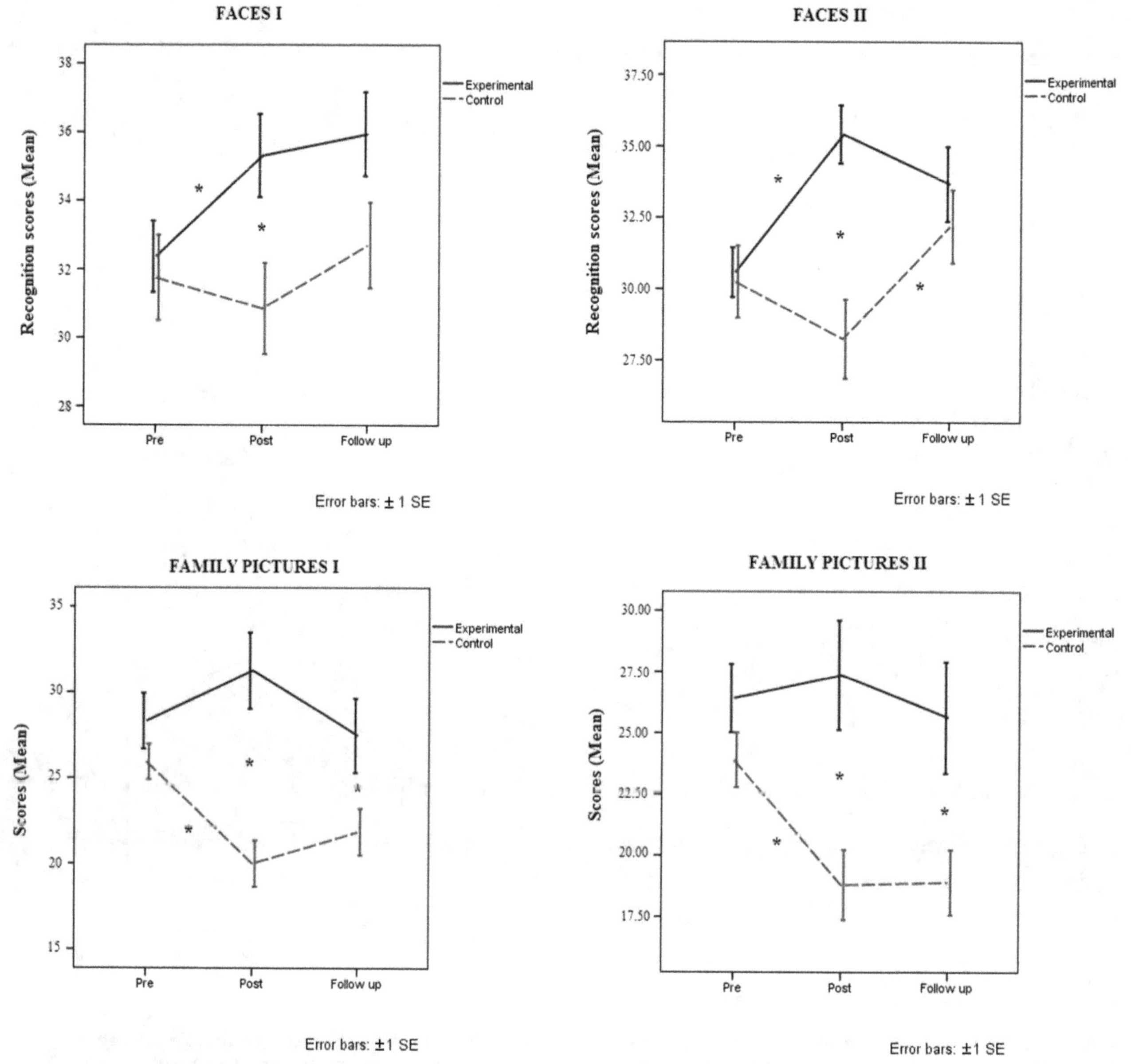

FIGURE 3 | Mean performance of trained and control groups at pre-test, post-test and follow-up in the episodic memory tasks. Top: Faces I (left) and Faces II (right). **Bottom:** Family Pictures I (left) and Family Pictures II (right). Error bars represent ± SE. *$p < 0.05$.

MSe = 50.11, p = 0.01, η_p^2 = 0.10) with better performance at the 3-month follow-up (mean = 34.32, SD = 5.42) than at pre-test (mean = 32.05, SD = 5.05). There were no significant differences (p = 0.55) between pre-test (mean = 32.05, SD = 5.05) and post-test (mean = 33.08, SD = 5.61), of between post-test (mean = 33.08, SD = 5.61) and 3-month follow-up (mean = 34.32, SD = 5.42). The two-way Group by Session interaction was significant ($F_{(2,74)}$ = 3.28, MSe = 37.67, p = 0.04, η_p^2 = 0.08). The analysis of this interaction showed that there were significant differences between groups at post-test (p = 0.01), but only a trend was found at 3-month follow-up (p = 0.07). The trained group performed better at post-test than at pre-test (p = 0.03), but with similar performance at post-test and 3-month follow-up evaluations (p = 1.00). By contrast, the control group performed similarly in the three evaluation sessions ($p > 0.05$).

Faces II

The ANOVA conducted with Group (2) and Session (3) on the recognition scores (Faces II) showed that the effect of Group was statistically significant ($F_{(1,37)}$ = 4.20, MSe = 262.15, p = 0.04, η_p^2 = 0.10). The trained group performed better (mean = 33.22, SD = 4.52) than the control group (mean = 30.23, SD = 4.55). Session was also significant ($F_{(2,74)}$ = 5.40, MSe = 62.57, p = 0.001, η_p^2 = 0.12). There were no differences between pre-

TABLE 3 | Pre-test, post-test and follow-up training performance on working memory and episodic memory tasks corresponding to the trained and the control groups. M (Mean), SD (Standard deviation).

Task	Experimental			Control		
	Pre M (SD)	*Post M (SD)*	*Follow up M (SD)*	*Pre M (SD)*	*Post M (SD)*	*Follow up M (SD)*
Corsi Blocks task						
2 Serial position (Proportion)	0.86 (0.20)	0.98 (0.03)	0.95 (0.07)	0.79 (0.17)	0.86 (0.12)	0.86 (0.13)
3 Serial position (Proportion)	0.68 (0.30)	0.86 (0.13)	0.81 (0.16)	0.59 (0.24)	0.53 (0.27)	0.55 (0.29)
4 Serial position (Proportion)	0.50 (0.33)	0.73 (0.26)	0.57 (0.30)	0.35 (0.35)	0.36 (0.35)	0.28 (0.32)
5 Serial position (Proportion)	0.14 (0.21)	0.23 (0.24)	0.15 (0.21)	0.08 (0.17)	0.07 (0.18)	0.08 (0.16)
Jigsaw puzzle task						
4 pieces (Proportion)	0.68 (0.32)	0.93 (0.11)	0.92 (0.15)	0.67 (0.28)	0.59 (0.27)	0.65 (0.23)
6 pieces (Proportion)	0.42 (0.36)	0.64 (0.21)	0.58 (0.27)	0.32 (0.34)	0.22 (0.27)	0.29 (0.35)
9 pieces (Proportion)	0.05 (0.18)	0.18 (0.21)	0.14 (0.24)	0.05 (0.14)	0.02 (0.08)	0.02 (0.06)
Digit forward						
Score	5.00 (0.81)	5.57 (0.96)	5.47 (0.84)	5.10 (0.78)	5.20 (0.83)	5.15 (0.74)
Digit backward						
Score	4.31 (0.82)	4.32 (0.74)	4.26 (0.82)	4.25 (0.85)	3.45 (1.14)	3.55 (0.82)
Faces I						
Score	32.37 (4.53)	35.31 (5.30)	35.94 (5.32)	31.75 (5.58)	30.85 (5.95)	32.70 (5.59)
Faces II						
Score	30.58 (3.79)	35.42 (4.43)	33.68 (5.71)	30.25 (5.67)	28.25 (6.19)	32.20 (5.71)
Family Pictures I						
Score	28.16 (7.15)	31.42 (9.13)	27.47 (9.43)	25.95 (4.63)	20.00 (6.03)	21.85 (6.07)
Family Pictures II						
Score	26.42 (6.08)	27.36 (9.74)	25.10 (9.42)	23.90 (4.98)	18.75 (6.36)	18.90 (5.91)

test and post-test scores ($p = 0.15$), or between post-test and 3-month follow-up scores ($p = 0.55$), but performance was better ($p = 0.001$) at 3-month follow-up (mean = 32.94, SD = 5.61) than at pre-test (mean = 30.41, SD = 4.80). The two-way Group by Session interaction was also statistically significant ($F_{(2,74)} = 11.29$, $MSe = 130.70$, $p = 0.001$, $\eta_p^2 = 0.23$), suggesting that groups differed at post-test ($p = 0.001$), but not at the 3-month follow-up assessment ($p = 0.42$). The trained group improved from pre-test to post-test ($p = 0.001$), but not between post-test and 3-month follow-up ($p = 0.43$). Moreover, there were significant differences ($p = 0.02$) between pre-test and 3-month follow-up, suggesting that performance at follow-up (mean = 33.68, SD = 5.69) was better than at pre-test (mean = 30.57, SD = 4.82). In the control group there were no significant differences between pre-test and post-test ($p = 0.14$), but participants in this group performed better at 3-month follow-up than at post-test ($p = 0.001$). Differences between pre-test and 3-month follow-up were not significant ($p = 0.25$).

Episodic Memory Tests (Family Pictures)

Family Pictures I

An ANOVA with Group (2) and Session (3) performed on the recall scores (Family Pictures I) showed a significant effect of Group ($F_{(1,37)} = 11.18$, $MSe = 1203.86$, $p = 0.001$, $\eta_p^2 = 0.23$), indicating that the trained group performed better (mean = 29.01, SD = 5.95) than the control group (mean = 22.60, SD = 5.94). Session was not significant ($p = 0.06$), but the Session × Group interaction was significant ($F_{(2,74)} = 8.47$, $MSe = 211.37$, $p = 0.001$, $\eta_p^2 = 0.18$). The analysis of this interaction suggests that there were significant differences between groups at post-test ($p = 0.001$) and 3-month follow-up ($p = 0.03$). Performance of the trained group did not differ between sessions ($p > 0.05$), but the control group performed worse at post-test than at pre-test ($p = 0.001$) with no difference between post-test and 3-month follow-up ($p = 0.88$). However, the control group performed worse at 3 month follow-up than at pre-test ($p = 0.01$).

Family Pictures II

The ANOVA Group (2) × Session (3) conducted on the recall scores (Family Pictures II) showed that the effect of group was significant ($F_{(1,37)} = 8.89$, $MSe = 977.08$, $p = 0.001$, $\eta_p^2 = 0.19$), suggesting that the trained group performed better (mean = 26.29, SD = 6.00) than the control group (mean = 20.51, SD = 6.03). The effect of Session was also statistically significant ($F_{(2,74)} = 4.09$, $MSe = 100.71$, $p = 0.02$, $\eta_p^2 = 0.10$). There were no significant differences between post-test and 3-month follow-up ($p = 1.00$) or between pre-test and post-test ($p = 0.27$), but scores differed significantly between pre-test and 3-month follow-up ($p = 0.01$). Performance was worse at 3-month follow-up (mean = 22.00, SD = 7.08) than at pre-test (mean = 25.16, SD = 4.90). The Group by Session interaction was significant ($F_{(2,74)} = 3.73$, $MSe = 91.87$, $p = 0.02$, $\eta_p^2 = 0.09$), showing that the trained group performed better than the control group at both post-test and 3-month follow-up assessments. The trained group did not differ between sessions ($p > 0.05$), but the control group performed worse at post-test than at pre-test ($p = 0.01$). Moreover, the control group performed similarly at post-test and 3-month follow-up ($p = 1.00$), but this group performed worse ($p = 0.001$) at the 3-month follow-up test (mean = 18.90, SD = 7.82) than at pre-test (mean = 23.90, SD = 5.54).

DISCUSSION

The study yielded three main findings. First, the trainees improved their video game performance across sessions. Second, and most important, the trainees performed the Jigsaw puzzle, Corsi Blocks, Digit forward, and Faces I and II tasks better than the control group. Third, the improved performance of the trained group was maintained from baseline to the 3-month follow-up for the Jigsaw puzzle task, which is a visuospatial WM task, and on the Digits forward, and Faces I and II tasks, but not on the Corsi Blocks, the other visuospatial WM task. These results are encouraging considering the age-related declines that occur in these memory functions.

Non-Action Video Games Training Transferred to Working Memory

The improvements found in the present study are in line with previous findings reported in other video game training studies conducted with older adults (e.g., Basak et al., 2008; Anguera et al., 2013). Basak et al. (2008) found improvements on working memory tasks after training older adults for 23.5 h with a real-time strategy video game (action video game). Anguera et al. (2013) trained older adults (60–75 years) for 4 weeks with an adaptive version of *Neuroracer*. Participants reduced multitasking costs at the post-training evaluation compared to an active control group and a no-contact control group. Moreover, the benefits of training were extended to an untrained WM task, and gains persisted for 6 months.

The results of this longitudinal study are in agreement with those of other researchers who trained older adults using computerized training programs. For example, Buschkuehl et al. (2008) conducted an adaptive visual WM training study with oldest-old adults (mean age = 80 years). They found substantial gains in the trained task and improvements immediately after training in visual WM, which disappeared at the 1-year follow-up. Li et al. (2008) also investigated the effects of WM training on performance improvement, transfer and short-term maintenance of practice gains. In their study, young and older adults practiced a spatial WM task for 45 days, about 15 min per day. In both age groups, these researchers found improvements on the practiced tasks, and near transfer to spatial and numerical *n*-back tasks. Moreover, practice gains and near transfer effects were maintained at 3-month follow-up, but performance after training was lower in older than in young adults. Dahlin et al. (2008) conducted a computer-based training study with young and older adults based on updating information in WM. The results showed that both trained groups showed significantly greater improvement on the letter memory criterion task than the control group. Interestingly, gains were maintained 18 months later in young adults but not in older adults. Recently, Zinke et al. (2014) trained WM in older adults in nine sessions over 3 weeks and found near transfer effects in a Corsi blocks task at post-test compared with pre-test.

The results of the present study also agree with findings of a recent meta-analysis (Karbach and Verhaeghen, 2014). The authors showed that executive functions and WM training led to significant improvements in performance in the trained tasks as well as large near transfer effects in older adults. However, the findings of the present study do not agree with the results of Maillot et al. (2012) who found that after a 24-h training program the trainees improved more than controls in measures of executive control and processing speed functions, but not in visuospatial measures. The present results conflict with those of Ballesteros et al. (2014), who did not find any improvement in visuospatial WM tasks (Corsi Blocks and Jigsaw puzzle tasks) or executive functions after 20 1-h training sessions with 10 non-action video games selected from the *Lumosity* platform, although the video game training intervention was effective for improving RT, attention, and episodic memory.

The trained group improved digit span forward performance after training while the control group performed similarly across the three assessment sessions. However, in digit span backward test (a more difficult task), the trained group did not improve after training while the performance of the control group declined. It is important to note that the age-related declines in digit span backward performance is greater than that in digit span forward. This result is in agreement with the meta-analysis of Babcock and Salthouse (1990). This result supports the idea that with advancing age, the digit span forward test tends to remain stable while the digit span backward task tends to decline (Lezak, 1995). This might explain the performance of our control group in the forward and backward span digit tests.

Video Game Training Enhanced Some Episodic Memory Tests

The present study also found improvements in some episodic memory tests after training, similar to the results of our previous study (Ballesteros et al., 2014), in which we found effects of training in episodic memory (Family Pictures I and II). However, in the present study we found improvements after training in Faces (I and II), which were maintained over a 3-month period without contact. We found improvements in Faces I and II (two recognition tests) after training but not in Family Pictures (two recall tests). This result might be explained because free recall requires greater resources than recognition and this effect increases with age (Craik and McDowd, 1987). In Faces, the recognition test, the information is present while performing the memory task. However, in Family Pictures, a recall test, very few cues are provided and participants have to initiate a series of mental operations, which require more effort. In the trained group, video game training could help participants to recall features although they did not improve after training. The results obtained in Faces suggest that the task was easy for both groups. The trained group improved after training and controls were able to maintain their performance over time.

Our results are in line with those of Buschkuehl et al. (2008) who conducted a WM training study with 80-year-old adults who trained twice a week for 3 months. Participants showed improvements in the trained tasks (visual WM tasks) and to a lesser degree, in a visual episodic memory task (visual free recall) in which they had to look for differences between two almost identical pictures.

Results at 3-Month Follow-Up

The usefulness of the intervention depends on both the occurrence of transfer effects and the durability of the training effects. Accordingly, it was important to ascertain whether the benefits found at post-training on some WM tasks and short- and long-term memory tests were maintained after a 3-month no-contact follow-up period. In this study, transfer effects were maintained in the Digit forward test, the Jigsaw puzzle task, and in the Faces I and Faces II tests. However, significant improvements in the Corsi blocks task were not maintained.

Our results are in line with those of Anguera et al. (2013) who trained older adults for 4 weeks with an adaptive version of *Neuroracer* and found benefits after training. Specifically, they reported reduced multitasking costs in the trained group compared to the control group. The benefits found after training extended to an untrained WM task, and gains persisted for 6 months. The 3-month maintenance found in the present study is in line with the results of Li et al. (2008) who found specific improvements in young and older adults in a WM task and maintenance of near transfer effects at 3-month follow-up.

The Video Games Training Debate

The conflicting results obtained in cognitive and brain-training studies with computerized cognitive exercises and video games have been explored in several recent meta-analyses (Karbach and Verhaeghen, 2014; Lampit et al., 2014; Toril et al., 2014). Specifically, we found that short training interventions conducted with older adults produced better results than long regimes (Toril et al., 2014). Training sessions are exciting at first, but older adults get tired and bored during the last sessions. Karbach and Kray (2009) found significant transfer effects in older adults after just four training sessions, as did Kramer et al. (1995) who provided a limited number of training sessions. Lampit et al. (2014) concluded that unsupervised at-home training regimes were less effective than group-based sessions, and that training more than three times a week was also ineffective. Another important variable was the number of video games used during the training sessions. Although not significant, Toril et al. (2014) found a trend in the analysis indicating that it is better to use a small set of video games than a large set.

It is important to stress that, on the basis of previous results (Ballesteros et al., 2014, 2015b; Lampit et al., 2014), we designed the present study as a group-based training program with the presence of the experimenter throughout. The presence/absence of the experimenter might affect the participants' interest in training (Borella et al., 2010). It is important to note that in our previous training study (Ballesteros et al., 2014) the experimenter was always present during each training session, but each session involved only 2–3 participants and not the whole group. The lack of improvement after training in visuospatial WM in our previous study (Ballesteros et al., 2014) and the positive results obtained in the present study might be due to the larger number of video games used in the earlier study (10) compared to just six specially selected to train visuospatial WM in the present study. The training regime of the present study was focused on enhancing WM, and this might explain the positive training effects obtained here.

Another important question regarding cognitive training concerns transfer. The evidence of transfer from video game training to untrained tasks is mixed, with both positive and negative results. Some researchers (Melby-Lervåg and Hulme, 2013) argue that WM training has positive effects on tasks close to the trained tasks (near transfer). However, in a more recent study the same authors did not find evidence that WM training was effective (Melby-Lervåg and Hulme, 2016). Owen et al. (2010) examined whether some training tasks would improve cognitive performance, and concluded that there was no transfer to untrained tasks. In our study, we found positive near transfer effects, as well as smaller transfer effects on other untrained episodic memory tasks. Moreover, it is important to stress that there is not an overlap between the training and the transfer tasks.

CONCLUSIONS, LIMITATIONS OF THE PRESENT STUDY AND FUTURE DIRECTIONS

To summarize, the results of the present study suggest that training older adults with non-action video games can be an effective way of improving visuospatial WM performance in tasks designed to assess this type of memory and episodic memory tests. Importantly, the effects were maintained over a 3-month no-contact follow-up period in the Jigsaw puzzle task, Digit forward (short-term memory), and Faces I and Faces II (episodic memory). Transfer effects were not maintained on Corsi blocks. These findings suggest that older brains retain plasticity, but that some periodic boosting sessions are needed to maintain the benefits.

The present study has several limitations. First, our sample was smaller than in other studies (e.g., Mozolic et al., 2011; Anguera et al., 2013). However, it is important to stress that we did not have any drop-outs, which is unusual in longitudinal training studies, which lose between 30 and 40% of participants at follow-up. This suggests that training programs carried out in places that older adults attend regularly, and training sessions attended by the whole group with the presence of the experimenter are more effective than training individually at home or in small groups. Secondly, we did not examine the effects of training older adults with video games on everyday life tasks. This is an important issue for future studies. Thirdly, the control group in the present study was passive. However, most studies have also used a passive control group (e.g., Goldstein et al., 1997; Basak et al., 2008; Maillot et al., 2012; Ballesteros et al., 2014) to compare with the trained group, only a few training studies involving both an active and a passive control group (e.g., Torres, 2008; Stern et al., 2011; Anguera et al., 2013; Boot et al., 2013a). However, it is worth mentioning that in their meta-analysis, Toril et al. (2014) calculated the effect sizes of the published studies that included both an active and a passive control group (5 out of the 20 studies in the meta-analysis). The mean effect size (Cohen's *d*) was 0.36 for the active control group and 0.37 for the passive group. The difference was not statistically significant. However, future studies would include active and passive control groups.

It would be interesting in future studies to include a questionnaire to assess expectation (anticipated cognitive gains from game play) and the effects of the social contact with the experimenter and the other older adults. Furthermore, video game designers need to work with researchers in aging to create attractive and useful games specifically designed for older adults. Video games have to be interesting to motivate older adults to play them.

Commercial brain-training programs are currently generating millions of dollars, with very large revenues for the brain-training industry. Video game training is a very active area of research, but there are still important intervention-based factors that require further research. Large-scale longitudinal studies with long follow-up assessments of trained and control groups are necessary before researchers can answer many important questions related to the effectiveness of video-games to improve cognition (Boot et al., 2013b; Boot and Kramer, 2014; Green et al., 2014; Anguera and Gazzaley, 2015).

In conclusion, future research should investigate ways of designing video game training regimes that produce and maintain training benefits in older adults. Further research should take into account multi-domain interventions that can be carried out in social settings, involving computerized cognitive training (e.g., video game training) and physical exercise (Ballesteros et al., 2015b). In sum, future studies would benefit from using well-supported neuroscience findings to design multi-domain, longitudinal intervention studies to investigate the possible benefits for older adults, and then validate the benefits of the intervention.

AUTHOR CONTRIBUTIONS

PT, JM, SB and JMR: conceived and designed the experiments, contributed reagents/material/analysis tools, wrote the article, and reviewed the manuscript. PT: performed the experiments, analyzed the data. JMR: reviewing the data. PT, SB, JM: reviewing literature.

ACKNOWLEDGMENTS

This work was supported by a predoctoral fellowship to PT awarded to the *Studies on Aging and Neurodegenerative Diseases* Consolidated Research Group (Universidad Nacional de Educación a Distancia) and grants from the Spanish Government (PSI2013-41409R) and the Madrid Community (S2010/BMD-2349). We are very grateful to the Senior Center (Pozuelo de Alarcón, Madrid) and to the volunteers who participated in this study.

REFERENCES

Ackerman, P. L., Kanfer, R., and Calderwood, C. (2010). Use or lose it? Wii Brain exercise practice and reading for domain knowledge. *Psychol. Aging* 25, 753–766. doi: 10.1037/a0019277

Anguera, J. A., Boccanfuso, J., Rintoul, J. L., Al-Hashimi, O., Faraji, F., Janowich, J., et al. (2013). Video game training enhances cognitive control in older adults. *Nature* 501, 97–101. doi: 10.1038/nature12486

Anguera, J. A., and Gazzaley, A. (2015). Video games, cognitive exercises and the enhancement of cognitive abilities. *Current. Opin. Behav. Sci* 4, 160–165. doi: 10.1016/j.cobeha.2015.06.002

Babcock, R. L., and Salthouse, T. A. (1990). Effects of increased processing demands on age differences in working memory. *Psychol. Aging* 5, 421–428. doi: 10.1037/0882-7974.5.3.421

Baddeley, A. D., and Hitch, G. (1974). "Working memory," in *The Psychology of Learning and Motivation*, ed. G. H. Bower (New York, NY: Academic Press), 47–89.

Ballesteros, S., Bischof, G. N., Goh, J. O., and Park, D. C. (2013). Neural correlates of conceptual object priming in young and older adults: an event-related fMRI study. *Neurobiol. Aging* 34, 1254–1264. doi: 10.1016/j.neurobiolaging.2012.09.019

Ballesteros, S., Kraft, E., Santana, S., and Tziraki, C. (2015a). Maintaining older brain functionality: a targeted review. *Neurosci. Biobehav. Rev.* 55, 453–457. doi: 10.1016/j.neubiorev.2015.06.008

Ballesteros, S., Mayas, J., Prieto, A., Toril, P., Pita, C., Ponce de León, L., et al. (2015b). A randomized controlled trial of brain training with non- action video games in older adults: results of the 3-month follow-up. *Front. Aging. Neurosci.* 7:45. doi: 10.3389/fnagi.2015.00045

Ballesteros, S., and Mayas, J. (2015). Selective attention affects conceptual object priming and recognition: a study with young and older adults. *Front. Psychol.* 5:1567. doi: 10.3389/fpsyg.2014.01567

Ballesteros, S., Prieto, A., Mayas, J., Toril, P., Pita, C., Ponce de León, L., et al. (2014). Brain training with non-action video games enhances cognitive functions that decline with aging: a randomized controlled trial. *Front. Aging. Neurosci.* 6:277. doi: 10.3389/fnagi.2014.00277

Baltes, P. B., and Lindenberger, U. (1997). Emergence of a powerful connection between sensory and cognitive functions across the adult life span: a new window to the study of cognitive aging? *Psychol. Aging* 12, 12–21. doi: 10.1037/0882-7974.12.1.12

Basak, C., Boot, W. R., Voss, M. W., and Kramer, A. F. (2008). Can training in a real time strategy video game attenuate cognitive decline in older adults? *Psychol. Aging* 23, 765–777. doi: 10.1037/a0013494

Belchior, P. D. C. (2008). Cognitive training with video games to improve driving skills and driving safety among older adults [dissertation]. *Pro Quest Information Learn.*

Berch, D. B., Krikorian, R., and Huha, E. M. (1998). The corsi block-tapping task: methodological and theoretical considerations. *Brain. Cogn.* 38, 317–338. doi: 10.1006/brcg.1998.1039

Bialystok, E., and Craik, F. I. M. (2006). *Lifespan Cognition: Mechanisms of Change.* Oxford: Oxford University Press.

Boot, W. R., Blakely, D. P., and Simons, D. (2011). Do action video games improve perception and cognition? *Front. Psychol.* 2:226. doi: 10.3389/fpsyg.2011.00226

Boot, W. R., Champion, M., Blakely, D. P., Wright, T., Souders, D. J., and Charness, N. (2013a). Video games as a means to reduce age-related cognitive decline: attitudes, compliance and effectiveness. *Front. Psychol.* 4:31. doi: 10.3389/fpsyg.2013.00031

Boot, W. R., and Kramer, A. F. (2014). The brain-games conundrum: does cognitive training really sharpen the mind? *Cerebrum* 2014:15.

Boot, W. R., Simons, D., Stothart, C., and Stutts, C. (2013b). The pervasive problem with placebos in Psychology. Why active control groups are not sufficient to rule out placebo effects? *Perspect. Psychol. Sci.* 8, 445–454. doi: 10.1177/1745691613491271

Bopp, K. L., and Verhaeghen, P. (2005). Aging and verbal memory span: a meta-analysis. *J. Gerontol. B Psychol. Sci. Soc. Sci.* 60, 223–233. doi: 10.1093/geronb/60.5.p223

Borella, E., Carreti, B., Riboldi, F., and De Beni, R. (2010). Working memory training in older adults: evidence of transfer and maintenance effects. *Psychol. Aging* 25, 767–778. doi: 10.1037/a0020683

Boyke, J., Driemeyer, J., Gaser, C., Büchel, C., and May, A. (2009). Training induced brain structure changes in the elderly. *J. Neurosci.* 28, 7031–7035. doi: 10.1523/JNEUROSCI.0742-08.2008

Buschkuehl, M., Jaeggi, S. M., Hutchison, S., Perrig-Chiello, P., Däpp, C., Müller, M., et al. (2008). Impact of working memory training on memory performance in old-old adults. *Psychol. Aging* 23, 743–753. doi: 10. 1037/a0014342

Clark, J. E., Lamphear, A. K., and Riddick, C. C. (1987). The effects of videogame playing on the response selection processing of elderly adults. *J. Gerontol.* 42, 82–85. doi: 10.1093/geronj/42.1.82

Craik, F. I. M., and Bialystok, E. (2006). Cognition through the lifespan: mechanisms of change. *Trends Cogn. Sci.* 10, 131–139. doi: 10.1016/j.tics.2006. 01.007

Craik, F. I. M., and McDowd, J. (1987). Age differences in recall and recognition. *J. Exp. Psychol. Learn.* 13, 474–479. doi: 10.1037/0278-7393.13.3.474

Craik, F. I. M., Winocur, G., Palmer, H., Binns, M. A., Edwards, M., Bridges, K., et al. (2007). Cognitive rehabilitation in the elderly: effects on memory. *J. Int. Neuropsych. Soc.* 13, 132–142. doi: 10.1017/s1355617707070166

Dahlin, E., Nyberg, L., Bäckman, L., and Neely, A. (2008). Plasticity of executive functions in young and older adults: immediate training gains, transfer and long term maintenance. *Psychol. Aging* 23, 720–730. doi: 10.1037/a0014296

Drew, D., and Waters, J. (1986). Video games: utilization of a novel strategy to improve perceptual motor skills and cognitive functioning in the non-institutionalized elderly. *Cogn. Rehabil.* 4, 26–31.

Dustman, R. E., Emmerson, R. Y., Steinhaus, L. A., Shearer, D. E., and Dustman, T. J. (1992). The effects of videogame playing on neuropsychological performance of elderly individuals. *J. Gerontol.* 47, 168–171. doi: 10. 1093/geronj/47.3.p168

Edwards, J. D., Wadley, V. G., Vance, D. E., Wood, K., Roenker, D. L., and Ball, K. K. (2005). The impact of speed of processing training on cognitive and everyday performance. *Aging Ment. Health* 9, 262–271. doi: 10. 1080/13607860412331336788

Erickson, K. I., Colcombe, S. J., Wadhwa, R., Bherer, L., Peterson, M. S., Scalf, P. E., et al. (2007). Training- induced plasticity in older adults: effects of training on hemispheric asymmetry. *Neurobiol. Aging* 28, 272–283. doi: 10.1016/j. neurobiolaging.2005.12.012

Feng, J., Spence, I., and Pratt, J. (2007). Playing an action video game reduces gender differences in spatial cognition. *Psychol. Sci.* 18, 850–855. doi: 10.1111/j. 1467-9280.2007.01990.x

Fisher, M., Holland, C., Subramaniam, K., and Vinogradov, S. (2010). Neuroplasticity-based cognitive training in schizophrenia: an interim report on the 6 months later. *Schizophr. Bull.* 36, 869–879. doi: 10.1093/schbul/sbn170

Folstein, M. F., Folstein, S. E., and McHugh, P. R. (1975). "Mini-mental state". A practical method for grading the cognitive state of patients for the clinician. *J. Psychiatr. Res.* 12, 189–198. doi: 10.1016/0022-3956(75)90026-6

Goldstein, J., Cajko, L., Oosterbroek, M., Michielsen, M., Van Houten, O., Saavedra, F., et al. (1997). Videogames and the elderly. *Soc. Behav. Pers.* 25, 345–352. doi: 10.2224/sbp.1997.25.4.345

Green, C. S., and Bavelier, D. (2003). Action video game modifies visual selective attention. *Nature* 423, 534–537. doi: 10.1038/nature01647

Green, C. S., Strobach, T., and Schubert, T. (2014). On methodological standars in training and transfer experiments. *Psychol. Res.* 78, 756–772. doi: 10. 1007/s00426-013-0535-3

Hampstead, B. M., Shatian, K., Phillips, P. A., Amaraneni, A., Delaune, W. R., and Stringer, A. Y. (2012). Mnemonic strategy training improves memory for object location associations in both healthy elderly and patients with amnestic mild cognitive impairment: a randomized, single-blind study. *Neuropsychology* 26, 385–399. doi: 10.1037/a0027545

Hertzog, C., Kramer, A. F., Wilson, R. S., and Lindenberger, U. (2008). Enrichment effects on adult cognitive development: can the functional capacity of older adults be preserved and enhanced? *Psychol. Sci. Public Interest* 9, 1–65. doi: 10. 1111/j.1539-6053.2009.01034.x

Hoyer, W. J., and Verhaeghen, P. (2006). "Memory aging," in *Handbook of the Psychology of Aging*, eds J. Birren and W. Schaie (Burlington, MA: Elsevier Academic Press), 209–232.

Karbach, J., and Kray, J. (2009). How useful is executive control training? Age differences in near and far transfer of task-switching training. *Dev. Sci.* 12, 978–990. doi: 10.1111/j.1467-7687.2009.00846.x

Karbach, J., and Schubert, T. (2013). Training induced cognitive and neural plasticity. *Front. Human. Neurosci.* 7:48. doi: 10.3389/fnhum.2013.00048

Karbach, J., and Verhaeghen, P. (2014). Making working memory work: a meta-analysis of executive-control and working memory training in older adults. *Psychol. Sci.* 25, 2027–2037. doi: 10.1177/0956797614548725

Kelly, M., Loughrey, D., Lawlor, B., Robertson, I., Walsh, C., and Brennan, S. (2014). The impact of cognitive training and mental stimulation on cognitive and everyday functioning of healthy older adults: a systematic review and meta-analysis. *Ageing Res. Rev.* 15, 28–43. doi: 10.1016/j.arr.2014.02.004

Klingberg, T. (2010). Training and plasticity of working memory. *Trends Cogn. Sci.* 14, 317–324. doi: 10.1016/j.tics.2010.05.002

Kramer, A., Larish, J., and Strayer, D. (1995). Training for attentional control in dual task setting: a comparison of young and older adults. *J. Exp. Psychol.* 1, 50–76. doi: 10.1037/1076-898x.1.1.50

Kueider, A. M., Parisi, J., Gross, A. L., and Rebok, G. W. (2012). Computerized cognitive training with older adults: a systematic review. *PLoS One* 7:e40588. doi: 10.1371/journal.pone.0040588

Lampit, A., Hallock, H., and Valenzuela, M. (2014). Computerized cognitive training in cognitively healthy older adults: a systematic review and meta-analysis of effect modifiers. *PLoS Med.* 11:e1001756. doi: 10.1371/journal.pmed. 1001756

Lezak, M. D. (1995). *Neuropsychological Assessment.* 3rd Edn. New York, NY: Oxford University Press.

Li, S. C., Brehmer, Y., Shing, Y. L., Werkle-Bergner, M., and Lindenberger, U. (2006). Neuromodulation of associative and organizational plasticity across the life span: empirical evidence and neurocomputational modeling. *Neurosci. Biobehav. Rev.* 30, 775–790. doi: 10.1016/j.neubiorev.2006.06.004

Li, S. C., Schmiedek, F., Huxhold, O., Röcke, C., Smith, J., and Lindenberger, U. (2008). Working memory plasticity in old age: practice, gain, transfer and maintenance. *Psychol. Aging* 23, 731–742. doi: 10.1037/a0014343

Maillot, P., Perrot, A., and Hartley, A. (2012). Effects of interactive physical activity videogame training on physical and cognitive function in older adults. *Psychol. Aging* 27, 589–600. doi: 10.1037/a0026268

Mayas, J., Parmentier, F. B. R., Andrés, P., and Ballesteros, S. (2014). Plasticity of attentional functions in older adults after non-action video game training. *PLoS One* 9:e92269. doi: 10.1371/journal.pone.0092269

Melby-Lervåg, M., and Hulme, C. (2013). Is working memory training effective? A meta-analytic review. *Dev. Psychol.* 49, 270–291. doi: 10.1037/a0028228

Melby-Lervåg, M., and Hulme, C. (2016). There is no convincing evidence that working memory training is effective: a reply to Au et al. (2014) and Karbach and Verhaeghen (2014). *Psychon. Bull. Rev.* 23, 324–330. doi: 10.3758/s13423-015-0862-z

Milner, B. (1971). Interhemispheric differences in the localization of psychological processes in man. *Br. Med. Bull.* 27, 272–277.

Mitchell, D. B., and Bruss, P. J. (2003). Age differences in implicit memory: conceptual, perceptual o methodological? *Psychol. Aging* 18, 807–822. doi: 10. 1037/0882-7974.18.4.807

Morrison, A., and Chein, J. (2011). Does working memory training work? The promise of challenges and enhancing cognition by training working memory. *Psychon. Bull. Rev.* 18, 46–60. doi: 10.3758/s13423-010-0034-0

Mozolic, J. L., Long, A. B., Morgan, A. R., Rawley-Payne, M., and Laurienti, P. J. (2011). A cognitive training intervention improves modality-specific attention in a randomized controlled trial of healthy older adults. *Neurobiol. Aging* 32, 655–668. doi: 10.1016/j.neurobiolaging.2009.04.013

Muiños, M., and Ballesteros, S. (2014). Peripheral vision and perceptual asymmetries in young and older martial arts athletes and non-athletes. *Atten. Percept. Psychophys.* 76, 2465–2676. doi: 10.3758/s13414-014-0719-y

Muiños, M., and Ballesteros, S. (2015). Sport can protect dynamic visual acuity from aging: a study with young and older judo and karate martial arts athletes. *Atten. Percept. Psychophys.* 77, 2061–2073. doi: 10.3758/s13414-015-0901-x

Nilsson, L. G. (2003). Memory function in normal aging. *Acta Neurol. Scand. Suppl.* 179, 7–13. doi: 10.1034/j.1600-0404.107.s179.5.x

Osorio, A., Pouthas, V., Fay, S., and Ballesteros, S. (2010). Ageing affects brain activity in highly educated older adults: an ERP study using a word-stem priming task. *Cortex* 46, 522–534. doi: 10.1016/j.cortex.2009.09.003

Owen, A. M., Hampshire, A., Grahn, J. A., Stenton, R., Dajani, S., Burns, A. S., et al. (2010). Putting brain training to test. *Nature* 465, 775–778. doi: 10.1038/nature09042

Park, D. C., and Bischof, G. (2013). The aging mind: neuroplasticity in response to cognitive training. *Dialogues Clin. Neurosci.* 15, 109–119.

Park, D. C., and Gutchess, A. H. (2002). Aging, cognition and culture: a neuroscientific perspective. *Neurosci. Biobehav. Rev.* 26, 859–867. doi: 10.1016/s0149-7634(02)00072-6

Park, D. C., Lautenschlager, G., Hedden, T., Davidson, N., Smith, A. D., and Smith, P. (2002). Models of visuo-spatial and verbal memory across the adult lifespan. *Psychol. Aging* 17, 299–320. doi: 10.1037/0882-7974.17.2.299

Park, D. C., and Reuter-Lorenz, P. (2009). The adaptive brain: aging and neurocognitive scaffolding. *Annu. Rev. Psychol.* 60, 173–196. doi: 10.1146/annurev.psych.59.103006.093656

Perrig, W. J., Hollenstein, M., and Oelhafen, S. (2009). Can we improve fluid intelligence with training on working memory in persons with intellectual disabilities? *J. Cogn. Educ. Psychol.* 8, 148–164. doi: 10.1891/1945-8959.8.2.148

Raz, N., and Lindenberger, U. (2013). Life-span plasticity of the brain and cognition: from questions to evidence and back. *Neurosci. Biobehav. Rev.* 37, 2195–2200. doi: 10.1016/j.neubiorev.2013.10.003

Raz, N., Lindenberger, U., Rodrigue, K. M., Kennedy, K. M., Head, D., Williamson, A., et al. (2005). Regional brain changes in aging healthy adults: general trends, individual differences and modifiers. *Cereb. Cortex* 15, 1676–1689. doi: 10.1093/cercor/bhi044

Redick, T. S., Shipstead, Z., Fried, D. E., Hambrick, D. Z., Kane, M. J., and Engle, R. W. (2013). No evidence of intelligence improvement after working memory training: a randomized, placebo-controlled study. *J. Exp. Psychol. Gen.* 142, 359–379. doi: 10.1037/a0029082

Reuter-Lorenz, P. A., and Park, D. C. (2014). How does it STAC up? Revisting the scaffolding theory of aging and cognition. *Neuropsychol. Rev.* 24, 355–370. doi: 10.1007/s11065-014-9270-9

Richardson, J. T. E., and Vecchi, T. (2002). A jigsaw-puzzle imagery task for assessing active visuospatial processes in old and young people. *Behav. Res. Methods Instrum. Comput.* 34, 69–82. doi: 10.3758/bf03195425

Rönnlund, M., Nyberg, L., Bäckman, L., and Nilsson, L. G. (2005). Stability, growth and decline in adult life span development of declarative memory: cross-sectional and longitudinal data from a population-based study. *Psychol. Aging* 20, 3–18. doi: 10.1037/0882-7974.20.1.3

Sacco, K., Cauda, F., D'Agata, F., Duca, S., Zettin, M., Virgilio, R., et al. (2011). A combined robotic and cognitive training for locomotor rehabilitation: evidences of cerebral functional reorganization in two chronic traumatic brain injured patients. *Front. Hum. Neurosci.* 5:146. doi: 10.3389/fnhum.2011.00146

Salthouse, T. A. (1996). The processing-speed theory of adult age differences in cognition. *Psychol. Rev.* 103, 403–428. doi: 10.1037/0033-295x.103.3.403

Shipstead, Z., Redick, T. S., and Engle, R. W. (2010). Does working memory training generalize? *Psychol. Belg.* 50, 245–276. doi: 10.5334/pb-50-3-4-245

Shipstead, Z., Redick, T. S., and Engle, R. W. (2012). Is working memory training effective? *Psychol. Bull.* 138, 628–654. doi: 10.1037/a0027473

Smith, G. E., Housen, P., Yaffe, K., Ruff, R., Kennison, R. F., Mahncke, H. W., et al. (2009). A cognitive training program based on principles of brain plasticity: results from the improvement in memory with plasticity-based adaptative cognitive training (IMPACT) study. *J. Am. Geriatr. Soc.* 57, 594–603. doi: 10.1111/j.1532-5415.2008.02167.x

Snodgrass, J. G., and Vanderwart, M. (1980). A standardized set of 260 pictures: norms for name agreement, image agreement, familiarity and visual complexity. *J. Exp. Psychol. Hum. Learn.* 6, 174–215. doi: 10.1037/0278-7393.6.2.174

Söderqvist, S., Nutley, S. B., Ottersen, J., Grill, K. M., and Klingberg, T. (2012). Computerized training of non-verbal reasoning and working memory in children with intellectual disability. *Front. Hum. Neurosci.* 6:271. doi: 10.3389/fnhum.2012.00271

Stern, Y., Blumen, H. M., Rich, L. W., Richards, A., Herzberg, G., and Gopher, D. (2011). Space Fortress game training and executive control in older adults: a pilot intervention. *Neuropsychol. Dev. Cogn. B Aging Neuropsychol. Cogn.* 18, 653–677. doi: 10.1080/13825585.2011.613450

Takeuchi, H., Taki, Y., and Kawashima, R. (2010). Effects of working memory training on cognitive functions and neural systems. *Rev. Neurosci.* 21, 427–449. doi: 10.1515/revneuro.2010.21.6.427

Toril, P., Reales, J. M., and Ballesteros, S. (2014). Video game training enhances cognition of older adults. A meta-analytic study. *Psychol. Aging* 29, 706–716. doi: 10.1037/a0037507

Torres, A. (2008). Cognitive effects of video games on older people. *ICDVRAT* 19, 191–198.

van Muijden, J., Band, G. P. H., and Hommel, B. (2012). Online game training aging brains:limited transfer to cognitive control functions. *Front. Hum. Neurosci.* 6:221. doi: 10.3389/fnhum.2012.00221

Wechsler, D. (1997). *Wechsler Memory Scale (WMS-III).* San Antonio, TX: Psychological Corporation and Harcourt Brace.

Wechsler, D. (1999). *WAIS-III: Wechsler Adult Intelligence Scale. Administration and Scoring Manual.* 3rd Edn. San Antonio, TX: Psychological Corporation, Harcourt Brace.

Zinke, K., Zeintl, M., Rose, N., Putzmann, J., Pydde, A., and Kliegel, M. (2014). Working memory training and transfer in older adults: effects of age, baseline performance and training gains. *Dev. Psychol.* 50, 304–315. doi: 10.1037/a0032982

16

Barriers, Benefits, and Beliefs of Brain Training Smartphone Apps: An Internet Survey of Younger US Consumers

John Torous[1*†], *Patrick Staples*[2†], *Elizabeth Fenstermacher*[1], *Jason Dean*[1] *and Matcheri Keshavan*[1]

[1] *Department of Psychiatry, Beth Israel Deaconess Medical Center, Boston, MA, USA,* [2] *Department of Biostatistics, Harvard T.H. Chan School of Public Health, Boston, MA, USA*

Edited by:
Soledad Ballesteros, Universidad Nacional de Educación a Distancia (UNED), Spain

Reviewed by:
José Manuel Reales, Universidad Nacional de Educación a Distancia (UNED), Spain
Chariklia Tziraki-Segal, MELABEV and Hebrew University, Jerusalem

***Correspondence:**
John Torous
jtorous@bidmc.harvard.edu

†*Co-first authors*

Background: While clinical evidence for the efficacy of brain training remains in question, numerous smartphone applications (apps) already offer brain training directly to consumers. Little is known about why consumers choose to download these apps, how they use them, and what benefits they perceive. Given the high rates of smartphone ownership in those with internet access and the younger demographics, we chose to approach this question first with a general population survey that would capture primarily this demographic.

Method: We conducted an online internet-based survey of the US population via mTurk regarding their use, experience, and perceptions of brain training apps. There were no exclusion criteria to partake although internet access was required. Respondents were paid 20 cents for completing each survey. The survey was offered for a 2-week period in September 2015.

Results: 3125 individuals completed the survey and over half of these were under age 30. Responses did not significantly vary by gender. The brain training app most frequently used was Lumosity. Belief that a brain-training app could help with thinking was strongly correlated with belief it could also help with attention, memory, and even mood. Beliefs of those who had never used brain-training apps were similar to those who had used them. Respondents felt that data security and lack of endorsement from a clinician were the two least important barriers to use.

Discussion: Results suggest a high level of interest in brain training apps among the US public, especially those in younger demographics. The stability of positive perception of these apps among app-naïve and app-exposed participants suggests an important role of user expectations in influencing use and experience of these apps. The low concern about data security and lack of clinician endorsement suggest apps are not being utilized in clinical settings. However, the public's interest in the effectiveness of apps suggests a common theme with the scientific community's concerns about direct to consumer brain training programs.

Keywords: brain, apps, smartphones, memory, technology assessment

INTRODUCTION

Over the last decade, consumer markets have seen a veritable explosion in products marketed for "brain training". "Brain training' entails the use of specific exercises, often games, which reputedly improve cognitive performance. While many companies advertise a neuroscientific basis for the efficacy of their brain training products, there is little peer-reviewed research to substantiate these claims. Nevertheless, brain training exercises have maintained broad appeal. Current estimates suggest that brain training has become a billion dollar annual industry, with over 70 million active users of Lumosity, one of the most popular brain training programs. (Sukel, 2015). A direct evaluation of these programs" efficacy is beyond the scope of this article, and we refer the reader to other work which has addressed this topic (Owen et al., 2010; Bavelier et al., 2012; Rabipour and Raz, 2012; A Consensus on the Brain Training Industry from the Scientific Community, 2014; Lampit et al., 2014; Toril et al., 2014; Ballesteros et al., 2015). This article seeks to assess consumer motivations and perceived benefits and attitudes towards of brain training exercise programs, with a particular focus on smartphone applications (apps). Smartphone apps offer an accessible, affordable, and convenient method for millions of consumers to access and engage in brain training. Understanding why consumers choose to download and use brain training apps is an important question that can help clinicians discuss and understand the role of these digital tools. As non-invasive, easily accessible, and affordable cognitive interventions, brain training apps are appealing consumer devices. From younger workers hoping to become more efficient (Borness et al., 2013), to older adults concerned about dementia (Corbett et al., 2015; Salthouse, 2015) and other psychiatric disorders (Keshavan et al., 2014), brain training holds tremendous promise.

There is little research or consensus regarding what drives consumers to use brain-training apps. One recent study investigated user expectations and noted that people who use these apps tend to have high expectations, even before using them (Rabipour and Davidson, 2015). In early 2016, the US Federal Trade Commission ordered one brain training app, Lumosity, to pay a two million dollar settlement regarding "deceptive advertising" stating the company "preyed on consumers" (Lumosity to Pay $2 Million to Settle FTC Deceptive Advertising Charges for Its "Brain Training" Program [Internet]., 2016). However, little is known about who uses brain training apps, which apps they are using, what they expect in terms of cognitive improvement, and what they perceive as barriers to use.

Although brain training apps are marketed across all ages, we chose to focus on a more tech-savvy demographic, which was highly correlated with a younger demographic, which has also been shown to be the largest group *per capita* of smartphone owners. National survey data suggests that 85% of US adults between ages 18–29 and 70% between ages 30–50 own a smartphone (Smith, 2015). Compared to those over the age of 50, this younger demographic is more than twice as likely to use their phones to find health related information online (Fox and Duggan, 2012). Survey data of outpatient psychiatric patients also found high rates of smartphone ownership and interest in apps among a similar demographic (Torous et al., 2014), though there is no survey data on smartphone ownership and app interest among those seeking brain training. We conducted the following survey study in order to better characterize consumer opinions and attitudes towards brain training apps specifically choosing a survey modality that would capture the largest tech-savvy group of consumers through an on-line survey format as this demographic is most likely to use these programs. This tech-savvy group of consumers is largely comprised of a younger demographic and the majority of our respondents were under the age of 50.

MATERIALS AND METHODS

In order to reach a large population, we conducted a survey study of the general United States population, using an online survey platform, Amazon's Mechanical Turk (mTurk). This platform has been validated for more complex behavioral research (Crump et al., 2013), though here we used it as a simple anonymous survey platform. The survey was conducted in September 2015 and was offered to 3125 subjects registered to take surveys on mTurk, with compensation of 20 cents per survey. The survey, shown below in **Figure 1**, received hospital IRB approval. Of note, we included a simple math question, "9 + 4 = ?" in order to ensure that subjects were actively engaged with the material and not simply "clicking" through the survey.

As our survey contained questions around which brain training apps subjects had used, we sought to identify the most popular brain training apps from both the Apple iTunes store and Android Google Play store. Considering that each app store ranks apps by different criteria and provides different information on number of downloads, reviews, and users, we combined the top ten apps from each marketplace (in June 2015) in a single top ten list, based on our judgment and consensus. We also sought to identify brain-training apps that have been clinically studied and identified six apps from an article that reviewed the evidence for brain training apps (Brooks, 2014). Lumosity was the only app the overlapped as it has been clinically studied and was in the top ten apps on the commercial marketplaces. Some questions (7, 8, 9, 10, 11) asked subjects for their perception on features of brain training regardless of use of these apps and this was intentional to be able to explore how perception varied with use. In creating the survey, we composed a list of possible concerns of the participants in the survey (see Question 16). We interpreted these concerns as possible barriers. While our survey was open to anyone and age was not an exclusion factor, the mTurk platform is skewed towards a more tech savvy and therefore younger demographic.

RESULTS

Over a 2-week period in September 2015, 3125 subjects completed the survey. 48.4% were female (age mean 33.9, SD 12.2), 51.3% were male (age mean 30.9, SD 9.2), and 0.3% of respondents did not answer this question. Of the 3125 subjects,

1. What is your gender?
   - o Male
   - o Female

2. What is your age?

3. Do you own a smartphone?
   - o Yes
   - o No

4. Do you download apps onto your smartphone?
   - o Yes
   - o No

5. Do you have health or fitness related apps on your smartphone?
   - o Yes
   - o No

6. Have you ever used an app that is meant to help improve or increase your memory, focus, attention, or other cognitive abilities? For the purpose of this survey, we will call these "brain training apps"?
   - o Yes
   - o No

7. Do you think brain training apps improve thinking?
   - o Yes
   - o No

8. Do you think brain training apps improve attention?
   - o Yes
   - o No

9. Do you think brain training apps improve memory?
   - o Yes
   - o No

10. Do you think brain training apps improve mood?
    - o Yes
    - o No

11. Do you think brain training apps can have side effects or be harmful in any way?
    - o Yes
    - o No

12. Please check the box with the correct answer to: 9+4 =
    - o 11 or 12 or 13 or 14

13. Which (if any) of the following brain training apps have you used? (Choose all that apply)
    - o Brain Games P.A.C., Brain Wars, Lumosity, Mind Games brain training, Elevate, Fit Brains Trainer, Neuronation brain training, Memory Trainer, Brain Workout, Peak, None of the above

14. Which (if any) of the following brain training apps have you used? (Choose all that apply)
    - o CogMed, Posit Science, Attention Process Training, Cognifit, Happy Neuron, None on the above

15. What is the longest duration you have ever used a brain training app for? If never used, pick 'Have never used'
    - o Have never used, less than one week, one week – 4 weeks, 1 month – 2 months, 2 months – 3 months, 3 months – 6 months, 6 months – 1 year, 1 year or longer

16. Which (if any) of the following concerns do you have about brain training apps (Choose all that apply:)
Cost of Apps, Time Required to Use, Unsure if they are effective, Not recommended by a healthcare provider, I am not interested in them, My health data is not secure, None of the above

FIGURE 1 | A copy of the survey questions reformatted to be displayed in a single figure.

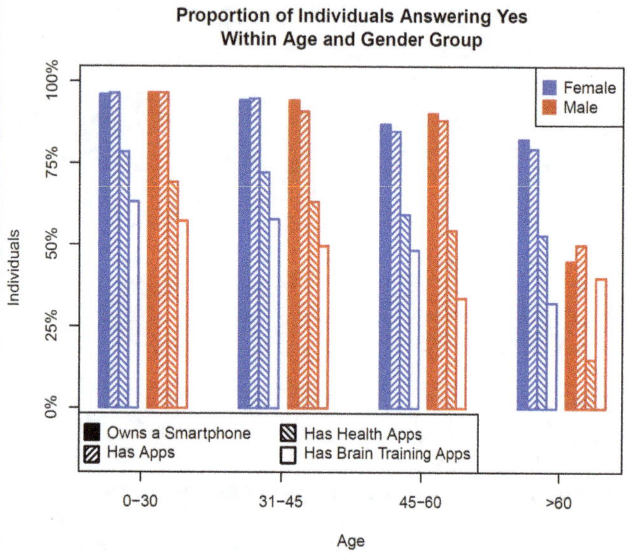

FIGURE 2 | A bar graph showing the proportion of survey respondents by age and sex who own a smartphone, have apps, have healthcare apps, and have brain training apps.

1558 (nearly 50%) were under age 30, 978 (just over 31%) were between ages 31 - 45, 276 (almost 9%) between ages 46 - 60, and 54 (nearly 2%) older than age 60. **Figure 2** below shows the a breakdown of smartphone ownership, having any apps, having health apps, and having brain training apps by age brackets. 93.7% of subjects report having apps, 69.2% having used health apps, and 55.7% having used brain training apps. 66.9% reported that brain training apps helped with thinking, 69.3% with attention, 53.3% with mood, 65% with memory, and 14.9% reported that they felt there may be dangers with app use. 98.2% answered the math question correctly. Demographic age and gender related information of subjects and there ownership/use of smartphones and apps is shown below in **Figure 2.**

Of the 16 apps subjects were asked if they had ever used, Lumosity was the most used with 70% of those who had used brain training apps having tried it. **Figure 3** below displays apps used by subjects in a polar plot showing the proportion of brain training apps used, stratified by reported gender.

Looking at **Figure 3**, we notice several trends. First, the largest correlations (0.77 - 0.82) exist between beliefs about the positive effects of brain training apps on cognitive abilities (memory, thinking, and attention). A strong but attenuated correlation also exists between these and the reported benefit of brain training apps on mood (0.34 - 0.40). However, it is instructive to observe that the correlation between using brain apps and reporting the positive effects above, while statistically significant, is very slight (0.09 - 0.14). This suggests two points: first, that those who use brain training apps do not observe the main benefits intended by the app; and second, those who do report benefits report many that are mostly independent of each other, and do not distinguish strongly between specific benefits.

In order to better understand correlations between individual survey responses, we calculated the correlation coefficients which are displayed below in **Figure 4.**

To understand the summary difference between those who have not used app vs. those who have used one or more, we created a score calculated by adding one each point for responding "yes" to any of Questions 7–10 (apps help with either attention, memory, thinking, or mood) and for responding "no" to Question 11 (there are dangers to app use). Thus the potential score range is between 0 and 5. The results are displayed below in **Figure 5** which presents perceptions of brain training apps in comparison to the number of brain training apps a subject has reported using, subjects were asked to report barriers toward brain training app use and results are shown below in **Figure 6.**

Figure 6 shows that our sample is not generally concerned about the security of the data gathered by a brain training app (4% males, 6% females), nor whether the brain training app was recommended by a healthcare provider (3% females, 2% males). In contrast, subjects were most likely to report concerns about the cost of apps (30% females, 25% males), as well as concerns about their effectiveness (25% females, 26% males). To understand the association between app ownership on perceptions of efficacy, we compared the distribution of the number of brain training apps used among those who responded that they have concerns about app efficacy to those who did not respond that they have these concerns. A t-test for a difference in the means of these distributions yielded a p-value of 0.12, failing to reject the hypothesis that those with or without concerns about app efficacy differ in the mean number of brain-training apps they use. We also conducted a similar t-test to understand if there is an association of app ownership with concerns about cost of apps, and again failed to find a significant difference ($p = 0.35$).

DISCUSSION

To date, this is the largest Internet survey of user perceptions of brain training apps, which provides a window into the use, barriers, and consumer attitudes towards these programs. The mean age of the 3125 respondents was 32.4 years old, which is consistent with the largest demographic of smartphone owners, app users, and internet survey participants. Our data elucidates strong positive perceptions of cognitive training apps, with roughly equal percentages of respondents reporting a belief that these apps improve thinking (66.9%), memory (70.3%), and attention (69.3%). A significant proportion (53.3%) of respondents also believed that brain training apps have a positive effect on mood.

While nearly 50% of survey respondents were under age 30, our results still provide an interesting window on who is using brain training apps. Rates of smartphone ownership, having health apps, and having brain training apps was very similar although slightly lower in the 31 - 45 age demographic as compared to those less than 30, suggesting a broader appeal of these apps beyond those less than age 30. Given that only 9% of respondents were in the 45 - 60 demographic

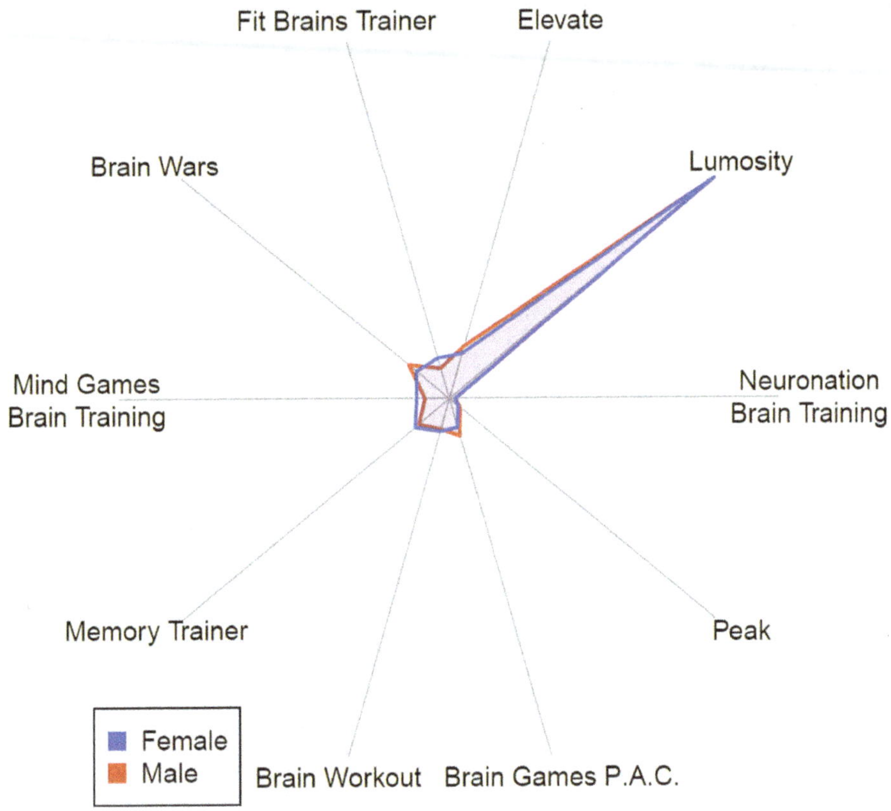

FIGURE 3 | A polar plot showing the proportion of brain training apps used, stratified by reported gender. Each gender is normalized to show the same total volume, and the magnitude is normalized to show the global maximum of reported proportion at the maximum radius. Lumosity is clearly reported as used more than any other brain training app.

and 2% in the above 60 years old demographic it is harder to interpret the results for these groups. This 2% result is interesting as it is in line with a recent survey study suggesting that only 1.2% of US adults over age 65 have ever used a handheld device to track their health (Shahrokni et al., 2015). Given national trends that smartphone ownership in younger generations is reaching saturation, and our results that ownership is also less in older demographics, it is possible that the next wave of growth in brain training apps may come from those who are older as they begin to further adopt smartphones Although our sample size is small for adults over age 60, it is interesting to note that in male subjects, brain training apps were reported downloaded more than health apps. While our study is not designed to answer why this may be so, it suggests that brain training apps may be of strong interest in this population.

Subjects' belief that these apps are beneficial for thinking is strongly correlated with the belief that they improve attention, memory and mood. However, this correlation was not as strong in users who reported prior use of a brain training app. This finding is in line with perceptions of barriers in that using a greater number of apps did not improve consumer attitudes. Those who had never used a brain training app reported a positive response score of 3.5. There was a small positive correlation between the number of apps used and positive responses, with the positive response score increasing only minimally for those who had used more apps, reaching 3.84 for those who had used up to five apps. Regardless of the number of apps used, the use of these programs was not strongly correlated with a change in the positive response score. These results are thus in agreement with a recent study, which found that consumers have high expectations for brain training apps before their use (Rabipour and Davidson, 2015). In addition, we have shown that consumer expectations and perceptions do not change after these apps have been used. It is possible that the positive attitude towards these programs may stem primarily from preexisting expectations, not positive experiences with the apps themselves. Or conversely, that strong preexisting positive expectations may be the primary driving force behind app ownership and usage. Our results also suggest that consumer opinions on barriers to app use, such as cost and perceived efficacy, are not statistically correlated with app ownership or number of apps used by subjects. These seemingly paradoxical results may reflect consumers' inconsistency in the recognition of their own preferences, and highlight the complexity in understanding why consumers choose to use or not use these apps.

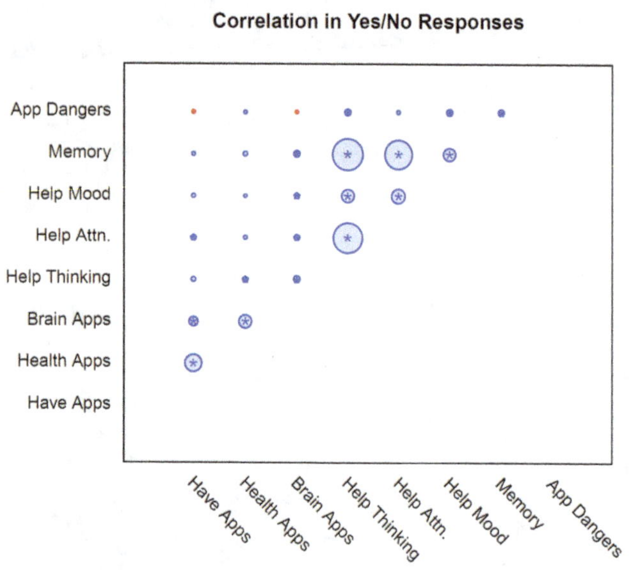

FIGURE 4 | The pairwise correlations between each response. Correlation is proportional to area and colored by valence (positive shown in blue, negative in red), with the maximum correlation being 0.82 (Memory and Help Thinking). Statistical significance (adjusted for multiple testing) is indicated with a star.

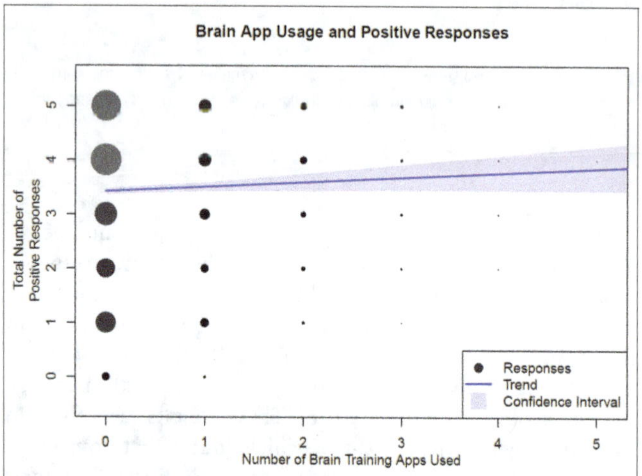

FIGURE 5 | Total number of brain training apps used by total number of responses. We consider a positive response to be an answer "Yes" to Questions 7–10, and "No" to Question 11. The blue line is a linear regression fit, with 95% confidence bands.

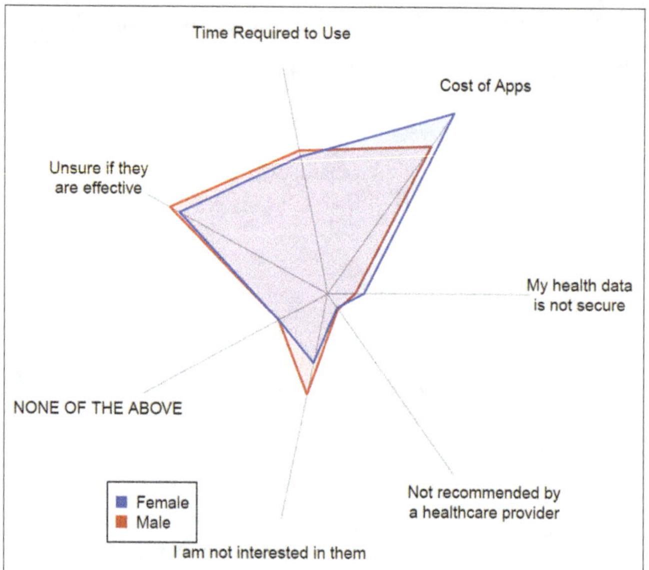

FIGURE 6 | A polar plot showing the proportion of barriers to use reported, stratified by reported gender. Each gender is normalized to show the same total volume, and the magnitude is normalized to show the global maximum of reported proportion at the maximum radius.

Whereas clinicians are concerned with privacy and clinical recommendations and evidence backing new technologies like apps (Huckvale et al., 2015) these features were of least concern to consumers, who cited cost as the primary barrier to use. Of note, consumers also listed uncertainty regarding the efficacy of these programs as a strong barrier to use. Overall, our results suggest that consumers prefer an app that is inexpensive, time efficient, and has an evidence base to support its efficacy. Although our survey did not specify what was meant by health data not being secure, further research could explore the overall lack of concern regarding data security. For instance, it is possible that consumers are unaware of how their healthcare data may be used when using these apps.

While our survey did not assess whether user perceptions of efficacy correlates with actual benefit, this topic has recently become a topic of debate (Brooks, 2014; Rabipour and Davidson, 2015). A recent consensus statement by numerous neuroscientists further underscores the lack of rigorous scientific evidence and the concern for misleading marketing (A Consensus on the Brain Training Industry from the Scientific Community, 2014). While many studies have shown positive results (Green and Bavelier, 2008; Anguera et al., 2013; Ballesteros et al., 2014; Hardy et al., 2015), there is concern that these improvements could also be related to improved skill at using the app, rather than an actual improvement in cognition (Owen et al., 2010; Burch, 2014). Our results, which suggest that positive consumer attitudes are related more to preexisting beliefs than to positive user experiences, could support the notion of a digital placebo effect. Our results also indicate a high demand for a more rigorous, scientific approach to these applications. Continued consumer demand for these applications, despite the current paucity of evidence, could present an opportunity for academic researchers, consumers, and industry to collaborate in an exploration of new approaches to brain training.

Like all survey research, our study has several limitations. Our results are self-reported and many questions, especially around barriers were subjective. We focused on correlations, and while we can speculate on potential links between these correlations, our survey was not designed to address causation. In addition, our data is inevitably skewed towards a younger and more digitally connected population, as our research was conducted online and targeted US residents. This limitation was expected, given our focus on tech-savvy internet users and the use of the mTurk platform. Our survey was not designed to assess if they were seeking brain training apps for a specific reason, e.g., ADHD symptoms. Although our respondents reported high rates of smartphone ownership, 96% for those below age 30, such numbers are close to the US national average which in 2015 was reported at 85% for this same demographic. While our survey may over represent younger connected individuals, it underrepresents older adults (age >65) as they only represented 54 of our 3125 subjects or 1.7%. Perceptions of brain training in an older demographic is an important future research direction, as many older adults may use brain training apps to address declining cognition. Another potential limitation of survey data in general is poor attention to the online survey task, but the fact that over 98% of respondents answered the distracter math question correctly suggests that they were attentive to the other survey questions as well. Of note, we included response from the slightly less than 2% of respondents who answered the math question incorrectly.

The future of brain training smartphone apps is at a crossroads. One path leads to further development of brain training apps, driven largely by marketing and expectations, rather than scientific evidence. The other route rests on further app development, with a focus on efficacy research and generalizable benefits. Based on our survey data of consumer perspectives and the current body of scientific literature, it appears that brain training app users would prefer the latter path. With the right scientific efforts, consumer education and empowerment, and partnerships with industry, this goal will hopefully be attainable in the near future.

AUTHOR CONTRIBUTIONS

JT and MK conceived the research idea. JT, EF, and JD wrote the protocol and IRB. PS analyzed the data and produced all figures. JT, EF, JD, and MK conducted background literature review. All authors helped in the writing and drafting on this manuscript. All authors edited the manuscript.

REFERENCES

A Consensus on the Brain Training Industry from the Scientific Community. (2014). *Max Planck Institute for Human Development and Stanford Center on Longevity.* Available online at: http://longevity3.stanford.edu.ezp-prod1.hul.harvard.edu/blog/2014/10/15/the-consensus-on-the-brain-training-industry-from-the-scientific-community/ (Accessed November 22, 2015).

Anguera, J. A., Boccanfuso, J., Rintoul, J. L., Al-Hashimi, O., Faraji, F., Janowich, J., et al. (2013). Video game training enhances cognitive control in older adults. *Nature* 501, 97–101. doi: 10.1038/nature12486

Ballesteros, S., Prieto, A., Mayas, J., Toril, P., Pita, C., Ponce de León, L., et al. (2014). Brain training with non action video games enhances aspects of cognition in older adults: a randomized controlled trial. *Front. Aging Neurosci.* 6:277. doi: 10.3389/fnagi.2014.00277

Ballesteros, S., Kraft, E., Santana, S., and Tziraki, C. (2015). Maintaining older brain functionality: a targeted review. *Neurosci. Biobehav. Rev.* 55, 453–477. doi: 10.1016/j.neubiorev.2015.06.008

Bavelier, D., Green, C. S., Pouget, A., and Schrater, P. (2012). Brain plasticity through the life span: learning to learn and action video games. *Annu. Rev. Neurosci.* 35, 391–416. doi: 10.1146/annurev-neuro-060909-152832

Borness, C., Proudfoot, J., Crawford, J., and Valenzuela, M. (2013). Putting brain training to the test in the workplace: a randomized, blinded, multisite, active-controlled trial. *PLoS One* 8:e59982. doi: 10.1371/journal.pone.0059982

Brooks, L. (2014). *Science or Sales? The Evidence and Application of Brain Training Games [Internet].* Available online at: http://www.psychiatrictimes.com/neuropsychiatry/science-sales-evidence-application-brain-training-games.

Burch, D. (2014). What could computerized brain training learn from evidence-based medicine? *PLoS Med.* 11:e1001758. doi: 10.1371/journal.pmed.1001758

Corbett, A., Owen, A., Hampshire, A., Grahn, J., Stenton, R., Dajani, S., et al. (2015). The effect of an online cognitive training package in healthy older adults: an online randomized controlled trial. *J. Am. Med. Dir. Associ.* 16, 990–997. doi: 10.1016/j.jamda.2015.06.014

Crump, M. C., McDonnell, J. V., and Gureckis, T. M. (2013). Evaluating amazon's mechanical turk as a tool for experimental behavioral research. *PLoS One* 8:e57410. doi: 10.1371/journal.pone.0057410

Fox, S., and Duggan, M. (2012). *Mobile Health 2012 [Internet]. Pew Research Center Internet Science Tech RSS.* Available online at: http://www.pewinternet.org/2012/11/08/mobile-health-2012/.

Green, C. S., and Bavelier, D. (2008). Exercising your brain: a review of human brain plasticity and training-induced learning. *Psychol. Aging* 23, 692–701. doi: 10.1037/a0014345

Hardy, J. L., Nelson, R. A., Thomason, M. E., Sternberg, D. A., Katovich, K., Farzin, F., et al. (2015). Enhancing cognitive abilities with comprehensive training: a large, online, randomized, active-controlled trial. *PLoS One* 10:e0134467. doi: 10.1371/journal.pone.0134467

Huckvale, K., Prieto, J. T., Tilney, M., Benghozi, P. J., and Car, J. (2015). Unaddressed privacy risks in accredited health and wellness apps: a cross-sectional systematic assessment. *BMC Med.* 13:214. doi: 10.1186/s12916-015-0444-y

Keshavan, M. S., Vinogradov, S., Rumsey, J., Sherrill, J., and Wagner, A. (2014). Cognitive training in mental disorders: update and future directions. *Am. J. Psychiatry* 171, 510–522. doi: 10.1176/appi.ajp.2013.13081075

Lampit, A., Hallock, H., and Valenzuela, M. (2014). Computerized cognitive training in cognitively healthy older adults: a systematic review and meta-analysis of effect modifiers. *PLoS Med.* 11:e1001756. doi: 10.1371/journal.pmed.1001756

Lumosity to Pay $2 Million to Settle FTC Deceptive Advertising Charges for Its "Brain Training" Program [Internet]. (2016). *Lumosity to Pay $2 Million to Settle FTC Deceptive Advertising Charges for Its "Brain Training" Program.* Available online at: https://www.ftc.gov/news-events/press-releases/2016/01/lumosity-pay-2-million-settle-ftc-deceptive-advertising-charges.

Owen, A. M., Hampshire, A., Grahn, J. A., Stenton, R., Dajani, S., Burns, A. S., et al. (2010). Putting brain training to the test. *Nature* 465, 775–778. doi: 10.1038/nature09042

Rabipour, S., and Davidson, P. S. (2015). Do you believe in brain training? A questionnaire about expectations of computerised cognitive training. *Behav. Brain Res.* 295, 64–70. doi: 10.1016/j.bbr.2015.01.002

Rabipour, S., and Raz, A. (2012). Training the brain: fact and fad in cognitive and behavioral remediation. *Brain Cogn.* 79, 159–179. doi: 10.1016/j.bandc.2012.02.006

Salthouse, T. A. (2015). Do cognitive interventions alter the rate of age-related cognitive change? *Intelligence* 53, 86–91. doi: 10.1016/j.intell.2015.09.004

Shahrokni, A., Mahmoudzadeh, S., Saeedi, R., and Ghasemzadeh, H. (2015). Older people with access to hand-held devices: who are they? *Telemed. J. E Health* 21, 550–556. doi: 10.1089/tmj.2014.0103

Smith, A. U. S. (2015). *Smartphone Use in 2015 [Internet]. Pew Research Center Internet Science Tech RSS.* Available online at: http://www.pewinternet.org/2015/04/01/us-smartphone-use-in-2015/.

Sukel, K. (2015). Does anyone care if "brain games" actually work? [Internet]. Fortune Magazine. Available from: http://fortune.com/2015/08/11/does-anyone-care-if-brain-games-actually-work/.

Toril, P., Reales, J. M., and Ballesteros, S. (2014). Video game training enhances cognition of older adults? A meta-analytic study. *Psychol. Aging* 29, 706–716. doi: 10.1037/a0037507

Torous, J., Chan, S. R., Yee-Marie Tan, S., Behrens, J., Mathew, I., Conrad, E. J., et al. (2014). Patient smartphone ownership and interest in mobile apps to monitor symptoms of mental health conditions: a survey in four geographically distinct psychiatric clinics. *JMIR Ment. Health* 1:e5. doi: 10.2196/mental.4004

Permissions

All chapters in this book were first published in CBPIPECTVGCI, by Frontiers; hereby published with permission under the Creative Commons Attribution License or equivalent. Every chapter published in this book has been scrutinized by our experts. Their significance has been extensively debated. The topics covered herein carry significant findings which will fuel the growth of the discipline. They may even be implemented as practical applications or may be referred to as a beginning point for another development.

The contributors of this book come from diverse backgrounds, making this book a truly international effort. This book will bring forth new frontiers with its revolutionizing research information and detailed analysis of the nascent developments around the world.

We would like to thank all the contributing authors for lending their expertise to make the book truly unique. They have played a crucial role in the development of this book. Without their invaluable contributions this book wouldn't have been possible. They have made vital efforts to compile up to date information on the varied aspects of this subject to make this book a valuable addition to the collection of many professionals and students.

This book was conceptualized with the vision of imparting up-to-date information and advanced data in this field. To ensure the same, a matchless editorial board was set up. Every individual on the board went through rigorous rounds of assessment to prove their worth. After which they invested a large part of their time researching and compiling the most relevant data for our readers.

The editorial board has been involved in producing this book since its inception. They have spent rigorous hours researching and exploring the diverse topics which have resulted in the successful publishing of this book. They have passed on their knowledge of decades through this book. To expedite this challenging task, the publisher supported the team at every step. A small team of assistant editors was also appointed to further simplify the editing procedure and attain best results for the readers.

Apart from the editorial board, the designing team has also invested a significant amount of their time in understanding the subject and creating the most relevant covers. They scrutinized every image to scout for the most suitable representation of the subject and create an appropriate cover for the book.

The publishing team has been an ardent support to the editorial, designing and production team. Their endless efforts to recruit the best for this project, has resulted in the accomplishment of this book. They are a veteran in the field of academics and their pool of knowledge is as vast as their experience in printing. Their expertise and guidance has proved useful at every step. Their uncompromising quality standards have made this book an exceptional effort. Their encouragement from time to time has been an inspiration for everyone.

The publisher and the editorial board hope that this book will prove to be a valuable piece of knowledge for researchers, students, practitioners and scholars across the globe.

List of Contributors

Renate M. van de Ven and Jaap M. J. Murre
Department of Psychology, Brain and Cognition, University of Amsterdam, Amsterdam, Netherlands

Dick J. Veltman
Department of Psychiatry, VU University Medical Center, Amsterdam, Netherlands

Ben A. Schmand
Department of Psychology, Brain and Cognition, University of Amsterdam, Amsterdam, Netherlands
Department of Medical Psychology, Academic Medical Centre, University of Amsterdam, Netherlands

Maria J. Maraver and M. Teresa Bajo
Department of Experimental Psychology - Research Center for Mind, Brain and Behavior, University of Granada, Granada, Spain

Carlos J. Gomez-Ariza
Department of Psychology, University of Jaen, Jaen, Spain

Iseult A. Cremen
Trinity College Institute of Neuroscience and School of Psychology, Trinity College Dublin, Dublin, Ireland

Richard G. Carson
Trinity College Institute of Neuroscience and School of Psychology, Trinity College Dublin, Dublin, Ireland
School of Psychology, Queen's University Belfast, Belfast, United Kingdom

Teri Lawton
Perception Dynamics Institute, Del Mar, CA, USA
Department of Computer Science and Engineering, University of California, San Diego, La Jolla, CA, USA

David Moreau, Ian J. Kirk and Karen E. Waldie
Centre for Brain Research and School of Psychology, University of Auckland, Auckland, New Zealand

Rui Nouchi
Creative Interdisciplinary Research Division, Frontier Research Institute for Interdisciplinary Science (FRIS), Tohoku University, Sendai, Japan
Human and Social Response Research Division, International Research Institute of Disaster Science, Tohoku University, Sendai, Japan
Smart Ageing International Research Centre, Institute of Development, Aging and Cancer, Tohoku University, Sendai, Japan

Yasuyuki Taki
Department of Nuclear Medicine and Radiology, Institute of Development, Aging and Cancer, Tohoku University, Sendai, Japan
Division of Medical Neuroimage Analysis, Department of Community Medical Supports, Tohoku Medical Megabank Organization, Tohoku University, Sendai, Japan
Division of Developmental Cognitive Neuroscience, Institute of Development, Aging and Cancer, Tohoku University, Sendai, Japan

Hikaru Takeuchi
Division of Developmental Cognitive Neuroscience, Institute of Development, Aging and Cancer, Tohoku University, Sendai, Japan

Takayuki Nozawa
Smart Ageing International Research Centre, Institute of Development, Aging and Cancer, Tohoku University, Sendai, Japan
Department of Ubiquitous Sensing, PreClinical Research Center, Institute of Development, Aging and Cancer, Tohoku University, Sendai, Japan

Atsushi Sekiguchi
Division of Medical Neuroimage Analysis, Department of Community Medical Supports, Tohoku Medical Megabank Organization, Tohoku University, Sendai, Japan
Department of Adult Mental Health, National Institute of Mental Health, National Center of Neurology and Psychiatry, Tokyo, Japan

Ryuta Kawashima
Smart Ageing International Research Centre, Institute of Development, Aging and Cancer, Tohoku University, Sendai, Japan
Division of Developmental Cognitive Neuroscience, Institute of Development, Aging and Cancer, Tohoku University, Sendai, Japan
Department of Ubiquitous Sensing, PreClinical Research Center, Institute of Development, Aging and Cancer, Tohoku University, Sendai, Japan
Department of Functional Brain Imaging, Institute of Development, Aging and Cancer, Tohoku University, Sendai, Japan

Marc Palaus, Elena M. Marron and Diego Redolar-Ripoll
Cognitive NeuroLab, Faculty of Health Sciences, Universitat Oberta de Catalunya, Barcelona, Spain

Raquel Viejo-Sobera
Cognitive NeuroLab, Faculty of Health Sciences, Universitat Oberta de Catalunya, Barcelona, Spain
Laboratory for Neuropsychiatry and Neuromodulation, Massachusetts General Hospital, Boston, MA, USA

Erika Borella, Elena Carbone, Rossana De Beni and Barbara Carretti
Department of General Psychology, University of Padova, Padova, Italy

Massimiliano Pastore
Department of Developmental and Social Psychology, University of Padova, Padova, Italy

Judith C. Peters
Department of Cognitive Neuroscience, Faculty of Psychology and Neuroscience, Maastricht University, Maastricht, Netherlands
Department of Neuroimaging and Neuromodeling, Netherlands Institute for Neuroscience, Institute of the Royal Netherlands Academy of Arts and Sciences (KNAW), Amsterdam, Netherlands

Carlijn van den Boomen and Chantal Kemner
Department of Experimental Psychology,Helmholtz Institute, Utrecht, Netherlands
Department of Developmental Psychology, Utrecht University, Utrecht, Netherlands

Patrick D. Gajewski
Ageing Research Group, Leibniz Research Centre for Working Environment and Human Factors (IfADo), Technical University of Dortmund, Dortmund, Germany

Gabriele Freude
Federal Institute for Occupational Safety and Health, Berlin, Germany

Michael Falkenstein
Ageing Research Group, Leibniz Research Centre for Working Environment and Human Factors (IfADo), Technical University of Dortmund, Dortmund, Germany
Institute for Working, Learning and Aging, Bochum, Germany

Valentin Bégel
Euromov Laboratory, University of Montpellier, Montpellier, France
NaturalPad, Montpellier, France

Ines Di Loreto
Homme, Environnement et Technologies de l'Information, Université de Technologie de Troyes, Troyes, France

Antoine Seilles
NaturalPad, Montpellier, France

Simone Dalla Bella
Euromov Laboratory, University of Montpellier, Montpellier, France
Institut Universitaire de France, Paris, France
International Laboratory for Brain, Music and Sound Research (BRAMS), Montreal, QC, Canada
Department of Cognitive Psychology, WyzPsza Szkoła Finansów i Zarzadzanią w Warszawie (WSFiZ), Warsaw, Poland

Soledad Ballesteros
Studies on Aging and Neurodegenerative Diseases Research Group, Universidad Nacional de Educación a Distancia (UNED), Madrid, Spain
Department of Basic Psychology II, Universidad Nacional de Educación a Distancia (UNED), Madrid, Spain

Claudia Voelcker-Rehage
Institute of Human Movement Science and Health, Technische Universität Chemnitz, Chemnitz, Germany

Louis Bherer
Department of Medicine, Université de Montréal, Montreal, QC, Canada
Montreal Heart Institute, Montreal, QC, Canada
Institut Universitaire de Gériatrie de Montréal, Montreal, QC, Canada

Wei Wei
Advanced Technology Innovation Center for Future Education, Beijing Normal University, Beijing, China
Department of Psychology and Behavioral Sciences, Zhejiang University, Hangzhou, China
State Key Laboratory of Cognitive Neuroscience and Learning, Beijing Normal University, Beijing, China

Chuansheng Chen
Department of Psychology and Social Behavior, University of California, Irvine, CA, USA

Qi Dong and Xinlin Zhou
State Key Laboratory of Cognitive Neuroscience and Learning, Beijing Normal University, Beijing, China

Marlen Schmicker, Patrick Müller and Melanie Schwefel
Neuroprotection Laboratory, German Center for Neurodegenerative Diseases (DZNE), Magdeburg, Germany
Otto von Guericke University, Magdeburg, Germany

John Torous, Elizabeth Fenstermacher, Jason Dean and Matcheri Keshavan
Department of Psychiatry, Beth Israel Deaconess Medical Center, Boston, MA, USA

Notger G. Müller
Neuroprotection Laboratory, German Center for Neurodegenerative Diseases (DZNE), Magdeburg, Germany
Otto von Guericke University, Magdeburg, Germany
Center for Behavioral Brain Sciences, Magdeburg, Germany

Pilar Toril, Julia Mayas and Soledad Ballesteros
Studies of Aging and Neurodegenerative Diseases Research Group, Universidad Nacional de Educación a Distancia (UNED), Madrid, Spain
Department of Basic Psychology II, Universidad Nacional de Educación a Distancia (UNED), Madrid, Spain

José M. Reales
Studies of Aging and Neurodegenerative Diseases Research Group, Universidad Nacional de Educación a Distancia (UNED), Madrid, Spain
Department of Methodology of the Behavioral Sciences, Universidad Nacional de Educación a Distancia (UNED), Madrid, Spain

Patrick Staples
Department of Biostatistics, Harvard T.H. Chan School of Public Health, Boston, MA, USA

Index

www.ingramcontent.com/pod-product-compliance
Lightning Source LLC
LaVergne TN
LVHW080954210926
848485LV00004B/835